Short Course Breast Radiotherapy

Douglas W. Arthur • Frank A. Vicini
David E. Wazer • Atif J. Khan
Editors

Short Course Breast Radiotherapy

A Comprehensive Review of Hypofractionation, Partial Breast, and Intra-Operative Irradiation

Springer

Editors
Douglas W. Arthur
Department of Radiation Oncology
Virginia Commonwealth University School of Medicine
Richmond
Virginia
USA

David E. Wazer
Department of Radiation Oncology
Tufts University School of Medicine
Alpert Medical School of Brown University
Boston
Massachusetts
USA

Frank A. Vicini
21st Century Oncology
Michigan Healthcare Professionals
Farmington Hills
Michigan
USA

Atif J. Khan
Department of Radiation Oncology
Rutgers Cancer Institute of New Jersey
School of Medicine
New Brunswick
New Jersey
USA

ISBN 978-3-319-24386-3 ISBN 978-3-319-24388-7 (eBook)
DOI 10.1007/978-3-319-24388-7

Library of Congress Control Number: 2015960184

Springer Cham Heidelberg New York Dordrecht London

Printed on acid-free paper

Springer International Publishing AG Switzerland is part of Springer Science+Business Media
(www.springer.com)

Preface

In this first edition of *Short Course Breast Radiotherapy: A Comprehensive Review of Hypofractionation, Partial Breast, and Intra-operative Irradiation,* we build upon our preceding book that focused solely on accelerated partial breast irradiation. Over the past 5–10 years, the field of radiation oncology has continued to introduce accelerated hypofractionated treatment approaches into clinical practice and the clinical research arena. Published clinical trial data and the introduction of new treatment technologies and concepts have continued to emerge and impact treatment decisions. For this new book, the content has been expanded beyond partial breast irradiation to include all aspects of accelerated radiotherapy for breast cancer treatment. With this expansion of focus, the content has been organized into sections concentrating on accelerated partial breast irradiation, intraoperative radiotherapy, and hypofractionated whole breast radiotherapy. Each section will include details of patient selection, physics, techniques, data, and toxicity. This book represents a comprehensive handbook that represents a needed resource for the clinician in the implementation of short-course radiotherapy for the treatment of breast cancer.

Richmond, VA, USA — Douglas W. Arthur
Farmington Hills, MI, USA — Frank A. Vicini
Boston, MA, USA — David E. Wazer
New Brunswick, NJ, USA — Atif J. Khan

Contents

Part I
Background and Supporting Concepts

Chapter 1
APBI: History, Rationale, and Controversies

Julia White

Contents

Breast conservation for early-stage breast cancer is one of the remarkable achievements of modern cancer care. Numerous randomized clinical trials initiated >30 years ago have reported 20-year durable results documenting that survival is equivalent to mastectomy when the breast is conserved by removal of the index cancer with wide excision followed by whole-breast radiotherapy [1–4]. Since then, there has been extensive clinical research focused on optimizing the results of breast conservation in terms of defining the ideal patient population, surgical resection margins, role of systemic therapy, etc. Improvements in surgical and radiation methods as well as more effective systemic therapy agents have now resulted in equivalent local regional control for those undergoing breast conservation as compared to mastectomy in modern series [5, 6]. Nearly simultaneous to the initial trials studying breast conservation instead of mastectomy, investigators began to study alternative approaches that could achieve comparable cancer outcomes while reducing the burden of care imposed by the 4–6 weeks of daily radiotherapy delivery post lumpectomy (Fig. 1.1). Partial breast irradiation, that is, radiotherapy confined exclusively to the breast tissue adjacent to the surgical cavity, was among the earliest alternatives studied. This underscores the long history of partial-breast irradiation with roots of origin that extend nearly concurrent to the development of breast conservation itself. Multiple influences have since contributed to the development and

J. White, MD
Department of Radiation Oncology, OSUCCC-James,
300w 10th Ave, Ste094D, Columbus, OH 43210, USA
e-mail: Julia.White@osumc.edu

D.W. Arthur et al. (eds.), *Short Course Breast Radiotherapy: A Comprehensive Review of Hypofractionation, Partial Breast, and Intra-Operative Irradiation*,
DOI 10.1007/978-3-319-24388-7_1

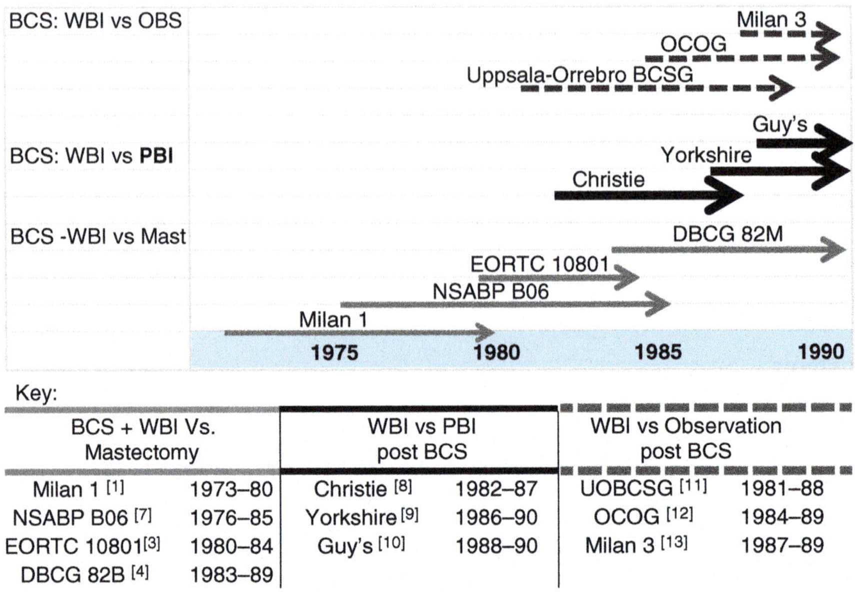

Fig. 1.1 Timeline of clinical trials evaluating breast conservation for early-stage disease prior to 1990

success of what is now modern accelerated partial-breast irradiation (APBI) to make it one of many effective approaches available today for radiotherapy post lumpectomy in selected early-stage breast cancer patients.

1.1 Rationale for Alternatives to Whole-Breast Radiotherapy

Since the 1980s, it has been well recognized that for selected early-stage breast cancer patients, breast-conserving therapy is a safe alternative to mastectomy [1–4]. The landmark clinical trials that established breast conservation therapy as equivalent treatment to mastectomy uniformly delivered whole-breast radiation post lumpectomy. In the four largest trials, the whole breast was consistently treated post lumpectomy with 50 Gy over 25 fractions [1–4], and in three of these trials, lumpectomy cavity boosts were delivered; another 10 Gy/5 fractions with orthovoltage in Milan 1 [1], 10–25 Gy in 5–12 fractions in the Danish Breast Cancer Group 82TM [4], and 25 Gy with an iridium-192 low-dose rate implant in EORTC 10801 [3]. Therefore, receipt of radiotherapy enabling breast preservation extended over several weeks. Not long after breast conservation became validated as an effective alternative treatment, heterogeneous adoption into clinical practice was documented in the United States and abroad [14–16]. A portion of this variability in clinical practice utilization was attributed to the burden of the protracted radiotherapy delivery. Women residing at an increased distance from a hospital with a radiotherapy facility had a decreased likelihood of undergoing breast conversation [17] and similarly those diagnosed in winter months were less likely to receive radiotherapy [18]. Distance from a radiation facility still remains a barrier to receipt of breast conservation as reported in a recent analysis of the National Cancer Database (NCDB) from 1998 to 2011 which demonstrated that utilization was greater if a woman's residence is within 27.8 km of a treatment facility [19]. The desire to reduce the burden of radiotherapy for breast conservation led to investigating alternatives to whole-breast irradiation. These alternatives included omission of radiotherapy post lumpectomy in selected populations, and once observations regarding relapse patterns post breast-conserving surgery emerged, investigation began into partial-breast irradiation.

Early adopters of breast conservation therapy who studied and reported subsequent patterns of in-breast recurrence suggested early on that most patients tended to relapse in the breast at the primary site [20–22]. Initial experiences with breast-conserving treatment that was delivered mostly in the late 1970s reported that the location of an in-breast failure when it occurred was at the primary site in roughly 87–90 % of cases [20, 21]. This observation was regularly reported despite a treatment era in which systemic therapy was inconsistently used and the extent of excision and breast radiotherapy doses varied significantly. This is illustrated well by a 1982 publication which relates that of 620 cases of stage I–II breast cancer treated with breast conservation at Princess Margaret Hospital between 1958 and 1978, of which 23 % received no radiotherapy, 29 % received breast radiotherapy, and the remainder breast and nodal treatment that, "it was exceptional to find recurrence in any other part of the breast remote from the original primary site" [22]. The in-breast recurrence rate at 5 years in those patients where only the breast was irradiated was 7.6 %, 12.3 % if the breast with any nodal site was irradiated, and 24.4 % where no radiation was given. This pattern of failure was further supported by findings from three randomized clinical trials that opened in the 1980s studying observation post lumpectomy as another alternative to radiotherapy for breast conservation in early-stage disease (Fig. 1.1). The Ontario Clinical Oncology Group (OCOG) trial randomized 837 axillary node-negative breast cancer patients post lumpectomy with primaries ≤4 cm in size between 1984 and 1989 to breast radiotherapy with 40 Gy/16 fractions with a 12.5 Gy/5 fraction boost versus observation [12]; the Uppsala-Orrebro Breast Cancer Study Group (UOBCSG) randomized 381 axillary node-negative patients post lumpectomy with tumor size ≤2 cm from 1981 to 1988 to whole-breast radiotherapy 54 Gy in 27 fractions of 2 Gy without a boost versus observation [11]; and Milan 3 randomized 579 breast cancer patients post quadrantectomy with tumors <2.5 cm from 1987 to 1989 to breast radiotherapy with 50 Gy/25 fractions followed by a 10 Gy/5 fraction primary site boost versus observation [13]. Each of these trials reported in-breast recurrences and the relapse patterns in both the radiotherapy and observation arms. As can be seen in Table 1.1, most in-breast recurrences occurred at the primary site irrespective of receipt of radiotherapy. Focusing on just the crude rate of recurrence outside the primary site, <1 % of those who were irradiated had an elsewhere in-breast recurrence, and in those who were observed post lumpectomy, the risk of elsewhere in-breast recurrences was somewhat higher ~ 1.5–3.5 % but substantially lower than the 4.1–22 % crude local recurrence rate seen at the primary site (Table 1.1). This supported that

Table 1.1 Patterns of failure in randomized controlled trials of lumpectomy *with* versus *without* breast radiotherapy

Trial	*n*	Fol. up Mo.	Ipsilateral in-breast cancer recurrence							
			All[a]		% at primary site in breast[b]		Crude failure primary site[b]		Crude failure elsewhere[b]	
			XRT	Obs.	XRT	Obs.	XRT	OBS	XRT	OBS
OCOG [12]	837	43	23/416 (5.5 %)	108/423 (25.7 %)	19/23 (82 %)	93/108 (86 %)	19/416 (4.6 %)	93/423 (22 %)	4/416 (0.96 %)	15/423 (3.5 %)
Milan 3 [13]	579	109	16/294 (5.4 %[c])	59/273 (23.5 %[c])	11/13 (85 %)	48/56 (86 %)	11/294 (3.7 %)	48/273 (17.5 %)	2/294 (0.68 %)	8/273 (2.9 %)
UOBCSG [11]	381	33	4[d]/187 (2.9 %)	11/194 (7.9 %)	3/4 (75 %)	8/11 (72.7 %)	3/187 (1.6 %)	8/194 (4.1 %)	1/187 (0.53 %)	3/194 (1.5 %)

XRT treated with radiotherapy post lumpectomy, *Obs* observed post lumpectomy

[a]Kaplan–Meier

[b]Crude rate

[c]Cumulative incidence

[d]Two recurrences in patients who did not receive breast RT

within the breast post lumpectomy, risk of recurrence varies and is the highest in breast tissue immediately adjacent to the surgical cavity. It also implied that the major effect of breast radiotherapy is predominantly at the primary site with less effect elsewhere in the breast.

1.2 Historical Experience with Partial Breast Irradiation and Lessons Learned

The initial randomized trials evaluating less than whole-breast irradiation for breast conservation primarily used external beam methods (Table 1.2). The Christie Hospital trial was the first randomized controlled trial that evaluated PBI versus whole-breast irradiation and remarkably began accruing in 1982 while the NSABP B06 and EORTC 10801 randomized control trials evaluating BCT versus mastectomy were still open (Fig. 1.1). The Christie Hospital trial sought to answer several questions prevalent in the early practice of breast conservation. One practical issue in that era was in anticipation of a rise in breast conversation that would require increasing use of existing radiation facilities so how the trial results could address the best use of scarce resources and available treatment times for breast cancer patients without detriment to their survival. However, the trial's primary question was based on initial observations that most patients after breast conservation with radiotherapy relapsed at the primary site [20–22] and that the recurrence rate in the untreated axilla was much lower than anticipated [23]. The trial aimed to answer whether the whole breast and ipsilateral axilla needed to be treated in all cases and what surgical and pathologic factors influenced the site and rate of local recurrence in the breast and nodal regions. Once enrolled, all women underwent excision of the

Table 1.2 Early attempts at PBI post-breast-conserving surgery

						% recurrence	
Clinical trial	Follow-up	Pop.	Arm	*n*	Dose	Breast	Axilla
Randomized:							
Christie [8, 24]	5.4 years	cT1-2, cN0	WBI	355	Breast nodes 40 Gy/15 F	11	10
		cT-2 cN0	PBI	353	42.5Gy/8 F 10-MeV electrons	19.4	23
Yorkshire [9]	8 years	pT1-2 31 % pN1	WBI	90	Breast 40 Gy/15 F Boost 15 Gy/5 F	4	4
		pT1-2 41 % pN1	PBI	84	55 Gy/20 F	12	12
Single arm:							
Guy's [10, 25]	6 years	44 % pN1	PBI	27	55 Gy/5 D/LDR	37	–
Ontario [26]	7.6 years	pT1-2, N0	PBI	39	37.2 Gy/10 F/BID HDR	16.2	–

primary alone without specific axillary surgery and then were randomized to either irradiation of the whole breast and nodes or localized high-dose electron therapy to the tumor bed only (PBI) over 10 days [8]. No adjuvant hormone or chemotherapy was to be administered. Eligible breast cancer patients were <70 years old, had negative axillae by clinical palpation, and had breast tumors ≤4 cm in size. All follow-up was also by clinical assessment with mammography done only if symptoms or signs of recurrence occurred. Partial breast irradiation included the quadrant of the breast where the tumor was clinically located and used an average field size of 8 cm×6 cm. Mean age of enrolled patients was 52.5 years, 64 % had a clinical tumor size <2 cm in size, and pathologically 30 % had a grade III tumor, and 80 % had a complete excision. At 37 months, there were a total of 30 (8 %) recurrences in the breast without distant metastases for the PBI treatment group versus 13 (4 %) in those who underwent breast-regional nodal RT. Notably, 50 patients (14 %) in the PBI only group had developed axillary recurrence with or without distant metastases, compared to 14 patients (4 %) in the whole-breast-nodal RT group. There was no statistically significant difference in distant recurrence-free or overall survival between the treatment arms. This trial was updated with 65-month median follow-up and overall survival remained the same in each treatment group, 83.7 % and 83.8 % at 5 years, respectively, for PBI and whole-breast–regional nodal RT [24]. At 7 years, 19.6 % experienced an in- breast recurrence in the PBI group compared to 11 % in the breast-nodal RT group, $p=0.0008$. This difference in breast recurrences between arms was partially attributed to the 9 % of cases with infiltrating lobular histology where at 7 years there was in-breast recurrence of 34 % in the PBI treatment arm versus 8 % for whole-breast-nodal RT arm. However, there was still a significant difference in the rate of breast recurrence when just the infiltrating ductal cancers were considered of 15 % versus 11 % ($p=0.01$) for PBI and whole-breast-nodal RT arms, respectively. As one would expect, a very high rate of axillary recurrence of 23 % was reported in the PBI arm where the axilla was neither dissected nor irradiated compared to 10 % in the other arm where the whole breast and axilla were both irradiated. In addition, the PBI arm was more likely to have marked fibrosis (14 % vs 5 %) and marked telangiectasia (33 % vs 12 %) compared to the whole-breast and nodal RT group.

A second randomized trial of PBI compared to whole-breast irradiation post lumpectomy was begun by the Yorkshire Breast Cancer Group in 1986 [9]. This study was intended to accrue a total of 400 breast cancer patients. Unlike the Christie Hospital trial, more stringent selection criteria were used and standardized surgical and systemic therapy was employed. The trial enrolled women with pathologic (p) T1-2, pN0-1 breast cancers that had local excision with negative margins and a level two axillary lymph-node dissection. All patients were to receive chemotherapy and 5 years of tamoxifen. Randomization was between standard whole-breast radiotherapy and PBI directed solely to the tumor bed with a 1 cm margin. A variety of extern beam methods were used for delivery of PBI based on clinician preference, including a direct cobalt or cesium beam, electrons, or an mV photon tangential pair. By 1990 only 174 women were randomized and the trial closed. The median age of those enrolled was 52 years, 36 % were node positive, and 25 % had grade 3 histology. At a median follow-up of 8 years, 4.4 % (4/90) of women treated with whole-breast RT developed an in-breast recurrence in the absence of regional or distant disease compared with 11.9 % (10/84) women in the PBI group ($P=0.07$). Similarly, four (4 %) women within the WBRT group developed ipsilateral axillary recurrence compared with 10 (12 %) in the PBI group ($P=0.05$). Total actuarial local/regional recurrence rates were thus 24 % in the PBI group compared with 9 % in the whole-breast RT group. There was no significant difference in distant metastatic rate or survival between the treatment arms. When looking closer at the patterns of failure in this trial, 7 of the 10 recurrences occurring within the PBI arm occurred within or near to the irradiated volume.

The initial PBI experience with brachytherapy is exemplified by two single-arm prospective trials that utilized temporary multi-catheter implants for treatment (Table 1.2). The first of these was conducted at Guy's Hospital in London in 1988–1990 and studied low-dose rate (LDR) brachytherapy with a temporary multi-catheter implant for PBI [10]. Eligibility included women less than 70 years of age with a tumor 4 cm or smaller in size by clinical palpation. All patients underwent an axillary dissection and had a gross tumor excision from the breast without attention to clearance of microscopic margins. Suitability for treatment was determined by the presence of sufficient breast tissue in the tumor-bearing quadrant after surgery, so that an implant was technically possible. Hollow stainless steel needles were then implanted into the tumor bed in a multiplane triangular array according to the Paris low-dose rate (LDR) system. Individual dose calculations were not performed in most cases but tables were used to calculate the activity of the iridium (Ir^{192}) wire and the LDR treatment time needed to give a dose of 55 Gy in 5.5 days to 85 % of the basal dose rate as defined by the Paris system. There were 27 patients included in the study. For 17 patients a two-plane implant was used with a median of 9 Ir^{192} wires and in 10 a three-plane implant was used with a median of 12 Ir^{192} wires. The mean patient age was 51 years, 9 were premenopausal, and 18 were postmenopausal. The mean tumor diameter measured clinically was 3 cm; 20 patients had infiltrating ductal and 5 had infiltrating lobular carcinomas. Axillary nodes were histologically positive in 12 cases (44 %). After a median follow-up of 6 years, in-breast recurrence (IBR) occurred in 10 (37 %) [25]. Clinical and pathologic features of IBR versus cases without IBR were compared. Of the patients who had an IBR, axillary nodal metastases were confirmed histologically in 70 % but in only 29 % of the non-relapsed group (Fisher's exact test, $P=0.057$). A younger median patient age of 48.4 years was noted in the IBR group compared to 53.2 years in those without relapse but this did not reach statistical significance. It is important to note that post-excision surgical margins were known to be positive in 55 %, clear in 37 %, and unknown in 8 %. Similar proportions of involved margins were reported, in fact 60 % and 53 %, respectively, for those with and without breast recurrence. In all except 1 case, the site of relapse was within the irradiated field.

An initial clinical trial with multi-catheter high-dose rate (HDR) brachytherapy for PBI post lumpectomy was conducted at the London Regional Cancer Centre, in Ontario, Canada from 1992 to 1996 [26]. Eligible patients had T1 or T2 and node-negative breast cancer with microscopic resection margins negative for both invasive and in situ cancer. Infiltrating lobular cancers were excluded. All 39 patients who enrolled underwent complete excision of the primary tumor and an axillary node dissection. Surgical clips outlining the lumpectomy cavity were required. An average of 7 (range: 3–11) brachytherapy needles were placed per patient. There were 11 single-plane implants, 25 double-plane implants, and 3 triple-plane implants. The total dose was 37.2Gy, 10 fractions of 3.72 Gy given twice daily with a minimum inter-fraction interval of 6 h over 5–7 days prescribed as a minimum peripheral dose to match or exceed the volume defined by the surgical clips as seen on CT scan. The median volume encompassed by the 37.2 Gy isodose shell was 30.35 cm^3 (range: 9.6–110.8 cm^3). Median follow-up of all patients is 91 months (range: 22–118 months) with a minimum follow-up of 6 years for the 33 women that are still alive (range: 77–118 months). The median patient age was 59 years, 82 % had tumors ≤2 cm in size, all had negative margins of excision, and 15 % had metastases to axillary nodes. Six of the 39 women (15.4 %) enrolled developed ipsilateral breast recurrences. Two women had in-field recurrences/marginal misses. Unlike the prior LDR brachytherapy PBI study from Guy's hospital, roughly 2/3rd or 67 % of patients had out-of-field recurrences that were 1.6 cm or greater from the nearest surgical clip marking the lumpectomy site. There were no regional nodal recurrences.

Three important lessons were learned from these early experiences with PBI that informed subsequent single and multiple institution clinical trials. First, the importance of adequate surgical excision of the primary tumor and accurate staging of the axilla is evident. In particular, the high rates of in-breast and axillary recurrence in both treatment arms of the Christie Hospital trial emphasize the deleterious effect of undertreatment by surgery and exclusion of systemic therapy in combination of underestimating the extent of disease with staging by clinical palpation only. The influence of incomplete excision of the breast primary is further evident in the Guy's Trial where 55 % had positive resection margins and the 37 % rate of in-breast recurrence after post-excision PBI with LDR brachytherapy is greater than ~23–25.7 % rate reported *without any* radiation in the observation only arms of OCOG and Milan 3 trials listed in Table 1.2. The second lesson from these early experiences is that there are adverse pathologic features associated with poorer outcome from PBI that should influence patient selection. For example, infiltrating lobular cancers were associated with very high rates of in-breast recurrence in the Christie Hospital trial and in the Guy's trial; those who experienced a recurrence post PBI were more likely axillary node positive. It is important to point out that none of these early attempts at PBI reported estrogen/progesterone receptor presence and HER2 Neu presence/amplification used standardly in current clinical practice as biomarkers for prognosis classification. Lastly, each of these early studies underscores the need for fidelity in defining the PBI clinical target volume (CTV) and quality assurance measures that the dose is being delivered adequately to the CTV. Specifically this means reliable identification of the post-excision surgical cavity, defining the extent of adjacent breast tissue that is at highest risk for recurrence that should be included in the CTV and then determining that an adequate radiation dose is then delivered. For example, the authors of the Yorkshire trial noted that their method of using scar location and other clinical information to identify the PBI target volume likely explained the higher than expected in-breast recurrence risk. Even when the surgical cavity is better defined, an excess risk of recurrence can exist if either the margin around the cavity for the CTV is insufficient in including the adjacent breast tissue at highest risk or if the PBI fails to dosimetrically cover the breast tissue in the CTV. This is a plausible contributing factor to the 16.2 % local recurrence rate reported in the Ontario HDR Brachytherapy APBI trial (Table 1.2). Many elements of the Ontario trial were well controlled, such as adequate surgical treatment, systemic therapy, careful pathologic selection criteria, as well as reliable methods for placing multi-catheter implants by either direct visualization intraoperatively or with the use of surgical clips that demarcated the cavity extent. However, the mean number of catheters used in the HDR implant was only 7. At treatment planning the 100 % isodose was chosen to, "match or exceed the volume defined by the surgical clips," without a consistent defined margin for CTV, and on average was fairly small at 30.35 cm^3. In comparison, the Radiation Therapy Oncology Group (RTOG) 9517 phase 1–2 trial of multi-catheter APBI in a similar patient population also required surgical clips to demarcate the lumpectomy cavity but the CTV was defined as a 2 cm margin peripheral to the cavity and 1 cm anteriorly and posteriorly. On average the number of catheters used was 17 [27], more than double of that in the Ontario trial. A recent updated analysis of the RTOG 95–17 trial at 12-year median follow-up revealed that at 10 years 5.2 % had an isolated in-breast recurrence without distant metastases as the first site of failure and 6.2 % overall when including those concurrent with distant metastases [28].

Building on the lessons learned, the next generation of clinical trials investigated primarily multi-catheter brachytherapy for APBI post lumpectomy and documented successful local regional cancer control in selected early-stage breast cancer patients (Table 1.3). Three trials that typify this era of APBI clinical trial investigation include a small randomized controlled trial from the National Institute of Oncology (NIO), Budapest, Hungary [29], and two single institution prospective trials from William Beaumont Hospital (WBH) in Royal Oak, Michigan [30], and the Ochsner Medical Center in New Orleans, Louisiana [31], that compared the APBI results to women treated with the institutional standard whole-breast irradiation by matched-pair analysis. These studies are characterized by having well-controlled surgery methods, systemic therapy, patient selection, and consistent targeting and dose delivery for APBI.

The NIO Budapest trial accrued 258 women from 1998 to 2004 with unifocal breast cancer ≤20 mm in size (pT1), pN0 or $pN1^{mic}$ (nodal micrometastasis ≤2 mm) axillary nodal status, and histological grades 1–2 [29]. All patients underwent lumpectomy with microscopic margin clearance and axillary node dissection and were randomized to receive either APBI with MCT brachytherapy or whole-breast irradiation without boost. The surgical cavity boundaries were marked with clips. The targeted accrual was 570 but the trial was closed after 258 were randomized as of June 2004 since all eligible patients were instead offered enrollment in the European multicenter GEC-ESTRO (Groupe Européen de Curiethérapie-European Society for Therapeutic Radiology and Oncology) phase III APBI trial. Of the 128

Table 1.3 Select next-generation clinical trials evaluating post-lumpectomy APBI with multi-catheter brachytherapy

Clinical trial	Follow-up	Pop.	Arm	n	Dose	% recurrence	
						Breast	Axilla/Ln
Randomized:							
NIO Budapest [29]	10.2 years	pT1, pN0-1[mic]	PBI	128	HDR 36.4 Gy, 5.2 Gy × 7	5.9	2.5
			WBI	130	50 Gy/25 F No boost or nodal RT	5.1	1.7
Single-arm APBI w/matched analysis:							
WBH [30]	9.4 years	pT1, pT2<3 cm pN0-1	PBI	199	LDR: 50 Gy, 0.52 Gy/h HDR: 32–34 Gy, 8–10 F	5	1.6
	13.7 years		WBI	199	45–50.4 Gy/25–28 F Boost 10 Gy/5 F	4	0.5
Ochsner [31]	6.2 years	pTis,1–2, pN0-1	PBI	51	LDR: 45 Gy/0.94 Gy/h HDR: 32 Gy, 4 Gy × 8 bid	2	6
	6.2 years		WBI	94	45–50.4 Gy/25–28 F Boost 10 Gy/5 F	5	0

randomized to the APBI arm, in 69 % an HDR MCT implant was successfully completed and in the other 31 % that were technically unsuitable for a MCT implant PBI was delivered with 50 Gy/25 fractions using 6–15 MeV electrons. For APBI the planning target volume (PTV) was defined as the excision cavity delineated by the surgical clips plus a margin of 2 cm. The patient population is characterized by many good risk features with a median breast tumor size of 13 mm, 94.5 % N0, 100 % grades1–2, 89 % estrogen receptor positive, and 78 % postmenopausal, and 71 % receive either adjuvant hormone or chemotherapy. The actuarial 10-year rate of in-breast recurrence was 5.9 % for the APBI versus 5.1 for the WBI and for regional recurrences the APBI arm was 2.5 % versus 1.7 % for the WBI arm.

At William Beaumont Hospital, 199 women were enrolled in 3 prospective trials evaluating post-lumpectomy APBI with MCT brachytherapy from 1993 to 2001 [30]. Eligibility criteria included having infiltrating ductal carcinomas less than 3.0 cm in diameter, having negative surgical margins (≥2 mm), being over 40 years of age, and having negative lymph nodes. The MCT brachytherapy APBI was LDR for 120 (60 %) and HDR for 79. The patient population enrolled included many low-risk features such as a median patient age of 65 years with 92 % being older than 50 years; 92 % had a pathologic tumor size ≤20 mm, the median tumor size was 13 mm, 100 % had negative resection margins, 88 % were N0, and 86 % were estrogen receptor positive. Adjuvant hormone or chemotherapy was delivered to 70 %. With a median follow-up of 9.6 years, there have been 8 in-breast recurrences for a 10-year actuarial rate of 5 % and a regional nodal recurrence rate of 1.6 %. When matched to breast cancer cases with similar clinical and pathologic features that underwent WBI post lumpectomy, a comparable rate of local recurrence rate at 4 % and the regional recurrence of 0.5 % was found.

Analogous findings were reported from a single-arm prospective trial from the Ochsner Medical Center that enrolled 51 early-stage breast cancer patients from 1992 to 1993, to receive multi-catheter APBI post lumpectomy and axillary node dissection [31]. Eligibility criteria included having stage 0–II breast cancer with a unifocal primary <4.0 cm in diameter, negative surgical margins, and pN0-1 nodal stage with 1–3 nodal metastases. The mean patient age was 63 years, 82 % had a pathologic tumor size ≤20 mm, and 100 % had negative resection margins. This trial included a slightly higher risk population with 18 % having axillary nodal metastases and 43 % with grade III cancers. At a median follow-up of 75 months, there were 1 in-breast recurrence (2 %) and 3 regional nodal recurrences (6 %). The matched analysis to breast cancer cases with similar clinical and pathologic features that underwent WBI post lumpectomy yielded statistically comparable findings with 5 (5 %) in-breast recurrences and no regional nodal recurrences.

The next set of investigations determined if the success with APBI within a single institution could be translated to the multi-institution setting. Three successive phase II studies demonstrated the feasibility of technically reproducible APBI being delivered across many institutions and confirmed the efficacy for other methods of APBI delivery: RTOG 9517 enrolled 100 patients from 1997 to 2000 confirming that multi-catheter APBI can be reliably and safely delivered [32]; an industry trial enrolled 70 and successfully treated 43 women post lumpectomy with the first single-entry balloon brachytherapy device (MammoSite®) between 2000 and 2001 [33]; and RTOG 0319 enrolled 58 from 2003 to 2004 to establish external beam three-dimensional conformal radiotherapy (3DCRT) methods for APBI [34] (Table 1.4). These phase II trials among others established a foundation of experience with APBI that helped launch several large phase III randomized trials that are powered to determine if APBI can yield equivalent local control to standard whole-breast irradiation post-lumpectomy (Table 1.5). Four trials have already enrolled

Table 1.4 Initial phase II multi-institution trials that further established APBI as sole radiotherapy modality post lumpectomy for BCT

Clinical trial	*n*	APBI type	Dose	Target definition	*Population (%)* T1	N0	ER+	Median F/u	% IBR[a]
RTOG 9517 [27, 28]	99	MCT Brachy	34 Gy, 10 F, BID	C/PTV: 2 cm radial 1 cm Ant/post	88	81	74	12.2 years	6.2
MammoSite Industry [33, 35]	43	Device Brachy	34 Gy, 10 F, BID	C/PTV: 1 cm expansion	100	100	–	5.5 years	0
RTOG 0319 [34, 36]	52	3DCRT	38.5 Gy, 10 F, BID	CTV: 1.5 cm PTV: 1.0 cm	94	92	83	8 years	7.7

[a]All IBR (in-breast recurrences) include isolated and with regional nodal and/or distant metastases

Table 1.5 Phase III randomized clinical trials evaluating post-lumpectomy APBI vs standard whole-breast radiotherapy with results pending

Clinical trial	Status	Accrual goal	PBI method	Eligibility
NSABP B-39/ RTOG 0413	Closed 2013	4214	3-DCRT MST MCT	>18 yo, stages 0–II, < 3 cm, pN-0 – N-1 (<3 LN+), negative margins
GEC-ESTRO	Closed 2009	1300	MCT	≥40 yo, stages 0–II, < 3 cm, pN0 – N^{mic}, negative margins (2 mm)
RAPID OCOG	Closed 2012	2135	3-DCRT	≥40 yo, stages 0–II, < 3 cm, pN-0, negative margins, excludes inf. lobular
IMPORT Low MRC	Closed 2011	1935	IMRT/3D	≥50 yo, stages I–II, < 3 cm, pN-0 – N-1 (<3 LN+), negative margins (2 mm), excludes inf. lobular
IRMA	Open	3302	3DCRT	≥49 yo, stages I–II, < 3 cm, pN-0 – N-1 (<3 LN+), negative margins (2 mm)
SHARE	Open	2796	3DCRT	≥50 yo, stage 1, < 2 cm, p N0-N^{i+} negative margins (2 mm)

and randomized nearly 10,000 early-stage breast cancer patients to receive APBI versus a standard course of whole-breast radiotherapy following lumpectomy with either sentinel node biopsy or axillary dissection (Table 1.5). Two other phase III trials are ongoing and collectively will accrue an additional 6,000 women: IRMA, an Italian multi-institution trial has enrolled 2520 of its intended 3303, and SHARE, a French multi-institution trial with a targeted accrual of 2796.

1.3 Factors That Supported the Advancement of Accelerated Partial Breast Irradiation

It has been nearly two decades since the initial clinical trials of more modern APBI reviewed above were begun. Numerous factors have contributed to the sustained research and growth of APBI into clinical practice. Three trends in particular over the past decade have been critical to the prevalence of APBI: 1. advances in technology and its integration into radiation treatment planning for breast cancer, 2. successful application of the linear quadratic equation to apply more novel fractionation schedules for breast cancer treatment, and 3. the emergence of the intrinsic subtyping of breast cancer by gene expression that reliably stratified patients by prognosis for cancer recurrence.

Technology integration has been a key factor in making APBI broadly accessible as an alternative to standard whole-breast radiotherapy post lumpectomy. Multi-catheter brachytherapy was the first method developed in modern APBI but is hampered by its technical complexity for it to have had widespread adoption into clinical practice. It was really the advent of the first single-entry brachytherapy device

(SEBD), MammoSite™, that enabled APBI to be more widely adopted into clinical practice [32]. Subsequently, technology advancement led to several other SEBD being developed and implemented improving on the limitations of the initial MammoSite device [37, 38]. In addition, the past decade has witnessed significant integration of innovative advanced technology into CT-based treatment planning methods for all of external beam radiation with both 3DCRT and intensity-modulated radiotherapy (IMRT), including breast cancer. Application of 3DCRT and IMRT methods for an external beam approach to APBI further supported its adoption into practice. This is illustrated in an analysis of a total of 574,835 non-neo-adjuvant American Joint Committee on Cancer (AJCC) stage 0 to II breast cancer patients in the National Cancer Database (NCDB) that were treated with lumpectomy and WBI or APBI during 2003–2010 [39]. Use of APBI for the entire cohort increased from 3.4 % in 2003 to 12.8 % ($p = 0.001$) in 2008 and then decreased to 12.4 % in 2010 (Fig. 1.2). Three-dimensional conformal APBI increased from 0.8 to 2.2 %, IMRT APBI increased from 0.7 to 1.3 %, and brachytherapy APBI increased from 2.0 to 8.9 %. In women >65, roughly 15 % were treated with APBI post lumpectomy for breast conservation.

Another significant factor supporting APBI has been the reconsideration of the alpha–beta ratio for breast cancer and normal tissue sensitivity led by the UK Standardization of Breast Radiotherapy (START) trials [40]. Spurred by historical use of a more hypo-fractionated regimen for breast radiotherapy in the UK initiated primarily for resource management, the START investigator reevaluated the data

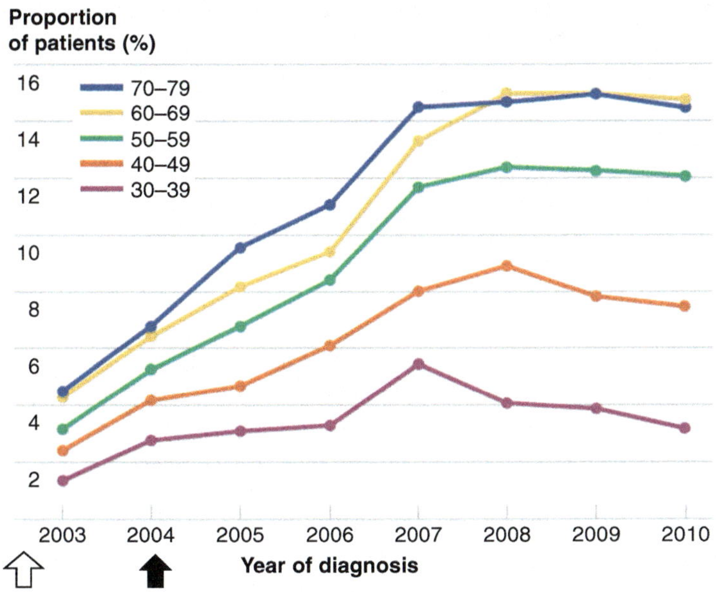

Fig. 1.2 Utilization of accelerated partial-breast irradiation by patient age, 2003–2010. 2002 (*open arrow*) – the first single-entry brachytherapy device, MammoSite™, is approved by the FDA. 2004 (*closed arrow*) – the Medicare reimbursement of APBI with brachytherapy begins

underlying the assumptions of a larger alpha–beta ratio for breast cancer and late-reacting normal tissue. They hypothesized that the alpha–beta ratio for breast cancer is lower and closer to the predominantly soft tissue normal tissue encountered during breast cancer irradiation such that the historically used UK breast radiotherapy fractionation may be optimal. Long-term outcomes from START A and B trials [40] and the OCOG hypo-fractionation trial [41] have demonstrated similar in breast local control and normal tissue damage in fewer fractions in comparison with 50 Gy in 25 of 2Gy fractionation schedule. These trials, along with additional analyses of other data sets, support that an alpha–beta ratio is low and, assuming the alpha–beta of normal breast tissue is also close to 3, then less complication for normal structures may be expected in hypo-fractionated schemes [42]. By inference, this has supported that the novel fractionation schedules used in APBI should yield comparable local control in the highest risk breast tissue encompassed in the CTV around the lumpectomy site with acceptable toxicity.

Lastly, since 2001, breast cancer has become classified based into at least 5 subtypes, luminal A, luminal B, basal, HER2 enriched, and claudin low/normal-like based on gene expression patterns that correlate with tumor characteristics and clinical outcome [43]. Specifically this subtyping has identified that the hormone-sensitive, HER2 Neu-negative luminal A subtype group that is characterized by high expression levels of estrogen receptors and lower histological grade and proliferation has a relatively favorable prognosis. After breast conservation with lumpectomy and radiotherapy, local regional recurrence has been demonstrated to be much lower for those categorized as luminal A by multi-gene assay or immunohistochemistry proxy [44]. In more modern clinical trials examining APBI, the majority of women treated have been hormone sensitive, Her2-neg, or luminal A-like such that there may be biological factors in addition to technical ones contributing to the success of APBI so far.

1.4 Controversies and Unanswered Questions

The numerous phase III randomized controlled trials listed in Table 1.5 will help address two key outstanding questions regarding APBI, i.e., for which breast cancer patients that undergo lumpectomy will it yield equivalent local control to standard whole-breast irradiation and are the toxicity and cosmetic outcomes comparable? So far, the population of breast cancer patients most frequently treated with APBI has included the following features: age greater than 50, T1 tumor size ($\leq$2 cm), node negative, and hormone sensitive. Other populations of breast cancer patients are much less frequently represented in the APBI outcome data. Several organizations and societies have developed consensus statements and guidelines regarding optimal patient selection for post-lumpectomy APBI until more robust level one evidence is available from the pending randomized controlled trials. This has included the American Brachytherapy Society (ABS) [45], American Society of Breast Surgeons (ASBS) [46], American Society of Radiation Oncology (ASTRO) [47], and Groupe

Européen de Curiethérapie-European Society for Therapeutic Radiology and Oncology (GEC-ESTRO) [48]. As can be seen in Table 1.6, there is some similarity in the characteristics identified by the various societies for whom APBI is currently considered a reasonable treatment option post lumpectomy. These guidelines have been a subject of ongoing debate. So far there have been two smaller phase III clinical trials that have reported comparable in-breast local cancer control from APBI versus WBI: the NIO Budapest trial [29] and the University of Florence trials (n=520) [49]. A closer look at the patient populations on these trials reveals that they are both characterized by the following in >90 % of cases: patient age >50 years, T-1, N-0, margin negative, and ER/PR positive or essentially fitting into the more rigorous of the good risk groups outlined in Table 1.6. Therefore, the results of the other randomized control trials (Table 1.5) will be crucial to determine if APBI can be applied to other less frequently studied risk groups with more adverse clinical and pathologic features and still yield similar good rates of in-breast cancer control. In addition, the randomized control trials are anticipated to answer the question of whether there is comparable toxicity and cosmetic outcome from APBI as compared to WBI for breast conservation. So far, two trials using external beam methods for APBI have reported opposite results; one finding APBI yielded more frequent fair or poor cosmetic results [49] and the other finding it did not [50]. If equivalent local control outcomes are found from APBI and WBI post lumpectomy, then cosmetic outcome may become the determining factor regarding further APBI clinical adoption.

Despite the greater than 10,000 women enrolled in the pending phase III randomized controlled trials, there are some clinically relevant questions surrounding APBI that they are not designed to answer. These include: 1. identifying the optimal dose-fractionation regimen for APBI, 2. determining if an in-breast recurrence after APBI can be successfully salvaged with a second breast-conserving treatment, and 3. whether APBI post lumpectomy improves local control over observation in biologically and clinically low-risk breast cancer populations.

The majority of the pending phase III randomized clinical trials are using a hypofractionated dose regimens delivered twice a day (BID) for 8–10 fractions with the goal of a minimum of 6 h between fractions. This can be burdensome for patients

Table 1.6 Comparison of ABS/ASBS recommended, ASTRO suitable, and GEC-ESTRO low-risk categories for APBI clinical use

Statement	Age (years)	T-size	pN Stage	ER/PR	Histology	Margins	DCIS
ABS [45]	>50	≤3 cm	N-0	–	No EIC/LVI	Negative	Yes
ASBS [46]	>45	≤3 cm	N-0	–	–	Negative	Yes
ASTRO [47]	>60	≤2 cm	N-0	Positive	No ILC/EIC/LVI	Negative	No
GEC-ESTRO [48]	>50	≤3 cm	N-0	–	No ILC/EIC/LVI	Negative	No

ABS American Brachytherapy Society, *ASBS* American Society of Breast Surgeons, *ASTRO* American Society of Radiation Oncology, *GEC-ESTRO* Groupe Européen de Curiethérapie-European Society for Therapeutic Radiology and Oncology, *ILC* infiltrating lobular cancer, *EIC* extensive intraductal component, *LVI* lymphatic or vascular space invasion and treatment facilities. Furthermore, there is concern that the 6 h inter-fraction interval is too brief to permit any significant repair of normal tissue injury and therefore the twice daily fractionation will lead to worse toxicity outcome [51]. This will likely be an important priority area for investigation once the population of breast cancer best suited to APBI for breast conservation is determined.

One of the proposed advantages of APBI over WBI is that a portion of the treated breast is spared from exposure to radiotherapy. This seems to suggest that additional attempts of breast conservation should be more feasible after APBI than WBI when there is an in-breast recurrence. However, so far mastectomy is the most common salvage for in-breast recurrence after APBI as is demonstrated in the ASBS MammoSite registry study where it was used for 75 % [52]. It may prove to be an overall advantage of APBI if it allows a better overall chance at breast conservation because salvage with a second breast conservation procedure is more feasible.

Increasingly, luminal A breast cancers, identified by immunohistochemistry or gene expression, are being studied to determine if breast radiotherapy can be omitted completely following lumpectomy given their favorable prognosis. For example, a recent analysis by luminal subtype of the Princess Margaret Clinical trial for women >50 years of age with hormone-sensitive, stage 1, breast cancer who were randomized to whole-breast radiotherapy versus observation post lumpectomy revealed that luminal A subtypes derived less benefit from radiation [53]. In an exploratory analysis of women >60 years of age with grade 1–2 disease combined with luminal A subtype, there was no significant benefit from radiotherapy in terms of local regional control at 10 years. In these groups of patients at very low risk for recurrence post lumpectomy, additional investigation will be needed to determine the role for APBI.

References

1. Veronesi U, Cascinelli N, Mariani L, et al. Twenty-year follow-up of a randomized study comparing breast-conserving surgery with radical mastectomy for early breast cancer. N Engl J Med. 2002;347:1227–32.
2. Fisher B, Anderson S, Bryant J, et al. Twenty-year follow-up of a randomized trial comparing total mastectomy, lumpectomy, and lumpectomy plus irradiation for the treatment of invasive breast cancer. N Engl J Med. 2002;347:1233–41.
3. Litiere S, Werutsky G, Fentiman I, et al. Breast conserving therapy versus mastectomy for stage I–II breast cancer: 20 year follow-up of the EORTC 10801 phase 3 randomized trial. Lancet Oncol. 2012;13:412–9.
4. Blichert-Toft M, Nielsen M, During M, et al. Long-term results of breast conserving surgery vs. mastectomy for early stage invasive breast cancer: 20-year follow-up of the Danish randomized DBCG-82TM protocol. Acta Oncol. 2008;47:672–81.
5. Coulombe G, Tyldesley S, Speers C, et al. Is mastectomy superior to breast-conserving treatment for young women? Int J Radiat Oncol Biol Phys. 2007;67(5):1282–90.
6. Adkins F, Gonzalez-Angulo A, Lei X, et al. Triple-negative breast cancer is not a contraindication for breast conservation. Ann Surg Oncol. 2011;18:3164–73.

7. Fisher B, Bauer M, Margolese R, et al. Five-year results of a randomized clinical trial comparing total mastectomy and segmental mastectomy with or without radiation in the treatment of breast cancer. N Engl J Med. 1985;312:665–73.
8. Riberio G, Dunn G, Swindell R, et al. Conservation of the breast using two different radiotherapy techniques: interim report of a clinical trial. Clin Oncol. 1990;2:27–34.
9. Dodwell D, Dyker K, Brwon J, et al. A randomized study of whole-breast vs tumour-bed irradiation after local excision and axillary dissection for early breast cancer. Clin Oncol. 2005;17:618–22.
10. Fentiman I, Poole C, Tong D, et al. Iridium implant treatment without external radiotherapy for operable breast cancer: a pilot study. Eur J Cancer. 1991;27(4):447–50.
11. Liljegren G, Holmberg L, Bergh J, et al. 10-year results after sector resection with or without postoperative radiotherapy for stage I breast cancer: a randomized trial. J Clin Oncol. 1999;17:2326–33.
12. Clark R, McCulloch P, Levine MT, et al. Randomized clinical trial to assess the effectiveness of breast irradiation following lumpectomy and axillary dissection for node-negative breast cancer. J Natl Cancer Inst. 1992;84:683–9.
13. Veronesi U, Marubini E, Mariani L, et al. Radiotherapy after breast-conserving surgery in small breast carcinoma: Long-term results of a randomized trial. Ann Oncol. 2001;12:997–1003.
14. Nattinger A, Gottlieb M, Veum J, et al. Geographic variation in the use of breast-conserving treatment for breast cancer. N Engl J Med. 1992;326:1102–7.
15. Chouillet AM, Bell CM, Hiscox JG. Management of breast cancer in southeast England. BMJ. 1994;308:168–71.
16. de Koning HJ, van Dongen JA, van der Maas PJ. Changes in use of breast conserving therapy in years 1978–2000. Br J Cancer. 1994;70:1165–70.
17. Nattinger A, Kneusel R, Hoffman R, Gilligan MA. Relationship of distance from a radiotherapy facility and initial breast cancer treatment. J Natl Cancer Inst. 2001;93(17):1344–6.
18. Celaya M, Rees J, Gibson J, et al. Travel distance and season of diagnosis affect treatment choices for women with early-stage breast cancer in a predominantly rural population (United States). Cancer Causes Control. 2006;17:851–6.
19. Lautner M, Lin H, Shen Y, et al. Disparities in the use of breast-conserving therapy among patients with early stage breast cancer. JAMA Surg. 2015;150(8):778–86. doi:10.1001/jamasurg.2015.1102.
20. Hellman S, Harris J, Levene M. Radiation therapy of early carcinoma of the breast without mastectomy. Cancer. 1980;46:988–94.
21. Kurtz J, Spitalier JM, Amalric R. Late breast recurrence after lumpectomy and irradiation. Int J Radiat Oncol Biol Phys. 1983;9:1191–4.
22. Clark R, Wilkinson R, Mahoney LJ, Mac DW. Breast cancer: a 21 year experience. Int J Radit Oncol Biol Phys. 1982;8:961–75.
23. Fisher B, Redmond C, Fisdher E, et al. Ten year results of a randomized clinical trial comparing radical mastectomy and total mastectomy with or without radiation. N Engl J Med. 1985;312:674–81.
24. Riberio G, Magee B, Swindell R, et al. The Christie hospital breast conservation trial: an update at 8 years from inception. Clin Oncol. 1993;5:278–83.
25. Fentiman I, Poole C, Tong D, et al. Inadequacy of iridium implant as sole radiation treatment for operable breast cancer. Eur J Cancer. 1996;32A(40):608–11.
26. Perera F, Yu E, Engel J, et al. Patterns of breast recurrence in a pilot study of brachytherapy confined to the lumpectomy site for early breast cancer with six years' minimum follow-up. Int J Radiat Oncol Biol Phys. 2003;57(5):1239–46.
27. Ibbott GS, Hanson WF, O'Meara E, et al. Dose specification and quality assurance of Radiation Therapy Oncology Group protocol 9517; a cooperative group study of iridium-192 breast implants as sole therapy. Int J Radiat Oncol Biol Phys. 2007;69(5):1572–8.
28. White J, Winter K, Kuske R et al. Long term cancer outcomes from NRG Oncology/RTOG 9517: a phase II study of accelerated partial breast irradiation with multicatheter brachytherapy

following lumpectomy for early stage breast cancer; ASCO Breast Cancer Symposium 2012, San Francisco, CA, http://meetinglibrary.asco.org/search/site/white?content_type[0]=fctContentType%3AAbstract&author=white&meeting_id[0]=125.
29. Polgar C, Fodor J, Major T, et al. Breast-conserving therapy with partial or whole breast irradiation: ten-year results of the Budapest randomized trial. Radiother Oncol. 2013;108:197–202.
30. Vicini F, Kestin L, Chen P, et al. Limited-field radiation therapy in the management of early-stage breast cancer. J Natl Cancer Inst. 2003;95:1205–11.
31. King T, Bolton J, Kuske R, et al. Long-term results of wide-field brachytherapy as the sole method of radiation therapy after segmental mastectomy for Tis,1,2 breast cancer. Am J Surg. 2000;180:299–304.
32. Kuske R, Winter K, Arthur D, et al. Phase II trial of brachytherapy alone after lumpectomy for select breast cancer: toxicity analysis of RTOG 95–17. Int J Radiat Oncol Biol Phys. 2006;65(1):45–51.
33. Keisch M, Vicini F, Kuske R, et al. Initial clinical experience with the mammosite breast brachytherapy applicator in women with early-stage breast cancer treated with breast-conserving therapy. Int J Radiat Oncol Biol Phys. 2003;55(2):289–93.
34. Vicini F, Winter K, Wong J, et al. Initial efficacy results of RTOG 0319: three-dimensional conformal radiation therapy (3D-CRT) confined to the region of the lumpectomy cavity for stage I/ II breast carcinoma. Int J Radiat Oncol Biol Phys. 2010;77(4):1120–7.
35. Benitez P, Keisch M, Vicini F, et al. Five-year results: the initial clinical trial of Mammosite balloon brachytherapy for partial breast irradiation in early-stage breast cancer. Am J Surg. 2007;194:456–62.
36. Rabinovitch R, Moughan J, Vicini F, et al. Long term update of RTOG 0319: a phase I/II trial to evaluate three dimensional conformal radiation therapy (3D-CRT) confined to the region of the lumpectomy cavity for stage I and II breast Carcinoma. 55th Annual meeting of the American Society of Therapeutic Radiation Oncology (ASTRO), Atlanta, GA, September 2013
37. Yashar C, Scanderberg D, Kuske R, et al. Initial clinical experience with the strut-adjusted volume implant (SAVI) breast brachytherapy device for accelerated partial-breast irradiation (APBI): first 100 patients with more than 1 year of follow-up. Int J Radiat Oncol Biol Phys. 2011;80(3):765–70.
38. Cuttino L, Arthru D, Vicini F, et al. Long-term results from the contura multilumen balloon breast brachytherapy catheter phase 4 registry trial. Int J Radiat Oncol Biol Phys. 2014;90(5): 1025–9.
39. Czechura T, Winchester D, Pesce C, et al. Accelerated partial-breast irradiation versus whole-breast irradiation for early-stage breast cancer patients undergoing breast conservation, 2003–2010: a report from the national cancer data base. Ann Surg Oncol. 2013;20:3223–32.
40. Haviland J, Owen J, Dewar J, et al. The UK Standardisation of Breast Radiotherapy (START) trials of radiotherapy hypofractionation for treatment of early breast cancer: 10-year follow-up results of two randomised controlled trials. Lancet Oncol. 2013;14:1086–94.
41. Whelan T, Pignol JP, Levine M, et al. Long-term results of hypofractionated radiation therapy for breast cancer. N Engl J Med. 2010;362:513–20.
42. Qi XS, White J, LI XA. Is alpha/ beta for breast cancer really low? Radiother Oncol. 2011;10:282–8.
43. Sorlie T, Perou C, Tibshirani R, et al. Gene expression patterns of breast carcinomas distinguish tumor subclasses with clinical implications. Proc Natl Acad Sci U S A. 2001;98(19): 10869–74.
44. Nguyen P, Taghian A, Katz M, et al. Breast cancer subtype approximated by estrogen receptor, progesterone receptor, and HER-2 is associated with local and distant recurrence after breast-conserving therapy. J Clin Oncol. 2008;26:2373–8.
45. Shah C, Vicini F, Wazer D, et al. The American Brachytherapy Society consensus statement for accelerated partial breast irradiation. Brachytherapy. 2013;12:267–77.

46. The American society of breast surgeons consensus statement for accelerated partial breast irradiation. 2011. https://www.breastsurgeons.org/new_layout/about/statements/PDF_Statements/APBI.pdf.
47. Smith B, Arthru D, Buchholz T, et al. Accelerated partial breast irradiation consensus statement from the American Society for Radiation Oncology (ASTRO). Int J Radiat Oncol Biol Phys. 2009;74(4):987–1001.
48. Polgar C, Van Limbergern E, Potter R, et al. Patient selection for accelerated partial-breast irradiation (APBI) after breast-conserving surgery: Recommendations of the Groupe Européen de Curiethérapie-European Society for Therapeutic Radiology and Oncology (GEC-ESTRO) breast cancer working group based on clinical evidence (2009). Radiother Oncol. 2010;94:264–73.
49. Olivotto I, Whelan T, Parpia S, et al. Interim cosmetic and toxicity results from RAPID: a randomized trial of accelerated partial breast irradiation using three-dimensional conformal external beam. J Clin Oncol. 2013;31(32):4038–45.
50. Livi L, Meattini I, Marrazzo L, et al. Accelerated partial breast irradiation using intensity modulated radiotherapy versus whole breast irradiation: 5-year survival analysis of a phase 3 randomised controlled trial. Eur J Cancer. 2015;51(4):451–63.
51. Bentzen S, Yarnold J. Reports of unexpected late side effects of accelerated partial breast irradiation – radiobiological considerations. Int J Radiat Oncol Biol Phys. 2010;77(4):969–73.
52. Shah C, Wilkinson J, Jawad M, et al. Outcome after ipsilateral breast tumor recurrence in patients with early-stage breast cancer treated with accelerated partial breast irradiation. Clin Breast Cancer. 2012;12(6):392–7.
53. Liu F, Wei S, Done SJ. Identification of a low-risk luminal a breast cancer cohort that may not benefit from breast radiotherapy. J Clin Oncol. 2015;33:2035–40.

Chapter 2
Pathological Anatomy of Early-Stage Breast Cancer: Defining the Target

Anna M. Kirby

Contents

Target volumes for radiotherapy have been defined by the International Commission on Radiation Units and Measurements (ICRU) (ICRU reports 50 and 62 [32, 33]). This chapter reviews the clinicopathological evidence for delineation and definition of the gross tumor volume (GTV) and clinical target volume (CTV) in the context of early-stage breast cancer [39].

2.1 Target Volume Definition for Breast Radiotherapy

2.1.1 Gross Tumor Volume

The ICRU defines gross tumor volume (GTV) as the gross demonstrable extent and location of a malignant growth [32]. In the context of radiotherapy for early-stage breast cancer, the GTV has usually been excised along with a variable margin of surrounding breast tissue leaving behind a cavity. This cavity does not exactly represent the GTV, but is related to it. The first step in target volume definition for most peri- or postoperative whole and partial breast radiotherapy techniques is therefore to identify the walls of this cavity. These cavity walls are referred to hereafter as the tumor bed (TB).

A.M. Kirby
Department of Academic Radiotherapy, Royal Marsden NHS Foundation Trust & Institute of Cancer Research, Sutton, UK
e-mail: anna.kirby@rmh.nhs.uk

D.W. Arthur et al. (eds.), *Short Course Breast Radiotherapy: A Comprehensive Review of Hypofractionation, Partial Breast, and Intra-Operative Irradiation*,
DOI 10.1007/978-3-319-24388-7_2

Where intraoperative brachytherapy techniques are being used, it is clearly straightforward to directly visualize the TB and thereby appose the brachytherapy device to the cavity walls (albeit that challenges remain regarding the definition of the clinical target volume as discussed later in the chapter). However, the identification of TB for radiotherapy techniques delivered postoperatively including external beam whole or partial breast radiotherapy and interstitial brachytherapy is more challenging. Clinical methods of TB delineation are still in common use particularly in the context of defining the target volume for the radiotherapy boost (Imogen Locke, personal communication, UK Royal College of Radiologists Audit of Breast Radiotherapy Practice, 2011), but while patient recollection, preoperative notes, presurgical imaging (including mammography, ultrasound, and magnetic resonance imaging (MRI)), surgical scar, and clinical palpation are all supporting evidence for TB location, they cannot locate the TB precisely. Studies testing the accuracy of clinical methods against orthogonal x-ray imaging localization of clips show that clinical methods result in a geographical miss and/or unnecessary normal tissue irradiation in up to 50 % of patients [6, 27, 42, 49].

To overcome the inaccuracies of clinical methods, postoperative imaging (including ultrasound, CT, PET-CT, and MRI) has increasingly been employed to identify the tumor bed for breast boost and partial breast irradiation. However, different imaging modalities may lead to delineation of quite different pathological structures yielding a difference in target volume size [39]. Most postoperative imaging techniques aim primarily to identify the fluid (or seroma) which has collected in the TB following wide local excision of the GTV. Where the seroma is of sufficient volume and under sufficient pressure, it might be assumed that, using kV-CT imaging or ultrasound (US), the interface between fluid and breast tissue might be clearly visible. The clinical reality however is not as straightforward. Firstly, large-volume, discrete seromas are unusual [45], such that the fluid-tissue interface is often difficult to identify. Furthermore, full-thickness closure of the excision cavity, which minimizes seroma formation, is becoming more widely practiced as studies have demonstrated advantages including reduced incidence of hematoma formation [59], reduced postoperative infection rates [35], improved cosmesis [30, 54], and increased sensitivity of mammography to detect local recurrence [35]. Secondly, two-dimensional [62] and three-dimensional (3D) ultrasound (US) techniques [11] consistently underestimate TB volume compared with CT and implanted tumor bed markers, suggesting that granulation tissue, which can't be distinguished from seroma fluid on CT, has been laid down within the cavity walls. Support for this hypothesis comes from post-lumpectomy MRI which has reported heterogeneous, irregular-bordered, fluid-filled cavities containing regular concentric rings of differing signals [84] with low-signal rings on T_1-weighted fat-suppressed MR sequences correlating histopathologically with granulation tissue [22]. Thirdly, following oncoplastic surgical procedures in which residual normal breast tissue is translocated and/or reduced in order to achieve better cosmesis [1], seroma may not represent TB at all. Fourthly, even where the immediate postoperative seroma is representative of TB, it may become less visible over time [37], reducing its reliability as a fiducial marker. Alternatives to seroma delineation include identification of postoperative peri-cavity inflammation on PET [18] or postsurgical changes on

MRI [65]. However, these techniques can lead to definition of larger TB volumes which are likely to overestimate the volume of the true excision cavity.

Insertion of radiopaque markers into the excision cavity walls overcomes some of the limitations described above. Tumor bed clips inserted according to protocol in pairs at the four radial and superficial and deep cavity margins according to a defined protocol [4, 12] provide additional localization information compared to kV-CT imaging alone, leading to modification of field borders in 43 % of patients [12]. Clips inserted under direct vision do not migrate [12], and serial CT imaging also suggests that clips serve as stable surrogates for the TB over time [83]. Nonetheless, questions over the accuracy of CT/clip-based TB delineation remain as clips can only define specific points on the breast tissue/excision cavity interface such that the remainder of the interface must be derived by interpolation, taking into account tissue density and distortion [11]. Limited soft-tissue contrast on CT makes it an unreliable modality for detecting small volumes of seroma between clips [87] and for distinguishing surgically induced densities from normal glandular breast tissue [45]. In light of this, TB delineation using CT alone has been compared with TB delineation based on fused MR plus CT (MRCT) in patients with 6–12 titanium TB clips [38]. MRCT defined larger TB volumes by identifying additional seroma, hemorrhage, and hematoma, but satisfactory coverage of the MRCT-defined CTV was achieved in all cases by tangential external beam PBI fields designed to cover the CT-defined CTV, suggesting that the addition of MRI to CT/clip-based TB delineation is unnecessary. For patients undergoing oncoplastic breast surgical techniques, guidelines specify placement of markers in the TB walls *prior* to tissue translocation in order that they be as representative as possible of original GTV location. Use of clips in this situation has been shown to extend the TB outside the index quadrant in over 70 % of cases [60].

2.1.2 Clinical Target Volume

Having identified as accurately as possible the TB (or GTV surrogate), the CTV must next be defined. This is defined by the ICRU as a volume containing demonstrable GTV and/or suspected subclinical malignant disease (ICRU report 62) [32]. In the context of breast radiotherapy, there is considerable debate regarding the volume and location of residual breast tissue at risk of local relapse (LR). The principle underlying whole breast radiotherapy is that, once a cancer or premalignant lesion has developed in one part of the breast tissue, the remaining breast tissue is at risk of developing further cancerous or premalignant changes in the future and that these can be sterilized by radiation therapy to help reduce the risk of local tumor relapse. One of the most important studies underpinning this principle is that undertaken by Holland et al. in which mastectomy specimens from over 300 women who fulfilled criteria for breast conservation surgery were subject to systematic histopathological examination [29]. Holland reported that 60 % of apparently unifocal tumors based on physical examination, mammography, and ultrasound were associated with foci of hitherto undetected multifocal and multicentric disease (or "satellite lesions"). In 16 % of cases, these satellite lesions were found to be more than

2 cm from the edge of the index lesion. More recently, Faverly et al. simulated breast conservation surgery in 135 mastectomy specimens and found satellite lesions beyond 1 cm from the edge of the index lesion in nearly 50 % of cases [15].

Meanwhile, the standard model of post-lumpectomy local relapse that underpins partial breast irradiation (PBI) assumes that most of the LR risk preventable by radiotherapy is causally related to residual foci of subclinical disease in the vicinity of the primary tumor following breast surgery. The assumption rests largely on spatial patterns of LR after breast conservation surgery [5, 10, 16, 21, 31, 41, 43, 47, 50, 63, 69, 76, 77]. However, the hypothesis is also supported by the mastectomy studies described above and by histopathological studies of re-excision specimens following breast conservation surgery [80]. These data are now reviewed in turn, before discussing alternative models of LR and then preliminary data from clinical studies of partial breast irradiation.

2.1.2.1 Clinical Data on Spatial Patterns of Relapse

Clinical data on spatial patterns of relapse from prospective randomized controlled trials [10, 16, 47, 50, 77] and retrospective analyses [5, 21, 31, 41, 43, 63, 69, 76] report widely varying percentages (55–90 %) of LR occurring in the vicinity of the primary tumor (see Table 2.1). Part of this variation is due to differing definitions of same-site relapse which range from the "scar area" [77] to "within the same quadrant" [41]. Only two studies quantify the distance from the primary site to the

Table 2.1 Spatial patterns of ipsilateral breast tumor relapse (IBTR) in patients enrolled in randomized controlled trials testing the effect of whole breast radiotherapy (WBRT) and in retrospective studies of patients treated with breast conservation surgery and WBRT

Author	n	Median FU (years)	% IBTR	Percentage and definition of same-site relapse
Randomized controlled trials				
Fisher, 1992	1108	3.3	9.9	86 % within or close to index quadrant
Liljegren, 1999	381	10.0	15.0	76 % in or around the surgical field
Clark, 1996	937	3.6	15.7	86 % at site of primary surgery
Veronesi, 2001	579	9	13.0	85 % in the scar area
Malmstrom, 2003	1178	5	8.8	90 % within index quadrant
Retrospective studies				
Kurtz, 1989	1593	11	11.2	79 % within 5 cm of original primary
Recht, 1988	597	6.3	11.2	72 % within the margins of/just outside the border of the boost
Veronesi, 1995	2233	8.5	6.8	79 % same-site relapse
Smith, 2000	1152	14.2	11.8	55 % same-quadrant relapse
Huang, 2002	1339	12.4	9.4	67 % within 3 cm of primary tumor bed
Freedman, 2005	1990	7.7	6.0	59 % same-quadrant relapse
Krauss, 2004	1448	8.5	5.5	75 % same-quadrant relapse
Bartelink, 2007	5318	10.8	10.2	57 % primary tumor bed or scar relapse

relapse [31, 43]. In summary, while the clinical data do not support quantitative conclusions regarding the magnitude of the TB-to-CTV margin, they qualitatively support the hypothesis that there is some degree of spatial relationship between LR and the index lesion.

2.1.2.2 Histopathological Examination of Mastectomy Specimens

Subgross whole organ sectioning of mastectomy specimens [29] also demonstrates a spatial relationship between index tumor and satellite lesions of multifocal and multicentric disease. Holland et al. found that 60 % of 264 apparently unifocal cancers of ≤4 cm in diameter (based on physical examination, mammography, and ultrasound) were associated with satellite lesions. In 90 % of these cases, satellite lesions of invasive disease were restricted to ≤30 mm from the edge of the index tumor. Given that surgeons aim to remove 10–20 mm of peritumoral tissue at wide local excision [24], a TB-to-CTV margin of 10–20 mm could therefore be inferred to be reasonable according to these data. However, criticisms of applying mastectomy data to current radiotherapy practice include firstly that, given advances in the quality of preoperative assessment imaging in recent decades, many women in Holland's study might have been ineligible for breast conservation surgery by modern standards and secondly that the 15 mm error in the extensive mapping procedure is significant in the context of the dimensions described.

More contemporary publications analyzing mastectomy and quadrantectomy specimens from women considered appropriate for BCT show that the microscopic extension of malignant cells beyond the edge of the index tumor is less than that reported by Holland et al. For example, Ohtake et al. used a subgross and stereomicroscopic technique to examine the extent of residual DCIS remaining in the breast after quadrantectomies in 20 patients with invasive cancers of mean diameter 17 mm [57]. By reconstructing the mammary duct-lobular system in three dimensions using computer graphics, they found that the average maximum distance of intraductal tumor extension was 12 mm for the whole group (and <8 mm in patients >50 years of age). In a related study, Imamura et al. measured the maximal DCIS extension in 253 mastectomy specimens in women with invasive breast cancer and reported a median extension of DCIS of only 9 mm beyond the edge of the invasive tumor. In patients ≥40 years of age, the maximum extension was <9 mm in all cases [34]. These studies are more likely to be applicable to contemporary populations whose breast cancers are largely screen detected.

2.1.2.3 Histopathological Examination of Re-excision Specimens

A study of re-excision specimens provides further support for a TB-to-CTV margin in a similar ballpark to that derived from the Holland data [80]. In this study, the maximal distance of residual disease from the initial excision margin was measured in 333 patients who had undergone an initial excisional resection with a rim of normal breast parenchyma around the clinically apparent tumor or the tissue at the tip of the needle localization wire and then re-excision of margins for inadequate surgical clearance or questionable postsurgical mammography results at the discretion of the surgeon or radiation oncologist. The re-excision specimens were reviewed for presence, type, amount, and linear (radial) extension of cancer cells from the edge of the original margin. Of the 214 cases with residual invasive carcinoma or DCIS in the re-excision specimen, 86 % had disease within 15 mm of the TB. A ≥3 mm width of invasive carcinoma and/or ≥13 DCIS ducts near the margin, and an initial excision specimen invasive carcinoma to specimen dimension ratio of ≥0.6 each correlated with disease beyond 10 mm, suggesting that a 10 mm margin may be sufficient for cases without these features. In the 134 cases with initially negative margins (i.e., the patient population who would have been eligible for PBI studies), 38 % had residual disease in the re-excision specimen, and in 90 % of these cases, the residual disease was within 10 mm from the edge of the original lumpectomy margin. Using a combination of more detailed pathological analyses of tumor burden close to the margins and the initial excision specimen invasive carcinoma to specimen dimension ratio, it was possible to identify all 13 (9.7 %) patients with disease extending ≥10 mm from the edge of the lumpectomy cavity. Limitations of applying this data to defining the TB-to-CTV margin for PBI include the fact that the actual extent of disease may be underestimated due to a variable width of breast tissue being lost through electrocautery and tissue processing. Furthermore the perpendicular extension distance of preinvasive and invasive disease within the re-excision specimen may not fully represent the overall residual tumor burden in the breast. In summary, however, for patients in whom the tumor is clear of ink in the primary excision specimen, this data suggests that a TB-to-CTV margin of 10 mm will encompass residual subclinical disease in the majority of cases.

2.1.2.4 Alternative Models for the Pathogenesis of Local Relapse following Breast Conservation Surgery

Differing interpretations of the clinical and pathological data, together with more recent pathological and genetic data, suggest that matching CTV to the reported distribution of satellite lesions of invasive and preinvasive disease may be misjudged [51]. First, we must deal with the fact that the percentage of cases in which lesions are found outside the vicinity of the primary has been reported to be as high as 45 % in the clinical studies listed in Table 2.1,and 50 % in studies of mastectomy specimens [15, 29, 73]. A proportion of these lesions are likely to be located in different ductal systems and to represent independent pathological entities (or "new primaries" as defined by Moffat and Going [53]). Indeed, a large randomized controlled clinical study has confirmed, on the basis of histopathological classification and timing of recurrence, that the majority of out-of-quadrant recurrences are new primaries [69]. Furthermore, a study of the spatial and temporal pattern of ipsilateral relapse in over 2500 patients treated with breast conservation surgery +/− radiotherapy found that, while nearly 75 % of ipsilateral relapses presented ≤2 cm from the surgical scar, the rate of recurrences outside the index quadrant was comparable to the rate of contralateral primary disease, suggesting that radiotherapy is ineffective against new primaries [66]. If this is the case, then restricting the CTV for adjuvant breast radiotherapy to the index quadrant would seem reasonable. However, other randomized controlled data report that WBRT is associated with a lower rate of elsewhere ipsilateral breast recurrence than of contralateral BC [17, 19, 47, 50, 61, 77, 85], suggesting that radiotherapy does have some effect upon out-of-quadrant recurrences whether or not they are new primaries. Among the randomized controlled trials of breast conservation surgery +/– whole breast RT, Veronesi et al. [77] reported site of LR by treatment group. 48/59 (85 %) LR in the unirradiated group and 11/13 (85 %) LR in the irradiated group occurred within the scar area, and 8/59 (15 %) (unirradiated) versus 2/13 (15 %) occurred outside the index quadrant, suggesting that RT might reduce within-quadrant and out-of-quadrant relapses to a similar extent. Indeed, image reconstruction [57, 58] and ductoscopy studies [14, 48] suggest that many out-of-quadrant recurrences are in fact arising from the same ductal system as the primary. The CTV may therefore be more appropriately defined according to ductal anatomy, rather than by index quadrant. As yet, however, there is no standard imaging technique by which ductal anatomy can be defined, despite previous studies of ultrasonographic [68] and MRI [28] methods.

Other investigators suggest, based on the high proportion of out-of-quadrant satellite lesions [73] together with the constant risk reduction in post-RT ipsilateral breast tumor relapse (IBTR) independent of excision margin [2, 81], that local recurrences do not necessarily arise from satellite lesions at all [74]. Instead, recent pathological studies have demonstrated that IBTR correlates with monomorphic epithelial proliferations [25] and loss of heterozygosity [44, 46] in morphologically normal cells close to the excision specimen margin. Goldstein et al. measured monomorphic epithelial proliferations (i.e., morphologically normal epithelium sharing genetic alterations with ipsilateral breast tumor relapse from the same patient) in 70 cases with IBTR and 140 matched controls and reported a significant relationship between the mean number of monomorphic epithelial proliferations near the initial excision specimen margin and the subsequent risk of IBTR [25]. Meanwhile, Li et al. reported a significant association between IBTR and the presence of an index tumor-specific loss of heterozygosity (a well-established method for determining the clonality of two breast carcinomas) in histologically normal terminal ductal lobular units. Loss of heterozygosity in normal breast tissue has also been observed at some distance from the index tumor [44] consistent with the abovementioned hypothesis that LR risk may be related to ductal anatomy.

Radiotherapy has also been reported to modify the stimulatory effects of seroma in the TB as discussed by Mannino and Yarnold [52]. A link between the wound-healing process and the risk of local relapse has been suggested by a study reporting that an activated (versus quiescent) wound-response gene expression signature is the most powerful predictor for local relapse (independent of age, tumor size, and use of a radiotherapy boost) [55]. A subsequent study has compared proliferation indices in sections of tumor from wide local excisions versus re-excision specimens from the same patient [72]. Increased expression of ERBB2 was reported in the re-excision specimens. Furthermore, the authors reported that wound fluids from these patients induced proliferation of breast cancer cell lines in vitro, particularly those with ERBB2 overexpression, and that the degree of induced cell proliferation was proportional to the amount of surgical damage as measured by seroma creatine phosphokinase levels. Perioperative TB irradiation (cavity plus 2 mm) has been found to be associated with a reduction in the stimulatory effects of surgical wound fluids upon proliferative, migratory, and invasive abilities of BC cell lines [8]. Radiotherapy may therefore be effective in altering the microenvironment of peri-cavity (pre)malignant cells in addition to any directly lethal damage to the DNA of these cells, but this may depend upon radiotherapy being given at the time of surgery, rather than weeks later.

2.1.2.5 Outcomes of Clinical Studies of Partial Breast Irradiation

The above hypotheses have been put to the test in several phase I–III clinical trials of partial breast irradiation. Favorable early outcomes of phase I and II accelerated partial breast irradiation (PBI) are supportive of a TB-to-CTV margin of 10–20 mm. For example, Vicini et al. reported a 5-year actuarial control rate of 98.8 % in a series of patients in whom interstitial brachytherapy was used to treat the lumpectomy cavity plus a 10–20 mm margin [79]. More recently, the Radiation Therapy Oncology Group (RTOG) 95–17 study evaluated multicatheter interstitial brachytherapy (using HDR or LDR) in 99 patients with tumors less than 3 cm in diameter, negative margins, and 0–3 axillary lymph nodes without extracapsular extension [3]. After a median follow-up of 74 months, the IBTR rate was 3 % in the HDR brachytherapy group and 6 % in the LDR brachytherapy group. Benitez et al. [9] prospectively evaluated the use of an intracavitary MammoSite brachytherapy device in 70 patients of age >45 years, with pT1N0 disease, and clear surgical margins. At a median follow-up of 5 years, there were no recurrences. In the American Society of Breast Surgeons (ASBS) MammoSite Registry Trial [7] involving 1449 patients, the 5-year IBTR rate was 3.5 %. One percent of recurrences were classified as true local recurrences and 2.5 % as elsewhere failures. Trends toward increased rates of elsewhere failures were seen with tumor size ($p=0.067$) and extensive intraductal component ($p=0.087$). External beam PBI is the most recently tested of the techniques. Shah et al. evaluated outcomes in 192 patients treated with 3D conformal external beam accelerated PBI (TB plus 10–15 mm) and reported an IBTR of 0 % at a median follow-up of 4.8 years (this result is particularly interesting given that 62.5 % of patients were classified as belonging to the ASTRO consensus "cautionary" and "unsuitable" groups for PBI) [67]. Rodriguez et al. treated 102 patients in a randomized trial of whole breast irradiation versus accelerated PBI (TB plus index quadrant) and, at a median follow-up of 5 years, reported no local recurrences [64]. Galland-Girodet et al. compared proton beam PBI against 3D conformal photon beam accelerated PBI treatment of the lumpectomy cavity plus 15–20 mm in 98 patients (19 of whom were treated with protons and 79 with photons). At a median follow-up of 7 years, the overall IBTR rate was 7 % (11 % in the proton group and 4 % in the photon group, $p=0.22$) [23].

Several phase III trials (either ongoing or in follow-up) are also comparing outcomes in patients in whom the CTV has, to some extent, been restricted to breast tissue in the vicinity of the TB versus those in whom the entirety (or almost all) of the ipsilateral breast tissue has been irradiated (Table 2.2). These trials differ significantly in terms of the RT techniques used and, more importantly, in terms of their definition of CTV such that their results may be helpful in explaining the mechanism(s) by which breast radiotherapy prevents LR. Only two of these phase III studies have published LR data thus far. The single-center ELIOT trial (electron intraoperative therapy) randomized 1305 patients between 2000 and 2007 to intraoperative radiotherapy (IORT) using electrons versus whole breast radiotherapy. The 5-year IBTR rate was 4.4 % in the IORT group versus 0.4 % in the whole breast irradiation group. Although these figures were within the pre-specified equivalence margin, the rate of IBTR in the IORT arm was significantly greater than for the whole breast radiotherapy approach. There was however no difference in overall survival between the groups (96.8 % in the IORT group versus 96.9 % in the external beam radiotherapy group). The international TARGIT-A trial randomized 3451 patients between 2000 and 2012 to whole breast external beam radiotherapy (EBRT) versus intraoperative radiotherapy (IORT) using the Intrabeam™ device [75]. Of the 3451 patients included in this study, 1153 were randomized postoperatively to tumor bed boost using IORT versus whole breast EBRT such that this subset did not truly test IORT. The remaining 2298 patients were randomized before surgery to IORT versus whole breast radiotherapy. Taking the trial population as a whole ($n=3451$), local recurrence following EBRT was lower than for those receiving partial breast radiotherapy (1.3 % versus 3.3 %, $p=0.042$). However, for the subset randomized presurgically to EBRT versus IORT, the difference in local recurrence was smaller and nonsignificant (EBRT = 1.1, IORT = 2.1 %, $p=0.31$). Again, there was no significant difference in breast cancer mortality or overall survival between the two groups. Lower local control rates in the intraoperative arms of these studies may suggest that the CTV has been inadequately treated due to the TB-to-CTV margin being too narrow.

Assuming all seven phase III trials of PBI are completed as planned, LR data will ultimately be available for nearly 16,000 women and are likely to contribute significantly to our understanding of how radiotherapy modifies LR relapse risk in women with early breast cancer. Alongside local recurrence rates, detailed three-dimensional mapping of IBTRs together with histopathological, molecular, and genetic characterization thereof will be crucial in distinguishing, for example, true LR from new primaries. It will also be important that follow-up continues long enough to detect out-of-quadrant relapses, the median time to which is longer than for same-quadrant relapse [20].

2.1.2.6 Patient and Pathological Factors Influencing Clinical Target Volume Definition for PBI

Based on the clinical and pathological data described above, the choice of a 10–15 mm TB-to-CTV margin in ongoing studies of external beam PBI and for off-trial accelerated external beam PBI seems reasonable. Patient and tumor factors

Table 2.2 Phase III studies of PBI in women at low risk of local relapse

Trial/ institution (ref)	N (eligibility)	Control arm	Experimental arm (and CTV)	Status
ELIOT[a], Milan [78]	824 (quadrantectomy, age > 48 years, any invasive ca ≤2.5 cm, pN0)	WBI 50 Gy/25# +/− boost 10 Gy	Intraoperative 21 Gy single fraction, 3–9 MeV electrons (80 % isodose varies from 13 mm (3 MeV) to 24 mm (9 MeV))	Median FU 5.8 years
TARGIT[b] [75]	1600 (suitable patients selected by institution, ILC or EIC proceed to adjuvant WBI)	WBI according to each institution's guidelines	20 Gy low-energy x-rays, 50 kV intraoperative single fraction (delivers 5–7 Gy at 10 mm from applicator surface)	Median FU 2.4 years
GEC-ESTRO [70]	1170 (lumpectomy, ≥40 years, T ≤ 3.0 cm, margins ≥2 mm (≥5 mm for lobular or pure DCIS), ≤1 axillary micrometastasis)	WBI 50–50.4 Gy/1.8–2.0 Gy fractions, +/− 10 Gy boost	Interstitial brachytherapy 32 Gy/8# or 30.3 Gy/7# high dose rate (HDR) or 50 Gy pulsed dose rate (PDR) (TB plus 10–20 mm)	In follow-up
NSABP B-39/ RTOG 0413 [86]	4300 (lumpectomy, any age, stage 0–II, T ≤ 3.0 cm, pN1, neg margins)	WBI 50–50.4 Gy/1.8–2.0 Gy fractions, +/− boost to 60–66 Gy	34 Gy/10# using MammoSite balloon catheter (dose prescribed to 10 mm from applicator surface), multicatheter brachytherapy or 38.5 Gy/10# using 3D conformal RT (TB plus 10–15 mm)	In follow-up
RAPID[c]/Ontario Oncology Group [56]	2128 (lumpectomy, ≥40 years, DCIS, pT < 3 cm, pN0, non-lobular). No BRCA 1/2	WBI 42.5 Gy/16#/22 days (small breasts), 50 Gy/25#/35d (large breasts) +/− 10 Gy/4–5# boost	3D conformal RT 38.5 Gy/10#/5–8 days. Minimum daily fraction separation 6–8 h (TB plus 10–15 mm)	In follow-up
Innovazioni nella Radioterapia della Mammella (IRMA) [36]	3302 (lumpectomy, ≥49 years, pT < 3 cm, pN0-1, margins ≥5 mm)	WBI 45 Gy/18# or 50 Gy/25# or 50.4 Gy/28# (daily RT for 4–5 weeks) +/− 10–16 Gy boost	3D conformal RT 38.5 Gy/10#/5 days. Minimum daily fraction separation = 6 h (TB plus 10–15 mm)	Recruiting
IMPORT Low[d], UK [88]	1935 (lumpectomy, ≥50 years, pT ≤ 2 cm, pN0 (isolated tumor cells ≤0.2 mm allowed), non-lobular, margins ≥2 mm)	WBI 40 Gy/15#/3 weeks	Arm 1: 36 Gy/15# to low-risk volume and 40 Gy/15# to region of primary; arm 2: 40 Gy/15# to region of primary tumor only (partial breast CTV = TB plus 15 mm)	In follow-up

[a] *ELIOT* electron intraoperative therapy trial
[b] *TARGIT* targeted intraoperative radiotherapy trial
[c] *RAPID* randomized trial of accelerated partial breast irradiation
[d] *IMPORT Low* intensity-modulated and partial organ radiotherapy following breast conservation surgery for early breast cancer

however should be borne in mind in refining future treatment and research protocols. While this chapter does not address the possible indications for PBI, some of the known prognostic factors for local recurrence (such as patient age [57], lymphovascular invasion [81], and tumor grade) may indicate that a wider TB-to-CTV margin should be employed [25]. For example, Ohtake et al. found that the distance of extension of intraductal tumor spread was inversely related to patient age, ranging from 8 mm in women ≥50 years to 23 mm in women aged 30–39 years, implying that a 15 mm TB-to-CTV margin is insufficient to cover residual disease in younger women. This data is consistent with the EORTC boost trial which reported a higher frequency of moderate and extensive DCIS in younger women [82]. It is thought that the reduced intraductal extension in older women could be due to physiological involution of the ductal system [13, 51, 52]. Although no studies have yet investigated the impact of involution on breast cancer relapse risk, it is possible that age-related morphometric and functional breast changes affect intraductal patterns of spread. Meanwhile in younger women, given that intraductal changes appear limited to a single duct system [58], it will be important to explore tailoring both breast conservation surgery and radiotherapy to single duct systems.

Furthermore, if the majority of LR does indeed originate from foci of residual invasive and/or intraductal disease in the vicinity of the TB after complete microscopic resection, the TB-to-CTV margin logically takes account of the position of primary tumor within the surgical resection specimen. Specimen radiographs suggest that the GTV is likely to be eccentrically placed within the excision specimen, and histopathological studies show that 3D excision margins are often asymmetrical [26, 40]. The current minimum UK histopathological data set requires that only the closest surgical clearance margin be defined, but by measuring the distance from edge of tumor (GTV) to the radial, superior, and inferior aspects of the excision specimen, it is possible to construct an anisotropic CTV that might more accurately encompass multifocal/centric disease. If, as Holland's data suggest, the majority of disease is within 30 mm of the edge of the index lesion, this would suggest that expanding the TB by 30 mm minus the surgical excision margin might be more appropriate than adding a symmetrical 15 mm margin. Where the surgical clearance margin is narrow, the TB-to-CTV margin would be wider and vice versa. Stroom et al. have compared boost volumes defined using a standard 15 mm margin with those defined using excision margins and have found that CTVs can frequently be reduced (on the basis of surgical excision margins of >15 mm) without compromising coverage of the at-risk volume [71]. However, meticulous orientation of the excision specimen is required.

2.2 Conclusions

Target volume definition for adjuvant breast radiotherapy begins with accurate identification of the tumor itself (for preoperative radiotherapy) or the surgical tumor bed. Clinicopathological data reporting distributions of residual disease in relation to the primary tumor support a TB-to-CTV margin of 10–15 mm as used in several phase III studies (either ongoing or in follow-up). Outcomes from these studies will contribute to our understanding of the pathogenesis of local relapse and will help in developing further research and treatment protocols for CTV definition in adjuvant breast radiotherapy.

References

1. Anderson BO, Masetti R, Silverstein MJ. Oncoplastic approaches to partial mastectomy: an overview of volume-displacement techniques. Lancet Oncol. 2005;l6(3):145–57.
2. Antonini N, Jones H, Horiot JC, et al. Effect of age and radiation dose on local control after breast conserving treatment: EORTC trial 22881–10882. Radiother Oncol. 2007;l82(3):265–71.
3. Arthur DW, Winter K, Kuske RR, et al. A Phase II trial of brachytherapy alone after lumpectomy for select breast cancer: tumor control and survival outcomes of RTOG 95–17. Int J Radiat Oncol Biol Phys. 2008;72(2):467–73.
4. Association of Breast Surgery at BASO 2009. Surgical guidelines for the management of breast cancer. Eur J Surg Oncol. 2009;35 Suppl 1:1–22.
5. Bartelink H, Horiot JC, Poortmans PM, et al. Impact of a higher radiation dose on local control and survival in breast-conserving therapy of early breast cancer: 10-year results of the randomized boost versus no boost EORTC 22881–10882 trial. J Clin Oncol. 2007;25(22):3259–65.
6. Bedwinek J. Breast conserving surgery and irradiation: the importance of demarcating the excision cavity with surgical clips. Int J Radiat Oncol Biol Phys. 1993;26(4):675–9.
7. Beitsch PD, Wilkinson JB, Vicini FA, et al. Tumor bed control with balloon-based accelerated partial breast irradiation: incidence of true recurrences versus elsewhere failures in the American Society of Breast Surgery MammoSite((R)) Registry Trial. Ann Surg Oncol. 2012;19(10):3165–70.
8. Belletti B, Vaidya JS, D'Andrea S, et al. Targeted intraoperative radiotherapy impairs the stimulation of breast cancer cell proliferation and invasion caused by surgical wounding. Clin Cancer Res. 2008;14(5):1325–32.
9. Benitez PR, Keisch ME, Vicini F, et al. Five-year results: the initial clinical trial of MammoSite balloon brachytherapy for partial breast irradiation in early-stage breast cancer. Am J Surg. 2007;194(4):456–62.
10. Clark RM, Whelan T, Levine M, et al. Randomized clinical trial of breast irradiation following lumpectomy and axillary dissection for node-negative breast cancer: an update. Ontario Clinical Oncology Group. J Natl Cancer Inst. 1996;88(22):1659–64.
11. Coles CE, Cash CJ, Treece GM, et al. High definition three-dimensional ultrasound to localise the tumour bed: a breast radiotherapy planning study. Radiother Oncol. 2007;84(3):233–41.
12. Coles CE, Wilson CB, Cumming J, et al. Titanium clip placement to allow accurate tumour bed localisation following breast conserving surgery: audit on behalf of the IMPORT Trial Management Group. Eur J Surg Oncol. 2009;35(6):578–82.
13. Cowan D, Herbet TA. Involution of the breast in women aged 50 to 104 years: a histopathological study of 102 cases. Surg Pathol. 1989;2(4):323–33.
14. Dooley WC. Routine operative breast endoscopy during lumpectomy. Ann Surg Oncol. 2003;10(1):38–42.
15. Faverly DR, Hendriks JH, Holland R. Breast carcinomas of limited extent: frequency, radiologic-pathologic characteristics, and surgical margin requirements. Cancer. 2001;91(4):647–59.
16. Fisher B, Anderson S, Bryant J, et al. Twenty-year follow-up of a randomized trial comparing total mastectomy, lumpectomy, and lumpectomy plus irradiation for the treatment of invasive breast cancer. N Engl J Med. 2002;347(16):1233–41.

17. Fisher B, Bryant J, Dignam JJ, et al. Tamoxifen, radiation therapy, or both for prevention of ipsilateral breast tumor recurrence after lumpectomy in women with invasive breast cancers of one centimeter or less. J Clin Oncol. 2002;20(20):4141–9.
18. Ford E, Lavely W, Frassica D, et al. Comparison of PET/CT and CT for delineation of lumpectomy cavity for partial breast irradiation. Int J Radiat Oncol Biol Phys. 2006;66:S225–226.
19. Forrest AP, Stewart HJ, Everington D, et al. Randomised controlled trial of conservation therapy for breast cancer: 6-year analysis of the Scottish trial. Scottish Cancer Trials Breast Group. Lancet. 1996;348(9029):708–13.
20. Fowble B, Solin LJ, Schultz DJ, et al. Breast recurrence following conservative surgery and radiation: patterns of failure, prognosis, and pathologic findings from mastectomy specimens with implications for treatment. Int J Radiat Oncol Biol Phys. 1990;19(4):833–42.
21. Freedman GM, Anderson PR, Hanlon AL, et al. Pattern of local recurrence after conservative surgery and whole-breast irradiation. Int J Radiat Oncol Biol Phys. 2005;61(5):1328–36.
22. Frei KA, Kinkel K, Bonel HM, et al. MR imaging of the breast in patients with positive margins after lumpectomy: influence of the time interval between lumpectomy and MR imaging. AJR Am J Roentgenol. 2000;175(6):1577–84.
23. Galland-Girodet S, Pashtan I, MacDonald SM, et al. Long-term cosmetic outcomes and toxicities of proton beam therapy compared with photon-based 3-dimensional conformal accelerated partial-breast irradiation: a phase 1 trial. Int J Radiat Oncol Biol Phys. 2014;90(3): 493–500.
24. Gennaro M, Ferraris C, Guida V, et al. Conservative surgery in breast cancer. Significance of resection margins. Breast. 2001;10(5):432–7.
25. Goldstein NS, Kestin LJ, Vicini FA. Monomorphic epithelial proliferations: characterization and evidence suggesting they are the pool of partially transformed lesions from which some invasive carcinomas arise. Am J Clin Pathol. 2007;128(6):1023–34.
26. Hanbeukers B, Borger J, van den Ende P, et al. Customized computed tomography-based boost volumes in breast-conserving therapy: use of three-dimensional histologic information for clinical target volume margins. Int J Radiat Oncol Biol Phys. 2009;75(3):757–63.
27. Harrington KJ, Harrison M, Bayle P, et al. Surgical clips in planning the electron boost in breast cancer: a qualitative and quantitative evaluation. Int J Radiat Oncol Biol Phys. 1996;34(3):579–84.
28. Hirose M, Otsuki N, Hayano D, et al. Multi-volume fusion imaging of MR ductography and MR mammography for patients with nipple discharge. Magn Reson Med Sci. 2006;5(2): 105–12.
29. Holland R, Veling SH, Mravunac M, et al. Histologic multifocality of Tis, T1-2 breast carcinomas. Implications for clinical trials of breast-conserving surgery. Cancer. 1985;56(5):979–90.
30. Holmberg L, Zaren E, Adami HO, et al. The patient's appraisal of the cosmetic result of segmental mastectomy in benign and malignant breast disease. Ann Surg. 1988;207(2):189–94.
31. Huang E, Buchholz TA, Meric F, et al. Classifying local disease recurrences after breast conservation therapy based on location and histology: new primary tumors have more favorable outcomes than true local disease recurrences. Cancer. 2002;95(10):2059–67.
32. ICRU. Prescribing, recording and reporting photon beam therapy. Bethsada: International Commission on Radiation Units and Measurements (ICRU), 1999.
33. ICRU. Prescribing, Recording and Reporting Photon Beam Therapy. Bethsada: International Commission on Radiation Units and Measurements (ICRU), 1993.
34. Imamura H, Haga S, Shimizu T, et al. Relationship between the morphological and biological characteristics of intraductal components accompanying invasive ductal breast carcinoma and patient age. Breast Cancer Res Treat. 2000;62(3):177–84.
35. Indelicato D, Grobmyer SR, Newlin H, et al. Association between operative closure type and acute infection, local recurrence, and disease surveillance in patients undergoing breast conserving therapy for early-stage breast cancer. Surgery. 2007;141(5):645–53.
36. IRMA Trial Protocol available from: http://groups.eortc.be/radio/res/irma/synopsis_trial_irma1.pdf.

37. Kader HA, Truong PT, Pai R, et al. When is CT-based postoperative seroma most useful to plan partial breast radiotherapy? Evaluation of clinical factors affecting seroma volume and clarity. Int J Radiat Oncol Biol Phys. 2008;72(4):1064–9.
38. Kirby AM, Yarnold JR, Evans PM, et al. Tumor bed delineation for partial breast and breast boost radiotherapy planned in the prone position: what does MRI add to X-ray CT localization of titanium clips placed in the excision cavity wall? Int J Radiat Oncol Biol Phys. 2009;74(4):1276–82.
39. Kirby AM, Coles CE, Yarnold JR. Target volume definition for external beam partial breast radiotherapy: clinical, pathological and technical studies informing current approaches. Radiother Oncol. 2010;94(3):255–63.
40. Kirby AM, Evans PM, Nerurkar AY, et al. How does knowledge of three-dimensional excision margins following breast conservation surgery impact upon clinical target volume definition for partial-breast radiotherapy? Radiother Oncol. 2010;94(3):292–9.
41. Krauss DJ, Kestin LL, Mitchell C, et al. Changes in temporal patterns of local failure after breast-conserving therapy and their prognostic implications. Int J Radiat Oncol Biol Phys. 2004;60(3):731–40.
42. Krawczyk JJ, Engel B. The importance of surgical clips for adequate tangential beam planning in breast conserving surgery and irradiation. Int J Radiat Oncol Biol Phys. 1999;43(2):347–50.
43. Kurtz JM, Amalric R, Brandone H, et al. Local recurrence after breast-conserving surgery and radiotherapy. Frequency, time course, and prognosis. Cancer. 1989;63(10):1912–7.
44. Lakhani SR, Chaggar R, Davies S, et al. Genetic alterations in 'normal' luminal and myoepithelial cells of the breast. J Pathol. 1999;189(4):496–503.
45. Landis DM, Luo W, Song J, et al. Variability among breast radiation oncologists in delineation of the postsurgical lumpectomy cavity. Int J Radiat Oncol Biol Phys. 2007;67(5):1299–308.
46. Li Z, Moore DH, Meng ZH, et al. Increased risk of local recurrence is associated with allelic loss in normal lobules of breast cancer patients. Cancer Res. 2002;62(4):1000–3.
47. Liljegren G, Holmberg L, Bergh J, et al. 10-Year results after sector resection with or without postoperative radiotherapy for stage I breast cancer: a randomized trial. J Clin Oncol. 1999;17(8):2326–33.
48. Love SM, Barsky SH. Breast-duct endoscopy to study stages of cancerous breast disease. Lancet. 1996;348(9033):997–9.
49. Machtay M, Lanciano R, Hoffman J, et al. Inaccuracies in using the lumpectomy scar for planning electron boosts in primary breast carcinoma. Int J Radiat Oncol Biol Phys. 1994;30(1):43–8.
50. Malmstrom P, Holmberg L, Anderson H, et al. Breast conservation surgery, with and without radiotherapy, in women with lymph node-negative breast cancer: a randomised clinical trial in a population with access to public mammography screening. Eur J Cancer. 2003;39(12):1690–7.
51. Mannino M, Yarnold J. Accelerated partial breast irradiation trials: diversity in rationale and design. Radiother Oncol. 2009;91(1):16–22.
52. Mannino M, Yarnold J. Effect of breast-duct anatomy and wound-healing responses on local tumour recurrence after primary surgery for early breast cancer. Lancet Oncol. 2009;10(4):425–9.
53. Moffat DF, Going JJ. Three dimensional anatomy of complete duct systems in human breast: pathological and developmental implications. J Clin Pathol. 1996;49(1):48–52.
54. Mukesh MB, Barnett G, Cumming J, et al. Association of breast tumour bed seroma with postoperative complications and late normal tissue toxicity: results from the Cambridge Breast IMRT trial. Eur J Surg Oncol. 2012;38(10):918–24.
55. Nuyten DS, Kreike B, Hart AA, et al. Predicting a local recurrence after breast-conserving therapy by gene expression profiling. Breast Cancer Res. 2006;8(5):R62.
56. OCOG. Ontario Clinical Oncology Group (OCOG), Canadian Institutes of Health Research (CIHR), Canadian Breast Cancer Research Alliance. RAPID: Randomized Trial of Accelerated Partial Breast Irradiation. http://clinicaltrials.gov/ct2/show/NCT00282035. 2008.

57. Ohtake T, Abe R, Kimijima I, et al. Intraductal extension of primary invasive breast carcinoma treated by breast-conservative surgery. Computer graphic three-dimensional reconstruction of the mammary duct-lobular systems. Cancer. 1995;76(1):32–45.
58. Ohtake T, Kimijima I, Fukushima T, et al. Computer-assisted complete three-dimensional reconstruction of the mammary ductal/lobular systems: implications of ductal anastomoses for breast-conserving surgery. Cancer. 2001;91(12):2263–72.
59. Paterson ML, Nathanson SD, Havstad S. Hematomas following excisional breast biopsies for invasive breast carcinoma: the influence of deep suture approximation of breast parenchyma. Am Surg. 1994;60(11):845–8.
60. Pezner RD, Tan MC, Clancy SL, et al. Radiation therapy for breast cancer patients who undergo oncoplastic surgery: localization of the tumor bed for the local boost. Am J Clin Oncol. 2013;36(6):535–9.
61. Potter R, Gnant M, Kwasny W, et al. Lumpectomy plus tamoxifen or anastrozole with or without whole breast irradiation in women with favorable early breast cancer. Int J Radiat Oncol Biol Phys. 2007;68(2):334–40.
62. Rabinovitch R, Finlayson C, Pan Z, et al. Radiographic evaluation of surgical clips is better than ultrasound for defining the lumpectomy cavity in breast boost treatment planning: a prospective clinical study. Int J Radiat Oncol Biol Phys. 2000;47(2):313–7.
63. Recht A, Silen W, Schnitt SJ, et al. Time-course of local recurrence following conservative surgery and radiotherapy for early stage breast cancer. Int J Radiat Oncol Biol Phys. 1988;15(2):255–61.
64. Rodriguez N, Sanz X, Dengra J, et al. Five-year outcomes, cosmesis, and toxicity with 3-dimensional conformal external beam radiation therapy to deliver accelerated partial breast irradiation. Int J Radiat Oncol Biol Phys. 2013;87(5):1051–7.
65. Sabine B, Giovanna D, Peter P, et al. Open low-field magnetic resonance (MR) versus CT Scanner (CT) imaging in breast radiotherapy treatment planning. Int J Radiat Oncol Biol Phys. 2005;63:S232–3.
66. Salvadori B, Marubini E, Miceli R, et al. Reoperation for locally recurrent breast cancer in patients previously treated with conservative surgery. Br J Surg. 1999;86(1):84–7.
67. Shah C, Wilkinson JB, Lanni T, et al. Five-year outcomes and toxicities using 3-dimensional conformal external beam radiation therapy to deliver accelerated partial breast irradiation. Clin Breast Cancer. 2013;13(3):206–11.
68. Simonetti F, Huang L, Duric N, et al. Diffraction and coherence in breast ultrasound tomography: a study with a toroidal array. Med Phys. 2009;36(7):2955–65.
69. Smith TE, Lee D, Turner BC, et al. True recurrence vs. new primary ipsilateral breast tumor relapse: an analysis of clinical and pathologic differences and their implications in natural history, prognoses, and therapeutic management. Int J Radiat Oncol Biol Phys. 2000;48(5):1281–9.
70. Strnad V, Polgar C. On behalf of the European Brachytherapy Breast Cancer GEC-ESTRO Working Group. GEC-ESTRO APBI Trial: Interstitial brachytherapy alone versus external beam radiation therapy after breast conserving surgery for low risk invasive carcinoma and low risk duct carcinoma in-situ (DCIS) of the female breast. http://www.apbi.uni-erlangen.de/outline/outline.html. 2006.
71. Stroom J, Schlief A, Alderliesten T, et al. Using histopathology breast cancer data to reduce clinical target volume margins at radiotherapy. Int J Radiat Oncol Biol Phys. 2009;74(3):898–905.
72. Tagliabue E, Agresti R, Carcangiu ML, et al. Role of HER2 in wound-induced breast carcinoma proliferation. Lancet. 2003;362(9383):527–33.
73. Vaidya JS, Vyas JJ, Chinoy RF, et al. Multicentricity of breast cancer: whole-organ analysis and clinical implications. Br J Cancer. 1996;74(5):820–4.
74. Vaidya JS, Tobias JS, Baum M, et al. TARGeted Intraoperative radiotherapy (TARGIT): an innovative approach to partial-breast irradiation. Semin Radiat Oncol. 2005;15(2):84–91.
75. Vaidya JS, Wenz F, Bulsara M, et al. Risk-adapted targeted intraoperative radiotherapy versus whole-breast radiotherapy for breast cancer: 5-year results for local control and overall survival from the TARGIT-A randomised trial. Lancet. 2014;383(9917):603–13.

76. Veronesi U, Marubini E, Del Vecchio M, et al. Local recurrences and distant metastases after conservative breast cancer treatments: partly independent events. J Natl Cancer Inst. 1995;87(1):19–27.
77. Veronesi U, Marubini E, Mariani L, et al. Radiotherapy after breast-conserving surgery in small breast carcinoma: long-term results of a randomized trial. Ann Oncol. 2001;12(7): 997–1003.
78. Veronesi U, Orecchia R, Maisonneuve P, et al. Intraoperative radiotherapy versus external radiotherapy for early breast cancer (ELIOT): a randomised controlled equivalence trial. Lancet Oncol. 2013;14(13):1269–77.
79. Vicini FA, Kestin L, Chen P, et al. Limited-field radiation therapy in the management of early-stage breast cancer. J Natl Cancer Inst. 2003;95(16):1205–10.
80. Vicini FA, Kestin LL, Goldstein NS. Defining the clinical target volume for patients with early-stage breast cancer treated with lumpectomy and accelerated partial breast irradiation: a pathologic analysis. Int J Radiat Oncol Biol Phys. 2004;60(3):722–30.
81. Voogd AC, Nielsen M, Peterse JL, et al. Differences in risk factors for local and distant recurrence after breast-conserving therapy or mastectomy for stage I and II breast cancer: pooled results of two large European randomized trials. J Clin Oncol. 2001;19(6):1688–97.
82. Vrieling C, Collette L, Fourquet A, et al. Can patient-, treatment- and pathology-related characteristics explain the high local recurrence rate following breast-conserving therapy in young patients? Eur J Cancer. 2003;39(7):932–44.
83. Weed DW, Yan D, Martinez AA, et al. The validity of surgical clips as a radiographic surrogate for the lumpectomy cavity in image-guided accelerated partial breast irradiation. Int J Radiat Oncol Biol Phys. 2004;60(2):484–92.
84. Whipp EC, Halliwell M. Magnetic resonance imaging appearances in the postoperative breast: the clinical target volume-tumor and its relationship to the chest wall. Int J Radiat Oncol Biol Phys. 2008;72(172):49–57.
85. Winzer KJ, Sauer R, Sauerbrei W, et al. Radiation therapy after breast-conserving surgery; first results of a randomised clinical trial in patients with low risk of recurrence. Eur J Cancer. 2004;40(7):998–1005.
86. Wolmark N, Curran WJ. Trial protocol March 13, 2007. On behalf of NSABP and RTOG of the American College of Radiology (ACR). NSABP Protocol B-39. RTOG Protocol 0413. A randomized phase III study of conventional whole breast irradiation versus partial breast irradiation for women with stage 0, I, or II breast cancer. National surgical adjuvant breast and bowel project (NSABP). 2007. p. 1–132.
87. Yang Z, Chen J, Hu W, et al. Planning the breast boost: how accurately do surgical clips represent the CT seroma? Radiother Oncol. 2010;97(3):530–4.
88. Yarnold J, Coles C. Trial Protocol, version 4, 19.02.2008. On behalf of the IMPORT LOW Trial Management Group: Intensity Modulated and Partial Organ Radiotherapy. Randomised trial testing intensity modulated and partial organ radiotherapy following breast conservation surgery for early breast cancer. Sutton, Surrey, UK: The Institute of Cancer Research: Royal Cancer Hospital; 2008. p. 1–74.

Chapter 3
The Radiobiology of Breast Radiotherapy

Atif J. Khan, Alexandra Stewart, and Roger Dale

Contents

In order to fully understand the possible impact of different radiotherapy techniques on a cancer, it is essential to have knowledge of the underlying radiobiology of both the cancer and the radiotherapeutic method. Without this, toxicity or control could be compromised when changing fractionation or delivery. The radiobiology of conventional external beam radiotherapy (EBRT) is relatively well understood, whereas the radiobiology of hypofractionated techniques is less clear. The challenge of integrating radiobiology into daily practice may perhaps become more straightforward as large randomized trials start to include radiobiology as a primary focus [1, 2].

A.J. Khan, MD (✉)
Department of Radiation Oncology, Robert Wood Johnson Medical School, Rutgers Cancer Institute of New Jersey, The State University of New Jersey, Piscataway, NJ 08854, USA
e-mail: khanat@cinj.rutgers.edu

A. Stewart, DM, MRCP, FRCR
Clinical Lead for Oncology, Consultant Clinical Oncologist, Royal Surrey County Hospital, Honorary Senior Lecturer, University of Surrey, Guildford, Surrey GU2 7XX, UK

R. Dale, PhD
Department of Surgery and Cancer, Faculty of Medicine, Imperial College, London, UK

D.W. Arthur et al. (eds.), *Short Course Breast Radiotherapy: A Comprehensive Review of Hypofractionation, Partial Breast, and Intra-Operative Irradiation*,
DOI 10.1007/978-3-319-24388-7_3

3.1 First Principles of Radiobiology

Early radiobiologists sought to mathematically characterize the observed relationship between radiation dose and the number of surviving "clonogens" (i.e., the number of observed colonies remaining vs. those expected in an irradiated cohort of cells). These early experiments were done in vitro on plates using cancer cells as well as in vivo on colony-forming assays such as formation of metastatic spleen colonies. Amidst two competing models, the linear-quadratic (or LQ) model [3, 4] appeared to hold true most consistently and was remarkably simple to understand and apply to clinical practice. Within this model, there are two components of radiation damage characterized by the radiosensitivity coefficients α and β. The α-mediated component results from a single ionizing radiation event, which simultaneously damages two individual targets. In a probable oversimplification, each strand of DNA is considered a discrete target. Thus, α-mediated damage crosses both strands resulting in a double-strand break. This non-repairable damage increases in a linear pattern with dose and is influenced by overall dose, rather than fractionation or dose rate.

The second, beta component (β) of radiation damage, is that resulting from two ionizing events, which separately and independently damage two targets. In the current (again likely oversimplified) model, the ionizing events are each causing a single-strand break. If these separate, damaged targets happen to be aligned correctly before repair can occur, a double-strand break may result, thus forming a lethal lesion. Although the final end point of β-damage is indistinguishable from that created via the α-process, its probability increases with the square of the instantaneous dose and is influenced by fractionation and dose rate as well as overall dose. Independent β-events may be temporally and/or spatially separated to allow for repair (sublethal damage repair) when the events are infrequent (i.e., in the low fractional dose or low-dose rate scenarios). However, as the dose increases, the probability of functional double-strand breaks resulting in lethal events increases dramatically (as a square when plotted on a log-linear graph). The repair of sublethal damage requires a full complement of DNA single- and double-strand break sensing and repair effectors.

The relative contribution of α and β modes of cell kill in a given test system can be characterized by the α/β ratio. The α/β ratio represents the dose at which single- and double-hit killing events are equal in number; at higher doses double-hit killing events start to progressively dominate. Cells with a low α/β ratio have an early transition to the "curvy" survival curve characteristic of β-mediated cell death. Systems with high α/β ratios tend to remain relatively straight. The clinical relevance of these empiric observations is discussed next.

In therapeutic irradiation, daily fraction sizes of 1.8 Gy or 2 Gy are commonly used and are described as "conventional." The rationale for conventional fractionation and the relationship between fraction size and tissue response are well described by the α/β ratio in the linear-quadratic model of fractionation sensitivity [5]. In this model, "late-reacting" normal tissues such as fibroblasts and terminally differentiated neurons have a low α/β ratio (2–5 Gy) and are very responsive to changes in fraction size, while "acutely reacting" normal tissues such as intestinal epithelium have a high α/β ratio (>7 Gy) and are less responsive to alterations in fraction size.

Cells with low α/β ratios have a relatively more "bendy" clonogenic survival curve which reflects the greater prominence of β-mediated cell killing and the increased capacity to repair sublethal damage when dose is fractionated. Cells with high α/β ratios have less capacity for sublethal damage repair. Estimates of the α/β ratio for squamous cell carcinomas of the head and neck and cervix uteri are >7 Gy [6]. In contrast, most normal, terminally differentiated tissues have low α/β ratios of 1–4 Gy. For this reason the generic α/β ratio for tumor control probability is usually taken to be 10 Gy, while the generic α/β ratio for late-responding normal tissue effects is usually taken as 3 Gy.

The biological effect of a given fractionation scheme is related to the α/β ratio by the equation:

$$\text{Effect} = \text{E} = \text{n}\left(\alpha \text{d} + \beta \text{d}^2\right)$$

where

d = dose/fraction
n = # well-spaced and identical fractions

Different fractionation schemes can be intercompared using the related concept of biologically effective dose (BED). In terms of n and d, BED may be written as

$$\text{BED} = \text{nd}\left[1 + \text{d}/(\alpha/\beta)\right]$$

Since the product ($n \times d$) is the total physical dose delivered, BED can be expressed in words as

$$\text{BED} = \text{Total physical dose} \times \text{Relative Effectiveness}\left(\text{RE}\right)$$

where RE is the factor which allows for the biological impact of the fractionation scheme in terms of the fraction size (d) and the specific α/β value of the irradiated tissue/organ being considered. For any given α/β, treatment schedules which produce identical BEDs are said to be radiobiologically isoeffective.

The BED for continuous low-dose rate brachytherapy can be calculated by the equation:

$$\text{BED} = \text{RT}\left[1 + 2\text{R}/\mu(\alpha/\beta)\right]$$

R = dose rate
T = treatment time
μ = sublethal damage repair constant (assuming mono-exponential repair)

This equation is valid provided the treatment time (T) is greater than about 12 h. For shorter treatment times a more complex expression is required [3]. Although relatively high cumulative doses of radiation are needed for tumor control, the daily fraction size (or dose rate) has to be respectful of the fraction sensitivity of normal tissues in the treated volume. As a result, for most epithelial tumors, daily fractions of 1.8–2 Gy are delivered over 4–8 weeks to reach a cumulative lethal dose of 45–85 Gy. In order to account for the greater fractionation sensitivity of late-responding tissues (low α/β), increases in fraction size have to be compensated for by reductions in cumulative radiation dose. However, this may result in a dose insufficient for tumor control.

The above discussion ignores a number of variables which may affect the probability of tumor control, for example, the potential effect of cellular proliferation that may occur during a course of fractionated radiation therapy. Although commonly ignored because of the uncertainty of this variable, a correction can be introduced into the above equation for this factor [7]:

$$\mathrm{BED} = \mathrm{nd}\left[1 + \mathrm{d}/(\alpha/\beta)\right] - 0.693\left(T - T_{\mathrm{lag}}\right)/\,\mathrm{a}T_{\mathrm{pot}}$$

T = overall treatment time
T_{lag} = lag time from beginning of treatment before fast repopulation begins
T_{pot} = potential tumor doubling time

In this formalism, it is postulated that after a certain initial period of time (i.e., the "kickoff time") from the start of radiotherapy, the remaining cells begin to proliferate, sometimes at an accelerated rate. Rosenstein et al. in their publication comparing several partial breast irradiation (PBI) fractionation schemes used a T_{pot} value of 13 days, an initial time lag of 14 days, and an α value of $0.3\mathrm{Gy}^{-17}$. Rew et al. suggest a T_{pot} of 10.4 days [8]. Both of these T_{pot} values are longer than those displayed by many other cancers and suggest some scope for using both hypofractionation and acceleration for breast tumors. An examination of tumor doubling time by Peer et al. suggests that doubling time may be age dependent and is smaller in women under 50 years of age [9], again indicating that a hypofractionated, accelerated approach may be of benefit in this group.

Another important consideration in linear-quadratic formalism is the "equal effect assumption" in which each fraction is assumed to produce the same fractional cell kill and with complete recovery of sublethal damage between fractions. With overnight interfraction intervals, the equal effect assumption tends to be mostly accurate because the half-life ($T_{1/2)}$ of sublethal damage repair, i.e., the molecular repair and resolution of DNA-strand breaks, is in the order of a few hours. For example, several groups have described the $T_{1/2}$ to be of the order of 1–1.5 h [10, 11], but others have reported it to be longer [12, 13]. Some studies suggest that repair processes in late-responding normal tissues may be biphasic with fast and slow components [14, 15]. The emerging view is that tumors and acute-responding normal tissues probably have a relatively short repair half-life (0.5–1.5 h), whereas late-responding tissues are indeed likely to exhibit biphasic repair, with respective fast and slow repair times of around 0.3 and 4 h [16].

3.2 The Radiobiology of Breast Cancer

In contrast to the standard assumptions for most epithelial tumors, the α/β ratio for breast tumors may be much lower than the usual assumption of 10 Gy. In vitro experiments in human breast carcinoma cell lines suggested an α/β ratio of about 4 Gy [17, 18]. An interesting set of clinical dose-response data for inoperable and locally recurrent breast cancer was published in 1952 [19] and reanalyzed to fit the linear-quadratic model [5, 20]. The point estimate for the α/β ratio from this data set was 4–5 Gy. Based on this information, the Royal Marsden Hospital and the Gloucestershire Oncology Centre (RMH/GOC) collaborated in a randomized clinical trial to evaluate the relative toxicity and efficacy of different whole-breast fractionation schemes [21, 22]. A total of 1410 women were randomized to one of three arms between 1986 and 1999:

1. 50 Gy in 25 fractions over 5 weeks
2. 39 Gy in 13 fractions (3.0 Gy/fx) over 5 weeks
3. 42.9 Gy in 13 fractions (3.3 Gy/fx) over 5 weeks

To interrogate the repair-related parameters (i.e., α and β), the overall treatment time was kept constant in all three arms. In the experimental arms, treatment was delivered using 5 fractions over a 2-week cycle. All patients were treated in the supine position. The primary end point was late breast change. Local control was a secondary end point. About 75 % of patients received a conventionally fractionated electron boost to the lumpectomy cavity. The protocol did allow treatment of regional lymph nodes (supraclavicular and axillary) with additional radiation fields, and these were used in 20 % of the patients. Fourteen percent of patients also received adjuvant CMF (cyclophosphamide, methotrexate, and fluorouracil) chemotherapy.

The 39 Gy arm was less likely to develop late radiation change compared to both 42.9 and 50 Gy [22] but also had worse local control than the 42.9 Gy arm [21]. However, the 42.9 Gy arm, which had 3.3 Gy fractions, was not significantly different from the 50 Gy arm for both development of late radiation change and local control. The α/β ratio for any late breast change was determined to be 3.6 Gy and the α/β ratio for tumor control was 4 Gy. The similarity of these two estimates is striking and served to validate the further study of hypofractionated regimens. This is because, when the tumor and late-reacting α/β values are broadly similar, no particular fractionation scheme is deemed to be markedly better in radiobiological terms, and, as a consequence, hypofractionation, which offers benefits in terms of patient convenience and economics, becomes the emergent choice. Finally, it must be noted that none of the 290 patients who were treated at the axillary and supraclavicular areas developed brachial plexopathy.

The results of the above RMH/GOC trial informed the design of the second generation of UK fractionation trials: the START A and START B trials. These trials represent the most robust collection of radiobiology parameters of any human malignancy to date.

In the START A trial [1], 2236 women with early breast cancer were randomized between 1998 and 2002 to either

1. 50 Gy in 25 fractions (2 Gy/fx)
2. 39 Gy in 13 fractions (3 Gy/fx)
3. 41.6 Gy in 13 fractions (3.2 Gy/fx)

The UK trialists kept the treatment schedules of the RMH/GOC trial with the exception of decreasing the third arm from 3.3 Gy/fraction to 3.2 Gy/fraction. This was done due to the slightly worse late effects in the 3.3 arm. Unlike the exploratory RMH/GOC trial, the primary end point was local-regional control. Also, unlike the RMH/GOC trial, 15 % of enrolled patients were treated to the chest wall after mastectomy. The thirteen-fraction schedules were treated using 5 fractions every 2 weeks as in the RMH/GOC trial. Approximately 60 % of women received a conventionally fractionated boost of 10 Gy with electrons. Regional nodal irradiation was delivered in 14 % of patients. Quality assurance of radiation technique included a site visit with phantom verification of technique and TLD measurements in a random sample of patients. With a median survival of 5.1 years, no significant differences in local control were detected. The 39 Gy arm had a lower likelihood of breast late effects on photographic and self-assessment. Toxicity events such as rib fractures and cardiac events were low in all arms. The START A trial determined the α/β ratio for local relapse to be 4.1 Gy, further validating the original RMH/GOC findings

In the START B trial [2], 2215 women with early-stage breast cancer were randomized between 1999 and 2001 to either

1. 50 Gy in 25 fractions (2 Gy/fx)
2. 40 Gy in 15 fractions (2.67 Gy/fx)

The primary end point of the trial was to exclude an increase of 5 % or more in 5-year locoregional relapse with 95 % power (and a one-sided $\alpha = 0.025$). Approximately, 8 % of patients were receiving postmastectomy radiation therapy. Approximately 40 % of intact breast patients received an electron boost to the lumpectomy bed of 10 Gy in 5 fractions. Approximately 7 % of patients received lymphatic irradiation. The trial found no detectable difference in local-regional control between the two arms of the study. Interestingly, both photographic scored assessments of change in breast appearance and patient-assessed quality of life questionnaires of late tissue effects revealed better results for the experimental arm. Toxicity events were low. All 82 patients who received regional irradiation with the hypofractionated schedule remained free of brachial plexopathy.

The UK trialists deserve tremendous credit for the meticulous and invaluable research efforts described above. Their findings have fundamentally challenged many underlying assumptions about adjuvant breast radiotherapy and have definitively established the relevant radiobiological parameters for future trials of altered fractionation.

Similar to the UK START B trial, the Canadian NCI randomized 1234 patients (1993–1996) with T1 and T2 tumors with negative margins and pathologically negative nodes (on level 1 and 2 dissection) to

1. 50 Gy in 25 fractions (2 Gy/fx) over 35 days
2. 42.5 Gy in 16 fractions (2.66 Gy/fx) over 22 days [23]

Notably, women with breast separations greater than 25 cm were excluded. Dose was prescribed to the 1/3 point, and homogeneity within 7 % was required. Lumpectomy bed boosts and treatment to regional draining lymph nodes were not allowed. With a median follow-up of 69 months, local recurrence-free survival (LFS) was equal (97.2 % vs. 96.8 %), and there was no difference in OS and DFS. Cosmesis was identical with excellent or good scores at 3 and 5 years in 77 % of patients in both groups. Toxicities were also comparable. Grade 2 and 3 toxicities were negligible. A limitation of the Canadian study is the lack of a lumpectomy boost, which has been subsequently found to significantly improve local control [24]. The patients eligible for the study had low risk for disease recurrence, limiting the general scope of the results.

3.2.1 *Molecular Classification*

Increasingly, treatment of individual cancers has transitioned from that of the general characteristics of a cell type (e.g., ductal carcinoma of the breast) to identification of the individual molecular characterization of a tumor with identification of its individual genetic profile. This molecular classification can be used to predict response to treatment, for example, tumors positive for interferon-related DNA damage resistance signature (IRDS) treated with adjuvant radiotherapy have a greater locoregional relapse rate than those that are IRDS negative [25]. In the way that molecular characterization has led to more personalized treatment with chemotherapy, it may also lead to more personalized radiotherapy, for example, subgroup analysis of the Canadian NCI trial suggested that grade III tumors were more sensitive to conventional fractionation, whereas grade I and II tumors were more suited to hypofractionation [26]. Though as this was not seen in post hoc analysis of the START trials [27], it warrants further prospective evaluation.

Investigation of individual molecular characteristics such as double-strand break (DSB) repair kinetics [28] as a predictor of normal tissue toxicity is an interesting area of study but has not yet provided definitive data that could be taken forward for treatment planning. In vitro examination of modified genetic expression [29] indicates that altered gene expression introduced by viral genetic vectors may affect the inherent radiosensitivity of a breast cancer cell and may be an avenue in the future to improve treatment response or decrease normal tissue toxicity. However, a cytotoxic effect was only achieved with fractional doses of 5 Gy or more which may indicate incomplete transfection of tumor cells or a requirement for more hypofractionated radiotherapy in this setting.

3.3 Partial Breast Radiotherapy

There are a variety of logistic reasons to consider partial breast radiotherapy such as improving access to breast-conserving surgery and increasing uptake of radiotherapy in poorly served geographic locations. However, there are also radiobiological indications that partial breast irradiation (PBI) may be preferable in certain situations. Current methods of PBI are marked by significant heterogeneity. Although all do focus on treatment of a partial volume of breast tissue around the index lumpectomy cavity, these methods are entirely dissimilar in their radiobiology. This is an important fact to consider when comparing techniques and when calculating dose and fractionation for a new technique. The radiobiological characteristics of the main techniques will briefly be contrasted in this section.

3.3.1 External Beam PBI

Three-dimensional conformal radiotherapy (3D CRT) for PBI is appealing because the technology of EBRT is well understood, and linear accelerators are more readily available than other PBI technologies. 3D CRT offers a more homogeneous dose distribution than intraoperative or brachytherapy PBI techniques, generally ranging from 95 to 107 % of the intended dose [30]. Again radiobiological principles must be considered in dose conversion. For example, the effect of improved homogeneity across the PBI target led to an increase in dose in the NSABP B39 study from 34 Gy in 10 fractions over 1 week for the brachytherapy APBI (accelerated PBI) cohort to 38.5 Gy in 10 fractions over 1 week for the 3D CRT APBI cohort. Formenti et al. predicted equivalent tumor control and late toxicity to 50 Gy in 25 fractions over 5 weeks if delivering 3D CRT APBI using 30 Gy in 5 fractions over 10 days (using an α/β ratio of 4 Gy for tumor and 2 Gy for fibrosis) [31]. This calculation assumed that full sublethal damage repair occurs between fractions and no significant cell proliferation occurs [32]. Many WBRT schedules receive an additional 16 Gy boost to the tumor bed in order to improve local control [33] which is not accounted for in many radiobiological comparisons. However, this additional dose may be less important in older patients [34] who are generally in the PBI cohort.

Since 3D CRT APBI with linac-generated X-ray beams often results in higher normal tissue doses than other APBI techniques [35, 36], other methods of EBRT delivery have been explored. Due to a higher RBE and a more rapid dose falloff, proton beams could decrease normal tissue irradiation [37]. Electrons may also have this effect. However, acute skin reactions may be increased due to higher entrance doses [38].

3.3.2 Interstitial Implant APBI

Three categories of brachytherapy were defined in the International Commission on Radiation Units and Measurements (ICRU) Report 38 [39]:

- Low dose rate (LDR) – a range of 0.4–2 Gy/h
- Medium dose rate (MDR) – a range of 2–12 Gy/h
- High dose rate (HDR) – over 12 Gy/h

Pulsed brachytherapy (PB) uses short pulses of brachytherapy every 1–4 h in an attempt to achieve the dose optimization available with a stepping source combined with the toxicity profile associated with the dose delivery of LDR brachytherapy.

The first experiences with APBI were of multi-catheter LDR implants typically prescribing 45–50 Gy to 100 % isodose at a dose rate of 0.5 Gy/h. The initially selected doses mimicked those used in EBRT; when the LDR dose was escalated to 60 Gy, there were no increase in tumor control and a trend toward increased fibrosis [40], suggesting that 50 Gy is adequate. A large variety of HDR interstitial implant treatment schedules exist, for example, the GEC-ESTRO trial of APBI vs. WBRT used 32 Gy in 8 fractions bid or 30.3 Gy in 7 fractions bid [41], and Polgar et al. used 36.4 Gy in 7 fractions bid [42]. One commonly used scheme used the LQ model to determine equivalence for tumor control and late toxicity. This generated the treatment schedule of 34 Gy in 10 fractions over 1 week [43]. This assumed a tumor $T_{1/2}$ for sublethal damage of 1.5 h which is longer than that assumed by other investigators [44]. Again radiobiological principles are important in dose conversion as this dose and fractionation scheme was used for the single-channel MammoSite catheter, without consideration of the differing dose homogeneity. This has been shown to result in a higher equivalent dose than using multiple interstitial catheters and may affect early and late toxicity [45, 46]. Although one advantage of an interstitial implant is the ability to deliver a hypofractionated course of radiotherapy quickly before chemotherapy, the timing of radiotherapy may be important as the administration of chemotherapy following the implant has been associated with significantly worse cosmesis in both the HDR and LDR setting [43, 47].

In contrast to brachytherapy in other areas of the body where dose inhomogeneity is favored, such as uterine cervix, the aim for a multi-catheter interstitial implant is to achieve as homogeneous a dose distribution as possible. This was easier with equal-activity LDR sources but when using HDR treatment plans optimized to a homogeneous dose distribution may not provide homogeneous cell killing, particularly at the implant periphery. Cell kill was also compromised with older, low-activity HDR sources [48]. Thus the dose homogeneity index (DHI) has been developed to indicate the homogeneity within an implant:

$$\mathrm{DHI} = \mathrm{V100} - \mathrm{V150} / \mathrm{V100}$$

where V100 and V150 are, respectively, the tissue volumes receiving 100 % and 150 % of the prescribed dose. The higher the DHI, the more uniform the dose distribution within an implant. A DHI of over 0.75 is recommended, with a value over 0.85 being ideal. The toxicity of multi-catheter interstitial implants is significantly lower if the dose is more homogeneous within the target volume [43, 47]. The volume of the individual high-dose regions also appears to be important with large areas receiving over 150 and 200 % of the prescribed dose contributing to increased rates of worse cosmesis and fat necrosis [47].

Balloon catheter techniques were developed in an attempt to make PBI using brachytherapy more available as they rely less on technical skill than interstitial implant placement and thus may be more universally applied. They are also cosmetically more appealing during the time of the implant. The first and simplest balloon catheter (MammoSite) utilizes a single catheter to deliver a uniform dose to a spherical cavity of depth 1 cm around the tumor bed. This treatment depth appears less than that normally assumed when planning interstitial implant techniques but has been shown to treat an effective thickness of tissue of up to 2 cm around the lumpectomy cavity [49, 50]. This is an important factor to bear in mind when selecting a target volume and using other balloon techniques which may not cause the same degree of tissue stretching, though the optimal target volume for PBI has not yet been established. The radiation may be delivered from a single dwell position in the center of the balloon or multiple dwell positions along the axis of the catheter. Using multiple positions decreases the effects of anisotropy from the HDR source, thereby improving dose coverage [50]. Both the dose distribution and equivalent uniform dose (EUD) may change when multiple dwell positions or different balloon diameters are used [50, 51]. Patients with unfavorable anatomic variations may receive higher doses to OAR (organs at risk) than others with a similar tumor bed position [36]. There is an association of increased EUD with hyperpigmentation and telangiectasia in a small series of MammoSite patients [51], and this may be a variable that should be used for dose comparison in future studies.

Other applicators with multiple channels are under investigation, and the differing radiobiology of these will be interesting to explore with an expectation of improved dose sculpting for organs at risk and therefore decreased EUD and thus decreased late toxicity due to the increased number of catheters [45, 52, 53].

3.3.3 *Single-Channel Electronic Brachytherapy*

3.3.3.1 Intraoperative PBI

Delivery of PBI at the time of surgery allows a large single fraction to be delivered under direct visualization while displacing or shielding uninvolved or dose-limiting tissues. This avoids a "geographical miss," a potential risk of EBRT techniques even with CT imaging techniques [54]. However, use of intraoperative radiotherapy

(IORT) at the time of surgery risks inappropriate patient selection when the full pathologic results are not available.

IORT is commonly delivered using a single fraction. Although one can approximately expect the same amount of tumor cell kill with about half to a third of the total dose used in conventionally fractionated radiotherapy [55], the predictive power of LQ-based radiobiological modeling may be much less reliable since the model is progressively less accurate for fraction sizes above about 8 Gy. Immediate administration may avoid the risk of tumor cell proliferation while awaiting radiotherapy as well as repopulation triggered by the growth factor-rich surgical cavity [56]. Although the overall treatment time effect may be modest in breast cancer, a detrimental effect (i.e., reduced local control) has been demonstrated following prolonged waits for whole-breast radiotherapy (WBRT) [57], implying that repopulation of any remaining clonogens does begin almost immediately after surgery [58].

Intraoperative electron therapy delivers a homogeneous dose using energy 3–12 MeV to the tumor bed, usually 21 Gy to the 90 % isodose surface, giving an average dose of 22.5 Gy [55]. This single dose is reported as equivalent to 56 Gy in conventional (1.8–2 Gy) fractionation, though this calculation used an incorrect α/β ratio of 10 Gy for tumor [55].

Intraoperative photon beams using 50 kV X-rays has been reported, most commonly using the Intrabeam device (Carl Zeiss Meditec, Dublin, CA, USA), though use of the Xoft Axxent device (Xoft, San Jose, CA, USA) is also reported. The tissue conforms to a spherical applicator delivering a high dose quickly to the tumor bed with rapid dose falloff. A prescription dose of 20 Gy to the tumor bed is typically used, falling to 5 Gy only 10 mm away. The dose delivered at depth with intraoperative photon therapy is much lower than with other PBI techniques; again it is noted that the ideal volume for PBI has not been defined; however pathologic studies do show cancer cells within 1–2 cm of a lumpectomy cavity. However the relative biological effect (RBE) of photons increases as the photon energy decreases. Initial assumptions used an RBE of 2.2, assuming an α/β ratio of 10 Gy for tumor cells [44]. These calculations were made assuming a $T_{1/2}$ for sublethal damage of 15 min; if in fact the $T_{1/2}$ is longer, then the RBE would be proportionally higher. The first publication of the TARGIT-A randomized trial designed to demonstrate non-inferiority of this technique showed no significant difference in local recurrence in the IORT or WBRT groups [59]. The update of this trial is discussed elsewhere.

Delivery of radiotherapy at the time of surgery may give an added biological advantage to immediate radiotherapy in addition to that solely of radiation-induced cell kill. It is known that EBRT induces changes in the extracellular matrix which persist for at least 30 years after radiotherapy [60]. Breast cancer cell growth may be accelerated by surgery; when surgical wound fluid was added to breast cancer cell lines, it was seen to stimulate growth, motility, and invasion [56]; this effect may be diminished or prevented by IORT. When surgical wound fluid from a patient who had undergone IORT was added to the same cell lines, these effects were no longer seen. Thus, IORT may cause wound microenvironment changes that directly affect cell growth and invasion, in addition to the direct cell-killing effects of radiation.

3.4 Conclusion

Thanks to well-designed clinical trials, the radiobiology of breast cancer is among the best understood of all cancers. The importance of radiobiology in the development of new techniques and new methods of dose delivery has been emphasized, and future research should continue to examine all radiobiological variables at an early stage.

References

1. The START Trialists Group. The UK standardisation of breast radiotherapy (START) trial A of radiotherapy hypofractionation for treatment of early breast cancer: a randomised trial. Lancet Oncol. 2008;9:331–41.
2. The START Trialists Group. The UK standardisation of breast radiotherapy (START) trial B of radiotherapy hypofractionation for treatment of early breast cancer: a randomised trial. Lancet. 2008;371:1098–107.
3. Dale RG. The application of the linear quadratic dose-effect equation to fractionated and protracted radiotherapy. Br J Radiol. 1985;58:515–28.
4. Joiner MC, van der Kogel AJ. In: Steel GG, editors. Basic clinical radiobiology. Arnold; 1997. p. 106–22.
5. Fowler J. The linear-quadratic formula and progress in fractionated radiotherapy. Br J Radiol. 1989;62:679–94.
6. Bentzen S, Baumann M. In: Steel GG, editors. Basic clinical radiobiology. Arnold; 2002. p. 134–46.
7. Rosenstein B, Lymberis S, Formenti S. Biologic comparison of partial breast irradiation protocols. Int J Radiat Oncol Biol Phys. 2004;60:1393–404.
8. Rew DA, Wilson GD. Cell production rates in human tissues and tumours and their significance. Part II: clinical data. Eur J Surg Oncol. 2000;26:405–17.
9. Peer PG, van Dijck JA, Hendriks JH, et al. Age-dependent growth rate of primary breast cancer. Cancer. 1993;71:3547–51.
10. Pop LA, van den Broek JF, Visser AG, et al. Constraints in the use of repair half times and mathematical modelling for the clinical application of HDR and PDR treatment schedules as an alternative for LDR brachytherapy. Radiother Oncol. 1996;38:153–62.
11. Dale RG. What minimum number of fractions is required with high dose rate remote afterloading? Br J Radiol. 1987;60:300–2.
12. Orton C. High dose rate brachytherapy may be radiobiologically superior to low dose rate due to slow repair of late responding normal tissue cells. Int J Radiat Oncol Biol Phys. 2001;49:183–9.
13. Bentzen SM, Saunders MI, Dische S. Repair halftimes estimated from observations of treatment-related morbidity after CHART or conventional radiotherapy in head and neck cancer. Radiother Oncol. 1999;53:219–26.
14. Fowler JF. Is repair of DNA strand break damage from ionizing radiation second-order rather than first-order? A simpler explanation of apparently multiexponential repair. Radiat Res. 1999;152:124–36.
15. Millar WT, Canney PA. Derivation and application of equations describing the effects of fractionated protracted irradiation, based on multiple and incomplete repair processes. Part 1L: derivation of equations. Int J Radio Biol. 1993;64:275–91.

16. Fowler JF. Half-times of irradiation recovery in accelerated partial breast irradiation: Incomplete recovery as a potentially dangerous enhancer of radiation damage. J Canc Res Ther. 2013;1:230–4.
17. Matthews J, Meeker B, Chapman J. Response of human tumor cell lines in vitro to fractionated irradiation. Int J Radiat Oncol Biol Phys. 1989;16:133–8.
18. Steel G, Deacon J, Duschesne G. The dose-rate effect in human tumour cells. Radiother Oncol. 1987;9:299–310.
19. Cohen L. Radiotherapy in breast cancer. The dose-time relationship: theoretical considerations. Br J Radiol. 1952;25:636–42.
20. Douglas B, Castro J. Novel fractionation schemes and high linear energy transfer. Prog Exp Tumor Res. 1984;28:152–65.
21. Owen J, et al. Effect of radiotherapy fraction size on tumor control in patients with early-stage breast cancer after local tumour excision: long-term results of a randomised trial. Lancet Oncol. 2006;7:467–71.
22. Yarnold J, et al. Fractionation sensitivity and dose response of late adverse effects in the breast after radiotherapy for early breast cancer: long-term results of a randomised trial. Radiother Oncol. 2005;75:9–17.
23. Whelan T, et al. Randomized trial of breast irradiation schedules after lumpectomy for women with lymph node-negative breast cancer. J Natl Cancer Inst. 2002;94:1143–50.
24. Bartelink H, et al. Recurrence rates after treatment of breast cancer with standard radiotherapy with or without additional radiation. N Engl J Med. 2001;345:1378–87.
25. Weichselbaum RR, et al. An interferon-related gene signature for DNA damage resistance is a predictive marker for chemotherapy and radiation for breast cancer. Proc Natl Acad Sci U S A. 2008;105:18490–5.
26. Whelan TJ, et al. Long-term results of hypofractionated radiation therapy for breast cancer. N Engl J Med. 2010;362:513–20.
27. Haviland JS, Yarnold JR, Bentzen SM. Hypofractionated radiotherapy for breast cancer. N Engl J Med. 2010;362:1843.
28. Mumbrekar KD, et al. Influence of double-strand break repair on radiation therapy-induced acute skin reactions in breast cancer patients. Int J Radiat Oncol Biol Phys. 2014;88:671–6.
29. Li ZL, et al. Expression of Smac induced by the Egr1 promoter enhances the radiosensitivity of breast cancer cells. Cancer Gene Ther. 2014;21:142–9.
30. ICRU 50. Prescribing, recording and reporting photon beam therapy. Report No. 50. International Commission on Radiation Units and Measurements, Bethesda, 1993.
31. Formenti SC. External-beam partial-breast irradiation. Semin Radiat Oncol. 2005;15:92–9.
32. Formenti SC, et al. Prone accelerated partial breast irradiation after breast conserving surgery: preliminary clinical results and dose-volume histogram analysis. Int J Radiat Oncol Biol Phys. 2004;60:493–504.
33. Bartelink H, et al. Impact of a higher radiation dose on local control and survival in breast-conserving therapy of early breast cancer: 10-year results of the randomized boost versus no boost EORTC 22881–10882 trial. J Clin Oncol. 2007;25:3259–65.
34. Veronesi U, Luini A, Del Vecchio M, et al. Radiotherapy after breast-preserving surgery in women with localised cancer of the breast. N Engl J Med. 1993;328:1587–91.
35. Stewart AJ, et al. Dose volume histogram analysis of normal structures associated with accelerated partial breast irradiation delivered by high dose rate brachytherapy and comparison with whole breast external beam radiotherapy fields. Radiother Oncol. 2008;19:38.
36. Khan AJ, et al. A dosimetric comparison of three-dimensional conformal, intensity-modulated radiation therapy and MammoSite partial-breast irradiation. Brachytherapy. 2006;5:183–8.
37. Kozak KR, et al. Accelerated partial-breast irradiation using proton beams: initial clinical experience. Int J Radiat Oncol Biol Phys. 2006;66:691–8.
38. Ribero GG, Magee B, Swindell R, Harris M, Banergee SS. The Christie hospital breast conservation trial: an update at 8 years from inception. Clin Oncol (R Coll Radiol). 1993;5:278–83.

39. International Commission on Radiation Units and Measurements. Dose and volume specifications for reporting intracavitary therapy in gynecology (report 38). International Commission on Radiation Units and Measurements, 1985.
40. Lawneda BD, et al. Dose-volume analysis of radiotherapy for T1N0 invasive breast cancer treated by local excision and partial breast irradiation by low-dose-rate interstitial implant. Int J Radiat Oncol Biol Phys. 2003;56:671–80.
41. http://www.apbi.uni-erlangen.de/outline/outline.html. Accessed 17 Aug 2007.
42. Polgár C, et al. High-dose-rate brachytherapy alone versus whole breast radiotherapy with or without tumor bed boost after breast-conserving surgery: seven year results of a comparative study. Int J Radiat Oncol Biol Phys. 2004;60:1173–81.
43. Arthur DW, Koo D, Zwicker RD, et al. Partial breast brachytherapy after lumpectomy: Low-dose-rate and high-dose-rate experience. Int J Radiat Oncol Biol Phys. 2003;56:681–9.
44. Herskind C, Steil V, Kraus-Tiefenbacher U, Wenz F. Radiobiological aspects of intraoperative radiotherapy (IORT) with isotropic low-energy X rays for early-stage breast cancer. Radiat Res. 2005;163:208–15.
45. Armpilia C, Dale RG, Sandilos P, Vlachos L. Radiobiological modelling of dose-gradient effects in low dose rate, high dose rate and pulsed brachytherapy. Phys Med Biol. 2006;51:4399–411.
46. Stewart AJ, et al. Does equivalent uniform dose affect toxicity for high dose rate brachytherapy using the MammoSite applicator? Brachytherapy. 2009;8:138.
47. Wazer DE, Kaufman S, Cuttino L, Dipetrillo T, Arthur DW. Accelerated partial breast irradiation: an analysis of variables associated with late toxicity and long-term cosmetic outcome after high-dose-rate interstitial brachytherapy. Int J Radiat Oncol Biol Phys. 2006;64:489–95.
48. Manning MA, Zwicker RD, Arthur DA, Arnfield M. Biologic treatment planning for high-dose-rate brachytherapy. Int J Radiat Oncol Biol Phys. 2001;49:839–45.
49. Edmundson GK, Vicini FA, Chen PY, et al. Dosimetric characteristics of the MammoSite RTS, a new breast brachytherapy applicator. Int J Radiat Oncol Biol Phys. 2002;52:1132–9.
50. Dickler A, Kirk M, Choo J, et al. Treatment volume and dose optimization of mammosite breast brachytherapy applicator. Int J Radiat Oncol Biol Phys. 2004;59:469–74.
51. Stewart AJ, et al. Equivalent uniform dose for accelerated partial breast irradiation using the MammoSite applicator. Radiother Oncol. 2013;108:232–5.
52. Dale RG, Coles IP, Deehan C, O'Donoghue JA. Calculation of integrated biological response in brachytherapy. Int J Radiat Oncol Biol Phys. 1997;38:633–42.
53. Niemierko A. Reporting and analyzing dose distributions: a concept of equivalent uniform dose. Med Phys. 2007;24:103–10.
54. Landis DM, et al. Variability among breast radiation oncologists in delineation of the postsurgical lumpectomy cavity. Int J Radiat Oncol Biol Phys. 2007;67:1299–308.
55. Orecchia R, Veronesi U. Intraoperative electrons. Semin Radiat Oncol. 2005;15:76–83.
56. Belletti B, et al. Targeted intraoperative radiotherapy impairs the stimulation of breast cancer cell proliferation and invasion caused by surgical wounding. Clin Cancer Res. 2008;14:1324–32.
57. Mikeljevic JS, Haward R, Johnston C, et al. Trends in post-operative radiotherapy delay and the effect on survival in breast cancer patients treated with conservation surgery. Br J Cancer. 2004;90:1343–8.
58. Wyatt RM, Beddoe AH, Dale RG. The effects of delays in radiotherapy treatment on tumour control. Phys Med Biol. 2003;48:139–55.
59. Vaidya JS, Joseph DJ, Tobias JS, et al. Targeted intraoperative radiotherapy versus whole breast radiotherapy for breast cancer (TARGIT-A trial): an international, prospective, randomised, non-inferiority phase 3 trial. Lancet. 2010;376:91–102.
60. Cordes N, Park CC. beta1 integrin as a molecular therapeutic target. Int J Radiat Biol. 2007;83:753–60.

Chapter 4
Quality Assurance and Radiation Safety for Breast Irradiation

Bruce Thomadsen and Rupak Das

Contents

Breast irradiation, be it whole-breast external-beam or brachytherapy, proves highly effective in the treatment of breast cancer. However, errors in treatment can have significant consequences for the patient. Quality management (QM) stands as the barrier preventing off the intended track and into hazardous situations.

QM consists of more than just following checklists and performing verifications, although those are major parts of a QM program. QM consists of all a facility's activities aimed at achieving a reliable, high-quality program. A new paradigm for QM, based on systems engineering principles, has been making its way into radiation oncology. The concept recognizes that while equipment does fail and puts patients at risk, more often the humans involved err, and the system in which the

B. Thomadsen (✉)
Department of Medical Physics, School of Medicine and Public Health, University of Wisconsin, 1005 Wisconsin Institute for Medical Research, Madison, WI 53705, USA
e-mail: brthomad@wisc.edu

R. Das
Department of Human Oncology, University of Wisconsin, School of Medicine and Public Health, K4/B100 Clinical Sciences Center, Madison, WI 53792, USA
e-mail: rkdas@humonc.wisc.edu

D.W. Arthur et al. (eds.), *Short Course Breast Radiotherapy: A Comprehensive Review of Hypofractionation, Partial Breast, and Intra-Operative Irradiation*,
DOI 10.1007/978-3-319-24388-7_4

treatments are delivered must protect from all failures. This approach has been common in many high-reliability, high-risk industries and has proven useful and relatively simple in many medical disciplines. A report from Task Group (TG) 100 of the American Association of Physicists in Medicine (AAPM) studied the use of these techniques for radiotherapy and wrote a report that serves as a primer for learning the techniques and provides an example application for intensity-modulated radiotherapy (IMRT) [2, 8, 9].

According to the systems methodology, establishing QM for a procedure, such as breast implantation, begins with a risk assessment: mapping the process, performing a failure modes and effects analysis, and making a fault tree to understand where the risks lie and how errors propagate. Addressing the risks starts with fixing any environmental or technical problems found. A program also needs to ensure that it has in place the key core components identified by TG 100:

- Adequate resources (staffing, equipment, support from administration) to perform the procedure.
- Adequate training for the staff.
- A program for maintenance of equipment and software.
- Established standardized procedures.
- Clear and effective lines of communication have been established.

If the analysis indicates problematic steps in the procedure, consideration should be given to redesigning the procedure to eliminate the problem step if possible. Care should be taken to reevaluate the risk following the change to see if the new procedure opens pathways for new and different problems.

Preparing for the procedure requires commissioning. Usually, commissioning is thought to apply to equipment – making sure it works properly, understanding its limitations, and gathering all the data needed for its use. Commissioning applies equally to procedures. Commissioning a procedure runs through the procedure without the patient but with all the staff involved slowing at first and working up to the expected speed. During these practice runs, attention is paid to ensuring availability of all the required equipment and supplies, all information needed is at hand, that the communication patterns are established and understood and each team member knows what all the other members do and what is expected of them.

Finally, for outstanding quality potential problems, QM activities need to be established. Quality management activities discussed here consist of quality assurance (QA) and quality control (QC). QA includes all activities intended to indicate whether an action was performed correctly or a device is operating as it should. A manual calculation of the total treatment time for a high-dose-rate breast implant is an example of QA because it provides a measure that the outcome of the treatment plan falls within normal, expected limits. QC activities act to keep the procedure operating correctly, such as using surgical clips to verify coverage of interstitial needles during an interstitial breast implant. Much of the QC for breast irradiation, for both brachytherapy and external-beam radiotherapy, has become part of the procedure. The focus of this chapter mostly will be the QA for breast irradiation.

The discussion in this chapter mostly assumes that a facility has a QA program operation that covers the brachytherapy infrastructure, covering such things as QA for source calibration and the performance of the treatment planning system. Thus, this chapter considers the QA necessary particularly for breast radiotherapy.

Overall, QA for any radiotherapy procedure needs to cover:

- Preparation and procedures
- Input information
- Planning
- Setup and execution

4.1 Quality Assurance for Breast Brachytherapy

Before considering QA for breast radiotherapy, a look at events that have occurred with breast brachytherapy can be instructive.

4.1.1 Breast Brachytherapy Events

While breast brachytherapy has proven to be safe and usually of high quality, some events have occurred. Table 4.1 presents a summary of events reported to the US Nuclear Regulatory Commission between 2007 and 2014. It is not known how many cases were treated during that time, but an average of roughly three events per year is a very low fraction of patients with a serious problem involving the therapy.

Some of the events in the table, such as the first three, could happen with any high-dose-rate (HDR) treatment. While the rest of the event types could happen with other treatment sites, breast brachytherapy is particularly susceptible. These

Table 4.1 Events involving breast brachytherapy reported to the US Nuclear Regulatory Commission between 2007 and 2014

Source did not retract
Computer software failure and plan check not performed
Wrong patient's plan used (2)
Wrong length measured (10)
Wrong transfer tubes
Wrong dose planning (2)
Incorrect target in planning
Applicator digitized in the wrong direction (2)
Balloon lost fluid (punctured) (2)
SAVI – catheter path punctured the catheter and moved along the skin

The numbers in parentheses indicate the number of events of the type noted if more than one events were not particular to a given manufacturer, and although the way a particular event unfolded may have been unit specific, very similar events occurred with other units. The following provides more information about these events.

4.1.1.1 Source Retraction Failure

Not much information on this event is available. The problem could occur with any type of HDR treatment, but this case happened to be a breast treatment with no particular patient-related cause for the source retraction failure.

Knowing nothing more about the event, it does highlight two very important points:

- There needs to be someone at the control panel to recognize a problem and go immediately and unhesitatingly into the room and assess what action to take, and execute it quickly.
- Take the emergency practice seriously.

In this case, the radiation oncologist went into the room and disconnected the patient, preventing serious consequences.

4.1.1.2 Computer Software Failure Compounded by Lack of a Plan Check

One event resulted from a software error. Such a failure rarely happens but can never be ruled impossible. Part of the goal of a QA program is to protect from the many unlikely and unexpected failures.

In this case, the event report notes that no QA was performed on the plan but it does not tell whether it was omitted from this case or if the facility had no procedure for performing any type of QA. Obviously, remedial actions at the facility would differ depending on which of those situations existed. Either way, this event resulted from a system failure, either not having procedures to check plans or not having barriers in the procedure that would prevent treatment of a patient without the QA of the plan. Examples of plan QA procedures come later in this chapter. Methods to prevent treatment of a patient without the execution of the plan QA include a pre-treatment time-out (useful of preventing other errors, as will be seen soon) with a checklist that includes a check for satisfactory completion of the plan QA.

The time-out solution for preventing treatment without QA of the plan may work effectively or it may just move the failure downstream where the person leading the time-out may not perform their duty, particularly probable if it would be the same person who did not perform the plan QA in the first place. This is one reason it is good to have different individuals responsible for QA than those who perform the planning and treatment. If omitting any of the QA steps occurs in a facility, it indicates a cultural problem where priorities may be more on moving patients through the treatments than on the concern for the quality and safety of those treatments.

Reinforcement of such a practice comes from repeated treatments that present no problems, creating the confidence that problems do not happen. Problems are unusual and likely almost all treatments would proceed through completion without anything unusual happening. This complacency often leads to the omission of QA steps when problems with a patient lead to running behind schedule and pressures from the treatment team to hurry. However, these are exactly the patients for whom the QA becomes very important since the delays may result from something unusual, difficult or problematic with the patient, all of which increase the probability of errors in the case; the QA may protect from those errors affecting the patient. Changes in culture require strong support from upper management to placing safety before productivity.[1] The radiation oncologist, being responsible for the patient's care, plays a major role in establishing the culture at a facility.

4.1.1.3 Wrong Patient's Plan

On two occasions, a patient was treated with a different patient's plan. Such events happen not infrequently and certainly are an embarrassment. In a department with more than one patient under treatment, particularly when using balloon catheters with little obvious difference between plans, such errors become hard to notice incidentally. Usually, there are good reasons why a particular plan is up on the treatment computer, for example, to check a plan. Sometimes a schedule change also plays into the event. Regardless of how the situation presents, the usual QA measure involves the time-out procedure, just as in the last section. The time-out would check the identity of the patient and the name associated with the plan ready for treatment in the treatment unit's computer.

4.1.1.4 Incorrect Distance, Length or Location

By far, sending the source to the wrong initial location is the most common error affecting HDR treatments. There are many ways this error occurs. One of the more common error pathways comes in measuring the distance to the end of a catheter, either interstitial or intracavitary. Such a measurement establishes the position of the first dwell position, whether actually used or not, and as such where the dose distribution will fall. One manufacturer provides a device to make measurement of the distance to the end of the catheter by attaching the device to the transfer tube with the catheter on the other end and sliding a wire out of the device to travel to the end of the catheter. Figure 4.1a shows the device. The tip of the cable has a simulated source capsule (Fig. 4.1b), and the capsule and the cable duplicate the source traveling along its intended path. The other end of the cable connects to an indicator that slides along a scale, directly reading the distance of the simulated source (Fig. 4.1c). When using this device, several events resulted when the tip of the cable

[1] Attention paid to quality usually results in increases in productivity in the long run.

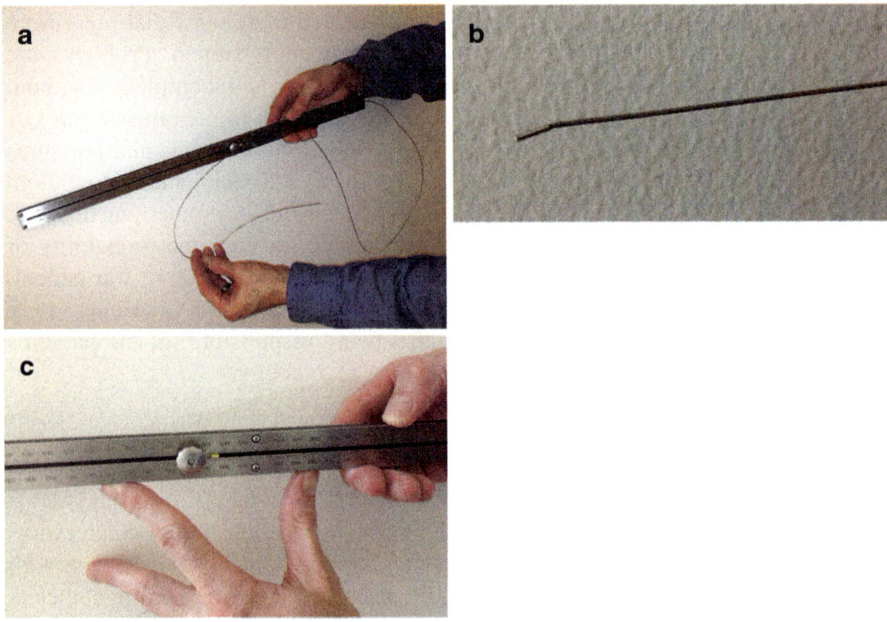

Fig. 4.1 (**a**) A device for measuring the distance to the end of a catheter or needle. (**b**) The simulated source capsule at the end of the cable that goes into the catheter. (**c**) The scale with the indication of the farthest possible first dwell position

got caught on the connection between the transfer tube and the catheter, giving a falsely short reading for the distance to the end of the catheter. These events follow a bending of the simulated source at the end of the cable, causing it to catch on junctions between the transfer tube and the catheter. When this erroneous value is used in the treatment program, the dose distribution shifts by the amount of the error in the direction of the treatment unit. Knowing an expected length for an applicator type would intercept these errors. Generally, the length to the end of applicator falls within a narrow range. Finding a measurement outside of the range would trigger an investigation *if* part of the treatment plan check includes comparison of the treatment distance to a known range. This type of comparison does not work for catheters that are cut to arbitrary lengths for patient comfort, and the facility needs to develop some different method of checking lengths.

Another way to treat the wrong location through incorrect lengths is using a different length transfer tube during treatment than assumed in the planning. This has happened with breast treatments and other anatomical sites as well. The switch of tubes usually is caught if erroneously short tubes are used for treatment because the check cable likely would run into the end of the catheter or applicator before reaching its intended distance, preventing initiation of treatment. However, if longer tubes are used, the check cable would not detect a problem and treatment would proceed with the dose distribution shifted by the difference in transfer-tube length in the direction of the treatment unit. Intercepting this type of error would require including the transfer-tube type in a time-out checklist. Because this is not an unusual failure type, such a check becomes important if it is possible at a facility. If a facility could manage, eliminating the use of transfer-tube types with different lengths would be a better solution and thus eliminate the possibility of an accidental switch. Another check that could detect many length errors would be performing pretreatment imaging with the check cable as shown in Fig. 4.2. Failure to visualize the tip of the check cable going to approximately the desired first position indicates a problem and gives a chance to correct the problem before treating the patient.

A related event occurred when a physicist responsible for connecting the transfer tubes to the applicator missed connecting a tube. During the treatment, the source apparently came out the transfer tube but had no pathway after that and irradiated the patient outside the treatment target. Usually, the transfer tubes have mechanisms to prevent the source from passing the tip unless a catheter or applicator is attached. These safety mechanisms wear out over time and are supposed to be checked periodically with replacement at their expiration date. Aside from including preventive maintenance for all the brachytherapy equipment and checking the operation as part of the ongoing QA program, some check of the patient setup, and device connection needs to be part of the pretreatment verifications. Such checks would include not only that the attachments have been made and secured but also that the transfer tubes properly connect the holes in the treatment unit indexer with the right catheters and the orientation of multi-lumen applicators duplicates that during the dosimetric imaging.

During treatment plan generation, the planner needs to enter a step size, that is, the distance between dwell positions. The dose distribution is tied to this value. Usually, when the treatment-planning computer sends the plan to the treatment-unit computer, the step size is part of the data. However, if some problem prevents the automatic transfer of the plan's delivery data, the personnel at the facility may have to enter the treatment parameters by hand. The data entry is tedious and prone to errors. Of particular concern would be if the unit has a default value for the step size but the plan used a different value. Often, the QA at the treatment unit includes a check of the treatment times and sometimes the distance for the first dwell position.

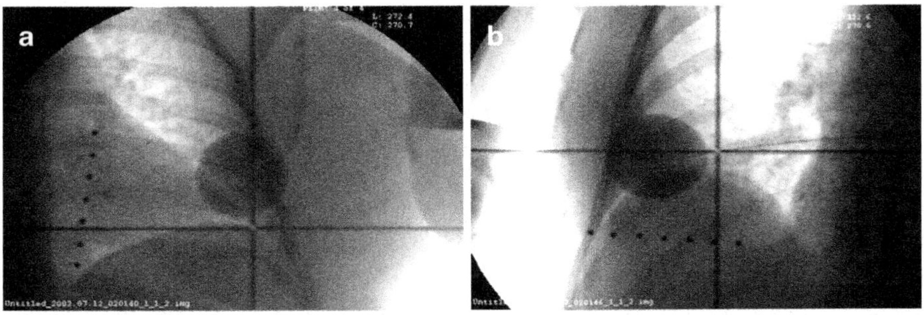

Fig. 4.2 Fluoroscopic images taken before treatment to verify the size of the balloon and the centering of the source position

The step size sometimes is not a parameter checked. An unnoticed difference in the step size not only distributes the dose along an applicator differently than intended but produces a different dose: closer dwell positions yield a higher dose over a shorter length and larger steps produce a lower dose over a longer swath of the applicator. While including the check of the step size in the final treatment-parameter QA should catch an error, no QA is perfect. If transfer of treatment data becomes a recurring problem, the causes for this failure need to be determined and eliminated since it forms a hazardous condition that could lead to many possible errors.

4.1.1.5 Treatment Planning Errors

Several events resulted from reconstruction of the applicator source tracks, in these cases, digitizing, backward. A common approach to reconstruct the source paths, and by inference, the dwell positions, allows localizing on images the first dwell position and the catheter path. Sometimes the first dwell position falls in a region containing several radiopaque objects, such as other catheter tips and a metallic nose cone that holds the catheters. Localizing the first dwell position in the image can be challenging. On the other hand, the catheters on the opposite end of the applicator may be easier to separate. A treatment planning system may allow reconstruction in either direction, tip to end or end to tip, but the planner has to indicate the direction. Usually, there is a default direction (and usually it is tip to end) unless otherwise stated. Since establishing the identity of a catheter and distinguishing it from others is sometimes easier end to tip, this may be the preferred direction in some cases. Two of the events result from the planning doing just that, reconstructing end to tip, but without changing the default, so the planning system thought the applicator faced the opposite direction. Thus, the dose distribution was backward from the intended. Were the applicator is symmetric, such as the single-lumen MammoSite (Hologic, Bedford MA), the error would have no effect on the patient, but with multicatheter applicators with differential loading to steer the dose distribution away from sensitive structures, the result may be to increase the dose where a decrease is desired or vice versa. This can be a very difficult error to detect. Treatment planning systems generally do indicate the direction of digitization, either with an arrow at the tip end of the reconstructed catheter or a number flag at the end. Unless one performing the QA on the plan explicitly looks for these subtle indicators as part of the QA check list, they are likely to be missed. Given that it is an easy error to commit and not normally detected, it is probable that the frequency of occurrence is much higher than that reported. To combat this error, an explicit check should be part of the pretreatment plan check.

Another planning error involved an incorrect target. The target in breast brachytherapy consists of the lumpectomy cavity and the margin. Sometimes the cavity has healed to the extent that it is difficult to determine and the CTV may be based on a few clips and a guess from the original mammogram. Other times, the cavity is difficult to find on the localization CT. Once drawn by the physician, if the target was difficult to delineate, it becomes unlikely that any but a very experienced physicist or dosimetrist would question the contour, making detection of an error in target contouring very unlikely. The most likely detection for such an error is peer review by another physician experienced in breast brachytherapy. At a facility with only one radiation oncologist experienced in the procedure, an arrangement with a colleague at another facility with the required expertise allows sending the images of the contoured targets for review.

One error in treatment planning involved specification of the wrong dose to the target. This is not a very likely error given that most facilities use only one dose protocol. Checking the dose in the treatment plan against the dose in the prescription and the dose in the protocol should spot an error of this type.

Breast brachytherapy is subject to several treatment planning errors common to all HDR treatments, and while this section was to exclude such common errors, because two commissioning errors have affected breast brachytherapy patients, they are mentioned here. Both involve source strength units. The first error type is entering the source strength into the treatment planning computer or the treatment unit computer with the wrong units, for example, Ci instead of U. The other is assigning the calibration factor for the well chamber used to assay the HDR source the wrong units. Events of this nature can affect a large number of patients and have devastating consequences. Because both errors result in the wrong source strength in at least one computer, a second, independent person who could work through the same calculations and evaluate the values for the source strength in all computers should check commissioning of a new source.

4.1.1.6 Applicator Failures

All applicators may be subject to failure, sometimes due to variations in manufacturing and other times due to inappropriate handling. In the period covered by this review, there were two event reports resulting from applicator failure.

One applicator failure was a balloon-based catheter that had a leak, resulting in the loss of the inflating saline which then resulted in extremely high doses to the breast tissues that should have been much farther from the source during treatment. Usually at this facility, the inflation of the applicator is checked using CT. For the seventh fraction of ten, the CT was not available and the applicator was checked for its inflated size using ultrasound shortly before treatment and the users noticed no problem. The staff did notice drainage around the applicator insertion site. Before the next fraction, a CT was again performed showing the applicator was deflated. The patient likely received about twice the intended dose at the seventh fraction. On the study of the applicator, the vendor determined that the balloon had been ruptured from the outside. No one could think of a reason for such an occurrence. The facility had no explanation for the staff misinterpreting the ultrasound image, if indeed they did. The balloon may have been at nearly its full inflation at the time of the seventh fraction and deflated afterward. Alternatively, the staff may have misinterpreted the ultrasound image, since such images are less distinct than the CT images they were used to seeing, and many seldom-used ultrasound units fail to have imaging QA performed regularly, which might exacerbate the potential problem. The staff seemed to have performed appropriately at each step. One might question not investigating further the drainage observed, but drainage is not unusual and they did just verify the inflation of the balloon immediately before noticing the drainage. This case illustrates a fundamental principle of quality and safety: failures will happen despite all the efforts made to prevent them.

The other applicator-base event involved a SAVI device. In this case, the source cable passed through the side of the catheter leading to the applicator and the source slid along the patient's skin during the treatment time for that catheter. There had been a kink in the end of one of the applicator's catheters near where it would connect with the transfer tube that resulted from improper connection techniques between the catheter and the transfer tube during previous fractions. The kink split and the staff at the facility made a repair using tape. During the treatment, the tape gave way and the source then left the catheter. After the kink, the facility was in a difficult situation. Removing the applicator and replacing it would add to the discomfort of the patient, take a considerable time for new localization imaging and dosimetry, and might result in missing a fraction that day leading to an additional weekend with the applicator in place. Given the possible consequences, fixing the catheter would sound worth a try. An event probably did not seem a likely outcome.

The SAVI event illustrates a generalization common in accident analysis: once out of the normal procedure, the situation often continues to move farther from normal, and bringing things back to normal keeps getting more difficult. The safe path may be clear but seems onerous and with undesirable aspects, while expedients appear to hold the promise of an easy, seductive resolution. Most of us have been there, and physicists often see their role as improvising in the difficult situations. Without considering the merits of the attempted fix, once a decision was made to continue with the same applicator, some method of monitoring the adequacy of the fix would be called for, such as surveillance of the site of the repair with the video monitor during treatment. Whatever monitoring method would be used would have to allow immediate termination of the treatment in case of a problem. Perhaps the staff felt that the check-cable run would detect a problem. It is difficult to analyze this event without hindsight bias that is looking at the outcome and thinking "What they should have done…" knowing that the solution would have prevented the event. We should all keep in mind that when we venture out from the normal procedures, we need to do so slowly, thinking about what could go wrong, and set up mitigation strategies to intercept a precipitation event as soon as possible. In this case, additional QA would not be warranted because there was nothing to detect that was not seen.

4.1.1.7 Learning from Events

When establishing a QM program, one step is establishing what could go wrong and assessing the risk. Little data exists for evaluating risk. Hopefully with the establishing of national radiotherapy event databases, data will accrue on probabilities of various types of failures. The events that have occurred give some glimpses into untoward possibilities, but the frequency of events is so low that any conclusion on relative hazards is severely skewed by the randomness of the events. That being said, the one lesson that transcends the details of the particular events is that QA on the treatment unit, the treatment plan and the treatment parameters stands as an effective barrier to events if they have been established based on risk. The report of Task Group 100 of the American Association of Physicists in Medicine provides detailed guidance for establishing a comprehensive quality management program [2].

4.1.2 Quality Assurance during Localization and Reconstruction

The discussion of localization and treatment planning in this chapter assumes the use of CT or MR imaging. Two-dimensional, radiographic imaging fails to delineate either the target or normal structures such as the skin or lungs. Larger volumes of the patient must be treated to give reasonable assurance of covering the target, and yet such coverage is not assured. This becomes especially true for intracavitary treatments, where radiographic images fail to identify situations that can cause injury to the patient.

As noted in the discussion of events in Section 4.1.1, great attention needs to focus on the direction of reconstructing the catheters. The length to the first dwell position sets all subsequent positions and must be correct for correct positioning of the dose distribution. On applicators where the transfer tubes connect directly to the catheters, and the catheters may be cut to arbitrary lengths, the distance to the end of the catheter must be measured. This can be measured by inserting a wire down the transfer tube with the catheter connected and measuring the length on the wire. However, in doing so one must know the offset from the end of the transfer tube to the zero point of the afterloader, as well as the distance from the tip of the source cable to the center of the activity and any margin required beyond the end position of the source cable to accommodate extra travel on the part of the check cable on some units. A better alternative is to use a tool such as that shown in Fig. 4.1. Alternatively, the Varian VariSource (Varian Medical Systems, Inc, Palo Alto CA) has an "end-seek" function that automatically finds the distance to the end of the catheter. Both units with "end-seek" functions and that use manual tools such as in Fig. 4.1 can be confused by kinks or unexpected resistance in the catheter. An approximate knowledge of the expected distance helps prevent misinterpreting readings in such cases, and the use of a check sheet, as shown in Fig. 4.3, helps note errors.

4.1.2.1 Intracavitary

Verification of Length

The length becomes a much more critical parameter for intracavitary treatments than with interstitial treatments. With interstitial treatments, one catheter with an erroneous length alters the dose distribution locally around that catheter but usually

Channel	Tip
1	
2	
3	
4	
5	
6	
7	
8	

Normal values for lengths:
1256–1261 mm

Fig. 4.3 Part of a quality assurance check sheet for Contura applications showing blanks for the entry of the length of each catheters and the expected range under the table

does not make a large difference in the overall dose distribution. With an intracavitary treatment, particularly one that uses a single dwell position, any shift in the position of the source causes an equal shift in the dose distribution. Even with multiple-lumen applicators, the number of catheters is so small that any catheter with a length error significantly alters the dose distribution, while an error in all lengths shifts the whole dose distribution. A 1-mm loss in diameter for a 4-cm balloon produces a 10 % variation in dose at the surface. A 1-mm misplacement in the length of a dwell position in a 4-cm diameter balloon also produces a 10 % variation in dose at the surface. Thus, verification of the length to send the source becomes of paramount importance, and the use of a special localization marker that indicates the location of the first dwell position becomes essential. At the time of treatment, coincidence between the dwell position and the center of the balloon again requires verification as discussed below.

4.1.2.2 Interstitial Implants

Regardless of the position of the patient during implantation, treatment is almost always delivered with the patient supine. Localization requires the patient to assume the same position as during treatment. Alternatively, if the bore of the imaging device (CT or MR) restricts the patient's position, treatment should be in the same position as localization. Whatever the patient's position, the position of the catheters will differ from the nice controlled array that existed during the implantation procedure, but through optimization during the treatment planning, the differences in catheter position seldom make any difference.

Preparing the Catheters for Imaging

Before imaging the patient, the catheters should have markers placed in them. The catheters do show on the images, CT or MR, as dark spots, although it is sometimes difficult to visualize the actual end of the catheter. The uncertainty in the end position is aggravated by the interslice resolution. Special markers for CT that indicate the end position of the source assist in obtaining the correct source positions for treatment planning. The limiting resolution of the slice thickness and interslice separation affects the accuracy of the calculation in all cases. If the catheters run perpendicular to the cuts, the position of the catheter is well defined, but the position of the dwells along the catheter becomes uncertain by half the slice thickness (assuming contiguous slices). If a catheter falls entirely in a slice (i.e., parallel to the axis of the scan), the dwell positions in the catheter can be well located, but the position of the catheter perpendicular to the slice becomes less certain. On MR images, the shadow cast by the catheter cavity or some markers can project beyond the true end of the catheter.

The thickness of the breast changes over the duration of the treatment. Initially, when a template is used, it takes some time after the removal of the template for the breast to relax from the compression and assume a normal shape. The breast also swells during, and for a time following, implantation. Because of these changes, the buttons fixing the catheters in place should not be placed too tightly immediately after the implantation. By the next day, a common time for localization imaging, the breast will have reduced toward its normal size. However, during the course of treatment, the breast usually swells again in response to the radiation, becoming noticeable about the third day of treatment. Thus, at the time of localization, the buttons should not be fastened too tightly either. Buttons that can slide along the catheter could be snugged at the time of localization and the pressure released as the breast swells. Buttons that fix solidly to the catheters must leave room for swelling. The changing contour or the breast during the course of treatment poses problems for correct localization of dwell positions. As the catheters sift in the breast, the distance to the center of the target remains constant to neither the entry nor the exit buttons – be they fixed or adjustable. Complicating the situation further, the target is seldom centered in the breast. Since there is no easy method to adjust for the change in the relative positions of the catheters with respect to the target, the margin in the direction of the catheter direction must include this uncertainty in expanding the clinical target volume to the planning target volume. The overall uncertainty can be approximately 1 cm. For consistency, it is probably best to keep the fixed end of the catheters (distalmost most with respect to the source travel) always against the skin, both during the localization and during treatments.

Catheter Numbering

Catheter identification, of course, becomes important both for input into the treatment planning and during catheter connection. We have already discussed labeling catheters in a previous section. During input into the treatment planning system, it

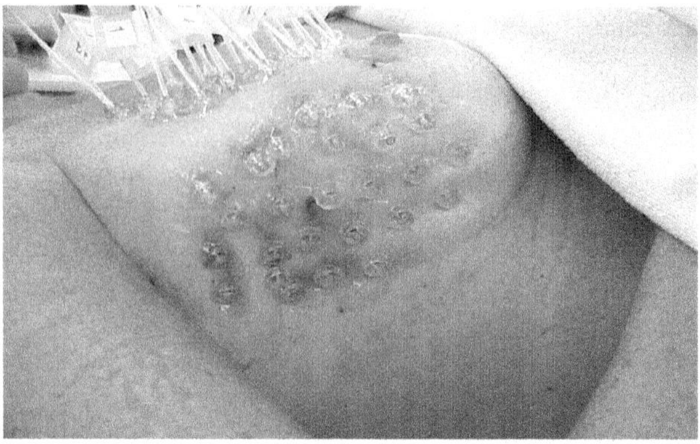

Fig. 4.4 A photograph of the exit side of an implant showing the catheter numbering as found from the entrance side

is useful to have photographs both from the tip end and the connector end. Figure 4.4 shows a photograph of the tip end. One of the easiest and surest ways to establish which exit button corresponds to which entrance catheter number is at the time of insertion of the imaging markers to both watch for the marker to show at the bottom of the catheter (most catheters allow seeing the shadow of the marker in the center of the button) or to feel the marker hit the bottom of the button on insertion. The photograph provides a check to compare against a three-dimensional end-on view to verify that the catheters were correctly identified.

Checking the Length of Catheters or Catheter Inserts

In an interstitial implant with many catheters of different lengths, great care should be taken in the measurement of the length of these catheters along with the transfer tubes. Accurate transfer of this measured length for each catheter to the treatment planning system is very crucial and requires a quality assurance check. Moreover maintaining a record of these lengths and verifying the recorded length with the programmed length before each treatment are essential, since any discrepancy results in a totally different dose distribution to the PTV. A different class of catheter systems has a fixed-length catheter system that uses special inserts attached to the transfer tubes that slide into the catheters (Comfort Catheter™, Elekta Nucletron AB, Stockholm) shown in Fig. 4.5. The inserts have a constant length so the length of the catheters becomes irrelevant. However, that moves the task of verification of the length from checking the catheters to checking the inserts. Performing this check, though, is easier than checking the length of the catheters. For the most part, checking the length of the inserts can simply be comparing the inserts to a standard insert that has been verified previously. Of course, the comparison only has meaning following verification of the length of the standard insert.

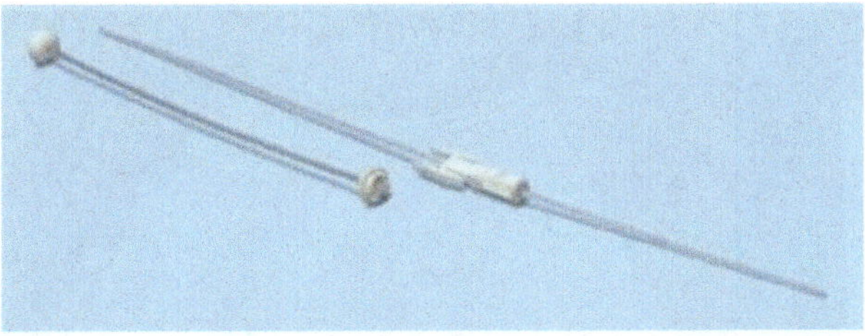

Fig. 4.5 Comfort Catheter™ (Courtesy of Nucletron BV, Veenendaal, Netherlands). The outer catheters form the implant as with conventional catheters, but the source track runs through the inserts that go into the catheters and lock in place. The inserts should all have the same length

Distances to the Skin and Other Structures

The minimum distance from the implant catheters to the skin does not pose the same problem as it does with intracavitary brachytherapy because the dwell positions near the skin usually can simply not be used without major deficits in the dose to the PTV. No particular distance need be kept between the skin and the catheters. The lack of guidance about lung doses, along with the ability to sculpt the dose with interstitial implants, leads to there being no recommendation for distance between catheters and the lung. However, for the heart, as with intracavitary treatments, the dose is dependent on proximity and, although is rarely an issue, should be considered in plan evaluation.

4.1.3 Quality Assurance at the Time of Treatment

For both interstitial and intracavitary treatments, the first step is to assure that the patient assumes the same position on the treatment table as during localization. Variations in position can produce variations in geometry of the catheters and then in the dose distribution.

4.1.3.1 Intracavitary

For intracavitary treatment, all the checks mentioned below for interstitial should be performed along with the following checks:

Volume Check

Before each treatment, an image of the balloon should be acquired to make sure that the volume of the balloon is the same and that the balloon has not collapsed or fluid from the balloon has leaked. Figure 4.2 shows fluoroscopic images of balloon

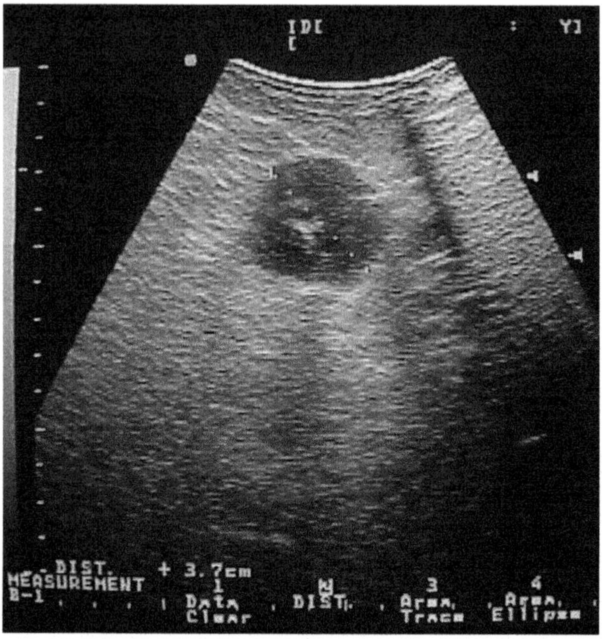

Fig. 4.6 Ultrasound images of a balloon-based catheter to verify the diameter. Such imaging is an alternative to the fluoroscopic approach shown in Fig. 4.2

catheters in two patients. A ruler with small opaque spheres separated by 1 cm is placed at the same level as the center of the balloon, helping to determine the diameter of the balloon. Assuring that the ruler falls at the same distance as the balloon can be difficult, and variations in the focus-to-ruler distance will give incorrect magnification factors for the image of the balloon and possibly mistakes in interpreting the balloon diameter. Figure 4.6 shows an ultrasound image of a Contura (SenoRX, Aliso Viejo, CA). The ultrasound verification takes about 1 min total.

Source Going to Correct Location

Figure 4.5 presented a table in a checklist for a Contura patient to help verify that the measured lengths for the catheters fall within the expected range. When checking the program in the treatment unit, a similar set of checks can be made using a table as in Fig. 4.7. The table has blanks for the measured length and the length in the program for each catheter. Manually writing the two values increases the likelihood of noticing a discrepancy. A check of the source traveling at the center of the balloon should also be confirmed. Figure 4.2 showed the programmed check cable run at the center of the balloon before the radioactive source run. This check would only be needed once, before the whole course of treatment begins.

Channel	Measured Length	Length on Program
1		
2		
3		
4		
5		
6		
7		
8		

Normal values for lengths:
1256–1261 mm

Fig. 4.7 A table used during verification of the treatment program in a treatment unit for a Contura patient. The table has blanks for the measured length and the length in the program for each catheter

4.1.3.2 Interstitial

Program Verification

Data from the treatment planning system to the treatment console station is either transported by LAN or by electronic memory devices. After the data has been transported, before the first treatment, the values in the program for patient name, total treatment time, step sizes or dwell locations, catheter lengths, and dwell times should be checked. For the most part, this check verifies that the correct plan has been imported into the treatment unit, since file corruption usually renders a file unusable rather than changing data in the file. However, checking the program is not unwise. For subsequent fractions, each dwell time need not be checked – only as many as necessary, or the overall time, to assure that the correct program is loaded.

Connection of the Catheters

Correct connection of the catheters, of course, is essential for a correct treatment. Errors in catheter connection can occur either while connecting the transfer tubes to the treatment unit or the connecting the catheters to the transfer tubes. If more than one set of transfer tubes is available for catheter connection (e.g., for different lengths to the first dwell position), selection of the correct set of tubes should be part of the verification procedures. Many errors in connecting the transfer tubes to the treatment unit tend to be protected by design, for example, skipping a hole when inserting the tubes into the indexer. Such a mistake would cause the unit to pause during treatment until the tubes were moved to fill the empty location. Mixing the tubes is not protected: any tube may go in any hole. However, any error in the order must actually be *two* errors, for example, inserting tube #12 in hole #2 would leave hole #12 without a corresponding tube unless tube #2 were placed there, making the error less likely.

Mistakes in connecting the transfer tubes to the catheters are more likely, particularly when more catheters are treated than transfer tubes (i.e., holes in the indexer). In such cases, the catheters from 1 through the highest number on the indexer are treated in a first set. Then, after disconnecting these catheters, the next numbers in line are connected. This process repeats until all the catheters are treated. With cases requiring multiple sets of connections, mistakes connecting catheters from different sets become a hazard. For example, while connecting the first set, catheter #32 could mistakenly be connected to hole #2 (or #3, depending on what the person connecting sees).

After connecting the catheters to the transfer tubes but before initiating treatment, the catheters must be moved so that the buttons on the exit side of the patient abut the skin, as they were for the localization imaging. Section 4.1.3.2.1 discussed this issue more completely.

Early in a breast brachytherapy program, a facility may wish to perform a patency check on all the catheters before starting the treatment, to assure that the treatment does not get stuck because of a catheter with a kink. However, as experience grows, confidence in the procedure probably will lead to skipping this step. In our experience, there has never been a catheter that the check cable detected as being kinked or blocked. (Frequently, the check cable detects connections that are not secured, but these are easily corrected.) Even without checking all the catheters before initiating treatment, the unit still checks each catheter immediately before sending the source.

4.1.4 Posttreatment Verification

Immediately after the end of treatment, the operator must check the patient with a radiation detector to verify complete retraction of the source. A source or part of a source remaining in the patient after treatment would deliver enough dose locally in 1 min to cause injury to the tissues. After the end of each treatment, the report of the treatment should be verified, including the length of each channel, the total irradiation time, and the individual dwell time.

4.2 Quality Management for External-Beam Patient Breast Irradiation

While whole breast irradiation has been practiced successfully (for the most part) for decades, with localization and positioning having become routine, for partial breast irradiation, the tolerances for positioning become greatly tightened (see Chap. 6). Unlike the brachytherapy approaches, where the applicator forces the dose distribution to conform to the target, for external-beam treatments, matching the dose to the target becomes a critical challenge. Thus, quality control for such treatments forms an indispensable link in the treatment chain.

4.2.1 Quality Control During Patient Positioning

4.2.1.1 Immobilization and Stability

Traditionally, the lasers in the treatment room have been the most important tool in the localization of the whole breast, while many radiation centers use breast boards for immobilization and stability. In partial breast irradiation, the planning target volume (PTV) is generated by the expansion of the clinical target volume (CTV) with a margin that includes the patient positioning error. Since setting up with lasers is not highly accurate, particularly for non-ridged parts of the body such as breasts, daily patient positioning error increases, thereby increasing the needed margin to expand the CTV to PTV (see Chap. 6). This leads to larger PTV, which ultimately defeats the aim of partial breast treatment. Breast boards do not reposition the patient as well as molds that support much of the upper and mid body. Imaging on the linear accelerator should be part of the repositioning, but requires some demarcation of the target, such as surgical clips.

4.2.1.2 Clearance

Clearance becomes a problem with external-beam breast patients at two steps. The first problem with clearance falls at the CT unit during imaging for treatment planning. When using a breast board, such as shown in Fig. 4.8, frequently the patient will not fit into the bore of the unit in the desired treatment position. Failure to have the correct position during this imaging results in poor conformance of the treatment plan to the execution. In mitigating the problem of positioning the patient on a breast board in the conventional treatment position (with the board raised), modern treatment planning usually allows good treatment plans with the patient completely supine. Problems with patient clearance at the CT become obvious during the imaging session and only propagate to degrade the treatment quality if the problems are ignored.

Clearance becomes an issue again when setting the fields developed during the planning phase. Particularly with multi-field conformal or IMRT plans, beam orientations that produce desirable dose distributions in the computer fall at combinations of angles that pose problems. Three common problems are as follows: (1) The beam passing through parts of the couch before the patient, attenuating the beam in unplanned (and often unknowable) ways. (2) The beam passing undesirably through part of the patient in the way to the target, for example, through or too near the contralateral breast, shoulder, or chin. (3) The beam exiting through an organ at risk,

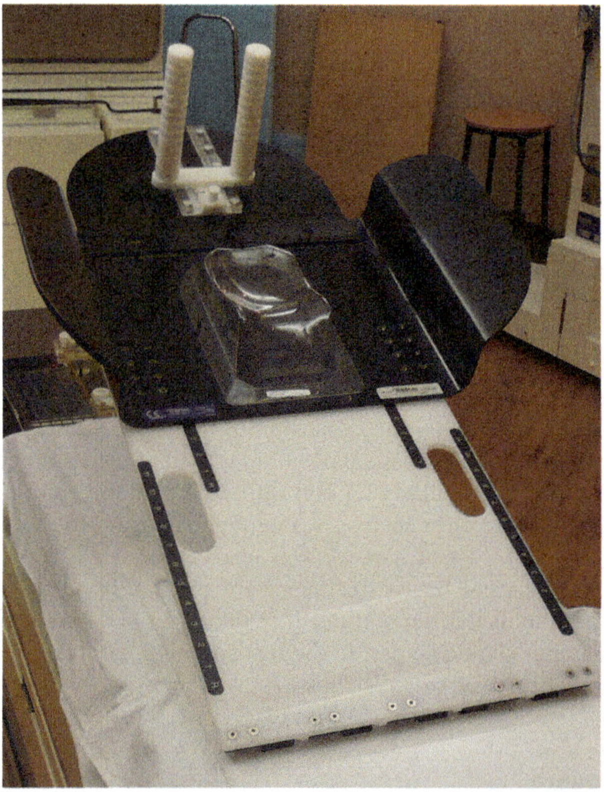

Fig. 4.8 A "breast board" used for positioning a breast patient for external-beam treatments

possibly outside of the CT image sets. Such problems usually only occur with novel beam orientations.

Clearance could be a problem with wedges or physical blocks, but with the common use of multileaf collimators and dynamic, or universal, wedges, those problems have become rare.

4.2.2 Quality Control During Treatment Planning

Regardless of the treatment approach, either three-dimensional conformal or intensity modulated, the quality assurance for the treatment plan remains the same:

1. Determine if the plan adequately satisfies the treatment objectives.
2. Test the plan for quality and errors.

Chapter 6 discusses the differences in treatment planning for the two modalities. The discussion here will assume that there is a conventional quality assurance program for external-beam treatment plans, as well as one for IMRT.

4.2.2.1 Evaluating Adequacy of the Plan

Most often, evaluation of external-beam treatment plans uses that parameters ${}_{PTV}V_{100\,\%}$, ${}_{PTV}V_{95\,\%}$ and ${}_{PTV}D_{95\,\%}$, and the corresponding quantities for normal-tissue structures, just as with brachytherapy. These quantities actually serve more for determining the treatment, particularly during the optimization for IMRT, then evaluating the plan. The first check considers if the treatment plan satisfies the requirements for the target volume. As discussed in Chap. 6, external-beam treatments require greater margins for expansion of the CTV to form the PTV than do brachytherapy plans; however, the desired dose distribution still has to cover the PTV to the extent specified by the "V" and "D" quantities in the prescription.

The second part of the evaluation entails avoiding excessive dose to the neighboring organs at risk, in the case of partial breast irradiation, the lung, heart and skin. The American Society for Radiology and Oncology published recommended specifications for external-beam breast treatments (see Table 4.2) [6].

4.2.2.2 Testing a Plan for Quality and Errors

Again, this chapter assumes that a facility has a quality management program for the treatment planning system and the treatment planning process, so only those aspects particularly of interest for partial breast irradiation will be addressed. The evaluation in the previous section simply asked if the plan did what was requested. Of the many possible plans for a given patient's treatment, some adequate plans may be markedly better than others in various respects, since most treatment planning involves compromises. Many evaluation quantities have been proposed for external-beam treatments but as of the time of writing, none have a strong body of support for their utility [1, 3]. An external-beam plan will have much greater dose uniformity than a brachytherapy plan, simply because it contains no radioactive sources where the dose approaches infinity. However, particularly for IMRT, the target dose uniformity may suffer greatly as the optimization program attempts to create a dose distribution that covers the entire periphery and avoids the organs at risk.

Table 4.2 Treatment planning targets for external-beam breast treatments recommended by the American Society for Radiation Oncology [7]

Target	Values
PTV coverage	${}_{PTV}V_{90\,\%} \geq 90\,\%$, ${}_{PTV}D_{max} \leq 120\,\%$
Lung doses	$V_{30\,\%} < 15\,\%$ for ipsilateral $V_{5\,\%} < 15\,\%$ for contralateral
Heart doses	$V_{5\,\%} < 5\,\%$ for right-sided treatments $V_{5\,\%} < 40\,\%$ for left-sided treatments
Thyroid doses	$D_{max} \leq 3\,\%$
Breast doses	$V_{\geq 50\,\%} \leq 60\,\%$ for ipsilateral $D_{max} \leq 3\,\%$ for contralateral

Using the indices can detect some errors in the treatment plan, but not those related to plans calling for performance that the treatment unit cannot provide. Examples of such problems include IMRT static (step-and-shoot) plans with segments exposed for too few monitor units to establish stable dose rate or dynamic (sliding window) plans that call for incompatible combinations of multileaf collimator blade movement or machine output. Establishing the performance limitations of an accelerator forms an important part of the commissioning. In the beginning of an IMRT program, or when beginning to use a new treatment unit for IMRT, testing the achievement of the planned fluence map provides assurance that planned treatments can be delivered. After validating the planning and delivery process, continued measurement of fluence maps serves little function.

4.2.3 Quality Management at the Time of Treatment

At the time of the setup of the patient for daily treatment, the in-room lasers can be used for initial alignment; however, once that is achieved, cone beam computed tomography (CBCT) should be used to align the patient with the treatment planning CT images. In the absence of CBCT, port films should be taken to confirm the alignment of the patient before the initiation of the treatment.

4.3 Regulations

The Nuclear Regulatory Commission (NRC) is a United States (US) government agency that oversees the civilian use of radioactive material. The NRC's mission is to regulate the US civilian use of by-product, source, and special nuclear materials to ensure adequate protection of public health and safety. The NRC oversees medical uses of nuclear material (by-product of reactors) through licensing, inspection, and enforcement programs. The NRC issues medical use licenses to medical facilities, authorizes physician and physicist users, develops guidance and regulations for use by licensees, and maintains a committee of medical experts to obtain advice about the use of by-product materials in medicine. The Advisory Committee on the Medical Uses of Isotopes, comprised of physicians, medical scientists, and other healthcare professionals, provides advice to the NRC staff on current initiatives in the medical uses of radioactive materials. The NRC (or the responsible agreement state[2]) also regulates the manufacture and distribution of these products. It also oversees the QA and quality management program of the institution using this product material for medical use. An often-discussed topic in the fractionated treatment

[2] Agreement states are those states that have entered into an agreement with the NRC to regulate by-product material in the stead of the NRC. The agreements stipulate that in most ways the state regulations conform to those of the NRC.

of breast with HDR RAL is the physical presence of personnel during the treatment. The regulations in title 10 of the Code of Federal Regulations, Part 35 paragraph 615, item (f) (2) (10 CFR 35.615(f) (2)) states that "for [HDR] units, require an [AU] and an [AMP] to be physically present during the initiation of all patient treatments involving the unit; and an [AMP] and either an [AU] or a physician, under the supervision of an [AU], who has been trained in the operation and emergency response for the unit, to be physically present during continuation of all patient treatments involving the unit" [4]. Details of the term "physically present" are clarified in details in the information notice 2012–08: High Dose-Rate Remote Afterloader (HDR) Physical Presence Requirements [5].

References

1. Feuvret L, Noel G, Mazeron JJ, Bey P. Conformity index: a review. Int J Radiat Oncol Biol Phys. 2006;64(2):333–42.
2. Huq S, Fraass BA, Dunscombe PB, Gibbons JP, Ibbott GS, Mundt AJ, Mutic S, Palta JR, Rath F, Thomadsen B, Williamson JF, Yorke ED. The report of Task Group 100 of the American Association of Physicists in Medicine: application of risk analysis methods to radiation therapy quality management. Med Phys. 2015. In press.
3. Kataria T, Sharma K, Subramani V, Karrthick KP, Bisht SS. Homogeneity index: an objective tool for assessment of conformal radiation treatments. J Med Phys. 2012;37(4):207–13.
4. NRCa, U.S. Nuclear Regulatory Commission. Code of Federal Regulations Title 10 Part 35.615 Safety precautions for remote afterloader units, teletherapy units, and gamma stereotactic radiosurgery units. Available at http://www.nrc.gov/reading-rm/doc-collections/cfr/part035/part035-0615.html
5. NRCb, U.S. Nuclear Regulatory Commission. NRC Information Notice 2012–08: High Dose-Rate Remote Afterloader (HDR) physical presence requirements. 2012. Available from http://pbadupws.nrc.gov/docs/ML1132/ML11320A228.pdf.
6. Smith BD, Arthur DW, Buchholz TA, Haffty BG, Hahn CA, Hardenbergh PH, Julian TB, Marks LB, Todor DA, Vicini FA, Whelan TJ, White J, Wo JY, Harris JR. Accelerated partial breast irradiation consensus statement from the American Society for Radiation Oncology (ASTRO). Int J Radiat Oncol Biol Phys. 2009;74(4):987–1001.
7. Shah C, Vicini F, Wazer DE, Arthur D, Patel RR. The American Brachytherapy Society consensus statement for accelerated partial breast irradiation. Brachytherapy. 2013;12 (4):267–77.
8. Thomadsen B. Elements of quality and safety in heath care. San Diego: Cognella Academic Publishing; 2015.
9. Thomadsen B, Dunscombe PB, Ford E, Huq S, Pawlicki T, Sutlief S. Quality and safety in radiotherapy: learning the new approaches in task group 100 and beyond, AAPM Medical Physics monograph no 36. Madison: Medical Physics Publishing; 2013.

Chapter 5
Surgical Considerations in Partial-Breast Irradiation

Peter D. Beitsch

Contents

5.1 Introduction

The relationship between breast surgeons and radiation oncologists has always been a close one since we are truly "kindred spirits." Our mutual goals are local and regional control while optimizing cosmesis without compromising overall cancer treatment. This relationship has grown since 2002 when the FDA cleared the MammoSite radiation therapy system (Hologic) which greatly simplified brachytherapy applicator placement. While previous interstitial brachytherapy required multiple catheter placements, the MammoSite balloon allowed the surgeon to place this single-lumen catheter into the lumpectomy cavity in their office or hospital (usually under ultrasound guidance). This greatly increased the need for communication between the specialties for optimal patient outcome. Discussion of proper

P.D. Beitsch, MD, FACS
Dallas Breast Center, 8140 Walnut Hill Lane Suite 800, Dallas, TX 75231, USA
e-mail: Beitsch@aol.com

D.W. Arthur et al. (eds.), *Short Course Breast Radiotherapy: A Comprehensive Review of Hypofractionation, Partial Breast, and Intra-Operative Irradiation*,
DOI 10.1007/978-3-319-24388-7_5

patient selection, type of device utilized, and timing of placement were all necessary before the device could be placed by the surgeon.

APBI treatments grew rapidly as surgeons developed and refined insertion techniques and radiation oncologists optimized treatment plans. Both specialties worked together to define appropriate use criteria including undertaking a large database – the American Society of Breast Surgeons MammoSite Registry Trial. This registry captured data from 1440 patients (almost 1/3 of all patients treated with balloon brachytherapy between May 2002 and July 2004). Numerous papers/presentations from registry data helped shape patient selection as well as reassure the oncology community of the safety and efficacy of partial-breast irradiation [1–3].

This chapter will focus on the surgical aspects of setting up a successful brachytherapy program.

5.2 Patient Selection

Patient selection guidelines have been suggested by the American Brachytherapy Society (ABS) and the American Society of Breast Surgeons. These are guidelines, and as such, there are patients and situations that fall outside of these guidelines that may be appropriately treated with brachytherapy. For example, a woman with large breasts and a 3.2 cm cancer could be well treated with partial-breast irradiation or a woman who is 44.9 years old with a 2 cm cancer even though she is just below the age "cutoff."

With APBI since only a portion of the breast undergoes radiation treatment, there are other issues that must be considered including multifocal/multicentric breast cancer and risk factors for ipsilateral breast tumor recurrence (IBTR).

Multifocal and multicentric breast cancers have various definitions and are often lumped together in many studies. Typically, multifocal disease is more than one cancer in the same quadrant or within some distance (often 2–3 cm) of the primary tumor, and multicentric disease is defined as more than one cancer in different quadrants of the breast or >3 cm from the primary. All definitions are somewhat arbitrary and depend on tumor location, breast size, ductal anatomy, etc. For this discussion, they will be considered together, and the issue for APBI is the occult (unknown to the physician) nature of a second (or more) cancer in the treating breast.

The incidence of multifocal/multicentric disease ranges from 5 to 70 % in the literature [4, 5] but is generally felt to be less than 20 %. With today's improved imaging, unrecognized multicentric/multifocal disease is much less of an issue – digital mammography, tomosynthesis, ultrasound, positron emission mammography (PEM), and breast MRI have all lead to better assurance that there is only one cancer to be treated. Not all women need advanced imaging (PEM or MRI), if their physical exam and basic imaging are easily interpretable. However, if the breast appears dense on mammogram (BIRADS 3–4 density) and physical exam is difficult due to fibrocystic changes, then consideration of advanced imaging to rule out additional cancers is indicated. All imaging abnormalities must be confirmed with tissue biopsy. The subsequent stress related to these additional potential lesions should not lead straight to mastectomy.

Risk factors for IBTR after standard breast-conserving therapy (BCT) with whole-breast irradiation (WBI) have included age <50, tumor size >5 cm, positive margins, lymphovascular invasion, estrogen receptor negativity, extensive intraductal component (EIC), positive nodes, high Oncotype DX score, and MammaPrint high-risk designation [6–8]. All of these factors are generally considered poor prognostic factors not just for IBTR after BCT but also for systemic recurrence – so-called bad cancers. These "bad cancers" may have higher local/regional recurrence rates after lumpectomy and APBI but also after lumpectomy and WBI or even after mastectomy. The same is true for systemic recurrences compared to less biologically aggressive cancers. Taken together, the risk factors associated with IBTR do raise the recurrence rates but do so after all types of local–regional treatments and therefore are not hard factors mitigating against APBI but are just one of the many variables to consider in an individual patient. Hopefully many of these patient selection criteria will be better defined by the several phase III trials (including NSABP B39) which have included them in their eligibility criteria.

With the above caveats, reasonable selection guidelines for off-protocol treatment have included:

Age ≥45 (or 50).
Histology: Invasive ductal or lobular; DCIS.
Margins: Clear – no ink on tumor.
Tumor size: ≤3 cm.
Biology: Oncotype DX low/intermediate risk or MammaPrint low risk has recently been looked at as potential selection criteria.

Two additional points about systemic therapy (chemotherapy and hormonal therapy) need to be addressed. First, any systemic therapy will lower the local/regional recurrence rate but should not be used to "clean up" poor surgery or inadequate radiation therapy. Second, in general patients who receive neoadjuvant chemotherapy should not receive partial-breast irradiation even though they may have clinical/pathologic complete responses. The breast may contain islands of cancer cells remote from the lumpectomy that were left behind as the tumor "shrank" with chemotherapy, so it is generally considered best to treat the whole breast with radiation. However, there are minimal published data addressing the issue.

5.3 Surgical Technique: Tumor Location

Intracavitary and interstitial brachytherapy techniques are easily accomplished when the lumpectomy cavity is located within the central aspect of the breast, away from the skin and chest wall. Of course breast cancers can occur anywhere within the breast, and the following will address some more difficult locations.

5.3.1 Subareolar Tumors

Tumors located in the subareolar region (Fig. 5.1) can be challenging when attempting to balance clear margins while maintaining a good cosmetic result. Trying to retain the nipple and a symmetrical areola usually results in thin skin flaps, making the use of intracavitary devices problematic. Removal of the nipple areolar complex for lesions abutting the base of the nipple/areola is a perfectly satisfactory approach and yields excellent outcomes [9]. In tumors where the nipple does not need to be removed, the use of radial incisions and removal of the skin overlying the lesion in an elliptical fashion is strongly advised. As opposed to periareolar incisions, radial incisions result in little distortion around the nipple–areola complex (Fig. 5.2). Because the use of intracavitary devices in the subareolar location may be difficult, multicatheter interstitial brachytherapy could be an alternative. This technique can be used in most instances and is an excellent alternative when considering partial-breast irradiation for patients with tumors in this location.

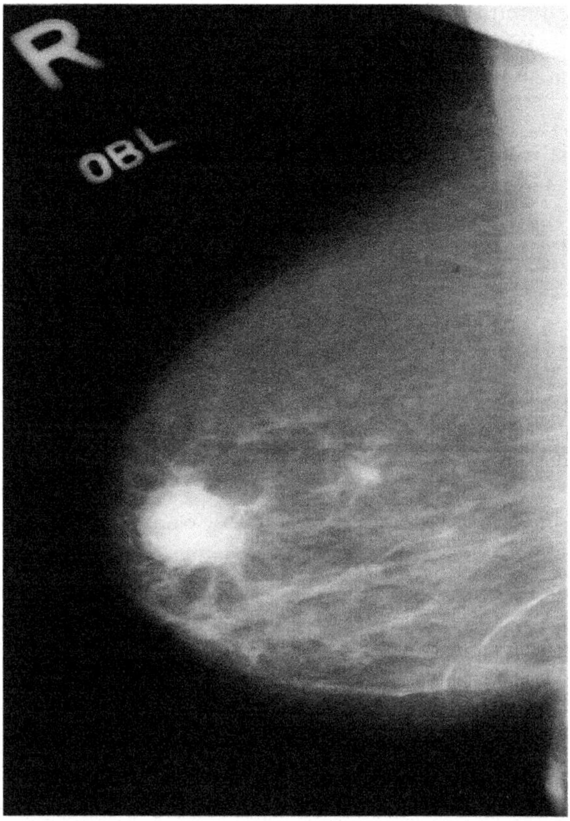

Fig. 5.1 Subareolar cancer

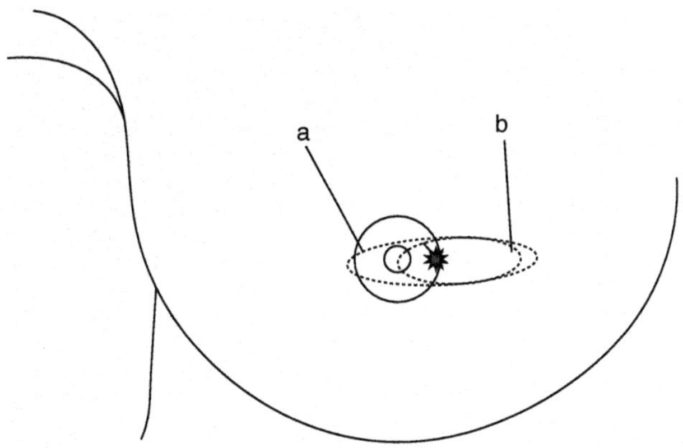

Fig. 5.2 *A* Removing the nipple areolar complex (NAC) or *B* radial incision excising part of the NAC

5.3.2 *Axillary Tail*

Tumors located in the axillary tail present special problems for the use of intracavitary devices. As can be seen in Fig. 5.3, breast fibroglandular tissue is on one side of the tumor, and the loose fibrofatty tissue of the axilla is on the other. Single-lumen balloon devices may deliver undesirable doses of irradiation to the axillary fat pad so multicatheter devices are optimal. Moreover, in patients who have undergone sentinel node biopsy, there will be little tissue left to support the axillary side of the device, and arm movement may also be an issue for devices placed laterally in the axillary tail, as devices may move in response to the pressure asserted by the overlying arm. Therefore, devices could be placed from the medial side stabilizing the device. In general, patients who have lesions located in the axillary tail may be difficult candidates for APBI using intracavitary devices. However, multicatheter interstitial therapy is quite suitable for this location and serves as a good alternative to intracavitary devices.

5.3.3 *Inframammary Fold*

Lumpectomy in this area may require either a radial incision from the NAC or an inframammary fold incision (Fig. 5.4). Either way, a cavity can be created that allows for a brachytherapy device to be placed from the lateral approach.

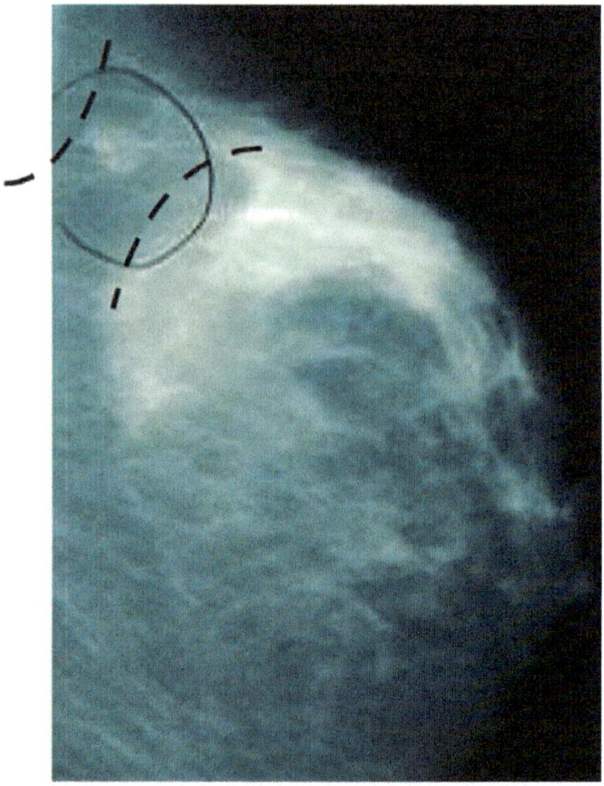

Fig. 5.3 Axillary tail cancer

5.3.4 Peripheral Locations

In the past, patients with tumors in other peripheral sites were not ideal candidates for APBI, except when achieved with interstitial implants. This is due to the smaller amounts of breast tissue in these areas in many women, resulting in thin skin flaps overlying the device. However, a non-balloon-based device has been developed that allows increased dosimetric control – SAVI (strut-adjusted volume implant from Cianna Medical, Inc.) – that has an "eggbeater" configuration with multiple intracavitary catheters, and occasionally even small multilumen balloon devices are able to be used.

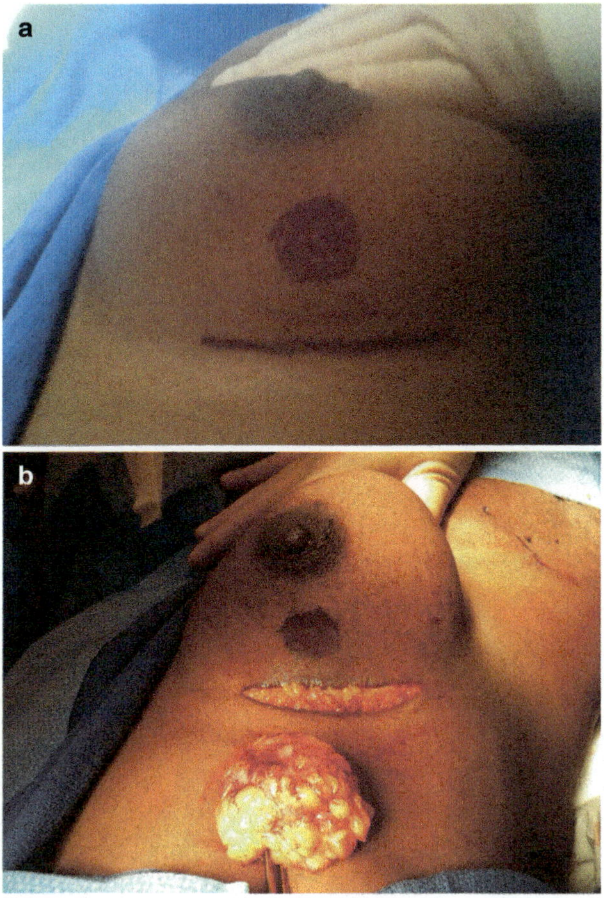

Fig. 5.4 (**a**) Inframammary cancer (*shaded area*) with planned incision. (**b**) Inframammary cancer with completed lumpectomy

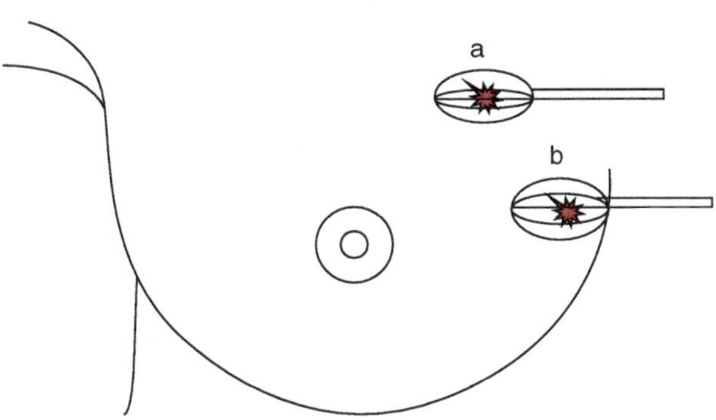

Fig. 5.5 Peripheral cancers (**a**) Superior (**b**) Medial

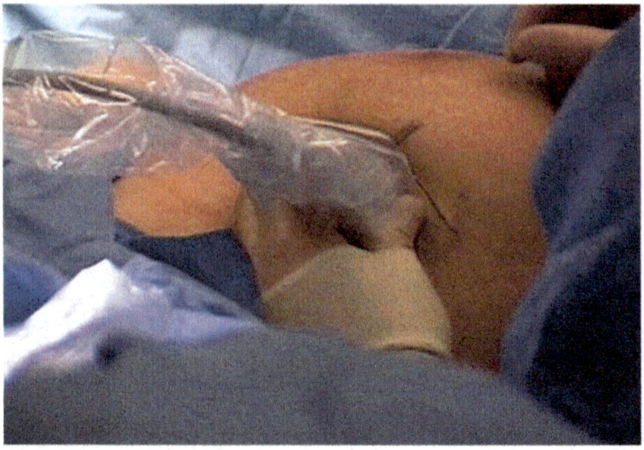

Fig. 5.6 Intraoperative ultrasound guidance

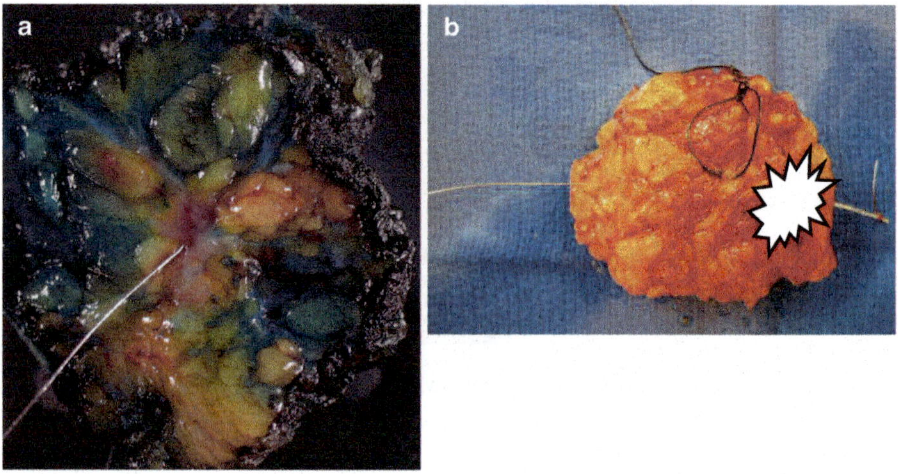

Fig. 5.7 (**a**) Excellent wire-localized lumpectomy. (**b**) Eccentric wire-localized lumpectomy

5.3.5 Surgical Technique: Lumpectomy

The goal of lumpectomy is to excise the cancer with a rim of normal breast tissue surrounding. This is usually best accomplished with ultrasound guidance (Fig. 5.6) even when the cancer is palpable (so the margins and extent of the cancer can be visualized). If the cancer is not palpable or visible on ultrasound, mammographic wire localization is utilized (can be combined with intraoperative ultrasound) with the goal of the cancer being in the middle of the lumpectomy (Fig. 5.7a) and not at the edge (Fig. 5.7b).

Cancers near the skin may require removing an ellipse of skin and subcutaneous tissue overlying the tumor which will allow a good skin/subcutaneous tissue buffer over the brachytherapy device (Fig. 5.8). Multilumen devices allow radiation oncologists to tailor the radiation dose away from the skin, making the device-to-skin distance less critical. However, in almost all circumstances, the device-to-skin distance is an extremely important factor in determining the ultimate cosmetic outcome.

Cavity size can, in many instances, determine whether it is possible for a patient who is otherwise a candidate to undergo APBI. Figure 5.9 shows a hypothetical patient with an infiltrating ductal carcinoma and intraductal extension. If the excision occurs as in "A," then the cavity will indeed be appropriate for an intracavitary device or interstitial catheters. However, if the surgeon elects excision "B," the cavity will be inappropriately large for all available devices and will require an unacceptable number of interstitial catheters for a good outcome. It is not unreasonable to assume that the ultimate cosmetic outcome is a function of cavity size. There is clearly a limit to lumpectomy volume in relation to breast size and shape where

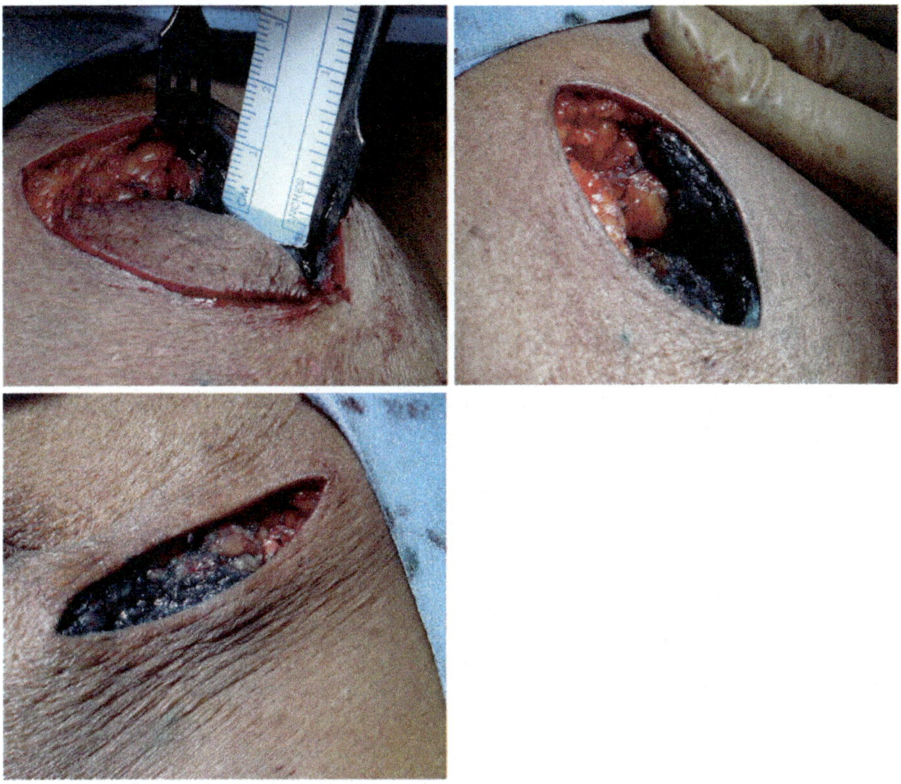

Fig. 5.8 Lumpectomy with excision of overlying skin

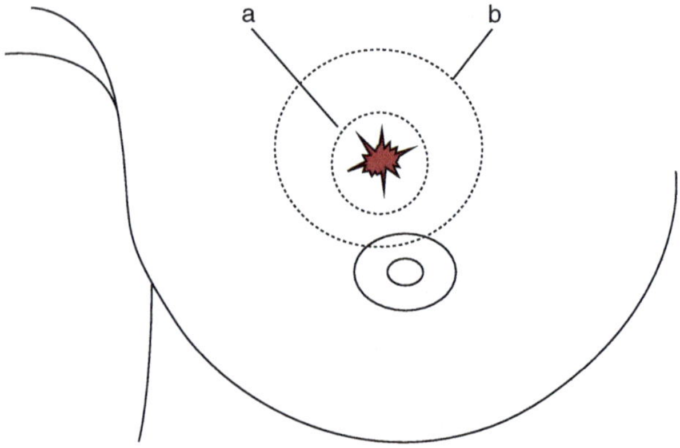

Fig. 5.9 Large lumpectomies may be difficult for intracavitary brachytherapy devices (**a**) Smaller lumpectomy (**b**) Larger lumpectomy

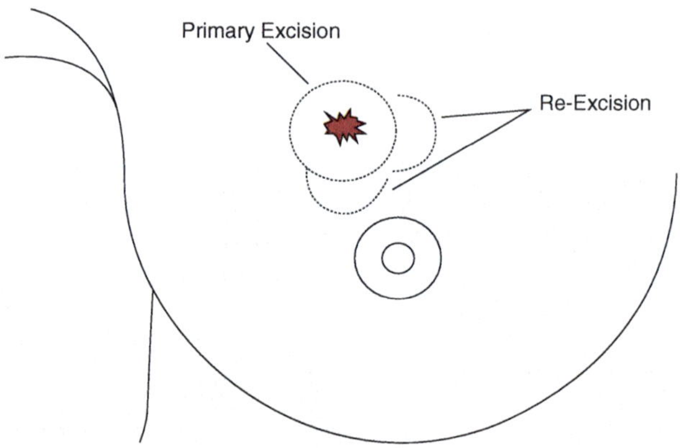

Fig. 5.10 Multiple re-excisions may make conformance of intracavitary devices more difficult

the resultant cosmetic outcome will be poor and breast conservation is therefore an inappropriate choice.

Re-excision of the lumpectomy cavity is often required to ensure that clear surgical margins are obtained. The need for re-excision varies widely, from 10 to 50 % [10, 11], and it is the removal of additional breast tissue that may present a conformance problem for intracavitary APBI devices. Although the increase in cavity size is a problem following re-excision, cavity shape irregularity may also be a challenge. Cavity shape irregularity usually results from the re-excision of one or two margins and not when the entire cavity is re-excised (Fig. 5.10). The re-excised cavity may result in an extremely irregular shape, reducing confidence in the ability to successfully place an intracavitary device. However, these devices can still be utilized in these irregular cavities since the device will expand and shapes the cavity to its own design (Figs. 5.11 and 5.12).

Ellipsoidal lumpectomy cavities commonly result from segmental mastectomies. This approach can be used in any patient with breast cancer but is more commonly encountered when treating patients with DCIS or in patients with an extensive

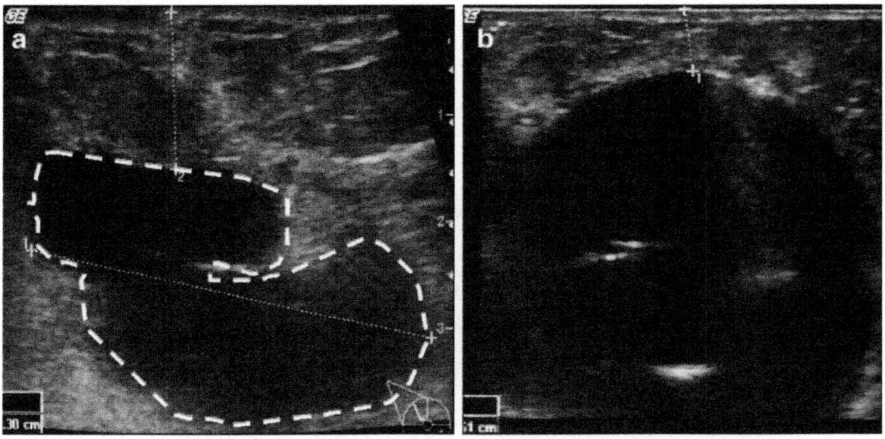

Fig. 5.11 (**a**) Postoperative breast ultrasound showing an irregular seroma cavity following re-excision. (**b**) Radiation balloon device expanded with good conformance in the seroma cavity

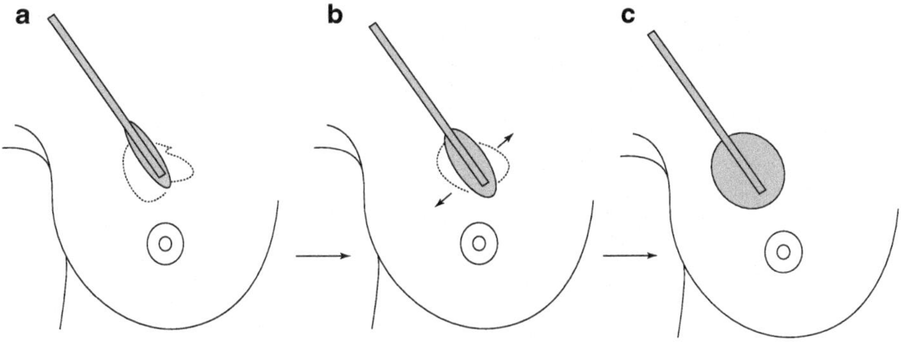

Fig. 5.12 Irregular lumpectomy cavities can in many instances be re-expanded by a balloon device, allowing for good tissue conformance. (**a**) Balloon device inserted, (**b**) partial expansion, and (**c**) complete expansion

intraductal component. Ellipsoidal devices such as SAVI or ellipsoidal balloons are available for cavities of this shape. Multicatheter interstitial therapy is also an option.

5.3.6 Lumpectomy Closure

Simple lumpectomies are usually performed directly over the tumor with relatively uniform flaps around the cancer. Closure of these wounds is straightforward but does require thinking about postoperative brachytherapy device placement at the

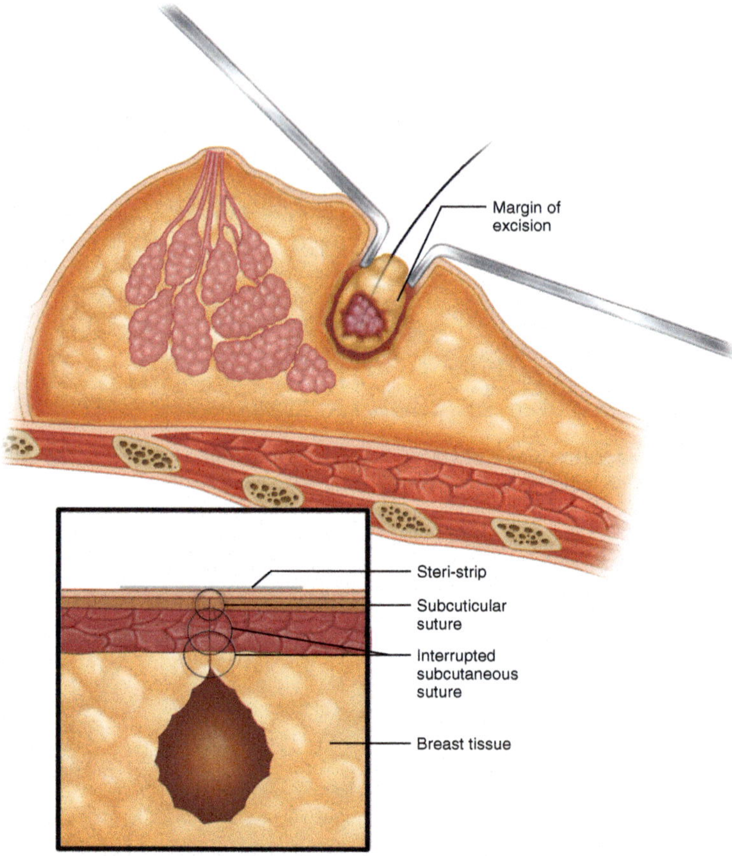

Fig. 5.13 Multilayered closure overlying the lumpectomy cavity

time of the lumpectomy and closure. This does not affect the extirpation of the cancer but may affect whether overlying skin is taken (often a good idea regardless of method of postoperative radiation) and the simple layered closure (Fig. 5.13) above the lumpectomy cavity (oncoplastic closures will be covered in the next section). It is important to remember to leave a cavity into which the device will be placed.

5.3.7 *Surgical Techniques: Oncoplasty*

In an attempt to maintain the natural shape of the breast or to improve a ptotic breast, oncoplastic lumpectomy techniques have become more common [12, 13]. The early adopters of these techniques applied cosmetic plastic surgical principles with

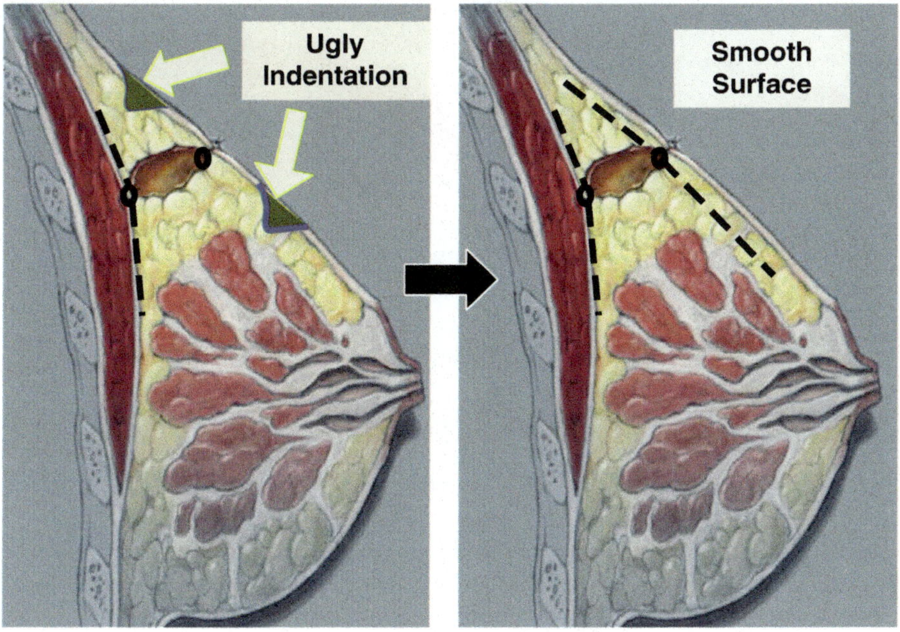

Fig. 5.14 Simple oncoplastic flap dissection to smooth out lumpectomy closure

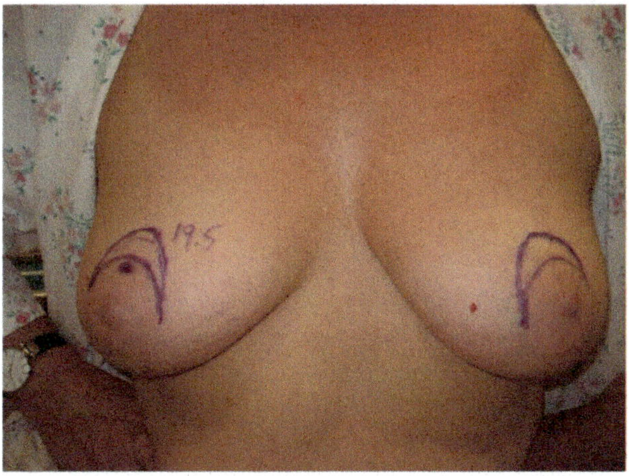

Fig. 5.15 Crescentic lumpectomy on the right with contralateral symmetry mastopexy

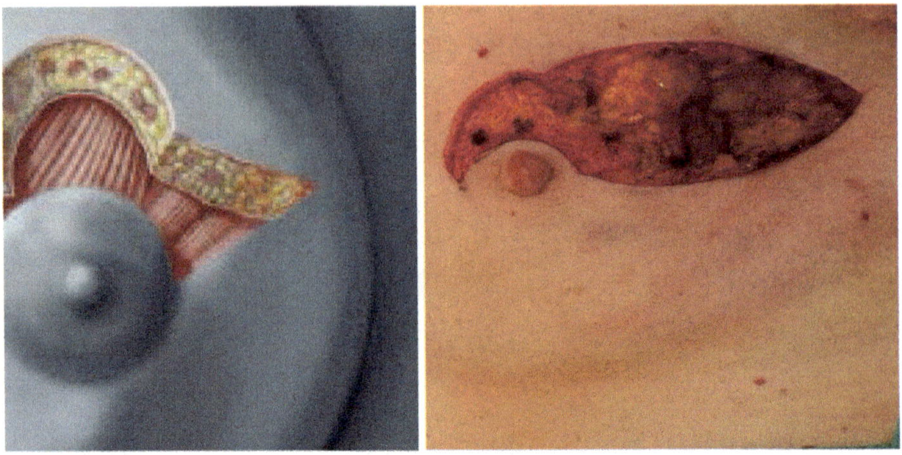

Fig. 5.16 Hemibatwing for lumpectomy and mastopexy

elimination of dead space and disallowing all seroma cavities. However, as others began developing oncoplastic techniques, it became apparent that leaving a lumpectomy cavity (seroma) did not compromise cosmetic outcome but did allow better targeting of whole-breast irradiation as well as allowing brachytherapy device placement. The most common oncoplastic lumpectomy techniques utilized today involve (1) simple advancement flap contouring overlying the lumpectomy (Fig. 5.14), (2) crescentic lumpectomy with mastopexy (Fig. 5.15), (3) hemibatwing (Fig. 5.16) (4) full batwing (Fig. 5.17), and (5) radial lumpectomy with crescentic mastopexy (for lower pole cancers) (Fig. 5.18). Mastopexy on the contralateral breast is commonly performed for symmetry. All of the techniques mentioned above allow for maintenance of a lumpectomy cavity into which brachytherapy devices can be placed.

In some instances, large segmental resections can be performed through reduction mammoplasty incisions (Fig. 5.19), with contralateral reductions for symmetry. These are usually done in conjunction with a breast plastic surgeon. These advanced lumpectomy techniques usually obliterate the lumpectomy cavity and rearrange the breast to such an extent that partial-breast irradiation of any kind is difficult.

5.3.8 *Insertion Techniques*

Postoperative brachytherapy device placement begins with preoperative anticipation that the patient is an appropriate candidate for APBI. This allows preliminary discussion with the patient regarding post-op radiation therapy and helps the surgeon plan the surgical techniques that will optimize in office device placement (see above). Patients with acceptable pathology (negative margins, <3 cm cancers, node negative) need to have a radiation oncology consult to discuss options, brachytherapy devices. and timing of implantation. Once the logistics have been worked out,

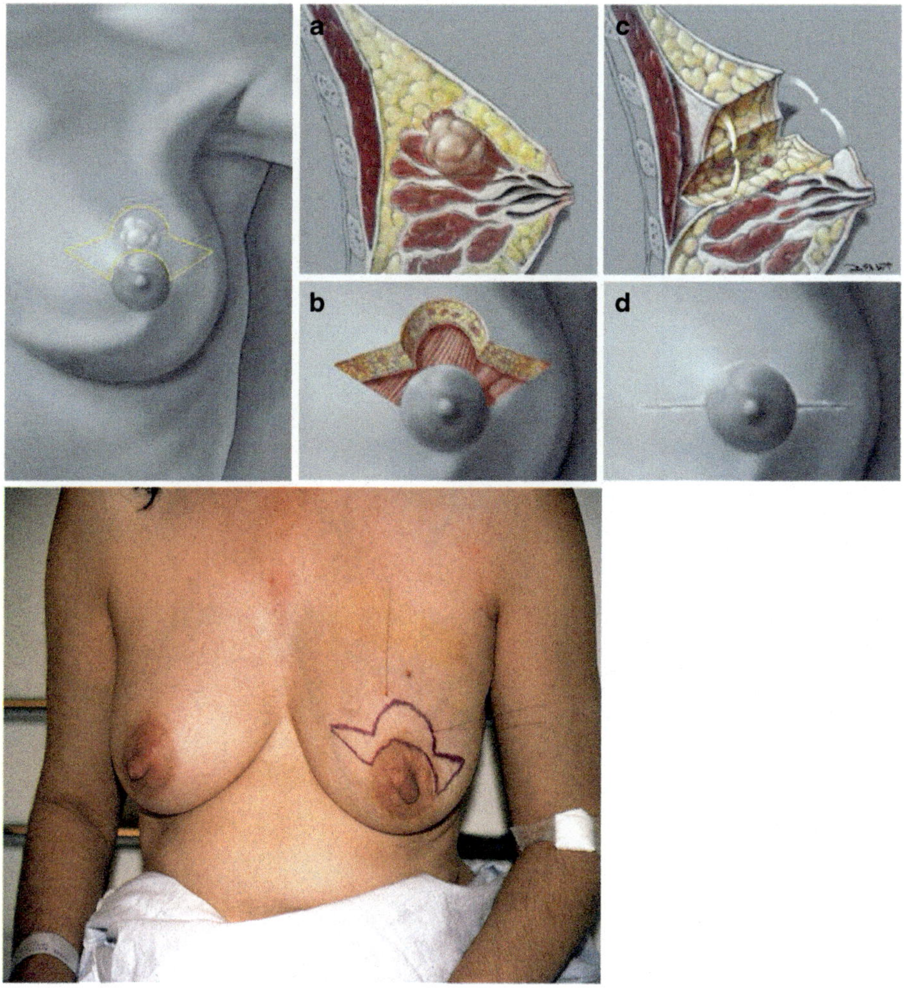

Fig. 5.17 Batwing technique (**a**) Tumor in breast (**b**) Tumor excised and reapproximation of breast tissue anteriorly and pectoralis fascia posteriorly (**c**) Batwing resection (**d**) Closure of Batwing

typical device placement is on a Thursday in the surgeon's office. Most implants will either be a (1) change out of a placeholder device (Fig. 5.20a) that was left at the time of surgery or (2) a de novo insertion through a lateral stab incision.

Patients with a placeholder device are usually changed out shortly (2–3 days) after surgery to minimize the length of time the device stays in the breast (as a potential source of infection). The patient is placed on an exam table, and local anesthesia is injected around the exit site of the placeholder and the track leading to the lumpectomy. The area of the lumpectomy and exit site of the placeholder device is prepped and draped with sterile towels (Fig. 5.20b). The appropriate-sized device is chosen and opened onto a sterile field. The placeholder is deflated and then removed, noting

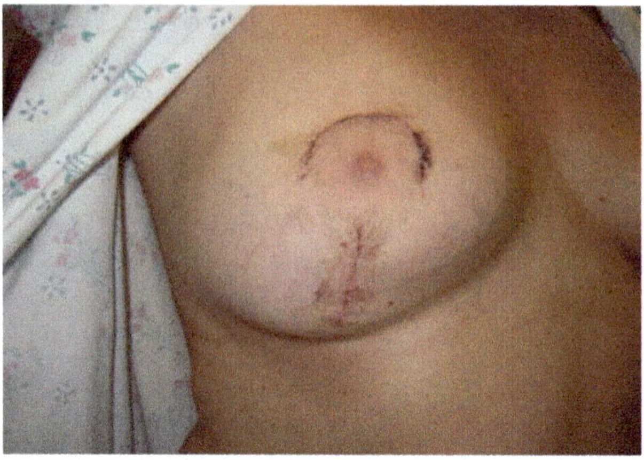

Fig. 5.18 Lower pole radial lumpectomy with crescentic mastopexy

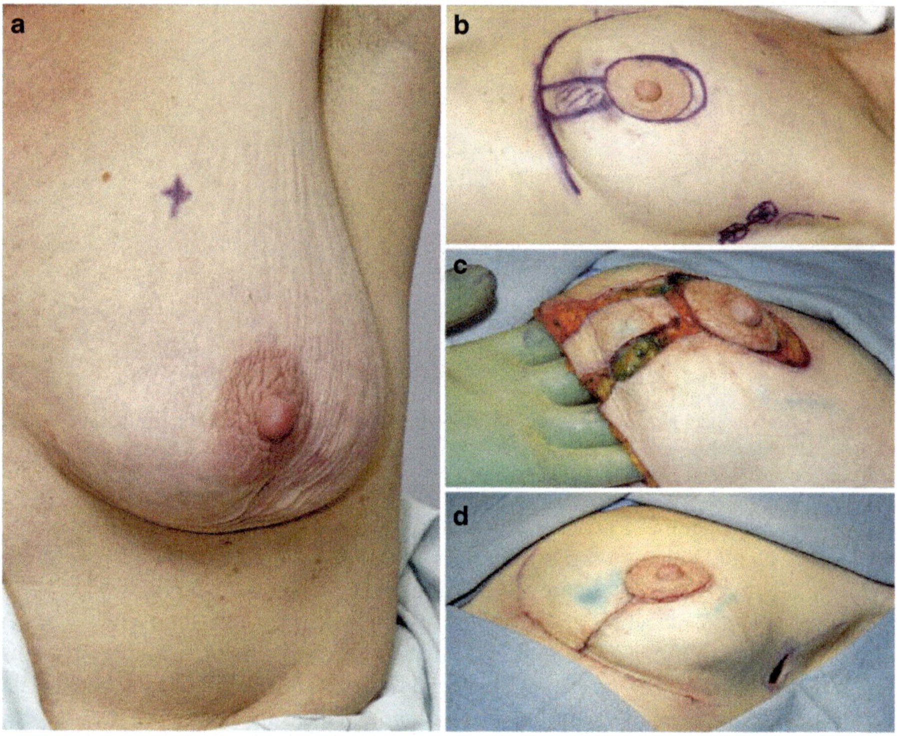

Fig. 5.19 Reduction mastopexy lumpectomy (**a**) Patient upright with inferior polp cancer (**b**) Reduction pattern drawn out (**c**) Incisions model pre-pectoral dissection (**d**) Closure of Reduction which includes removal of cancer

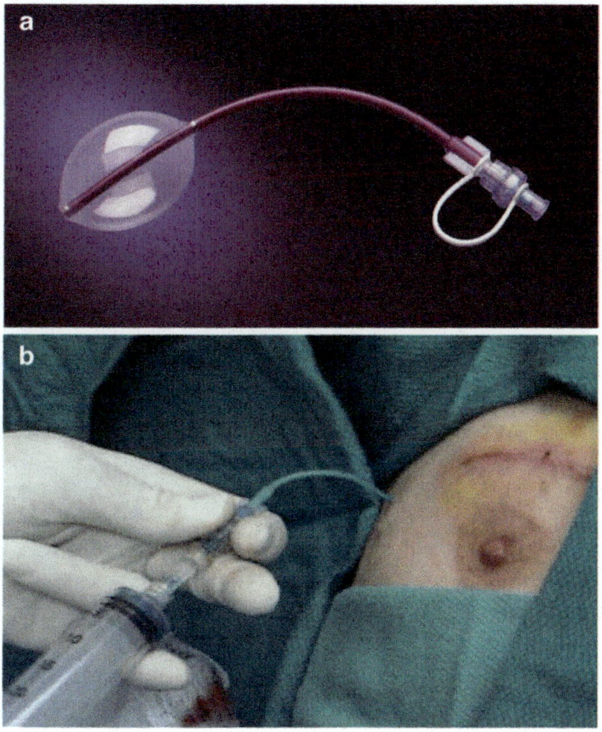

Fig. 5.20 (**a**) Placeholder device. (**b**) Deflating the placeholder device prior to inserting the brachytherapy device

the direction of the track leading to the lumpectomy. The device is then placed through the track and inflated or deployed depending on the device. If the surgeon has ultrasound available, the deployed device is checked to ensure proper placement; otherwise, this will be done at the time of CT for treatment planning.

Patients without a placeholder device will have their device placed under ultrasound guidance through a lateral stab incision. The patient is placed on an exam table and the cavity and surrounding breast tissue is examined using ultrasound. Once the appropriate site for the lateral stab incision is determined (typically 2–3 cm from the edge of the lumpectomy seroma), local anesthesia is injected at the site of the small incision and the track leading to the lumpectomy cavity. The area of the lumpectomy and lateral stab incision is prepped and draped with sterile towels. The appropriate-sized device is chosen and opened onto a sterile field. A small (typically 10–12 mm) incision is made with a #11 blade (Fig. 5.21a). The trocar is introduced through the incision (Fig. 5.21b) and advanced under sono guidance into the lumpectomy cavity to create the track for the device. Usually some or most of the seroma is evacuated as the trocar is removed. The device is placed through the trocar track into the lumpectomy cavity and deployed (Fig. 5.21c). Ultrasound is used to confirm appropriate placement (Fig. 5.21d).

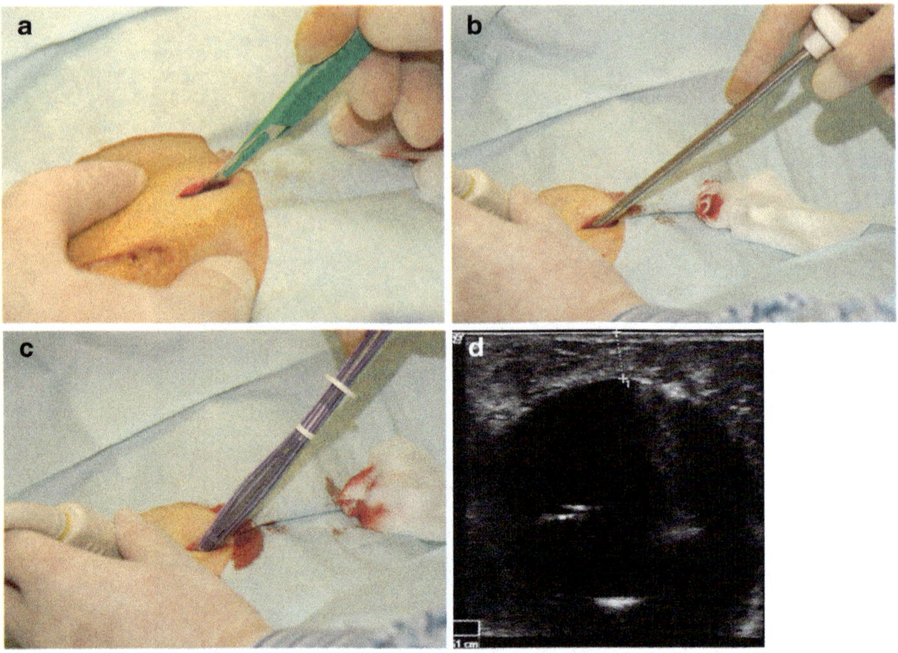

Fig. 5.21 (**a**) Lateral stab incision. (**b**) Trocar advancement into lumpectomy cavity. (**c**) Brachytherapy device placement through trocar track. (**d**) Ultrasound evaluation of deployed brachytherapy device

After the device is placed with either method, the exit site is dressed with sterile bandages (usually more for lateral stab technique due to the presence of the lumpectomy seroma). Typically patients are placed on an antibiotic (Bactrim DS, Keflex, clindamycin, Levaquin, etc) until the device is removed after the last treatment. The patient undergoes CT simulation either that day or the next day with treatment beginning thereafter.

Patients are instructed to keep the dressing clean and dry, to wear their bra, to change the dressing (or have it changed at the radiation center) if it becomes wet, to not to shower, or to remove any caps on the catheters.

Once the treatments are completed, the device is un-deployed/deflated and removed. Steri-Strips are applied to the small incision, or the wound is just left open and dressed with sterile bandages.

5.4 Summary

The most important concept to building a successful program is to realize this is a team approach to optimizing local treatment through coordinated care. Proper patient selection is paramount and that brachytherapy is not a substitute for inadequate surgery to "clean up" the margins. It is important to remember there are multiple ways to deliver APBI so multiple techniques should be available.

References

1. Beitsch P, Wilkinson JB, Vicini F, Haffty B, Fine R, Whitworth P, Kuerer H, Zannis V, Lyden M. Tumor bed control with balloon-based accelerated partial breast irradiation: incidence of true recurrences versus elsewhere failures in the American Society of Breast Surgery MammoSite Registry Trial. Ann Surg Oncol. 2012;19(10):3165–70 [Epub 2012 Jul 29].
2. Vicini F, Beitsch P, Quiet C, Keleher A, Garcia D, Snider H, Gittleman M, Zannis V, Haffty B, Kuerer H, Lyden M. Five year analysis of treatment efficacy and cosmesis by the American Society of Breast Surgeons MammoSite Breast Brachytherapy Registry Trial in patients treated with accelerated partial breast irradiation (APBI). Int J Oncol Biol Phys. 2010;79:808–17 [Epub ahead of print].
3. Beitsch PD, Vicini F, Keisch M, Haffty B, Shaitelman S, Lyden M. Five-year outcome of patients classified in the "unsuitable" category using the American Society of Therapeutic Radiology and Oncology (ASTRO) Consensus Panel guidelines for the application of accelerated partial breast irradiation: an analysis of patients treated on the American Society of Breast Surgeons/Mammosite Registry trial. Ann Surg Oncol. 2010;17(3):S219–25.
4. Bendifallah S, Werkoff G, Borie-Moutafoff C, Antoine M, Chopier J, Gligorov J, Uzan S, Coutant C, Rouzier R. Multiple synchronous (multifocal and multicentric) breast cancer: clinical implications. Surg Oncol. 2010;19(4):e115–123.
5. Yerushalmi R, Kennecke H, Woods R, et al. Does multicentric/multifocal breast cancer differ from unifocal breast cancer? An analysis of survival and contralateral breast cancer incidence. Breast Cancer Res Treat. 2009;117:365–70.
6. Mamounas EP, Tang G, Fisher B, Paik S, Shak S, Costantino JP, Watson D, Geyer Jr CE, Wickerham DL, Wolmark N. Association between the 21-gene recurrence score assay and risk of locoregional recurrence in node-negative, estrogen receptor–positive breast cancer: results from NSABP B-14 and NSABP B-20. J Clin Oncol. 2010;28:1677–83. published online on January 11, 2010.
7. Nguyen PL, Taghian AG, Katz MS, et al. Breast cancer subtype approximated by estrogen receptor, progesterone receptor, and HER-2 is associated with local and distant recurrence after breast-conserving therapy. J Clin Oncol. 2008;26:2373–8.
8. Drukker CA, Elias SG, Nijenhuis MV, Wesseling J, Bartelink H, Elkhuizen P, Fowble B, Whitworth PW, Patel RR, de Snoo FA, van 't Veer LJ, Beitsch PD, Rutgers EJ. Gene expression profiling to predict the risk of locoregional recurrence in breast cancer: a pooled analysis. Breast Cancer Res Treat. 2014;148(3):599–613. doi:10.1007/s10549-014-3188-z. Epub 2014 Nov 21.
9. Wagner E, Schrenk P, Huemer GM, Sir A, et al. Central quadrantectomy with resection of the nipple-areola complex compared with mastectomy in patients with retroareolar breast cancer. Breast J. 2007;13(6):557–63.
10. Waljee JF, Hu ES, Newman LA, Alderman AK. Predictors of re-excision among women undergoing breast-conserving surgery for cancer. Ann Surg Oncol. 2008;15:1287–303.
11. McCahill LE, Single RM, Aiello Bowles EJ, et al. Variability in reexcision following breast conservation surgery. JAMA. 2012;307:467–75.
12. Kollias J, Davies G, Bochner MA, Gill PG. Clinical impact of oncoplastic surgery in a specialist breast practice. ANZ J Surg. 2008;78(4):269–72.
13. Clough KB, Lewis JS, Couturaud B, Fitoussi A, Nos C, Falcou MC. Oncoplastic techniques allow extensive resections for breast-conserving therapy of breast carcinomas. Ann Surg. 2003;237:26–34.

Chapter 6
Impact of Oncoplastic Surgery on Adjuvant Radiation Therapy

Nayana L. Vora, Sharon L. Clancy, and Richard D. Pezner

Contents

Oncoplastic surgery of the breast is a combination of plastic surgery reconstructive techniques with optimal oncology procedures to maximize the aesthetic result in women undergoing breast conservation and has increased in use in recent years [1–4]. The incidence of poor aesthetic results after breast conservation with either

N.L. Vora, MD (✉)
Radiation Oncology, City of Hope National Medical Center, 1500 E Duarte Rd, Duarte, CA 91010, USA
e-mail: NVora@coh.org

S.L. Clancy, MD
Division of Plastic and Reconstructive Surgery, City of Hope National Medical Center, Duarte, USA

R.D. Pezner, MD
Radiation Oncology, City of Hope National Medical Center, Duarte, USA

D.W. Arthur et al. (eds.), *Short Course Breast Radiotherapy: A Comprehensive Review of Hypofractionation, Partial Breast, and Intra-Operative Irradiation*, DOI 10.1007/978-3-319-24388-7_6

lumpectomy or segmentectomy has been reported as high as 30 %, particularly for patients undergoing resection volumes of greater than 20 % of the breast volume [5]. Specific regions of the breast that yield poor aesthetic results after resection and are good candidates for oncoplastic surgery include the retroareolar, medial, or superior medial locations. Oncoplastic surgery can afford the oncologic surgeon greater margins around the tumor bed to assure adequate resection and minimize the chances of positive or close margin excisions while minimizing the cosmetic impact [6]. Surgery to combine the ablative resection and reconstruction in the same setting prior to radiation can achieve better aesthetic results [7].

6.1 Reconstructive Options

Components of successful oncoplastic procedures of the breast include adequate oncologic surgical excision, reshaping the breast accounting for skin and parenchymal glandular remodeling, and potential symmetrizing surgery of the contralateral breast to improve the aesthetic results. Optimal candidates for breast conservation are patients who have small- to moderate-size tumors (T1-2). This type of surgery requires significant cooperation and planning between plastic and oncologic surgeons to insure a successful and aesthetic result. If there is any concern about the margin status after the extirpative portion of the surgery, then the reconstruction should be delayed until confirmation of negative margins. The occurrence of this particular problem has been reported in one series to be 5 % in patients undergoing immediate reconstructive repair after partial mastectomy [8]. There are three general reconstructive techniques available to consider. The first is *postablative mammaplasty* with either a reduction in volume or rearrangement of the breast parenchyma. A second, technique used is *volume redistribution* either with or without skin alteration with a mastopexy or breast lift. Lastly, the third option is *volume replacement* that employs the movement of tissue flaps t to remodel the breast volume after excision.

6.2 Postablative Mammaplasty

Postablative mammaplasty is done in combination with the oncologic resection. The ideal candidates are patients with either a moderate- to large-size breast or significant ptosis. A large breast has historically been a moderate contraindication for breast conservation due to higher radiation dose inhomogeneity. A reduction of breast volume potentially affords a lower frequency of late radiation-induced toxicities [7]. The breast is marked for either a vertical pattern or inverted T or Wise pattern breast reduction or mastopexy (see Fig. 6.1). Preoperative consideration of tumor location, size, and quadrant is utilized in determining the pattern of skin excision and dermoglandular pedicle for the nipple-areolar complex. Ideally, resection of less than 20 % of the breast parenchyma leads to the most successful result

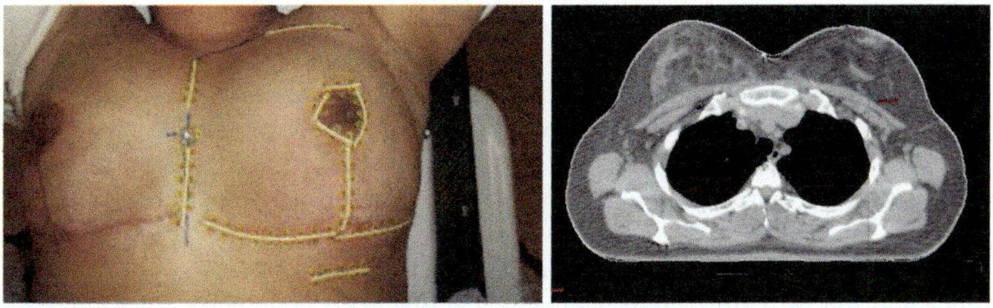

Fig. 6.1 A patient who had oncoplastic surgery. Yellow wires mark inverted T oncoplastic incision, surgically repositioned nipple-areola complex, and palpable boundaries of breast tissue. CT simulation films at level of clavicular heads shows presence of breast tissue which would cause difficulty in designing a separate standard supraclavicular nodal field

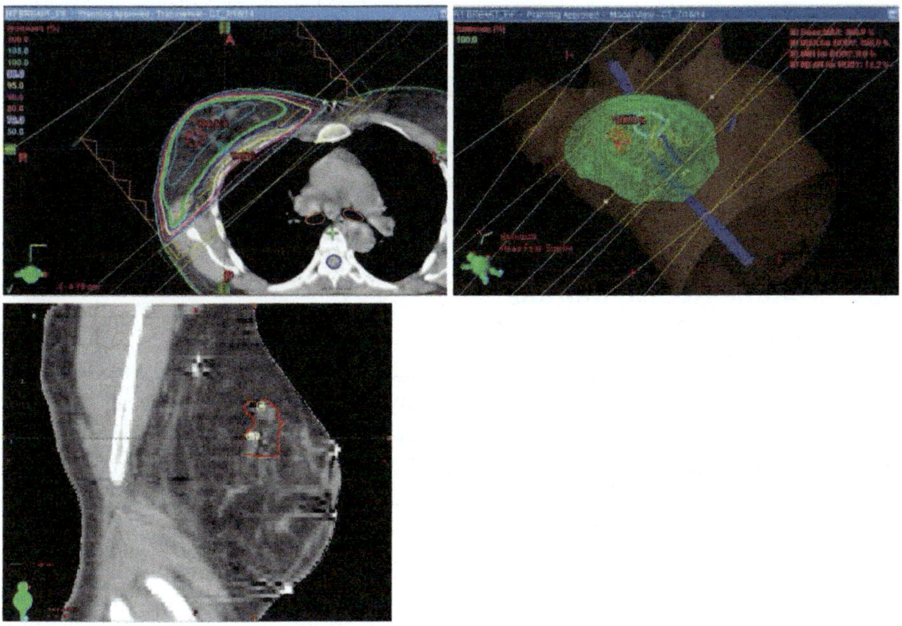

Fig. 6.2 CT simulation films with surgical clips placed in tumor bed following oncologic surgery and before oncoplastic reconstruction. Treatment planning study shows whole-breast and tumor bed volumes

in terms of aesthetic appearance; however, larger volumes can certainly be considered if the patient has significant macromastia. The patient typically undergoes needle localization of the tumor bed guiding tumor resection by the oncologic surgeon. This is ideally performed within the skin excision areas as marked while avoiding transection or violation of the planned pedicle for the nipple-areolar complex. The defect is then evaluated, and surgical clips are placed within the sides of the tumor bed cavity for future planning of targeted radiation to this area (see Fig. 6.2). The nipple-areolar complex is repositioned on a breast parenchymal flap, and the skin is excised or deepithelialized to accommodate the reduction or mastopexy pattern. Occasionally additional parenchymal breast flaps need to be created to fill the defect and may require advancement, rotation, or transposition. As much as possible, care is taken to avoid altering the location of the tumor bed, so it may remain in the same location and quadrant allowing acceptable delineation of the tumor cavity for improved radiation to the accelerated partial-breast or boost volume.

At the same procedure or at a future surgery, a contralateral breast symmetrizing procedure can be performed to maintain an aesthetic and symmetric breast appearance [9]. Anecdotally, there occasionally is parenchymal breast volume depletion after the radiation treatment. This needs to be taken into consideration when planning symmetrizing procedures in terms of volume removal or timing of the contralateral symmetrizing procedure. It is typically preferred to have the tumor-affected breast be about 10 % larger in volume compared with the contralateral breast to accommodate the parenchymal shrinkage and volume depletion of the affected reconstructed breast due to radiation [3]. It is our practice to typically perform the postablative mammaplasty and contralateral reduction mammaplasty at the same surgical setting to avoid two surgical procedures for the patient. However, delaying the symmetrizing procedure until after the final effects of the radiation are assessed sometimes allows a better result because the final size of the irradiated breast can be more accurately matched.

6.3 Volume Redistribution

Volume redistribution is an oncoplastic procedure where the internal breast parenchymal flaps are elevated to obliterate the defect from the lumpectomy or segmentectomy. This typically includes advancement of tissue without elevation of flaps that distort the architecture of the breast. Without the disruption of the architecture, the location of the tumor bed generally remains in its original location allowing easier delineation of the partial-breast or tumor boost treatment site. Typically this does not require a symmetrizing procedure of the contralateral breast being that the only volume difference is in the segmentectomy volume. Variations of this type of reconstructive technique include the "batwing" rearrangement, which may be utilized in central breast defects [2], and the breast remodeling technique, which utilizes a circumareolar incision with skin envelope elevation and application of the breast parenchyma to recreate the contour of the breast mound [9].

6.4 Volume Replacement

Volume replacement is an oncoplastic surgical technique that typically utilizes remote tissue from the breast glandular tissue. Instead of internal parenchymal flaps, this technique takes advantage of the plastic surgeon's armamentarium of flap procedures. This technique focuses on replacement of volume to maintain shape and existing volume of the breast with tissue transferred from the chest wall or truncal regions. Examples of these types of procedures include, but are not limited to, pedicle flaps such as a thoracodorsal artery perforator flap, muscle-sparing latissimus myocutaneous flap, or latissimus dorsi myocutaneous flap. Free tissue microsurgically transferred such as a deep inferior epigastric artery perforator flap or transverse rectus abdominis myocutaneous flap is an additional technique that can also be employed.

These volume replacement techniques typically maintain the location of the tumor bed without disruption. One of the concerns with this type of technique is that the surgery is usually larger and more extensive than just parenchymal rearrangement. It not only leaves scarring in additional areas of the body with scarring at the donor site location but then eliminates those flap options for potential total breast reconstruction in the setting of recurrence and need for future mastectomy with complete breast reconstruction [9]. Also, if the flap is performed at the time of the oncologic resection, then it will be subjected to radiation that may lead to volume depletion and a negative impact on the aesthetic result. However, the benefit using this technique in the immediate setting is that it may also avoid the need for a skin island that would decrease the aesthetic result. The overall aesthetic results of the oncoplastic surgery may change over time due to the often unpredictable effects of the radiation treatment.

6.5 Oncoplastic Surgery and External-Beam Radiation Therapy

The delivery of radiation therapy for oncoplastic patients may be more problematic for the radiation oncologist, particularly for designing of the local radiation boost after whole-breast irradiation or the target volume for APBI. The actual tumor bed may not be easily localized given the rearrangement of the breast tissue. The oncoplastic incision location may have no relationship to the tumor bed [1–3]. The presence of a seroma pocket palpable on examination or visualized on computed tomography (CT) simulation may be related to the plastic surgery reconstruction rather than the tumor bed that is typical in lumpectomy defects.

Pezner et al. [10] have reported difficulties in defining the tumor bed after oncoplastic surgery. CT simulation scans of patients with more than four clips placed in the tumor bed at the time of segmentectomy and oncoplastic reconstruction disclosed that the tumor bed was frequently located in a larger region of the breast or a completely different region than the initial tumor bed location. This must be taken into consideration when planning the postoperative radiation target volume.

Schaverien et al. reviewed 24 studies with 1933 patients who had oncoplastic surgery and radiation treatment [11]. They observed that the use of boost radiotherapy was not reported in the majority of published studies.

Furet et al. have reported on the comparison of preoperative and postoperative treatment-planning CT scans in a series of 31 conservation surgery patients [12]. They concluded that a minimum of three surgical clips were needed to define the tumor bed volume with accuracy. They also noted that 72 % of the 18 oncoplastic surgery patients had five titanium clips placed in the surgical cavity walls.

It is crucial that at the time of oncoplastic surgery, surgical oncologists, plastic surgeons, and radiation oncologists communicate and mark the tumor bed with an adequate number of surgical clips so that the boost volume can be clearly defined [13].

6.5.1 Oncoplastic Breast Conservation Combined with Intraoperative Radiation Therapy (IORT)

IORT techniques can deliver a single high dose of radiation to the visualized surgical tumor bed at the time of tumor resection. Radiation is delivered intraoperatively to the glandular tissue around the tumor bed while minimizing dose to the skin and subcutaneous tissue.

Experience with IORT for patients who have undergone oncoplastic surgery is very limited. Munhoz et al. and Silverstein et al. have reported the use of IORT at the time of oncoplastic surgery for selected low-risk patients [14, 15]. The selection criteria described included patients who had negative nodes, tumor size less than 3 cm, and surgical margins negative by at least 2 mm.

6.5.2 Oncoplastic Surgery with IORT Boost + External Radiation Treatment

This may be another approach for patients with advanced stage disease, post neoadjuvant chemotherapy, who undergo oncoplastic surgery at the time of lumpectomy. In this group of patients, direct visualization of the tumor bed may reduce the size of radiation boost volume. There have been several studies in the use of IORT as the tumor bed boost in patients who have not had oncoplastic surgery. Sedlmayer et al. have reported data from ISIORT, the International Society of Intraoperative Radiotherapy [16]. Their review included a total number of 1109 patients who were given IORT tumor bed boost dose of 10 Gy followed by WBRT 50–54 Gy. Of these patients, 60 % had at least one adverse prognostic feature such as tumor >2 cm, high grade, age <45 years, and/or positive lymph nodes. At a median follow-up of 72.4 months, 99.2 % had local control of tumor. Only 2 % of patients developed G3 toxicity. Lemanski et al. reported 50 patients with early breast cancer were treated with IORT 10 Gy using 9 MeV electron beam and WBRT 50 GY in 2 GY fraction [17]. After a median follow-up of 9.1 years (range 5–15 years), two local recurrences were observed. They observed that 14 % experienced grade 2 subcutaneous fibrosis. There was no grade 3 toxicity. Wong et al. have reported 6 years outcome in 52 patients with IORT of 10 Gy with 6–12 MeV electron beam and 48 Gy WBRT [18]. With a median follow-up of 79 months, there were two local recurrences. At the last follow-up, cosmesis was graded as excellent or good in 87 %, fair in 10 %, and poor in 4 %.

Other methods of radiation treatment such as 3-D conformal APBI treatment could also be used with proper identification and delineation of the target volume with the communication and procedures discussed above. In this setting, accurate localization of lumpectomy cavity becomes essential to local control success.

6.5.3 Accelerated Partial-Breast Radiation Treatment (APBI) Using the Interstitial Multicatheter Brachytherapy in Oncoplastic Breast Surgery

Roth et al. have reported on the use of interstitial brachytherapy following oncoplastic surgery for 136 breast cancers in 134 patients [19]. A multicatheter implant encompassing the volume defined by surgical clips with additional margin was performed approximately 3 weeks following surgery. APBI was given with either pulse dose rate of 50.4 Gy or high-dose rate (HDR) of 32 Gy over 4 days. The median follow-up time was 39 months (range 4–106 months). They reported three ipsilateral breast recurrences. Toxicities included mild fibrosis in 27, breast telangiectasia in 6, and hyperpigmentation in 14 cases. The authors noted that surgical clips were not visualized in 15 of 136 cases. In APBI, it cannot be overstated that that tumor bed visualization as a part of determining patient eligibility for this approach is essential so that treatment is effectively delivered to the required volume yielding less toxicity and higher local control.

6.6 In Summary

Oncoplastic breast surgery has in recent years significantly increased in use. This allows a larger breast excision to achieve the needed negative margins with more acceptable cosmetic and thus avoiding mastectomy in selected groups of patients.

The tumor bed needs to be marked properly for appropriate delineation and accurate delivery of targeted radiotherapy. We recommend placement of a minimum of six surgical clips in the tumor bed cavity walls following tumor resection and before oncoplastic surgical closure. IORT and APBI techniques as a local boost or as the sole radiation modality are potentially very appealing for oncoplastic surgery patients, but published experience to date is very limited.

References

1. Clough KB, Kaufman GJ, Nos C, et al. Improving breast cancer surgery: a classification and quadrant atlas for oncoplastic surgery. Ann Surg Oncol. 2010;17:1375–91.
2. Anderson BO, Masetti R, Silverstein MJ. Oncoplastic approaches to partial mastectomy: an overview of volume displacement techniques. Lancet Oncol. 2005;6:145–57.
3. Kronowitz SJ, Hunt KK, Kuerer HM, et therapy. Plast Reconstr Surg. 2007; 120:1755–68.
4. Rietjens M, Urban CA, Rey PC, et al. Long-term oncological results of breast conservation treatment with oncoplastic surgery. Breast. 2007;16:387–95.
5. Clough KB. Cosmetic sequelae after conservative treatment for breast cancer. Ann Plast Surg. 1998;41:471–81.
6. Hamdi M, Sinove Y, DePypere H, et al. The role of oncoplastic surgery in breast cancer. Acta Chir Belg. 2008;108(6):666–72.
7. Hamdi M. Oncoplastic and reconstructive surgery of the breast. Breast. 2013;22:S100–5.
8. Kronowitz S, Feledy J, Hunt K, et al. Determining the optimal approach to breast reconstruction after partial mastectomy. Plast Reconstr Surg. 2006;117:1–11.
9. Kronowitz S, Kuerer H, Buchholz T, et al. A management algorithm and practical oncoplastic surgical technique for repairing partial mastectomy defects. Plast Reconstr Surg. 2008;122: 1631–47.
10. Pezner RD, Tan MC, Clancy SL, et al. Radiation therapy for breast cancer patients who undergo oncoplastic surgery: localization of the tumor bed for the local boost. Am J Clin Oncol. 2013;36:535–9.
11. Schaverien MV, Stallard S, Dodwell D, Doughty JC. Use of boost radiotherapy in oncoplastic breast-conserving surgery – a systematic review. Eur J Surg Oncol. 2013;39:1179–85. doi:10.1016/j.ejso.2013.07.240. Epub 2013 Aug 26. Review.
12. Furet E, Peurien D, Fournier-Bidoz N, Servois V, Reyal F, Fourquet A, Rouzier R, Kirova YM. Plastic surgery for breast conservation therapy: how to define the volume of the tumor bed for the boost? Eur J Surg Oncol. 2014;40(7):830–4. doi:10.1016/ j.ejso. 2014.03.009. Epub 2014 Mar 28.
13. Coles CE, Wilson CB, Cumming J, et al. Titanium clip placement to allow accurate tumor bed localisation following breast conserving surgery: audit on behalf of the IMPORT Trial Management Group. Eur J Surg Oncol. 2009;35:578–82.
14. Munhoz AM, Filassi JR, Aldrighi C, et al. Bilateral reduction mammaplasty for immediate breast conservation surgery reconstruction and intraoperative radiotherapy: a preliminary report. Aesthetic Plast Surg. 2007;31(1):94–100.
15. Silverstein MJ, Tam M, Savalia N, Vaince F, Guerra L. Oncoplastic breast conservation surgery: the new paradigm. J Surg Oncol. 2014;110:82–9.
16. Sedlmayer F, Reitsamer R, Fussl C, Ziegler I, Zehentmayr F, Deutschmann H, et al. Boost IORT in breast cancer: body of evidence. Int J Breast Cancer. 2014;2014:472516. doi:10.1155/2014/472516. Epub 2014 Sep 2.
17. Lemanski C, Azria D, Thezenas S, Gutowski M, Saint-Aubert B, Rouanet P, et al. Intraoperative radiotherapy given as a boost for early breast cancer: long-term clinical and cosmetic results. Int J Radiat Oncol Biol Phys. 2006;64:1410–5. Epub 2006 Jan 25.
18. Wong WW, Pockaj BA, Vora SA, Halyard MY, Gray RJ, Schild SE. Six-year outcome of a prospective study evaluating tumor bed boost with intra-operative electron irradiation followed by whole-breast irradiation for early-stage breast cancer. Breast J. 2014;20:125–30. doi:10.1111/tbj.12235. Epub 2013 Dec 26.
19. Roth AM, Kauer-Dorner D, Resch A, Schmid A, Thill M, Niehoff P, Melchert C, et al. Groupe Europeen de Curietherapie-European Society for Therapeutic Radiology and Oncology (GEC-ESTRO) Breast Working Group. Is oncoplastic surgery a contraindication for accelerated partial breast radiation using the interstitial multicatheter brachytherapy method? Brachytherapy. 2014;13:394–9. doi:10.1016/j.brachy.2013.09.003.

Chapter 7
Comparison of True Cost Between Modalities in a Changing American Healthcare System

Matthew E. Schutzer, Noah S. Kalman, Sewit Teckie, and Louis Potters

Contents

7.1 Introduction

In the United States, healthcare expenditure per capita significantly exceeds that of other developed nations and continues to show a steadily increasing trend. This amount exceeded $8300 per person in 2012 and represented 16.2 % of our gross domestic product [1]. If this growth in spending continues as projected, the negative impact on our economy could be substantial [2]. Furthermore, this increase in expenditure has not led to superior outcomes. Changes to our current trajectory are therefore essential to the sustainability of our healthcare system.

Cancer care presents a unique challenge to efforts intended to curb rising medical costs. Rapid technological advances in medical, surgical, and radiation oncology are accompanied by equally rapid increases in expense. When considering this increasing trend along with the aging demographic in this country, the cost of cancer

M.E. Schutzer, MD • N.S. Kalman, MD
Department of Radiation Oncology, Virginia Commonwealth University Medical Center, Richmond, VA, USA

S. Teckie, MD • L. Potters, MD, FACR, FASTRO (✉)
Department of Radiation Medicine, North Shore-LIJ Health System and Hofstra North Shore-LIJ School of Medicine, New Hyde Park, NY, USA
e-mail: lpotters@nshs.edu

D.W. Arthur et al. (eds.), *Short Course Breast Radiotherapy: A Comprehensive Review of Hypofractionation, Partial Breast, and Intra-Operative Irradiation*, DOI 10.1007/978-3-319-24388-7_7

care is projected to increase by 39 % from the year 2010 to 2020 [3]. Advanced technologies such as targeted therapeutics not only cost more to deliver, but they are often applicable to a wider patient population given the improved toxicity profile. These broader indications for use of new technologies can escalate spending through increases in both cost and quantity of care [4]. The field of radiation oncology has certainly contributed to this pattern. In an analysis of growth in Medicare expenditure from 2002 to 2009, radiation oncology was found to exceed its sustainable growth rate target more than any other specialty, despite comprising a small portion of overall expenditure [5]. Notably, the burden of increasing costs falls not only on large organizations such as Medicare but also on individual patients and their families. In the National Survey of Households Affected by Cancer, 25 % of patients reported using all or most of their savings, and 11 % were unable to pay for necessities such as food, heat, or housing [6].

Cancer of the female breast was the malignancy with the highest total national expenditure in 2010, amounting to $16.5 billion [3]. Breast-conserving therapy is the most common treatment modality among women with early-stage disease. While advances in cancer care are typically associated with increasing cost, numerous trials have demonstrated that shortened adjuvant radiotherapy courses can be delivered with safety and efficacy comparable to conventional regimens for selected patients [7–15]. Such courses have the potential to significantly reduce cost. Moreover, in a survey of 5000 women with or without cancer, 90 % expressed a preference for an accelerated regimen if medically appropriate [16]. In 2013, the Choosing Wisely initiative formulated recommendations aimed to reduce unnecessary expenditure in radiation oncology [17]. The first of these guidelines asserts that shortened treatment schedules should be considered for all women over 50 with early-stage breast cancer after breast-conserving surgery. However, in an analysis of claims data for patients enrolled in commercial health plans, hypofractionated radiotherapy was used in only 34.5 % of patients for whom such treatment is endorsed by the American Society for Radiation Oncology (ASTRO) guidelines [18].

The reasons for the limited uptake of short-course radiotherapy are complex and are primarily related to physician biases and the financial incentive structure of the American healthcare system. In this chapter, an overview of this system is outlined, and the cost implications of accelerated radiotherapy regimens are reviewed. Finally, the concept of value in healthcare is introduced, and suggestions for promoting the use of short-course radiation through alignment of patient and physician incentives are discussed.

7.2 Payment in the Current Healthcare System

In the United States, medical care compensation is based on the specific services provided to patients, commonly referred to as "fee for service." With rare exception, every office visit and radiation treatment in radiation oncology is billed for and compensated separately.

Payment rates vary depending on patients' insurance, but most private payers follow Medicare's payment structure and policies, which are set by the Centers for Medicare and Medicaid Services (CMS). In the case of a hospital-based clinic, payment for medical services is divided into a professional component (physician activity) and a technical component (equipment or ancillary staff activity). Physicians receive the professional fee, and the hospital or nonphysician entity that owns the equipment/employs the ancillary staff receives the technical or facility component. In the case of a physician-owned practice, a global fee is provided that accounts for both physician and equipment/ancillary staff activity.

Billing for services is done via Current Procedural Terminology (CPT) codes [19]. There are separate codes for "evaluation and management" services such as consult and follow-up visits and "procedural" services such as simulation and treatment delivery. CPT codes are maintained by the American Medical Association (AMA). The AMA's CPT Editorial Panel adjusts current CPT codes, retires codes no longer in use, and establishes new CPT codes. An example of a recently created CPT code for radiation oncology is 77293: respiratory motion management during simulation.

An example is instructive. At initial consultation, the physician bills the payer for an evaluation and management visit. The visit is assigned a CPT code based on the complexity and duration of the visit. For patients with Medicare insurance, the CPT code is used to determine the reimbursement amount through the Medicare Physician Fee Schedule (PFS) payment rate formula [20]. In this formula, the CPT code is assigned relative value units (RVUs) based on three factors: (1) work RVUs account for the time required and complexity of the provided service; (2) practice expense (PE) RVUs account for practice costs such as office space, staff, and supplies; and (3) malpractice (MP) RVUs account for the expense of malpractice insurance. Each RVU component is adjusted by geographic practice cost indices (GPCIs), which account for geographic differences in practice costs. To obtain the specific reimbursement amount, the sum of the adjusted RVUs is multiplied by a conversion factor. In Federal Fiscal Year 2015, the conversion factor is $35.7547 per RVU [21].

The CMS issues yearly updates for the RVU values associated with CPT codes. The AMA's Relative Value Scale Update Committee (RUC) advises the CMS on updates to the RVU amounts for existing CPT codes and on establishing RVU amounts for new CPT codes [22]. In recent years, there has been some controversy whether current RVU evaluations favor specialty care [23]. However, the current system has been in place for over 20 years and remains today.

Similar to billing at initial consult, physicians assign CPT codes and bill for all aspects of patients' treatment: simulation (including immobilization and respiratory management), treatment planning (isodose planning, dosimetry calculations, and tissue-sparing devices such as wedges or MLCs), brachytherapy catheter placement (if part of treatment), on-treatment management (billed for every 5 days of treatment), and follow-up visits. For Medicare patients, these CPT codes are assigned RVU values which are then converted to reimbursement amounts.

Except in the case of a physician-owned practice, technical charges are compensated separately from physician professional charges. Technical charges also use CPT codes for billing. In many cases, a given CPT code has both a professional and technical component (e.g., simulation and treatment planning). Technical charges account for the simulation scan and immobilization devices used, as well as the work done by the radiation therapists, dosimetrists, and physicists. In the case of treatment delivery, a technical charge is generated for each treatment, which is separate from the professional fee for on-treatment management. In the case of external beam radiation delivery, one technical charge is generated. In the case of brachytherapy, two charges are generated: one for treatment delivery and one for source use (this accounts for depletion of the HDR source or use of LDR sources).

In Medicare, technical charges for CPT codes are assigned reimbursement values similar to physician billing through Medicare's outpatient prospective payment system (OPPS) [24]. In the OPPS, many CPT codes have been grouped into ambulatory payment classifications (APCs). For example, different CPT codes exist for simple, intermediate, and complex radiation treatment delivery. These related CPT codes are grouped by Medicare into APC 301, and Medicare reimburses the same amount for all CPT codes included in this APC.

During treatment delivery, every treatment generates its own technical charge. However, new in 2015, Medicare reimbursement for the technical fees for partial breast irradiation bundles the CPT codes of treatment delivery over the 1–2-week span of treatment into a single APC that receives a single payment amount [25]. Currently, this change applies only to partial breast irradiation. However, it is likely that over time, Medicare will bundle technical charges into single APCs for other discrete treatments, whether brachytherapy or external beam.

Some commercial payers and radiation oncology practices have experimented with bundling payments over an episode of care, from consult through follow-up and surveillance. These bundled payments encompass all services over the entire cycle of care for the given condition, as opposed to reimbursing individual services provided over the course of treatment. The reimbursement for such bundles is established to compensate for an average patient case. Such billing arrangements streamline reimbursement and reduce the financial incentive to choose treatment procedures that generate higher reimbursement but may not improve patient outcomes.

Given differences in appropriate treatment based on disease stage, patient age, and anatomy within a diagnosis, the appropriate reimbursement level depends on practices' case mix. For example, a recent study of 155 breast patients treated over a 14-month period at North Shore-Long Island Jewish Cancer Center showed significant variation in treatment: 37 % Canadian fractionation, 37 % standard fractionation, 4 % standard fractionation with comprehensive nodal irradiation plus boost, 9 % postmastectomy, 2 % treated on RTOG 1005 protocol, 8 % MammoSite, and 3 % others [26]. A bundled payment would pay more than the traditional fee for service model for some patients and less for others, due to the variability in treatment courses.

7.3 Comparison of Cost between Modalities for Adjuvant Breast Radiotherapy

Improved patient convenience and decreased costs are among the most commonly cited advantages of short-course radiotherapy over conventionally fractionated regimens. Numerous studies have been published in efforts to quantitatively analyze the cost differential between such modalities. A variety of methodologies have been employed in these investigations, and an equally variable range of results has been reported (Table 7.1). In this section, these results are reviewed, and the methods critically evaluated.

In a 2005 publication, Suh et al. modeled the cost incurred for a hypothetical 60-year-old patient with stage I invasive breast cancer undergoing adjuvant radiotherapy following breast-conserving surgery [27]. For eight distinct radiotherapy regimens, treatment planning and delivery utilization were estimated and costs were calculated as the sum of all direct medical costs to the payer and non-medical costs to the patient. Treatment modalities analyzed included (1) whole breast radiotherapy (WBRT) to 50 Gy in 25 fractions, (2) WBRT plus a boost (60 Gy in 30 fractions), (3) accelerated WBRT (42.5 Gy in 16 fractions), (4) WBRT using intensity-modulated radiotherapy (IMRT), accelerated partial breast irradiation (APBI) to 34 Gy in 10 fractions twice daily using (5) intracavitary (IC) or (6) interstitial (IT) brachytherapy, or APBI to 38.5 Gy in 10 fractions twice daily using (7) 3D conformal

Table 7.1 Estimated charges for various radiotherapy regimens

Publication	Fee schedule	Conventional WBRT ($)	Hypofractionated WBRT ($)	External beam APBI ($)	Brachytherapy APBI ($)	IORT
Suh et al. 2005 [27]	2003 Medicare	10,900 (30 Fx)	6100 (16 Fx)	7700 (10 Fx)	18,300 (10 Fx)	NR
Greenup et al. 2012 [28]	2011 Medicare	13,358 (30 Fx)	9122 (20 Fx)	5342 (9 Fx)	NR	NR
Grobmyer et al. 2012 [15]	NR	16,778	NR	NR	25,011	3094
Alvarado et al. 2013 [29]	2010 Medicare	10,464 (33 Fx)	6640 (16 Fx)	NR	NR	5547 (1 Fx)
Lanni et al. 2013 [30]	2011 Medicare	13,829 (33 Fx)	7826 (16 Fx)	6578 (10 Fx)	12,602 (10 Fx)	NR
Shah et al. 2013 [31]	2003 Medicare	11,726 (28 Fx)	NR	6578 (10 Fx)	12,602 (10 Fx)	NR

Values for external beam radiotherapy assume 3D conformal technique, and for brachytherapy assume use of a single-lumen intracavitary balloon

Abbreviations: *WBRT* whole breast radiotherapy, *APBI* accelerated partial breast irradiation, *IORT* intraoperative radiotherapy, *Fx* fractions, *NR* not reported radiotherapy (3D-CRT) or (8) IMRT. Costs to the payer were based on the 2003 Medicare Fee Schedule.

The total direct cost of conventional WBRT with boost was found to be $10,900 ($8500 without boost). By comparison, accelerated WBRT had the lowest estimated direct cost of $6100, corresponding to 44 % reduction. The most expensive modality was WBRT using IMRT ($19,300). APBI costs were $18,300 and $17,300 when using IC and IT brachytherapy, respectively; external beam APBI costs were $7700 and $9700 when using 3D-CRT and IMRT, respectively. The vast majority of cost variation resulted from differences between technical charges.

A similar analysis was conducted by Greenup et al. using the 2011 Medicare Fee Schedule to estimate potential cost savings when alternatives to conventional dose and fractionation (50 Gy plus a 10 Gy boost over 6 weeks) are utilized [28]. These alternatives included hypofractionation (42.5 Gy in 16 fractions plus a 4-fraction boost) and external beam APBI (36 Gy in 9 fractions twice daily). Radiotherapy costs were determined based on average current CPT codes billed per regimen. Conventional WBRT was estimated to cost $13,358.37, compared to $9121.98 for hypofractionated WBRT, and $5341.81 for external beam APBI. Additionally, a cost-minimizing model was created for a theoretical cohort of 1000 patients in which each patient was treated using the least expensive modality permitted by published guidelines, and adjuvant radiotherapy was omitted for patients meeting eligibility criteria for Cancer and Leukemia Group B 9343 [32]. Based on this cost-minimizing strategy, a theoretical savings of 43 % or $5.69 million per 1000 patients could be achieved compared to the uniform use of conventionally fractionated WBRT.

A study by Lanni et al. compared direct medical costs incurred by the payer for ten different breast radiotherapy techniques based on the 2011 Medicare Fee Schedule [30]. This study analyzed six different methods for WBRT and four methods for APBI. Conventional WBRT was estimated to cost $11,725 without boost and $13,829 with boost. Hypofractionated WBRT (16 fractions) costs were $7826, corresponding to a 43 % cost reduction compared to WBRT plus boost. In contrast to earlier reports, brachytherapy-based APBI was slightly less expensive in comparison to standard WBRT plus boost; single-channel and multichannel balloon-based brachytherapy cost $12,602 and $13,506, respectively. The least expensive regimen was found to be 3D-CRT APBI ($6578), and the most expensive regimen was WBRT plus boost using IMRT at $22,130.

In another analysis by Bekelman et al., patterns of healthcare utilization were evaluated using the HealthCore Integrated Research Database, which includes claims data from patients enrolled in one of 14 commercial health plans [18]. The study included 15,643 women who underwent breast-conserving surgery for breast cancer followed by adjuvant WBRT. Patients meeting the criteria for endorsement by the 2011 ASTRO guidelines (age >50, stage pT1-2 N0, no prior chemotherapy) [33] were classified as "hypofractionation endorsed" ($n=8924$). Because the guidelines do not prohibit the use of hypofractionated regimens in patients not meeting these criteria, such patients were classified as "hypofractionation permitted" ($n=6719$). Lastly, out-of-pocket patient expenses were examined and included deductibles, co-payments, and coinsurance.

While the primary analysis examined patterns of use for hypofractionation, the secondary analysis evaluated total health expenditure within 1 year of diagnosis of breast cancer as well as radiotherapy expenditures defined as the sum of all claims for radiotherapy simulation, planning physics, delivery, and management over a 3.5-month period. In comparing radiotherapy expenditure between hypofractionated (11–24 fractions) and standard WBRT (25–40 fractions), cost savings per patient was $4338 in the hypofractionation-endorsed cohort and $4785 in the hypofractionation-permitted cohort. Similarly, savings in total health expenditure were $2894 and $8587 for the respective cohorts. The relatively large difference seen within the hypofractionation-permitted cohort is likely explained in part by the use of chemotherapy, given the more advanced disease in the population. Out-of-pocket expenses did not differ significantly between hypofractionated and standard WBRT for either cohort.

Similar analyses have been conducted to assess potential cost savings associated with single-fraction intraoperative radiotherapy (IORT). Using the 2011 Medicare Fee Schedule, Alvarado et al. analyzed cost-effectiveness for IORT following breast-conserving surgery [29]. Their model estimated a cost of $5547 for IORT, which is 47 % less than 6-week WBRT ($10,464) and 16 % less than 3-week WBRT ($6640). Additionally, an up-front IORT boost followed by 5 weeks of WBRT was found to be the most expensive regimen ($13,640). In another series of 78 patients treated with lumpectomy followed by IORT, Grobmyer et al. include a cost analysis based on facility and professional charges [15]. Their estimate for IORT, $3094, is considerably less than for conventional WBRT ($16,778).

Each of these studies analyzes cost in terms of what is billed to the payer and is typically based on the Medicare Fee Schedule. These data therefore reflect charges from CPT codes, which, as described in the previous section, are determined by the Centers for Medicare and Medicaid Services. The reporting of such data is therefore limited in its ability to report the underlying cost required to provide a service [34, 35]. This concept of fundamental cost as a quantity distinct from charges billed is reviewed in further detail in the following section, and various methods to measure this quantity are discussed.

7.4 Understanding True Costs in Healthcare

While the sum of all charges associated with the delivery of a healthcare service such as adjuvant radiotherapy can be compiled with relative simplicity, estimating the underlying cost to a department is a more complex task. The numerous individual, equipment, and facilities expenses will all contribute to this summation in varying degrees and can be challenging to measure. Over time, increasingly granular costing methods have evolved, improving the accuracy and confidence in our approximations.

Among the simplest costing metrics is the ratio of cost to charges (RCC) method. First, a department's expenses over a given time period (typically 1 year) are totaled [36]. These costs include personnel, equipment, facilities, information technology, billing, utilities, housekeeping, etc. This quantity is divided by the department's total charges over that period to calculate the RCC. This ratio can then be applied to an individual service by multiplying its total charges by the RCC. For example, if a radiation oncology department's total costs are 60 % of their total charges, the RCC would be 0.6. Hypothetically, if the total charges to provide WBRT amounted to $10,000, then the estimated cost would be $6000. While this method is straightforward in nature, it relies on the assumption that this ratio is constant across all services. In reality, the ratio can be highly inconsistent, representing a shortcoming of the RCC method.

The RVU method is a modification of the RCC method and aims to account for the variable complexity among different treatments. Similar to RCC, the RVU method involves the summation of a department's total costs and divides this by their total number of RVUs to determine a cost per RVU ratio. This is then multiplied by the number of RVUs for an individual service to estimate its cost. Because the RVU is intended to reflect the difficulty and intricacy of a given task, this method theoretically improves upon the imprecision of the RCC approach. However, it is ultimately reliant on the same assumption of a constant ratio of cost to RVU for all services provided.

As a departure from the RCC and RVU methods, costing techniques such as activity-based costing (ABC) and more recently time-driven activity-based costing (TDABC) have been developed [36–39]. These approaches evaluate cost based on the resources consumed in the delivery of a service, including the personnel, space and equipment, and disposable materials. Because these methods measure the fundamental source of healthcare costs, they are considered bottom-up methodologies.

TDABC is a highly granular costing approach and has recently been applied to healthcare to an increasing extent [40–45]. In this technique, a process map is first created to outline every step (referred to as "activity") required over an entire episode of care. Through interviews with staff and/or tracking of patient flow, estimates are formulated of the amount of time that each activity requires of all involved resources, including personnel, equipment, and physical space. The capacity cost rate (CCR), defined as cost per minute, is then calculated for the above resources. For personnel, this represents the total annual cost, comprising salary, benefits, and supervision, divided by the total capacity of clinical minutes worked per year. For space and equipment, the CCR represents the annual maintenance and depreciation costs divided by annual capacity in minutes. In the final step, the total cost of the service is calculated by multiplying the total time required of each resource by its CCR and combining the sum of such costs with the expense of disposable materials. Further, note is made of variables that can influence activity times, thereby affecting cost. For example, the use of active breathing control to spare heart dose for selected women undergoing WBRT would require additional resources and result in an increased expense.

While TDABC is the most accurate tool for assessing cost in healthcare, no such analysis has been published within the field of radiation oncology to date. At Virginia Commonwealth University, TDABC was utilized to compare cost between conventional WBRT (25 fractions plus 5-fraction boost) and APBI using balloon-based brachytherapy (10 fractions twice daily), and the results are awaiting publication [46]. APBI was found to cost 30 % more than WBRT, largely due to increased use of personnel and materials. Specifically, the cost for APBI comprised 51 % personnel costs, 6 % space/equipment costs, and 43 % consumable material costs. Compared to WBRT, personnel costs were 17 % higher for APBI, which also necessitates additional cost for the device and surgical supplies.

Lievens et al. have published results of an ABC cost analysis for patients undergoing WBRT in the Belgian healthcare system [47, 48]. As a predecessor to TDABC, the ABC methodology estimates cost based on the activities required to provide a service and the resources consumed in each activity. However, rather than measuring time and CCR, the ABC model requires a more complex allocation of cost to each activity based on cost drivers. In the Belgian study, the ABC model estimated that the cost of conventionally fractionated WBRT plus boost can be reduced by about 20 % by omitting the boost and by 30 % when a hypofractionated regimen (13–16 fractions) is utilized. They further estimate that cost can be reduced by 60 % when the ultra-hypofractionated 5-fraction regimen from the UK FAST trial is used [49].

Unfortunately, until we have a reliable, agreed upon way of measuring and understanding costs of treatment, payers will continue to limit spending by reducing reimbursements and deciding what type of radiotherapy treatments they will cover. Payers employ radiation oncology business managers (ROBMs) to assess each prescribed radiotherapy treatment before deciding if they will reimburse the treatment course. By requiring prior authorization, peer-to-peer discussions, and completion of stock forms about disease stage and treatment intent, ROBMs function to limit approval and reimbursement of IMRT, radiosurgery, and other "expensive" radiotherapy treatments [50]. However, the resulting pressure upon physicians to choose a lower reimbursing treatment option may not always translate into cost savings, since cost and reimbursement are poorly correlated. As shown above by investigators at Virginia Commonwealth University, what would initially be considering a lower cost hypofractionated treatment option, such as APBI, may actually cost more when accounting for personnel, space, and equipment.

7.5 The Concept of Value in Healthcare

As outlined above, the current fee for service model financially rewards physicians based on volume. In radiation oncology, this creates an incentive toward more protracted treatment courses and is likely in part accountable for the use of hypofractionated WBRT regimens in only 35.4 % of patients meeting the ASTRO criteria [18]. Thus, the financial incentives for the physician and the best interests of the patients are often misaligned with the unintended consequences of prolonged treatment courses for the patient and increased cost to the healthcare system.

Harvard Business School professor Michael Porter and colleagues have introduced the concept of *value* in healthcare, which they define as the ratio of the quality of health outcomes for a specific medical condition to dollars spent to achieve these outcomes [51–54]. Shifting to a value-based healthcare system would therefore promote delivery of the greatest benefit to the patient while decreasing the financial strain on society.

The transition to a healthcare model that rewards value would entail a paradigm shift from our current system. To achieve this, Porter and colleagues have proposed a set of essential structural components. First, instead of reimbursement based on individual procedures and office visits, payment would be centered around specific medical conditions. Bundled payments have been proposed to create the financial incentive for improved efficiency and cost reduction, provided there are care pathways in place to ensure appropriate treatment. In the design of bundled payments, the detailed understanding of fundamental healthcare costs based on methods such as TDABC would become critical. Within radiation oncology, Teckie, McCloskey, and Steinberg have suggested that value be defined as a function of quality and cost, where quality is determined not only by outcomes but also by process and structure [55]. Additionally, ASTRO has commissioned a payment reform task force with the objective to investigate alternative payment models in order to incentivize value [56].

In addition, economists also assert the need for rigorous measurement and reporting of condition-specific health outcomes. Porter has proposed a three-tiered outcomes paradigm, in which quality is judged first by the health status attained (e.g., survival outcomes, tier I), then by time to recovery (tier II), and lastly by the long-term durability (tier III) of the intended results. While our present system incentivizes compliance with guidelines, his model asserts that a truly effective system would place more importance on the downstream results that directly affect patients while minimizing short-term and long-term costs.

7.6 The Value of Short-Course Radiotherapy

With value defined as outcomes achieved per dollar spent, it is evident that short-course radiotherapy can provide significant value to the patient. Hypofractionated WBRT has been shown in multiple randomized trials to offer comparable local control and toxicity when compared to conventionally fractionated WBRT [7–11]. The improved patient convenience offers a shorter time to recovery, thereby improving tier II on the outcomes hierarchy. Furthermore, the charges to the payer are consistently lower when fewer fractions are delivered [18, 27, 28, 30], and an ABC analysis reported similar results [47, 48]. Thus, for appropriately selected patients, hypofractionation clearly affords superior value to conventional fractionation through improved convenience and decreased cost.

Similarly, external beam APBI offers a convenient treatment schedule and has consistently been found to result in decreased charges [27, 28, 30]. However, the interim publication of a randomized trial has shown this therapy to be associated with increased rates of adverse cosmesis, telangiectasia, and breast induration [57]. In contrast, brachytherapy-based APBI has been shown to carry comparable toxicity rates in comparison to conventional adjuvant therapy [12–14]. While this modality can offer patients improved convenience and equivalent cosmetic outcomes, comparative cost analyses have demonstrated mixed results. Compared to WBRT, published charges for brachytherapy-based APBI range from equivalent [30] to significantly increased [27]. Additionally, a TDABC analysis performed at VCU showed balloon-based brachytherapy to consume 30 % more departmental resources than conventional WBRT, largely due to personnel and materials costs [46]. While APBI has potential to offer value to patients, further cost-effectiveness research is necessary to weigh the improvement in convenience against additional treatment expenses.

7.7 Conclusion

For selected patients, short-course radiotherapy offers improved convenience with comparable clinical outcomes. Modalities such as hypofractionated WBRT, external beam APBI, and IORT are associated with decreased charges to the payer when compared to conventional radiotherapy [15, 27–30], while cost estimates of brachytherapy-based APBI range from comparable to increased [27, 30]. An important distinction should be made between the charges to the payer and the underlying cost to provide a service. The latter is most accurately measured using bottom-up methodologies such as ABC or TDABC, which assess cost based on resources consumed.

While the use of short-course radiotherapy has increased in recent years, it is still utilized in only a minority of patients meeting criteria for its use [18]. Our current healthcare system reimburses physicians based on volume and lacks incentive for providing cost-effective care. In healthcare, the concept of value is defined as the quality of outcomes achieved per dollar spent. To incentivize value, changes to our healthcare system have been proposed and include transparent reporting of outcomes and conversion to a bundled payment model. Given the improved convenience and decreased cost, short-course radiotherapy has great potential to provide patients with value. Thus, in a system that rewards cost efficiency while promoting quality outcomes, the use of short-course radiotherapy would likely expand significantly.

References

1. Organization for Economic Cooperation and Development. OECD statistics: health expenditure since. 2000. http://www.oecd.org/els/health-systems/health-data.htm. Accessed 13 Mar 2015.
2. Chernew ME, Baicker K, Hsu J. The specter of financial Armageddon – health care and federal debt in the United States. N Engl J Med. 2010;362(13):1166–8.
3. Mariotto AB, Yabroff KR, Shao Y, Feuer EJ, Brown ML. Projections of the cost of cancer care in the United States: 2010–2020. J Natl Cancer Inst. 2011;103(2):117–28.

4. Elkin EB, Bach PB. Cancer's next frontier: addressing high and increasing costs. JAMA. 2010;303(11):1086–7.
5. Alhassani A, Chandra A, Chernew ME. The sources of the SGR "hole". N Engl J Med. 2012; 366(4):289–91.
6. Health TUTKFFHSoP. National survey of households affected by cancer. November 2006.
7. Whelan T, MacKenzie R, Julian J, et al. Randomized trial of breast irradiation schedules after lumpectomy for women with lymph node-negative breast cancer. J Natl Cancer Inst. 2002;94(15):1143–50.
8. Whelan TJ, Pignol JP, Levine MN, et al. Long-term results of hypofractionated radiation therapy for breast cancer. N Engl J Med. 2010;362(6):513–20.
9. Bentzen SM, Agrawal RK, Aird EG, et al. The UK Standardisation of Breast Radiotherapy (START) Trial A of radiotherapy hypofractionation for treatment of early breast cancer: a randomised trial. Lancet Oncol. 2008;9(4):331–41.
10. Bentzen SM, Agrawal RK, Aird EG, et al. The UK Standardisation of Breast Radiotherapy (START) Trial B of radiotherapy hypofractionation for treatment of early breast cancer: a randomised trial. Lancet. 2008;371(9618):1098–107.
11. Haviland JS, Owen JR, Dewar JA, et al. The UK Standardisation of Breast Radiotherapy (START) trials of radiotherapy hypofractionation for treatment of early breast cancer: 10-year follow-up results of two randomised controlled trials. Lancet Oncol. 2013;14(11):1086–94.
12. Polgar C, Sulyok Z, Fodor J, et al. Sole brachytherapy of the tumor bed after conservative surgery for T1 breast cancer: five-year results of a phase I-II study and initial findings of a randomized phase III trial. J Surg Oncol. 2002;80(3):121–8; discussion 129.
13. Polgar C, Fodor J, Major T, et al. Breast-conserving treatment with partial or whole breast irradiation for low-risk invasive breast carcinoma – 5-year results of a randomized trial. Int J Radiat Oncol Biol Phys. 2007;69(3):694–702.
14. Lovey K, Fodor J, Major T, et al. Fat necrosis after partial-breast irradiation with brachytherapy or electron irradiation versus standard whole-breast radiotherapy – 4-year results of a randomized trial. Int J Radiat Oncol Biol Phys. 2007;69(3):724–31.
15. Grobmyer SR, Lightsey JL, Bryant CM, et al. Low-kilovoltage, single-dose intraoperative radiation therapy for breast cancer: results and impact on a multidisciplinary breast cancer program. J Am Coll Surg. 2013;216(4):617–23; discussion 623–614.
16. Hoopes DJ, Kaziska D, Chapin P, et al. Patient preferences and physician practice patterns regarding breast radiotherapy. Int J Radiat Oncol Biol Phys. 2012;82(2):674–81.
17. Hahn C, Kavanagh B, Bhatnagar A, et al. Choosing wisely: the American Society for Radiation Oncology's top 5 list. Pract Radiat Oncol. 2014;4(6):349–55.
18. Bekelman JE, Sylwestrzak G, Barron J, et al. Uptake and costs of hypofractionated vs conventional whole breast irradiation after breast conserving surgery in the United States, 2008–2013. JAMA. 2014;312(23):2542–50.
19. Pinkawa M, Corral NE, Caffaro M, et al. Application of a spacer gel to optimize three-dimensional conformal and intensity modulated radiotherapy for prostate cancer. Radiother Oncol. 2011;100(3):436–41.
20. Medicare. Medicare physician fee schedule.
21. AMA. Medicare physician fee schedule.
22. AMA. Resource based relative value scale.
23. Commission MPA. Report to the congress: medicare payment policy. 2006.
24. Services CfMM. Outpatient prospective payment system.
25. Services CfMM. Outpatient prospective payment final rule FY 2015. 2014.
26. Potters L, Raince J, Chou H, et al. Development, implementation, and compliance of treatment pathways in radiation medicine. Front Oncol. 2013;3:105.
27. Suh WW, Pierce LJ, Vicini FA, Hayman JA. A cost comparison analysis of partial versus whole-breast irradiation after breast-conserving surgery for early-stage breast cancer. Int J Radiat Oncol Biol Phys. 2005;62(3):790–6.
28. Greenup RA, Camp MS, Taghian AG, et al. Cost comparison of radiation treatment options after lumpectomy for breast cancer. Ann Surg Oncol. 2012;19(10):3275–81.

29. Alvarado MD, Mohan AJ, Esserman LJ, et al. Cost-effectiveness analysis of intraoperative radiation therapy for early-stage breast cancer. Ann Surg Oncol. 2013;20(9):2873–80.
30. Lanni T, Keisch M, Shah C, Wobb J, Kestin L, Vicini F. A cost comparison analysis of adjuvant radiation therapy techniques after breast-conserving surgery. Breast J. 2013;19(2):162–7.
31. Shah C, Lanni TB, Saini H, et al. Cost-efficacy of acceleration partial-breast irradiation compared with whole-breast irradiation. Breast Cancer Res Treat. 2013;138(1):127–35.
32. Hughes KS, Schnaper LA, Berry D, et al. Lumpectomy plus tamoxifen with or without irradiation in women 70 years of age or older with early breast cancer. N Engl J Med. 2004; 351(10):971–7.
33. Smith BD, Bentzen SM, Correa CR, et al. Fractionation for whole breast irradiation: an American Society for Radiation Oncology (ASTRO) evidence-based guideline. Int J Radiat Oncol Biol Phys. 2011;81(1):59–68.
34. Finkler SA. The distinction between cost and charges. Ann Intern Med. 1982;96(1):102–9.
35. Perez CA, Kobeissi B, Smith BD, et al. Cost accounting in radiation oncology: a computer-based model for reimbursement. Int J Radiat Oncol Biol Phys. 1993;25(5):895–906.
36. Kaplan RS, Witkowski ML, Hohman JA. Boston Children's hospital: measuring patient costs (V). Harvard Business Review. 2012; Harvard Business School Case 113–057.
37. Kaplan R, Anderson S. Time-driven activity-based costing. Harv Bus Rev. 2004;82(11): 131–8.
38. Kaplan RS, Anderson SR. Time-driven activity-based costing: a simpler and more powerful path to higher profits. Boston: Harvard Business School Press; 2007.
39. Kaplan RS. Improving value with TDABC. Healthc Financ Manage. 2014;68(6):76–83.
40. Demeere N, Stouthuysen K, Roodhooft F. Time-driven activity-based costing in an outpatient clinic environment: development, relevance and managerial impact. Health Policy. 2009;92(2–3):296–304.
41. Oker F, Ozyapici H. A new costing model in hospital management: time-driven activity-based costing system. Health Care Manag (Frederick). 2013;32(1):23–36.
42. Inverso G, Lappi MD, Flath-Sporn SJ, Heald R, Kim DC, Meara JG. Increasing value in plagiocephaly care: a time-driven activity-based costing pilot study. Ann Plast Surg. 2015;74: 672–6.
43. Donovan CJ, Hopkins M, Kimmel BM, Koberna S, Montie CA. How Cleveland clinic used TDABC to improve value. Healthc Financ Manage. 2014;68(6):84–8.
44. French KE, Albright HW, Frenzel JC, et al. Measuring the value of process improvement initiatives in a preoperative assessment center using time-driven activity-based costing. Healthcare. 2013;1(3–4):136–42.
45. Kaplan RS, Porter ME. How to solve the cost crisis in health care. Harv Bus Rev. 2011;89(9): 46–52, 54, 56–61 passim. http://www.ncbi.nlm.nih.gov/pubmed/21939127.
46. Schutzer ME, Arthur DW, Anscher MS. Time driven activity based costing: a comparative cost analysis of whole breast radiotherapy versus balloon-based brachytherapy in the management of early stage breast cancer. Unpublished Manuscript. 2015.
47. Lievens Y. Hypofractionated breast radiotherapy: financial and economic consequences. Breast. 2010;19(3):192–7.
48. Lievens Y, van den Bogaert W, Kesteloot K. Activity-based costing: a practical model for cost calculation in radiotherapy. Int J Radiat Oncol Biol Phys. 2003;57(2):522–35.
49. Agrawal RK, Alhasso A, Barrett-Lee PJ, et al. First results of the randomised UK FAST trial of radiotherapy hypofractionation for treatment of early breast cancer (CRUKE/04/015). Radiother Oncol. 2011;100(1):93–100.
50. Teckie S, Potters L. The dangers of incorporating reimbursement data into clinical decision making. Pract Radiat Oncol. 2015;5(4):274–6.
51. Porter ME, Teisberg EO. Redefining health care: creating value-based competition on results. Boston: Harvard Business School Press; 2006.
52. Porter ME. A strategy for health care reform – toward a value-based system. N Engl J Med. 2009;361(2):109–12.
53. Porter ME. What is value in health care? N Engl J Med. 2010;363(26):2477–81.

54. Porter ME, Lee TH. The strategy that will fix health care. Harv Bus Rev. 2013;91(10):50–70.
55. Teckie S, McCloskey SA, Steinberg ML. Value: a framework for radiation oncology. J Clin Oncol. 2014;32(26):2864–70.
56. Butcher L. ASTRO developing payment reform plan. Oncol Times. 2013;35(11):18–9.
57. Olivotto IA, Whelan TJ, Parpia S, et al. Interim cosmetic and toxicity results from RAPID: a randomized trial of accelerated partial breast irradiation using three-dimensional conformal external beam radiation therapy. J Clin Oncol. 2013;31(32):4038–45.

Part II
Hypofractionated Whole Breast Irradiation

Chapter 8
Patient Selection for Hypofractionated Whole Breast Radiation Therapy for Treatment of Early-Stage Breast Cancer

Gary M. Freedman

Contents

8.1 Introduction

The establishment of postlumpectomy whole breast irradiation (WBI) as an alternative to mastectomy was a process that occurred over two to three decades. There was an origin in small retrospective series that led to the development of confirmatory

G.M. Freedman, MD
Department of Radiation Oncology, Perelman Center for Advanced Medicine,
Perelman School of Medicine of the University of Pennsylvania,
TRC 4 West 3400 Civic Center Blvd, Philadelphia, PA 19104, USA
e-mail: gary.freedman@uphs.upenn.edu

D.W. Arthur et al. (eds.), *Short Course Breast Radiotherapy: A Comprehensive Review of Hypofractionation, Partial Breast, and Intra-Operative Irradiation*,
DOI 10.1007/978-3-319-24388-7_8

large prospective randomized trials. However, even though breast conservation and radiation (BCT) rates increased in utilization above 0 % as compared to mastectomy, it remains significantly lower than 100 %, despite phase III data. The percentage of patients undergoing BCT with WBI in clinical practice varies widely depending on demographics, eligibility criteria, and patient preference.

This same process is occurring today in the adoption of hypofractionated whole breast irradiation (HWBI). Randomized trials may serve as a useful starting point to determining patient eligibility for HWBI, but each point of inclusion or exclusion criteria used in phase III studies may lend itself to further scrutiny and debate about subgroups that might be excluded from the overall results. For example, young age, lobular histology, extensive intraductal carcinoma, or involved margins were all studied extensively in the decades after phase III trials to determine whether they represented exceptions to the rule of BCT being equal to mastectomy. Even if not specifically excluded from the phase III trials, nonetheless they represented subgroups not well represented in the patients enrolled on most trials or not specifically studied prospectively by those trials. Similarly, it is to be expected in the decade after initial phase III results that subgroups such as young age, high grade, use of chemotherapy, or use of boost would be further scrutinized and debated to determine whether or not they are possible exceptions to the new rule of HWBI.

This chapter examines the criteria for patient selection for HWBI following breast-conserving surgery for early-stage breast cancer. HWBI will be considered the use of larger dose (>2 Gy) radiation fraction sizes compared to conventional radiation fraction sizes of 1.8–2 Gy per day. The chapter will examine the historical experience with hypofractionated WBI that culminated in the existing prospective phase III clinical trials. Sections of the chapter cover the evidence for current concepts in selection of patients for HWBI based upon clinical, pathologic, or treatment-related factors. Regional, economic, or practice environment factors affecting use of HWBI will not be discussed. Hypofractionation in the setting of partial breast and intraoperative radiation will be discussed in other chapters.

8.2 Hypofractionated WBI for Early-Stage Breast Cancer

Hypofractionation for breast cancer generally resulted in greater late tissue effects in early clinical experiences. Three fractions per week were associated with more severe late sequelae compared to 5-day a week treatment [1]. A daily fraction size of 2.5 Gy was associated with greater fibrosis, soft tissue atrophy, skin telangiectasias, and worse cosmetic outcome compared to 2 Gy [2, 3]. Once a week fractionation in breast cancer was generally only used for palliation or short-term local control, in elderly patients [4–7]. The outcomes after HWBI markedly improved in later studies, even with 2.5 Gy or larger fraction sizes, but only after the *total* radiation dose was lowered to doses of approximately 40–44 Gy [8–11]. However, based upon the early negative clinical experiences, hypofractionation was strongly discouraged by experts in the United States [12, 13]. Even years later, after publication of promising 5-year phase III data for HWBI, there remained many concerns about patient eligibility, technical factors, and possible long-term cosmetic and tissue effects of HWBI [14, 15]. This kept HWBI from being a part of most clinical practice and training of residents in the United States before 2010.

There have now been four prospective randomized phase III clinical trials of HWBI conducted in the United Kingdom and Canada that have long-term 10-year results (Table 8.1). These studies were paramount in establishing HWBI as a standard of practice and alternative to conventional fractionation worldwide. The trials also form the starting point for any discussion about which patients are now eligible for HWBI in today's clinical practice.

8.2.1 2011 American Society of Radiation Oncology Consensus Statement

As a response to the publication of phase III data with 5–10 year results, the American Society of Radiation Oncology (ASTRO) convened a task force of experts to make consensus recommendations on the use of HWBI in early-stage breast cancer [16]. A review of the literature and randomized trials was done to create a guideline for four specific questions regarding HWBI. First, there was consensus that HWBI resulted in equivalent results as conventional fractionation but for a relatively narrow definition of patients meeting the criteria on the randomized trials and accrued in large numbers on those trials. This was generally women 50 or older, T1–2, N0, breast-conserving surgery, no systemic chemotherapy, radiation to the breast only, and radiation dose heterogeneity of ±7 %. There was no consensus for or against high-grade tumors. There was consensus against HWBI for patients not included in the trials, such as DCIS, or underrepresented on the trials such as age <50 or needing regional node irradiation. Second, in regard to the use of a tumor bed boost, the task force concluded that there were "few data to define the indications for and toxicity of a tumor bed boost" in patients treated with HWBI. The task force recommended that HWBI not be used when a tumor bed boost was thought to be indicated. Third, 42.5 Gy in 16 fractions was recommended for patients treated with HWBI without a boost as was used on the OCOG trial. Fourth, optimization of dose homogeneity was recommended, with a strong recommendation for three-dimensional dose compensation and exclusion of the heart from the primary treatment fields with HWBI.

8.2.2 2012 Choosing Wisely Campaign

In 2012 ASTRO selected HWBI for their first out of five recommendations for the Choosing Wisely campaign, an initiative to foster conversations between patients and physicians about treatments that may be overused, unnecessary, or potentially harmful [17]. The recommendation made was "Don't initiate whole breast radiation therapy as a part of breast conservation therapy in women age ≥50 with early-stage invasive breast cancer without considering shorter treatment schedules." HWBI was

Table 8.1 Four prospective phase III randomized trials of hypofractionated whole breast irradiation versus conventional fractionation in early-stage breast cancer

Trial	Years conducted	Patients (number)	Fractionation (Gy/fractions)	Age <50 (%)	Boost (%)	Chemotherapy (%)	Regional node irradiation (%)
RMH/GOC	1986–1998	1,410	50/25 42.9/13 39/13	30	75	14	21
OCOG	1993–1996	1,234	50/25 42.5/16	25	0	11	0
START A	1998–2002	2,236	50/25 41.6/13 39/13	23	61	36	14
START B	1999–2001	2,215	50/25 40/15	21	43	22	7

RMH/GOC Royal Marsden Hospital, Sutton and Gloucestershire Oncology Centre, *START* Standardization of Breast Radiotherapy, *OCOG* Ontario Clinical Oncology Group selected for this campaign due to the high prevalence of radiation for early-stage breast cancer in clinical practice, the potential convenience to patients, the reduced cost of care, the strength of the medical evidence, and the previously published ASTRO consensus guideline. The text of the recommendation makes note that physicians could discuss with patients that HWBI is appropriate for selected women (but does not go into further detail about selection factors). Physicians could also make it known to their patients that there is relatively shorter 10-year follow-up data compared to longer results of 20 years or more for conventional WBI fractionation.

8.3 Patient Selection Factors for Hypofractionated Whole Breast Irradiation

8.3.1 Age

In the four major randomized trials of HWBI, the patient populations were 21–30 % aged <50 years (Table 8.1). Of 7,095 patients on these trials, 1,694 (24 %) were <50. Of patients on the RMH/GOC and START A and B trials, 343 of 5,861 (6 %) were <40 years. ASTRO had found consensus in their task force to recommend HWBI only for women ≥50, due in part to the lower percentage of this subgroup within the overall population on the trials. However, this is relatively subjective since 1,694 (24 %) <50 on four phase III trials is a substantial number of patients. The consensus for the acceptability of BCT itself was based on 2,067 women of whom less than 40–50 % were <50 treated on six randomized trials versus mastectomy [18–20].

The most recent local control and outcomes data from these trials of HWBI suggest women that are <50 years of age may be appropriate to include. The OCOG trial reported no significant difference in local control by age ≥50 versus <50 [21]. The OCOG trial also found that age <50 years had an odds ratio of 1.64 (1.26–21.5, $p<0.001$) compared to ≥50 for having a good or excellent cosmetic result, thus generally better than older women, and there was no interaction by treatment with either HWBI or conventional fractionation. A meta-analysis of the long-term START pilot, A and B trials also found no significant difference in 10-year local control for ages <40, 40–49, or ≥50 years [22]. The analysis of moderate to marked physician-assessed normal tissue effects on the breast (shrinkage, edema, induration or telangiectasia) was also either not significantly different or actually favored hypofractionation by age in the subgroup analysis.

8.3.2 Breast Size/Homogeneity

The OCOG trial specifically excluded patients with a breast "deemed too large to permit satisfactory radiation therapy (i.e., the maximum width of breast tissue >25 cm)" [23]. Radiation was given with tangential radiation fields with wedges used to improve dose homogeneity so that on a single central axis isodose plan, the dose was within 7 % of the prescribed dose (±7 %). The UK START A and B trials did not specifically exclude patients for a large breast size, but also placed a limitation on the dose inhomogeneity allowed on the central axis during radiation planning of 5 % of the prescribed dose (±5 %) [24, 25].

Although the four randomized trials are considered modern, it should be noted that patient enrollment was in the era of the 1990s when 2-dimensional planning, fluoroscopic simulation, and simple wedged tangents were standard practice. This technique can be associated with significant dose inhomogeneities to large portions of the breast tissue of >5–10 % of the radiation prescription [26, 27]. Radiation dermatitis and late fibrosis have been linked to whole breast radiation dose inhomogeneity particularly in women with a large breast size due to their greater dose inhomogeneity and tendency to larger skin folds [27–32]. More specifically to hypofractionation, the dose inhomogeneity and hot spots need to be restricted even more than with conventional fractionation in order to minimize risks for complications due to the steep late effects curve associated with equivalent tissue effects from altered dose fractionation. Keeping the dose homogeneity within 105 % should keep the isoeffective dose for late effects comparable between 2 and 3 Gy fraction sizes [33].

There have been significant advances in radiation planning that have been able to improve dose homogeneity and reduce complications. Today, 3-dimensional planning by CT simulator, and either field-in-field 3D conformal (forward planning) or intensity-modulated radiation therapy (inverse planning), can reduce dose inhomogeneity and reduce complications such as edema or negative cosmetic effects on the breast [31, 32, 34–37]. In addition to these measures, even a large chest wall separation >25 cm that was used as exclusion in the OCOG trial in the past may be mitigated by differences in patient positioning, such as prone, that can reduce the central axis separation and dose inhomogeneity of large-breasted women [38–40]. Therefore, the breast size of the patient should not be a contraindication to HWBI, as long as the dose homogeneity can be kept to acceptable levels <105–107 % during 3D treatment planning.

8.3.3 Left-Sided Breast Cancer

Left breast cancer was not specifically excluded from the randomized clinical trials of HWBI. The START A and B trials specifically did not show an increase in cardiac events for left-sided patients at 10 years with hypofractionation compared to conventional fractionation [22]. However, cardiac disease, and specifically coronary artery disease, in left-sided patients was responsible for a reduction in the overall potential survival benefit from radiation in older trials of postmastectomy and postlumpectomy radiation [41, 42]. Cardiac disease from radiation has a particularly late interval to onset of a mean 10–15 years. In the Surveillance

Epidemiology and End Results (SEER) database from 1973 to 1992, there was an excess rate of fatal myocardial infarction of 1–2 % over the course of 8–18 years from treatment for patients receiving left-sided versus right-sided adjuvant radiation [43]. Therefore, there may be a concern among physicians and patients that the 10-year results of clinical trials of HWBI have not ruled out possible differences in very late >10 year cardiac effects and longer follow-up is necessary. This may be a particular negative selection factor against HWBI in young patients and patients who have received potentially cardiotoxic chemotherapy or targeted therapy.

Regardless of fractionation used, modern developments in radiation therapy planning have resulted in significant improvements in cardiac dose. The ASTRO task force recommended for HWBI exclusion of the heart from the treatment field using basic 3-dimensional treatment planning, a good recommendation for any fractionation [16]. Field-in-field 3D conformal (forward planning) or intensity-modulated radiation therapy (inverse planning), prone position, and deep inspiration breath holding are all standard measures that may be employed today to reduce cardiac dose [44–48]. Left-sided breast cancer should not be a contraindication to HWBI with dose and fractionation schedules used in the phase III trials (267 cGy in OCOG and START B trials).

8.3.4 Grade

There was a great concern about the results of HWBI in patients with high-grade invasive cancer due to an unplanned subgroup analysis of the OCOG trial [21]. About 20 % of patients (233) on that trial were grade 3. The local recurrence was 15.6 % with HWBI compared to 4.7 % in high-grade patients. The hazard ratio for local recurrence in high-grade patients was 3.08 (1.22–7.76, $p=0.01$) in favor of conventional fractionation. Results were noninferior with HWBI in low- and intermediate-grade patients. This led to some initial reservations about offering HWBI to patients with grade 3 breast cancer.

However, since this initial report in 2010, there have been other publications that suggest that grade should not influence eligibility for HWBI. In 2012, a large Canadian population-based study of grade 3 patients treated with radiation, 1,083 treated with HWBI compared to 252 with conventional fractionation, showed no difference in the 10-year local control [49]. In 2014, in a meta-analysis of the long-term START pilot, A and B trials showed no difference in the local-regional relapse by grade as well, with a hazard ratio in 1,272 patients of 0.86 (0.59–1.25) trending in favor of HWBI over conventional fractionation, but not statistically significant [22]. Lastly, in 2014 an update of the OCOG trial was done with a central pathologic review of 989 of 1,234 patients enrolled on the original trial [50]. In contrast to the original subgroup analysis published in 2010, this report from the same trial showed that grade 3 was not a predictor of local recurrence with HWBI or conventional fractionation.

8.3.5 Use of a Boost

In prospective randomized studies in invasive breast cancer, the use of a tumor bed boost after WBI reduced the risk of local recurrence but also increased the risk for soft tissue side effects such as fibrosis [51, 52]. The prospective phase III trials of HWBI (Table 8.1) either did not use a boost [21] or used it only at the discretion of the treating department policy in a nonrandomized fashion [22, 53, 54]. The ASTRO task force was unable to reach consensus on whether or not to recommend a boost with HWBI [16]. Since then, a meta-analysis of the long-term START pilot, A and B trials showed no difference in the local-regional relapse by use of a tumor bed boost, with a hazard ratio of 0.99. However, there was a significant reduction in the occurrence of a moderate to marked tissue effect from radiation on the breast, with a hazard ratio of 0.86 (0.76–0.96) in patients treated with a boost, for HWBI versus conventional fractionation [22]. This difference in favor of HWBI was also seen in patients treated without a boost. However, as is the case with conventional radiation, it is likely that addition of a boost may increase late effects of HWBI. In one study of 312 women returning questionnaires for patient-reported outcomes, HWBI with a boost was associated with a modest increase in pain or negative cosmetic results compared to HWBI alone [55].

In the START trials, the boost was sequential with HWBI and given with conventional fractionation of 2 Gy per day in 5 fractions for a total of 10 Gy. In other studies, a sequential boost of 5 Gy in 2 fractions, 9 Gy in 3 fractions, 10 Gy in 4 fractions, or 12.5 Gy in 5 fractions has been used with HWBI [10, 49, 56–59]. There have been promising results of combining HWBI given over 3–4 weeks with a concurrent tumor bed boost as well [60–64]. Two prospective randomized trials testing HWBI with a concurrent versus sequential boost have been completed (see Sect. 8.4 below). In both, a sequential boost with HWBI was used for the control group. In light of the existing data, a sequential boost with conventional fractionation is acceptable after HWBI. As with conventional fractionation, patient selection is needed as to which patients may safely have the boost omitted – for low-risk patients, consideration must be given to the balance between a small magnitude of reduction in local recurrence and risks for added late toxicity.

8.3.6 Use of Chemotherapy

11–36 % of patients in the four major studies of HWBI (Table 8.1) had systemic chemotherapy. The chemotherapy used in the phase III trials was not specified by protocol but a reflection of the years of study from 1986 to 2002. In the RMH/GOC and OCOG trials, the chemotherapy was predominantly CMF (cyclophosphamide, methotrexate, and fluorouracil), and in the START A and B trials, 70 % of patients treated with chemotherapy received an anthracycline-based regimen, 29 % CMF, and 1 % a taxane-containing regimen. A meta-analysis of the long-term RMH/GOC, START A and B trials showed no difference in the local-regional relapse by use of chemotherapy [22]. In patients treated with chemotherapy, there was a nonsignificant trend in favor of HWBI with a hazard ratio of 0.81 (0.57–1.14) compared to conventional fractionation. In addition, there was a nonsignificant trend to lower occurrence of a moderate to marked tissue effect from radiation on the breast in patients treated with chemotherapy, with a hazard ratio of 0.88 (0.71–1.08). Subgroup analysis of the OCOG trial showed no difference in local control, or association with a good or excellent cosmetic result, between HWBI and conventional fractionation for the use of systemic therapy in general (chemo and/or endocrine therapy).

In a randomized trial, the use of concurrent CMF chemotherapy and radiation has been associated with increased risks for subcutaneous fibrosis, telangiectasias, skin pigment changes, and atrophy compared to sequential treatment based on physician assessment, but did not impact patient satisfaction [65]. Sequential chemotherapy and radiation, in a modern era of 2007–2010 that also included targeted agents in about 10 % of patients, were not found to be associated with patient-reported cosmetic outcomes [66]. Present data suggests that sequential administration of chemotherapy prior to or following radiation may not be a contraindication to delivering HWBI. Due to the possible increased soft tissue and cosmetic effects and lack of data in the setting of HWBI, concurrent administration of chemotherapy is not recommended.

8.3.7 Regional Nodal Irradiation

Regional node irradiation was either not permitted in the OCOG or used in 7–21 % of patients treated on the other prospective trials of HWBI (Table 8.1). In the 10-year results of the START A and B trials, there were no significant differences in shoulder stiffness or arm edema between HWBI and conventional fractionation [22]. The incidence of symptomatic lung fibrosis and brachial plexopathy was rare <1 %. However, supraclavicular and axillary radiation can treat an additional 12 % or more of lung volume compared to the breast alone [67]. It is known that regional irradiation increases the risk for lymphedema of the upper extremity, pneumonitis, and brachial plexopathy [68, 69]. Hypofractionation given in alternating days may increase the risk for plexopathy compared to daily fractionation [68]. Changes in pulmonary function however may occur even 8–10 years beyond receiving radiation [70]. And very late radiation injury from regional node treatment with hypofractionation, including brachial plexopathy, can occur from 10 to 20 years after treatment [71]. Given the severe nature of the potential complications, the poor response to treatment of plexopathy, and the potential for very late onset, regional node irradiation is recommended only with conventional fractionation.

8.3.8 Ductal Carcinoma In Situ

The randomized prospective trials of HWBI (Table 8.1) did not include patients with pure ductal carcinoma in situ (DCIS). However, it can be noted that the response to WBI, in terms of long-term local control, was the same in similarly treated patients by lumpectomy in the NSABP B-06 for invasive breast cancer and the NSABP B-17 for DCIS [18, 72]. Microinvasion in the setting of DCIS also has a similar natural history to pure DCIS when treated with WBI [73]. Williamson et al. [58] studied 266 women with DCIS, 162 treated with HWBI and 104 treated with conventional fractionation, and found a 4-year local recurrence of 6 % vs. 7 %, respectively ($p=0.9$). Ciervide et al. [74] found a 4.1 % local recurrence in 145 patients with DCIS treated with HWBI. Hathout et al. [75] reported in patients treated by HWBI a 3 % local recurrence at 5 years in 440 patients with DCIS. Lalani et al. [76] studied 1,609 women with DCIS, 638 patients treated with HWBI and 971 with conventional fractionation, and found a 10-year local recurrence rate of 11 % vs. 14 %, respectively ($p=0.03$), that was not significant on multivariate analyses. Therefore, present data suggests that DCIS treated by lumpectomy could be considered appropriately treated with adjuvant HWBI.

8.4 Future Phase III Clinical Trials of Hypofractionation Whole Breast Irradiation

One of the issues regarding more widespread acceptance of HWBI has been the relative low accrual of certain subgroups of patients onto the four major trials (Table 8.1) such as patients considered at a higher risk for in-breast failure, those under age 50, requiring a boost or systemic chemotherapy. There have been two additional randomized phase III trials conducted that had as a goal further expanding the acceptance of HWBI for these patient subgroups.

The Radiation Therapy Oncology Group completed a phase III randomized trial (RTOG 1005) of HWBI with a concurrent boost versus conventional or HWBI with a sequential boost [77]. The goal was to enroll a broader and higher-risk patient population than enrolled in the existing WBI hypofractionation studies. All patients in the study received a boost. Patient inclusion criteria were defined to include patients at higher than average risk for local recurrence and more likely to be treated with chemotherapy – age less than 50 years, node positive breast cancer, lymphovascular space invasion, presence of an extensive in situ ductal component (EIC), close resection margins, focally positive resection margins, and/or nonhormone-sensitive breast cancer. The control arm was WBI, with a standard sequential tumor bed boost using a conventional 2 Gy radiation fraction size. The WBI fractionation for the control arm was either conventional 50 Gy in 25 fractions or hypofractionated 42.7 Gy in 16 fractions. In the experimental arm, the overall length of treatment is fixed at 3 weeks with a WBI dose fractionation of 40 Gy in 15 fractions and a concurrent tumor bed boost of a total of 48 Gy. The IMPORT (Intensity Modulation and Partial Organ) High trial in the United Kingdom also enrolled women with early-stage breast cancer and an average or above average risk of local recurrence [78]. Eligibility for the trial also required 1 or more factor that would make the women considered at increased risk for local recurrence. The 3-arm trial had a control arm of 40 Gy WBI in 15 fractions with a sequential boost of 16 Gy in 8 fractions over 4½ weeks. The two experimental arms both deliver 36 Gy WBI in 15 fractions (escalated to 40 Gy in a higher-risk partial breast region in one of the arms) and two different dose levels of a concomitant tumor bed boost to 48 Gy or 53 Gy all in the same 15 fractions over 3 weeks.

8.5 Conclusions

Prospective phase III randomized trials have established the principle that HWBI in early-stage breast cancer may be used for WBI with acceptable toxicity and equal local control as conventional fractionation. There are many potential benefits including patient convenience and reduced cost of care. Local control has been equal and cosmetic results and complications equal or better, with HWBI compared to conventional fractionation with 10-year follow-up. For these reasons, HWBI is now a standard option as an alternative to conventional fractionation for most women. However, there has been some limitation in the extension of the overall positive results of HWBI to specific subgroups that were less well represented in these phase III trials.

Based on the available data, HWBI may be safely offered to most women with DCIS or early-stage invasive breast cancer treated by WBI. This includes women with age <50 years, high-grade cancer, requiring a sequential tumor bed boost or chemotherapy before or after radiation. Even a large breast size or large chest wall separation may no longer be contraindications due to the improvements in radiation therapy equipment and planning techniques since the conduct of earlier HWBI studies. Conventional fractionation remains standard for women who during planning have dose inhomogeneity >7 % of the prescribed dose and require concurrent chemotherapy or regional node irradiation.

Conflict of Interest Statement None.

References

1. Montague ED. Experience with altered fractionation in radiation therapy of breast cancer. Radiology. 1968;90(5):962–6.
2. Fehlauer F, Tribius S, Höller U, et al. Long-term radiation sequelae after breast-conserving therapy in women with early-stage breast cancer: an observational study using the LENT-SOMA scoring system. Int J Radiat Oncol Biol Phys. 2003;55:651–8.
3. Fehlauer F, Tribius S, Alberti W, Rades D. Late effects and cosmetic results of conventional versus hypofractionated irradiation in breast-conserving therapy. Strahlenther Onkol. 2005;181(10):625–31.

4. Rostom AY, Pradhan DG, White WF. Once weekly irradiation in breast cancer. Int J Radiat Oncol Biol Phys. 1987;13(4):551–5.
5. Ortholan C, Hannoun-Levi JM, Ferrero JM, Largillier R, Courdi A. Long-term results of adjuvant hypofractionated radiotherapy for breast cancer in elderly patients. Int J Radiat Oncol Biol Phys. 2005;61(1):154–62.
6. Courdi A, Ortholan C, Hannoun-Levi JM, et al. Long-term results of hypofractionated radiotherapy and hormonal therapy without surgery for breast cancer in elderly patients. Radiother Oncol. 2006;79(2):156–61.
7. Kirova YM, Campana F, Savignoni A, et al. Breast-conserving treatment in the elderly: long-term results of adjuvant hypofractionated and normofractionated radiotherapy. Int J Radiat Oncol Biol Phys. 2009;75(1):76–81.
8. Clark RM, Wilkinson RH, Miceli PN, MacDonald WD. Breast cancer. Experiences with conservation therapy. Am J Clin Oncol. 1987;10(6):461–8.
9. Ash DV, Benson EA, Sainsbury JR, Round C, Head C. Seven-year follow-up on 334 patients treated by breast conserving surgery and short course radical postoperative radiotherapy: a report of the Yorkshire Breast Cancer Group. Clin Oncol (R Coll Radiol). 1995;7(2):93–6.
10. Olivotto IA, Weir LM, Kim-Sing C, et al. Late cosmetic results of short fractionation for breast conservation. Radiother Oncol. 1996;41(1):7–13.
11. Shelley W, Brundage M, Hayter C, Paszat L, Zhou S, Mackillop W. A shorter fractionation schedule for postlumpectomy breast cancer patients. Int J Radiat Oncol Biol Phys. 2000;47(5):1219–28.
12. Cox JD. Large-dose fractionation (hypofractionation). Cancer. 1985;55(9 Suppl):2105–11.
13. Fletcher GH. Hypofractionation: lessons from complications. Radiother Oncol. 1991;20(1): 10–5.
14. Sartor CI, Tepper JE. Is less more? Lessons in radiation schedules in breast cancer. J Natl Cancer Inst. 2002;94(15):1114–5.
15. Goffman TE, Glatstein E. Hypofractionation redux? J Clin Oncol. 2004;22(4):589–91.
16. Smith BD, Bentzen SM, Correa CR, et al. Fractionation for whole breast irradiation: an American Society for Radiation Oncology (ASTRO) evidence-based guideline. Int J Radiat Oncol Biol Phys. 2011;81(1):59–68.
17. Hahn C, Kavanagh B, Bhatnagar A, et al. Choosing wisely: the American Society for Radiation Oncology's top 5 list. Pract Radiat Oncol. 2014;4(6):349–55.
18. Fisher B, Anderson S, Bryant J, et al. Twenty-year follow-up of a randomized trial comparing total mastectomy, lumpectomy, and lumpectomy plus irradiation for the treatment of invasive breast cancer. N Engl J Med. 2002;347:1233–41.
19. Veronesi U, Cascinelli N, Mariani L, et al. Twenty-year follow-up of a randomized study comparing breast-conserving surgery with radical mastectomy for early breast cancer. N Engl J Med. 2002;347:1227–32.
20. Jatoi I, Proschan MA. Randomized trials of breast-conserving therapy versus mastectomy for primary breast cancer: a pooled analysis of updated results. Am J Clin Oncol. 2005;28(3): 289–94.
21. Whelan TJ, Pignol J-P, Levine MN, et al. Long-term results of hypofractionated radiation therapy for breast cancer. N Engl J Med. 2010;362(6):513–20.
22. Haviland JS, Owen JR, Dewar JA, et al. The UK Standardisation of Breast Radiotherapy (START) trials of radiotherapy hypofractionation for treatment of early breast cancer: 10-year follow-up results of two randomised controlled trials. Lancet Oncol. 2013;14(11):1086–94.
23. Whelan T, MacKenzie R, Julian J, et al. Randomized trial of breast irradiation schedules after lumpectomy for women with lymph node-negative breast cancer. J Natl Cancer Inst. 2002;94(15):1143–50.
24. The START Trialists' Group. The UK Standardisation of Breast Radiotherapy (START) Trial A of radiotherapy hypofractionation for treatment of early breast cancer: a randomised trial. Lancet Oncol. 2008;9:331–41.
25. The START Trialists' Group. The UK Standardisation of Breast Radiotherapy (START) Trial B of radiotherapy hypofractionation for treatment of early breast cancer: a randomised trial. Lancet. 2008;371:1098–107.

26. Bucholz TAGE, Bice WS, et al. Dosimetric analysis of intact breast irradiation in off-axis planes. Int J Radiat Oncol Biol Phys. 1997;39:261–7.
27. Das IJCC, Fein DA, et al. Patterns of dose variability in radiation prescription of breast cancer. Radiother Oncol. 1997;44:83–9.
28. Neal AJ, Torr M, Helyer S, Yarnold JR. Correlation of breast dose heterogeneity with breast size using 3D CT planning and dose-volume histograms. Radiother Oncol. 1995;34(3): 210–8.
29. Fisher J, Scott C, Stevens R, et al. Randomized phase III study comparing best supportive care to Biafine as a prophylactic agent for radiation-induced skin toxicity for women undergoing breast irradiation: Radiation Therapy Oncology Group (RTOG) 97–13. Int J Radiat Oncol Biol Phys. 2000;48:1307–10.
30. Back M, Guerrieri M, Wratten C, Steigler A. Impact of radiation therapy on acute toxicity in breast conservation therapy for early breast cancer. Clin Oncol. 2004;16(1):12–6.
31. Pignol JP, Olivotto I, Rakovitch E, et al. A multicenter randomized trial of breast intensity-modulated radiation therapy to reduce acute radiation dermatitis. J Clin Oncol. 2008;26(13): 2085–92.
32. Freedman G, Li T, Nicolaou N, Anderson P. Breast intensity modulated radiation therapy reduces time spent with acute dermatitis for women of all breast sizes during radiation. Int J Radiat Oncol Biol Phys. 2009;74:689–94.
33. Yarnold J, Bentzen SM, Coles C, Haviland J. Hypofractionated whole-breast radiotherapy for women with early breast cancer: myths and realities. Int J Radiat Oncol Biol Phys. 2011;79(1): 1–9.
34. Vicini FA, Sharpe M, Kestin L, et al. Optimizing breast cancer treatment efficacy with intensity-modulated radiotherapy. Int J Radiat Oncol Biol Phys. 2002;54(5):1336–44.
35. Donovan E, Bleakley N, Denholm E, et al. Randomised trial of standard 2D radiotherapy (RT) versus intensity modulated radiotherapy (IMRT) in patients prescribed breast radiotherapy. Radiother Oncol. 2007;82(3):254–64.
36. Harsolia A, Kestin L, Grills I, et al. In clinical toxicities compared with conventional wedge-based breast radiotherapy. Int J Radiat Oncol Biol Phys. 2007;68:1375–80.
37. Keller LM, Sopka DM, Li T, et al. Five-year results of whole breast intensity modulated radiation therapy for the treatment of early stage breast cancer: the Fox Chase Cancer Center experience. Int J Radiat Oncol Biol Phys. 2012;84(4):881–7.
38. Merchant TE, McCormick B. Prone position breast irradiation. Int J Radiat Oncol Biol Phys. 1994;30(1):197–203.
39. Hardee ME, Raza S, Becker SJ, et al. Prone hypofractionated whole-breast radiotherapy without a boost to the tumor bed: comparable toxicity of IMRT versus a 3D conformal technique. Int J Radiat Oncol Biol Phys. 2012;82(3):e415–23.
40. Dorn PL, Corbin KS, Al-Hallaq H, Hasan Y, Chmura SJ. Feasibility and acute toxicity of hypofractionated radiation in large-breasted patients. Int J Radiat Oncol Biol Phys. 2012;83(1): 79–83.
41. Cuzick J, Stewart H, Rutqvist L, et al. Cause-specific mortality in long-term survivors of breast cancer who participated in trials of radiotherapy. J Clin Oncol. 1994;12:447–53.
42. Darby S, McGale P, Correa C, et al. Effect of radiotherapy after breast-conserving surgery on 10-year recurrence and 15-year breast cancer death: meta-analysis of individual patient data for 10,801 women in 17 randomised trials. Lancet. 2011;378(9804):1707–16.
43. Paszat LF, Mackillop WJ, Groome PA, Boyd C, Schulze K, Holowaty E. Mortality from myocardial infarction after adjuvant radiotherapy for breast cancer in the Surveillance, Epidemiology, and End-Results cancer registries. J Clin Oncol. 1998;16:2625–31.
44. Hurkmans CW, Cho BC, Damen E, Zijp L, Mijnheer BJ. Reduction of cardiac and lung complication probabilities after breast irradiation using conformal radiotherapy with or without intensity modulation. Radiother Oncol. 2002;62(2):163–71.
45. Chui CS, Hong L, Hunt M, McCormick B. A simplified intensity modulated radiation therapy technique for the breast. Med Phys. 2002;29(4):522–9.
46. Li JS, Freedman GM, Price R, et al. Clinical implementation of intensity-modulated tangential beam irradiation for breast cancer. Med Phys. 2004;31(5):1023–31.

47. Formenti SC, DeWyngaert JK, Jozsef G, Goldberg JD. Prone vs supine positioning for breast cancer radiotherapy. JAMA. 2012;308(9):861–3.
48. Eldredge-Hindy H, Lockamy V, Crawford A, et al. Active Breathing Coordinator reduces radiation dose to the heart and preserves local control in patients with left breast cancer: report of a prospective trial. Pract Radiat Oncol. 2015;5(1):4–10.
49. Herbert C, Nichol A, Olivotto I, et al. The impact of hypofractionated whole breast radiotherapy on local relapse in patients with Grade 3 early breast cancer: a population-based cohort study. Int J Radiat Oncol Biol Phys. 2012;82(5):2086–92.
50. Bane AL, Whelan TJ, Pond GR, et al. Tumor factors predictive of response to hypofractionated radiotherapy in a randomized trial following breast conserving therapy. Ann Oncol. 2014;25(5):992–8.
51. Romestaing P, Lehingue Y, Carrie C, et al. Role of a 10-Gy boost in the conservative treatment of early breast cancer: results of a randomized clinical trial in Lyon, France. J Clin Oncol. 1997;15:963–8.
52. Bartelink H, Horiot J-C, Poortmans PM, et al. Impact of a higher radiation dose on local control and survival in breast-conserving therapy of early breast cancer: 10-year results of the randomized boost versus no boost EORTC 22881–10882 trial. J Clin Oncol. 2007;25:3259–65.
53. Yarnold J, Ashton A, Bliss J, et al. Fractionation sensitivity and dose response of late adverse effects in the breast after radiotherapy for early breast cancer: long-term results of a randomised trial. Radiother Oncol. 2005;75:9–17.
54. Owen JR, Ashton A, Bliss JM, et al. Effect of radiotherapy fraction size on tumour control in patients with early-stage breast cancer after local tumour excision: long-term results of a randomised trial. Lancet Oncol. 2006;7(6):467–71.
55. Chan EK, Tabarsi N, Tyldesley S, et al. Patient-reported long-term cosmetic outcomes following short fractionation whole breast radiotherapy with boost. Am J Clin Oncol. 2014 May 12. [Epub ahead of print].
56. Clark RM, Whelan T, Levine M, et al. Randomized clinical trial of breast irradiation following lumpectomy and axillary dissection for node-negative breast cancer: an update. J Natl Cancer Inst. 1996;88:1659–64.
57. Fyles A, Manchul L, McCready D, et al. Updated results of a randomized trial of tamoxifen with or without radiation in women over 50 years of age with T1/2 N0 breast cancer. Radiother Oncol. 2006;80:S1.
58. Williamson D, Dinniwell R, Fung S, Pintilie M, Done SJ, Fyles AW. Local control with conventional and hypofractionated adjuvant radiotherapy after breast-conserving surgery for ductal carcinoma in-situ. Radiother Oncol. 2010;95(3):317–20.
59. Kim JY, Jung SY, Lee S, et al. Phase 2 trial of accelerated, hypofractionated whole-breast irradiation of 39 Gy in 13 fractions followed by a tumor bed boost sequentially delivering 9 Gy in 3 fractions in early-stage breast cancer. Int J Radiat Oncol Biol Phys. 2013;87(5):1037–42.
60. Formenti SC, Gidea-Addeo D, Goldberg JD, et al. Phase I-II trial of prone accelerated intensity modulated radiation therapy to the breast to optimally spare normal tissue. J Clin Oncol. 2007;25(16):2236–42.
61. Chadha M, Woode R, Sillanpaa J, et al. Results using 3-week accelerated whole-breast (WB) radiation therapy (RT) and concomitant boost for early-stage node negative breast cancer. Int J Radiat Oncol Biol Phys. 2009;75:S77.
62. Freedman GM, Anderson PR, Bleicher RJ, et al. Five-year local control in a phase II study of hypofractionated intensity modulated radiation therapy with an incorporated boost for early stage breast cancer. Int J Radiat Oncol Biol Phys. 2012;84(4):888–93.
63. Scorsetti M, Alongi F, Fogliata A, et al. Phase I-II study of hypofractionated simultaneous integrated boost using volumetric modulated arc therapy for adjuvant radiation therapy in breast cancer patients: a report of feasibility and early toxicity results in the first 50 treatments. Radiat Oncol. 2012;7:145.
64. Chadha M, Woode R, Sillanpaa J, et al. Early-stage breast cancer treated with 3-week accelerated whole-breast radiation therapy and concomitant boost. Int J Radiat Oncol Biol Phys. 2013;86(1):40–4.

65. Toledano AH, Bollet MA, Fourquet A, et al. Does concurrent radiochemotherapy affect cosmetic results in the adjuvant setting after breast-conserving surgery? Results of the ARCOSEIN multicenter, phase III study: patients' and doctors' views. Int J Radiat Oncol Biol Phys. 2007;68(1):66–72.
66. Hill-Kayser CE, Vachani C, Hampshire MK, Di Lullo GA, Metz JM. Cosmetic outcomes and complications reported by patients having undergone breast-conserving treatment. Int J Radiat Oncol Biol Phys. 2012;83(3):839–44.
67. Das IJ, Cheng EC, Freedman G, Fowble B. Lung and heart dose volume analyses with CT simulator in tangential field irradiation of breast cancer. Int J Radiat Oncol Biol Phys. 1998;42:11–9.
68. Bates T, Evans R. Report of the independent review commissioned by the Royal College of Radiologists into brachial plexus neuropathy following radiotherapy for breast carcinoma. London: Royal College of Radiologists; 1995.
69. Whelan T, Olivotto I, Ackerman I, et al. NCIC-CTG MA.20: An intergroup trial of regional nodal irradiation in early breast cancer. Journal of clinical oncology. 2011;29(18):suppl LBA1003.
70. Erven K, Weltens C, Nackaerts K, Fieuws S, Decramer M, Lievens Y. Changes in pulmonary function up to 10 years after locoregional breast irradiation. Int J Radiat Oncol Biol Phys. 2012;82(2):701–7.
71. Johansson S, Svensson H, Denekamp J. Dose response and latency for radiation-induced fibrosis, edema, and neuropathy in breast cancer patients. Int J Radiat Oncol Biol Phys. 2002;52:1207–19.
72. Fisher B, Dignam J, Wolmark N, et al. Lumpectomy and radiation therapy for the treatment of intraductal breast cancer: findings from National Surgical Adjuvant Breast and Bowel Project B-17. J Clin Oncol. 1998;16:441–52.
73. Parikh RR, Haffty BG, Lannin D, Moran MS. Ductal carcinoma in situ with microinvasion: prognostic implications, long-term outcomes, and role of axillary evaluation. Int J Radiat Oncol Biol Phys. 2012;82(1):7–13.
74. Ciervide R, Dhage S, Guth A, et al. Five year outcome of 145 patients with ductal carcinoma in situ (DCIS) after accelerated breast radiotherapy. Int J Radiat Oncol Biol Phys. 2012;83(2):e159–64.
75. Hathout L, Hijal T, Theberge V, et al. Hypofractionated radiation therapy for breast ductal carcinoma in situ. Int J Radiat Oncol Biol Phys. 2013;87(5):1058–63.
76. Lalani N, Paszat L, Sutradhar R, et al. Long-term outcomes of hypofractionation versus conventional radiation therapy after breast-conserving surgery for ductal carcinoma in situ of the breast. Int J Radiat Oncol Biol Phys. 2014;90(5):1017–24.
77. Radiation Therapy Oncology Group. A phase III trial of accelerated whole breast irradiation with hypofracitonation plus concurrent boost versus standard whole breast irradiation plus sequential boost for early-stage breast cancer. Available from URL: www.rtog.org/clinicaltrials/protocoltable/studydetails.aspx?study=1005. Accessed 1 Apr 2015.
78. IMPORT Trial Management Group. IMPORT HIGH: randomised trial testing dose escalated intensity modulated radiotherapy for women treated by breast conservation surgery and appropriate systemic therapy for early breast cancer. Available from URL: www.cancer.gov/clinicaltrials/search/view?cdrid=629770&version=healthprofessional. Accessed 1 Apr 2015.

Chapter 9
Physics of Hypofractionated Whole Breast Irradiation

Kristofer Kainz and X. Allen Li

Contents

K. Kainz • X.A. Li (✉)
Department of Radiation Oncology, Medical College of Wisconsin, Milwaukee, WI, USA
e-mail: kkainz@mcw.edu; ali@mcw.edu

D.W. Arthur et al. (eds.), *Short Course Breast Radiotherapy: A Comprehensive Review of Hypofractionation, Partial Breast, and Intra-Operative Irradiation*,
DOI 10.1007/978-3-319-24388-7_9

9.1 Overview of Hypofractionated Whole Breast Irradiation

Whole breast irradiation (WBI) is routinely used in the management of early-stage breast cancer, when coordinated with surgical removal of the gross tumor volume (GTV) (lumpectomy) along with a possible chemotherapy regimen. Whereas lumpectomy addresses the palpable breast lesion and chemotherapy is intended to address possible systemic disease, WBI is intended to respond to any possible subclinical disease within the ipsilateral breast that is otherwise not apparent in a surgical or imaging exam. The "conventional" WBI scheme of 50 Gy administered in 25 fractions (2 Gy per fraction) is a remnant of its application in the NSABP B-06 protocol (Circa 1985) which originally demonstrated the effectiveness of the role of WBI in breast conservation therapy.

However, several WBI fractionation schemes have been investigated, each of them exhibiting consistent efficacy. Thus, a hypofractionated regimen should provide equivalent control of local, regional, and distal disease as does the conventional regimen, provided that the radiobiological effects of increased dose per fraction are taken into account. Hypofractionated whole breast irradiation (HWBI) offers advantages to the patient such as reduced out-of-pocket costs (e.g., due to travel to and from clinic appointments) as well as to radiation oncology departments such as the ability to schedule and treat more patients per year on a given linear accelerator [12].

9.2 General Considerations for Hypofractionated Radiotherapy

The higher dose per fraction for HWBI compared with conventional WBI has some consequences with regard to how a conventional megavoltage linear accelerator will be applied for treatment. If the standard dose rate of the linear accelerator (typically approximately 200–300 cGy per minute at isocenter for lower-energy photons and approximately 600 cGy per minute for higher-energy beams) is applied to HWBI, the delivery time per fraction will be longer. This will require better control of the patient's motion during delivery. The delivery time per fraction could be reduced by increasing the dose rate and a practical way to do this is to remove the flattening filter from the treatment head. Although this will achieve dose rates of the order of several thousand cGy per minute, the flattening filter-free (FFF) beam profile will require the application of more complex inverse planning techniques such as intensity-modulated radiation therapy (IMRT), tomotherapy, and volumetric modulated arc therapy (VMAT).

The reduced number of fractions in HWBI offers the potential advantage of less time for interfractional changes to arise during the treatment course, such as breast or tumor bed shrinkage or postsurgical clip migration; thus, it is less likely that adaptive planning would be required. However, with fewer fractions, the consequences of a geometric miss of the tumor and ipsilateral breast are greater, among these consequences being lack of local or regional disease control and more severe complications due to dose to the lung or heart. More precise and accurate patient positioning is essential for HWBI. Image-guided radiation therapy (IGRT) may be useful, although the additional imaging procedures would increase dose to the contralateral breast and other organs at risk (OARs). Intrafractional motion of the breast due to breathing may require either a reproducible breath-hold or a respiration-correlated (gated) treatment. It should be noted that a gated treatment would further increase the overall delivery time per fraction.

9.3 Hypofractionation and Radiobiology

The most commonly used radiobiologic model to predict the response of acutely responding and late-responding tissue types is the linear quadratic model, such that, for a dose D, the parameter α characterizes the linear component (cell killing is proportional to D) and the parameter β characterizes the quadratic component (cell killing is proportional to D^2). The ratio α/β corresponds to the dose for which the linear and quadratic components are equal. The biological effectiveness of a given fractionation scheme, such that the dose per fraction *d* is administered in *n* fractions, can be predicted by the expression for biological effective dose (BED), which is derived from the linear quadratic formula and depends upon α/β as follows (Eq. 9.1):

$$\alpha\left(\frac{BED}{n}\right) = \alpha d + \beta d^2 \Rightarrow BED = nd\left(1 + d/(\alpha/\beta)\right) \tag{9.1}$$

If the effects of potential doubling time of the tumor (T_{pot}) and the overall duration of the treatment course are taken into account, the BED formalism becomes (Eq. 9.2)

$$BED = nd\left(1 + d/(\alpha/\beta)\right) - (ln2/\alpha)\left((T - T_K)/T_{pot}\right) \tag{9.2}$$

where T is the overall time from the start of treatment and T_K is the start-up time for tumor proliferation.

Tissue or tumor types with lower α/β are more sensitive to the dose per fraction than are tissue or tumor types with higher α/β; as $\alpha/\beta \rightarrow \infty$, BED approaches the physical total dose $n \times d$. Thus, in general, a lower α/β ratio is conducive to hypofractionation. Breast tumors and normal breast tissue may have adequately low α/β. Further, they may also have comparable α/β; for breast tumors, α/β was estimated to be approximately 4 from a retrospective analysis [20], and for normal breast tissue, α/β might be approximately 3.4 [12]. Thus, applying a hypofractionation scheme to WBI may not lead to substantially greater damage to normal breast tissue relative to tumor cell killing. It is expected that, for a hypofractionation scheme, normal breast tissue toxicity should be acceptable provided that the BED does not exceed that for a 50 Gy, 25 fraction treatment course [12]. Also, with hypofractionation, a reduced overall time for the treatment course should reduce the potential for cancer cells to repopulate, thus improving local control [20].

9.4 Treatment Planning Considerations

For simulation, kilovoltage CT imaging is standard practice, as it enables precise clinical target volume (CTV) delineation and dose calculation. Supplemental magnetic resonance or nuclear medicine images (registered to the CT, deformably if necessary) may aid in CTV delineation. For planning, the planning target volumes and organs at risk can be obtained as follows [21] (RTOG Contouring Atlas – http://www.rtog.org/CoreLab/ContouringAtlases/BreastCancerAtlas.aspx).

9.4.1 Intact Breast Radiation

The anatomic ipsilateral breast tissue, as apparent on the planning CT, is delineated. The lumpectomy cavity is contoured with an appropriate margin expansion to form the CTV to account for suspected subclinical disease. An additional expansion to a planning target volume (PTV) is performed to account for positioning uncertainty, uncertainty in beam geometry, patient intrafraction motion, or interfraction changes. The lumpectomy bed may be correctly identified using surgical clips [23]. Thus, daily IGRT based on surgical clips has utility in patient positioning.

9.4.2 Postmastectomy Radiation

The anatomic chest wall, as apparent on the planning CT, is delineated. The mastectomy scar is contoured and expanded accordingly into a CTV and a PTV.

9.4.3 Regional Lymph Nodes

The axillary, supraclavicular, and internal mammary chain lymph nodes are contoured, with appropriate expansions to PTVs, as deemed clinically relevant.

It should be noted that regional nodal irradiation may be characteristic of more advanced breast disease, and thus would likely not be incorporated in a HWBI regimen. Nodal irradiation leads to increased dose to OARs that are not otherwise of concern for WBI alone, such as the spinal cord, esophagus, thyroid, ribs, and brachial plexus. It may be necessary to account for the differing α/β ratios for these OARs.

9.4.4 Avoidance Structures and Organs at Risk

The contralateral breast tissue, ipsilateral and contralateral lungs, and heart are contoured as apparent on the planning CT. In order to visualize the left anterior descending coronary artery (LADA), the infusion of iodine contrast agent during planning CT acquisition may be required.

The treatment plan quality may be assessed using metrics such as homogeneity index (HI), uniformity index (UI), conformity index (CI), or conformation number (CN). These metrics are defined as follows (Eq. 9.3):

$$HI = \frac{D_{Rx}}{D_{\max}} \tag{9.3}$$

where D_{Rx} is the prescribed dose and $D_{\max}$ is the maximum point dose within the target volume. A higher HI conforms to more favorable dose uniformity (Eq. 9.4) [29].

$$UI = \frac{D_5}{D_{95}} \tag{9.4}$$

where D_5 and D_{95} are doses covering at least 5 % and at least 95 %, respectively, of the target volume. UI is always greater than or equal to unity; UI = 1 corresponds to ideal target dose uniformity (Eq. 9.5) [25].

$$CI = \frac{V_{95\%}}{V_{PTV}} \tag{9.5}$$

where $V_{95\,\%}$ is the volume covered by 95 % of the prescribed dose and V_{PTV} is the volume of the target [14]. Conformity index > 1 suggests the presence of dose outside the target volume. Although for perfect target volume conformity CI is equal to unity, it should be noted that prescription isodose volume need not overlap completely with the PTV for CI = 1 (Eq. 9.6).

$$CN = \left(\frac{V_{T,Rx}}{V_T}\right)\left(\frac{V_{T,Rx}}{V_{Rx}}\right) \tag{9.6}$$

where V_T is the volume of the target region of interest (ROI), V_{Rx} is the volume encompassed by the prescribed isodose surface, and $V_{T,Rx}$ is the volume of the target ROI that receives 95 % or more of the prescribed dose [1, 24]. Conformation number = 1 corresponds to perfect conformity of the prescribed isodose curve to the target ROI. Conformation number is reduced by underdosage of the target ROI or by a geometric miss (which reduces $V_{T,Rx}$ relative to V_T) or by unnecessary dose outside the target ROI (increasing V_{Rx} relative to $V_{T,Rx}$).

9.5 Organ at Risk Tolerances with Hypofractionation

The BED formalism of equations can be used, along with reasonable assumptions for α/β and potential tumor doubling time T_{pot}, to obtain the physical dose prescriptions for the ipsilateral breast and breast boost volume, along with dose-volume limits for the OARs; Table 9.1 shows the results of such calculations and may be used as a basis for various HWBI fractionation schemes. One can show that, using Eq. (9.2) and assuming from Qi et al. [20] the values of $\alpha/\beta = 2.88$, $\alpha = 0.08$, and $T_{pot} = 14.4$ days, the standard 25 fraction, 2 Gy per fraction regimen over 33 days is biologically equivalent to a common HWBI regimen of 16 fractions, 2.66 Gy per fraction over a 29-day time frame.

The dose-volume objectives for the lung and heart given in Table 9.1 for the standard 2 Gy per fraction scheme are below those recommended by QUANTEC. QUANTEC recommends restricting the volume of the lung receiving 20 Gy to less than 30–35 % to keep the risk of radiation pneumonitis below 20 % [18] and restricting the volume of the heart receiving 25 Gy to less than 10 % to keep the probability of cardiac mortality within 15 years to below 1 % [11].

Table 9.1 Summarized for several physical dose per fraction schemes are the prescribed physical doses to the ipsilateral breast and lumpectomy-site boost volumes, along with recommended physical dose-volume limits to the lungs and heart

Structure	Relative Volume at dose	Physical dose per fraction (Gy)							
		1.5	1.8	2.0	2.2	2.5	3.0	4.0	5.0
PTV boost	≥95 %	64.5	61.2	60.0	59.4	57.5	54.0	48.0	45.0
Ipsilateral breast	≥95 %	54.0	52.2	50.0	48.4	47.5	45.0	40.0	35.0
Ipsilateral lung	<25 %	5.3	5.2	5.0	4.8	4.5	4.2	3.6	3.1
	<10 %	21.3	20.8	20.0	19.2	18.2	16.7	14.3	12.5
Heart	<5 %	26.7	26.0	25.0	24.0	22.7	20.8	17.9	15.6

The 2 Gy per fraction values correspond to conventional WBI; the dose-volume objectives for other physical dose per fraction schemes were obtained using the BED formalism of Eq. (9.1)

9.6 Hypofractionated Whole Breast Irradiation Dose Delivery Techniques

9.6.1 Conventional 3D Conformal Radiation Therapy External Beam Techniques

The conventional opposed tangent-field arrangements should serve hypofractionated whole breast irradiation (HWBI) cases as well as they serve conventional WBI fractionation. Dose gradients to account for thicker breast tissue posteriorly or superiorly may be achieved using either wedges (physical or virtual) or by using subfields (the so-called "field-in-field" technique). The MLC leaf positions, angle and heel-orientation of wedges, collimator angle, and relative number of monitor units (MU) per beam can be determined via a trial-and-error technique or via an automated optimization [4]. To account for penumbra at the field edges, apertures extending 5 mm beyond the PTV are defined, with reductions as deemed appropriate to minimize the heart and lung [5]. If wedges are planned, virtual wedges (with the wedged dose profile generated by the motion of one of the linear accelerator's collimating jaws) should be used instead of physical wedges, especially for younger patients, as the increased scatter from a physical wedge has been suggested to increase the likelihood of inducing a secondary cancer years after the WBI treatment. For patients with larger breasts, the use of wedged fields may not be sufficient to achieve dose homogeneity to the breast [12], and a field-in-field technique may be necessary.

9.6.2 Hypofractionated Whole Breast Irradiation and Boost Irradiation

If a boost to the post-lumpectomy site is prescribed, a concurrent, concomitant, or simultaneous integrated boost (SIB) is preferable to a sequential boost, as the former retains the overall fraction-reducing and time-saving benefit of a hypofractionated radiotherapy course. An SIB treatment is practical provided that the lumpectomy bed does not change volume or migrate during the treatment course. Within a given fraction, the boost may be administered in the form of a dedicated electron field, a set of dedicated 3DCRT photon fields, or as part of an overall IMRT administration. For an electron boost, the energy of the electron beam is determined by the maximum depth of the lumpectomy PTV. For 3DCRT or IMRT boosts, the GTV-to-PTV margin will be receded to 5 mm distal to the skin surface so as to avoid skin reactions from the boost fields. In practice, for a SIB plan, the WBI portion of the plan creation is the most time consuming, since additional effort to reduce dose to the lungs, heart, and contralateral breast is often required for the WBI portion of the plan, whereas planning for the boost volume is usually straightforward [5]. If non-SIB plans are created separately for the WBI and boost volumes, the boost can be delivered either sequentially or simultaneously with appropriate MU scaling [5], subject to the limits of virtual-wedge minimum MU, MU per IMRT segment, or MU per control point for VMAT.

9.6.3 Inverse-Planned Radiation Therapy (Intensity-Modulated Radiation Therapy, Helical Tomotherapy, and Volumetric Modulated Arc Therapy)

Intensity-modulated radiation therapy (IMRT) techniques are expected to provide better dose uniformity than conventional wedged-field treatments [12]. Indeed, dose *uniformity* to the ipsilateral breast is better using IMRT techniques than using conventional 3DCRT techniques, although the dose *conformity* from both techniques is not significantly different [5]. For SIB treatments, hypofractionated or otherwise, the inherently nonuniform intensity profiles from IMRT may facilitate conformal boost-volume coverage and uniform dose distribution outside the boost volume.

In practice, for IMRT planning, it is more difficult to spare the heart from larger volumes of lower dose for left-sided breast cases than for right-sided cases, and it is more difficult to spare the lungs from larger volumes of lower doses. This is of concern since larger relative volumes of the lung receiving doses even as low as 5 Gy correlate with the incidence of radiation pneumonitis [26, 27], a condition that tends to become apparent several months after irradiation. However, there are indications that IMRT can lead to reduced skin dose and thus a reduced likelihood of radiation dermatitis [19].

For IMRT techniques, the field orientations are still typically tangent-like, as this is effective in reducing the OAR doses; however, protocols such as RTOG 1005 allow for non-tangential IMRT beams to be used [5]. Tangential IMRT planning was found to yield reduced V_{20Gy} to the lung in comparison to conventional wedged 3DCRT tangent fields [6, 10, 16].

Lower-energy photons, of the order of 6 MV, are typically used for IMRT treatments [5], although energies up to 10 MV are also considered depending upon the chest wall separation [10]. For 10 MV photons, a beam spoiler may be used to accommodate the increased buildup depth from the skin surface to the depth of maximum dose (d_{max}), which for 10 MV photons is approximately 2 cm. Higher-energy photon beams (15 MV and above) are not recommended for IMRT, given the increased peripheral photoneutron production inside the head of the linac.

Helical tomotherapy, a photon IMRT technique in which the gantry and radiation source rotate continuously around the patient while the patient couch moves through the gantry bore, has been applied to HWBI incorporating a SIB [21]. The TomoTherapy Hi-Art system (Accuray, Inc., Madison, Wisconsin) also includes an on-board fan-beam megavoltage CT (MVCT). While a non-flat 6 MV photon beam is used for treatment, the beam energy used for MVCT imaging is reduced to 3.25 MV, which is intended to slightly improve the contrast resolution. Although distinguishing the post-lumpectomy seroma from the surrounding breast tissue can be challenging with MVCT, if radio-opaque postsurgical clips are present, they can be readily seen in MVCT without the streaking artifacts that can arise in kilovoltage CT (kVCT).

As with fixed-gantry IMRT techniques, a challenge for tomotherapy is to reduce the large volumes of integral dose throughout the lungs, heart, and contralateral breast. One way to achieve this during the planning process is to designate these

OARs as either "directional blocks," such that the direct beam cannot pass through the OAR before reaching the target volume, although the opposite trajectory is allowed, or as "complete blocks," such that the direct beam cannot pass through the OAR under any circumstance. For complete blocking, in principle the OAR would receive only scatter dose; however, the ability to cover the PTV conformally and uniformly may be severely constrained.

The primary determinants of the treatment time per fraction for a tomotherapy plan are the longitudinal (table motion) extent of the PTV (which depends upon the specific patient), the dose rate at isocenter (approximately 900 cGy per minute for most TomoTherapy Hi-Art systems), the dose per fraction (which will be higher for hypofractionated treatments), and the longitudinal jaw size. A larger jaw size (e.g., 5 cm) will reduce the treatment time, since a larger volume of the PTV will be irradiated per gantry rotation; however, a smaller jaw size allows for better dose conformity to the PTV. The pitch, which is defined as the ratio of the distance the couch travels during one gantry rotation to the longitudinal width of the jaw at isocenter, does not have as much effect upon the delivery time; if a smaller pitch is used, more gantry rotations are required to cover the PTV but less dose is required per rotation; thus, the tomotherapy system can compensate for reduced pitch by increasing the gantry rotation speed. Obviously the pitch must be less than 1; a larger pitch would require a scatter dose contribution to in order to cover the PTV, which may not be deliverable by the tomotherapy system. To minimize the "threading" artifact (the dose ripple that arises at the patient's periphery due to beam divergence), a pitch of 0.86/n, where n is a positive integer, is recommended [13]. For most WBI and HWBI plans, a pitch of 0.287 works well.

The TomoTherapy planning system requires that, in the instance of multiple planning target volumes (PTVs) receiving different prescribed doses (as is the case with SIB), only one of the target structures can be designated as a "hard constraint," such that the planning system forces the dose-volume histogram (DVH) through that constraint. In practice, for a SIB plan, designating the lumpectomy PTV (the higher-dose target volume) as the hard constraint generally yielded good dose uniformity to both the lumpectomy PTV and the rest of the ipsilateral breast [21].

Volumetric modulated arc therapy (VMAT) is a photon IMRT delivery technique similar to helical tomotherapy, except that the couch is stationary during delivery and multiple modulated arcs may be superimposed upon each other. As with helical tomotherapy, VMAT is also capable of delivering HWBI with SIB. Scorsetti et al. [22] reported their experiences with using the Varian RapidArc system (Varian Medical Systems, Palo Alto, California). VMAT plans were comprised of two partial arcs, straddling the "classical" medical tangent direction and the posterior entrances through the boost-PTV side. Minimizing the gantry angle range over which the arc is delivered is expected to reduce the dose to the contralateral breast, lungs, and heart, as well as reduce the treatment delivery time per fraction. Using the Varian RapidArc system has the additional advantage of on-board kilovoltage cone beam CT (kVCBCT) for IGRT.

With regard to the use of IMRT for gated HWBI delivery, at this time this can be done in conjunction with static-gantry step-and-shoot IMRT (as with Siemens systems), but not for dynamic arc therapy procedures such as Siemens mARC, Elekta VMAT, or TomoTherapy.

9.6.4 Non-flat Photon Beams

Removing the flattening filter from a linac-produced photon beam's path results in increased photon fluence near the beam's central axis, which may enable a reduced treatment time per fraction; this is a consideration for larger prescribed dose per fraction, as is the case with HWBI. Although the delivery time may be reduced, it might not necessarily lead to a reduced number of MU per fraction. Wang et al. [29] compared WBI plans using only flat photon beams with those that include a non-flat component, where the reference doses for both flat and non-flat beams were set to 1 cGy per MU. They reported that the plans using entirely non-flat beams required 63 % more MU per fraction than did the conventional plans using only flat beams. An increased number of MU corresponds to an increased amount of scatter from the linac's MLCs, which could potentially increase the amount of peripheral scatter radiation upon the patient. It should be noted that the increased scatter from the MLCs could be offset in part by a reduction in scatter, penumbra, and out-of-field dose from the linac treatment head that would have otherwise arisen from the flattening filter [2, 7]. Also, given that neutron production is reduced for high-energy FFF beams [15], such beams might be applicable to breast planning in instances where increased penetration depth is needed.

Without a flattening filter, achieving a uniform dose distribution within the whole breast requires some form of beam profile modulation, using either compensating filters or multiple field segments. Forward planning, using wedges or field-in-field techniques, may be impractical for FFF beams; thus inverse planning techniques are more commonly used instead. Note that the 6 MV photon beam from the TomoTherapy Hi-Art system is inherently non-flat. It is possible to combine classical tangent fields using photon beams (as open fields) with IMRT-planned non-flat tangent beams to correct for dose inhomogeneities present when using the open tangent fields alone [29]. The IMRT component can be optimized using the dose distributions of the primary tangent fields as a background. Note that the open tangent fields could utilize either flat or non-flat photon beams.

9.7 Managing Patient Position and Organ Motion for Hypofractionated Whole Breast Irradiation

Since the delivery time per fraction for HWBI treatments can be expected to be longer, additional measures to ensure reproducible patient setup and reduction (or accommodation) of organ motion are essential.

9.7.1 Immobilization

For supine patient positioning, orienting the patient's arms superiorly is essential to keep the arm clear of the proposed treatment fields, whether classical tangent-like fields or more generalized step-and-shoot IMRT or arc therapy fields are used. If only a single-sided breast treatment is planned, it may be sufficient to place only the ipsilateral arm superiorly. An alpha cradle with a 10–15° wedged breast board placed underneath is usually sufficient for classical tangent 3DCRT HWBI treatments [10]. For tomotherapy treatments, however, Rong et al. [21] reported that the breast-board tilt was unnecessary and that the reproducibility of such devices may not be ideal. Vac-Loc or Body Fix immobilizers, similar to what is used for stereotactic body radiation therapy (SBRT), may allow better setup reproducibility [21].

9.7.2 Prone Versus Supine Positioning

Having the patient lie in a prone position with the ipsilateral breast allowed to suspend downward increases the distance between the ipsilateral breast and the chest wall, which should improve the sparing of the lung and heart [5, 8, 17]. Separation of the ipsilateral breast from the heart is especially important for treatment of the left breast. Prone positioning may also reduce the motion of the breast due to breathing that would otherwise arise for supine-positioned patients.

Formenti et al. [9] compared treatment plans for patients for whom simulation CT scans were acquired in both the prone and supine positions. They defined the posterior (chest wall) edge of the field along a line connecting the patient midline with the anterior extent of the ipsilateral latissimus dorsi muscle. For their prone plans, they reported that the volume of irradiated lung was less among all patients and that the volume of irradiated heart was less for 85 % of all left-breast patients.

There are some contingencies to consider with regard to prone positioning. Electron boosts may not be possible for prone-positioned patients, due to a lack of clearance of the electron applicator with the couch or transmission of the electron beam through the couch top or the prone breast board [5]. Also, prone positioning may displace the ipsilateral breast farther from the center of the patient, thus requiring a greater shift from the initial setup position if CT-based IGRT is used. If the ipsilateral breast is placed at either the CT or tomotherapy isocenter, however, the patient may not clear the gantry bore.

9.7.3 Motion-Correlated Treatment Techniques

Intrafraction motion of the breast due to breathing may be accommodated by having the patient perform a breath-hold (either voluntarily or using spirometry) while the beam is on or by gating the beam-on time to coincide with a specific organ geometry condition (corresponding to a specific respiratory phase). As breath-hold or gated radiotherapy requires additional treatment time per fraction, the additional time increase may be offset in part by increasing the dose rate via removal of the flattening filter [29]. The success of any motion-correlated simulation or treatment depends upon the repeatability and reproducibility of the respiratory motion, both intrafractional and interfractional.

Thoracic motion may be quantified within the simulation image acquired for planning, using cine image acquisition (e.g., 4D-CT) or gated image acquisition (e.g., respiratory-gated or cardiac-gated CT scanning). Respiratory-gated image acquisition can use the motion of an external marker whose motion correlates with respiration; an example is a reflective marker placed on the patient's anterior surface, as is done with the Varian RPM system (Varian Medical Systems, Palo Alto, California). Also, the expansion and contraction of an elastic band encircling the patient's thorax or abdomen can also correlated with patient motion; this technique is used with the Anzai system (Anzai Medical Company, Limited, Tokyo, Japan). Cardiac-gated image acquisition can use an electrocardiographic (ECG) signal.

An advantage of breath-hold techniques is the reduction of dose to the heart, especially for left-breast cases. For supine-positioned patients, the heart (and thus the LADA) can be spatially separated from the breast at the end-inhalation phase of respiration, hence an interest in breast patient simulation and planning using deep inspiration breath-hold (DIBH). Wang et al. [28] reported that the separation between the proximal edge of the heart and the breast tangents' distal edge varied negligibly during a DIBH, but the LADA's position relative to the fields varied substantially over the cardiac cycle. Based upon the observation that less than 10 % of the LADA volume moved by more than 5 mm among half of DIBH patients, a margin of ≥5 mm between the LADA and the treatment fields' posterior edge is recommended in clinical practice.

9.7.4 Image-Guided Radiation Therapy

Image-guided radiation therapy (IGRT) techniques such as cone beam computed tomography (CBCT) may play a role in motion management for HWBI. IGRT beams will contribute an additional low dose to the entire contralateral breast, lung, and heart; however, reducing the number of fractions will reduce the contribution of dose due to IGRT imaging. Non-radiographic IGRT techniques such as magnetic resonance (MR) or ultrasound will contribute no additional radiation dose. However, MR is contraindicated if there are metallic postsurgical clips from the lumpectomy procedure, limiting the utility of MR-guided IGRT for SIB treatments. Also, correct registration between the coordinate systems of the MR scanner and the linac is essential, although the advent of integrated MR-linac systems will resolve this in part. Ultrasound-guided IGRT may be an option if either the postsurgical clips or the interface between the chest wall and the lung can be readily identified.

Given the substantial lateral displacement of the breast, the patient will likely need to receive an IGRT scan in a different location from the treatment position. The requirement for such a large shift beyond that indicated by the IGRT scan itself may potentially introduce systematic error. If IMRT techniques are used, IGRT is essential to assure the clinicians that the highly conformal planned dose distributions are correctly and reliably delivered.

9.7.5 Adaptive Radiation Therapy

An advantage of a shorter treatment course due to fewer fractions is that there is less time for interfractional changes to arise during the treatment course. Thus, for HWBI there is less likelihood for the need for adaptive planning. If an adaptive plan is required, non-rigid image registration and dose deformation techniques are needed, as is IMRT planning to account for dose heterogeneities from the previous fractions.

9.8 Comparisons of Hypofractionated Whole Breast Irradiation with Partial Breast Irradiation

Partial breast irradiation (PBI) also offers shorter overall treatment duration, with the added advantage of reduced dose to regional OARs relative to WBI. However, the long-term results of PBI are still pending, and currently the enrollment criteria for patients undergoing PBI are still rather strict [10]. The question remains whether there is subclinical disease in the ipsilateral breast outside the lumpectomy cavity which, if not addressed with radiation therapy, may lead to a recurrence. Aside from additional skin reactions and increased dose to OARs, HWBI with a fractionation scheme similar to PBI is not expected to be more burdensome to the patient than PBI, with regard to positioning or immobilization.

9.9 Physics Aspects of Various Hypofractionated Whole Breast Irradiation Clinical Trials

Among the earliest HWBI techniques was the Canadian protocol which prescribed a total physical dose of 4256 cGy to the breast in 16 fractions. One possible reason why the Canadian protocol was originally not widely adopted in the United States and Europe is the absence of a boost [10]. Eighty-five percent of radiation oncologists surveyed in the United States and 75 % of radiation oncologists surveyed in Europe during 2001 and 2002 responded that they prescribe additional dose to a boost volume following WBI, even if the lumpectomy resection margins were negative [3]. Both the United Kingdom START A and START B trials allowed participants to prescribe a standard-fractionation sequential boost treatment following HWBI; however, the boost was not part of the protocol therapy.

9.9.1 Radiation Therapy Oncology Group Protocol 1005

In May, 2011, the Radiation Therapy Oncology Group (RTOG) protocol RTOG 1005 began enrolling patients to compare standard WBI followed by a sequential boost with HWBI including a simultaneous boost. Patients randomized to Arm I were prescribed conventional WBI of 50 Gy in 25 fractions (2 Gy per fraction) or hypofractionated WBI 42.7 Gy in 16 fractions to the whole breast followed by a sequential boost volume receiving an additional 2 Gy per fraction over 6 or 7 fractions (total physical boost dose of 12 Gy or 14 Gy). Patients randomized to Arm II were prescribed HWBI of 40.05 Gy in 15 fractions (2.67 Gy per fraction) with a SIB of 3.2 Gy per fraction to the boost volume; the boost volume would thus receive a total physical dose of 48 Gy.

Chen et al. [5] compared several combinations of WBI and boost-volume plan techniques that could be applied to patients enrolled in RTOG 1005. These combinations are as follows:

(1) 3DCRT WBI + 3DCRT boost
(2) 3DCRT WBI + electron boost
(3) 3DCRT WBI + IMRT boost
(4) IMRT WBI + 3DCRT boost
(5) IMRT WBI + electron boost
(6) IMRT WBI + IMRT boost
(7) IMRT SIB

Techniques (1) through (6) could be applied for patients in either Arm I or Arm II, whereas technique (7) was applicable for Arm II plans only. The protocol allows non-tangential beams. For the ipsilateral breast, the breast PTV was obtained from a 7 mm expansion of the breast CTV, excluding the heart and not crossing midline. The breast PTV-Eval volume was obtained by editing the breast PTV to exclude regions exterior to the patient surface, 5 mm distal to the skin surface, and the anterior surface of the ribs.

With regard to dose to the heart, Chen et al. [5] reported that although the mean dose to the heart tended to be higher for left-breast cases, there were no obvious differences among the seven different planning techniques investigated within RTOG 1005.

9.10 Conclusion

Hypofractionated WBI offering socioeconomic benefits is increasingly used in the clinic. Physics issues specific to HWBI include the need of 3D imaging-based conformal treatment planning, the changes of normal tissue dose-volume constraints, the consideration of motion management for intrafraction variations, and the use of IGRT to account for interfractional variations. Considerations of these issues would eventually improve treatment outcome of HWBI.

References

1. Baltas D, Kolotas C, Geramani K, et al. A conformal index (COIN) to evaluate implant quality and dose specification in brachytherapy. Int J Radiat Oncol Biol Phys. 1998;40:515–24.
2. Cashmore J. The characterization of unflattened photon beams from a 6 MV linear accelerator. Phys Med Biol. 2008;53:1933–46.
3. Ceilley E, Jagsi R, Goldberg S, et al. Radiotherapy for invasive breast cancer in North America and Europe: results of a survey. Int J Radiat Oncol Biol Phys. 2005;61:365–73.
4. Chen GP, Ahunbay E, Li XA. Automated computer optimization for 3D treatment planning of breast irradiation. Med Phys. 2008;35:2253–8.
5. Chen GP, Liu F, White J, et al. A planning comparison of 7 irradiation options allowed in RTOG 1005 for early-stage breast cancer. Med Dosim. 2015;40:21–5.
6. Chui C, Hong L, Hunt M, et al. A simplified intensity modulated radiation therapy technique for the breast. Med Phys. 2002;29:522–9.
7. Dalaryd M, Kragl G, Ceberg C, et al. A Monte Carlo study of a flattening filter-free linear accelerator verified with measurements. Phys Med Biol. 2010;55:7333–44.
8. Formenti SC, Gidea-Addeo D, Goldberg JD, et al. Phase I-II trial of prone accelerated intensity modulated radiation therapy to the breast to optimally spare normal tissue. J Clin Oncol. 2007;25:2236–42.
9. Formenti SC, DeWyngaert JK, Jozsef G, et al. Prone vs supine positioning for breast cancer radiotherapy. J Am Med Assoc. 2012;308:861–3.
10. Freedman GM, Anderson PR, Bleicher RJ, et al. Five-year local control in a phase II study of hypofractionated intensity modulated radiation therapy with an incorporated boost for early stage breast cancer. Int J Radiat Oncol Biol Phys. 2012;84:888–93.
11. Gagliardi G, Constine LS, Moiseenko V, et al. Radiation dose-volume effects in the heart. Int J Radiat Oncol Biol Phys. 2010;76:S77–85.
12. Holloway CL, Panet-Raymond V, et al. Hypofractionation should be the new 'standard' for radiation therapy after breast conserving surgery. Breast. 2010;19:163–7.
13. Kissick MW, Fenwick J, James JA, et al. The helical tomotherapy thread effect. Med Phys. 2005;32:1414–23.
14. Knöös T, Kristensen I, Nilsson P. Volumetric and dosimetric evaluation of radiation treatment plans: radiation conformity index. Int J Radiat Oncol Biol Phys. 1998;42:1169–76.
15. Kry SF, Titt U, Ponisch F, et al. Reduced neutron production through use of a flattening-filter-free accelerator. Int J Radiat Oncol Biol Phys. 2007;68:1260–4.
16. Li JS, Freedman GM, Price R, et al. Clinical implementation of intensity-modulated tangential beam irradiation for breast cancer. Med Phys. 2004;31:1023–31.
17. Lymberis SC, Dewyngaert JK, Parhar P, et al. Prospective assessment of optimal individual position (prone versus supine) for breast radiotherapy: volumetric and dosimetric correlations in 100 patients. Int J Radiat Oncol Biol Phys. 2012;84:902–9.
18. Marks LB, Bentzen SM, Deasy JO, et al. Radiation dose-volume effects in the lung. Int J Radiat Oncol Biol Phys. 2010;76:S70–6.
19. Pignol JP, Olivotto I, Rakovitch E, et al. A multicenter randomized trial of breast intensity-modulated radiation therapy to reduce acute radiation dermatitis. J Clin Oncol. 2008;26:2085.
20. Qi XS, White J, Li XA. Is α/β for breast cancer really low? Radiother Oncol. 2011;100:282–8.
21. Rong Y, Fahner T, Welsh JS. Hypofractionated breast and chest wall irradiation using simultaneous in-field boost IMRT delivered via helical tomotherapy. Tech Cancer Res Treat. 2008;7:433–9.
22. Scorsetti M, Alongi F, Fogliata A, et al. Phase I-II study of hypofractionated simultaneous integrated boost using volumetric modulated arc therapy for adjuvant radiation therapy in breast cancer patients: a report of feasibility and early toxicity results in the first 50 treatments. Radiat Oncol. 2012;7:145–52.
23. Solin LJ, Danoff BF, Schwartz GF, et al. A practical technique for the localization of the tumour volume in definitive irradiation of the breast. Int J Radiat Oncol Biol Phys. 1985;11:1215–20.

24. van't Riet A, Mak ACA, Moerland MA, et al. Conformation number to quantify the degree of conformality in brachytherapy and external beam irradiation: application to the prostate. Int J Radiat Oncol Biol Phys. 1996;37:731–6.
25. Wang X, Zhang X, Dong L, et al. Effectiveness of noncoplanar IMRT planning using a parallelized multiresolution beam angle optimization method for paranasal sinus carcinoma. Int J Radiat Oncol Biol Phys. 2005;63:594–601.
26. Wang S-L, Liao Z, Vaporciyan AA, et al. Investigation of clinical and dosimetric factors associated with postoperative pulmonary complications in esophageal cancer patients treated with concurrent chemoradiotherapy followed by surgery. Int J Radiat Oncol Biol Phys. 2006;64:692–9.
27. Wang S, Liao Z, Wei X, et al. Analysis of clinical and dosimetric factors associated with treatment-related pneumonitis (TRP) in patients with non-small-cell lung cancer (NSCLC) treated with concurrent chemotherapy and three-dimensional conformal radiotherapy (3D-CRT). Int J Radiat Oncol Biol Phys. 2006;66:1399–407.
28. Wang X, Pan T, Pinnix C, et al. Cardiac motion during deep-inspiration breath-hold: implications for breast cancer radiotherapy. Int J Radiat Oncol Biol Phys. 2012;82:708–14.
29. Wang Y, Vassil A, Tendulkar R, et al. Feasibility of using nonflat photon beams for whole-breast irradiation with breath hold. J Appl Clin Med Phys. 2014;15:57–64.

Chapter 10
New York University Experience and Prone Positioning

Onyinye Balogun and Silvia Formenti

Contents

O. Balogun • S. Formenti (✉)
Department of Radiation Oncology, Weill Cornell Medicine/
New York Presbyterian Hospital,
525 E 68th St, New York, NY 10065, USA
e-mail: onyi.balogun@gmail.com; formenti@med.cornell.edu

D.W. Arthur et al. (eds.), *Short Course Breast Radiotherapy: A Comprehensive Review of Hypofractionation, Partial Breast, and Intra-Operative Irradiation*,
DOI 10.1007/978-3-319-24388-7_10

10.1 Introduction

Prone positioning presents several advantages over standard supine positioning for breast irradiation. First, treatment in the prone position drastically reduces the respiratory excursion of the chest and enables better exclusion of the heart and lung from the trajectory of the tangent beams, resulting in consistent dosimetric advantages in sparing normal tissue. Moreover, with gravity displacing the breast from the prone chest wall, the incidence and severity of acute and late adverse skin effects at the inframammary fold are reduced, particularly for women with large and/or pendulous breasts. Originally devised at the University of Southern California [1], the prone breast irradiation program has been studied and further defined at New York University [2]. The rapidly identified dosimetric advantages of prone breast treatment facilitated methodic testing of the feasibility and efficacy of hypofractionated regimens. Over more than a decade, several prospective trials have investigated the optimal prescription dose/fractionation to the whole breast, the timing of lumpectomy bed boost, and the efficacy of prone partial breast irradiation.

10.2 Rationale for Prone Patient Positioning

Beginning in the 1990s, several attempts were made to improve dose homogeneity and thereby mitigate the skin toxicity and poor cosmesis associated with radiation therapy for patients with large breasts. Some of these approaches included treating patients in the lateral decubitus position [3] and using thermoplastic molds to shift lateral breast tissue anteriorly and superiorly [4]. An alternative was to treat patients in the prone position. Prone positioning exploits gravity's ability to displace the tissue of the index breast away from the chest. This decreases breast separation and dose inhomogeneity. In addition, once displaced from wrapping around the chest, the whole breast can be targeted using opposed tangent fields that avoid the lungs and heart. Preliminary studies of prone positioning confirmed its feasibility and tolerability. Also, dose homogeneity was improved and cosmetic and clinical outcomes of local control and overall survival were comparable to traditional supine treatment [5].

10.2.1 NYU 05–181: A Prospective Trial Comparing Supine and Prone Positions

During a trial of prone accelerated intensity-modulated radiotherapy [6], preliminary evidence emerged that prone positioning could achieve unprecedented exclusion of the heart and lung from the radiation field. Therefore, prone positioning could be the optimal way to irradiate most breast cancer patients. From 2006 to

2008, NYU 05–181, a prospective trial, was undertaken to test this hypothesis. In order to determine the optimal radiation treatment position for each individual, 400 women with stage 0–IIA breast cancer and negative margins after lumpectomy were accrued. Patients consented to undergo two CT planning sessions, one in the prone and one in the supine position [7]. The optimal position was defined as that which best encompassed the contoured breast volume and tumor bed while minimizing the volume of heart and lung tissue in the treatment field. Patients who had received previous radiation therapy to the ipsilateral breast, more than 3 positive lymph nodes or active connective tissue disorders, were excluded.

Based on the assessment of both sets of CT images, the majority of patients (91 %) were treated prone. Among the 200 right breast cancer patients, the prone position was superior in sparing lung volume in 98 % (195/200) and reduced the volume of lung in the treatment field on average by 107 cc (SD 75, range 0–463 cc) (Fig. 10.1a–b). In the five patients treated supine, the choice for supine treatment

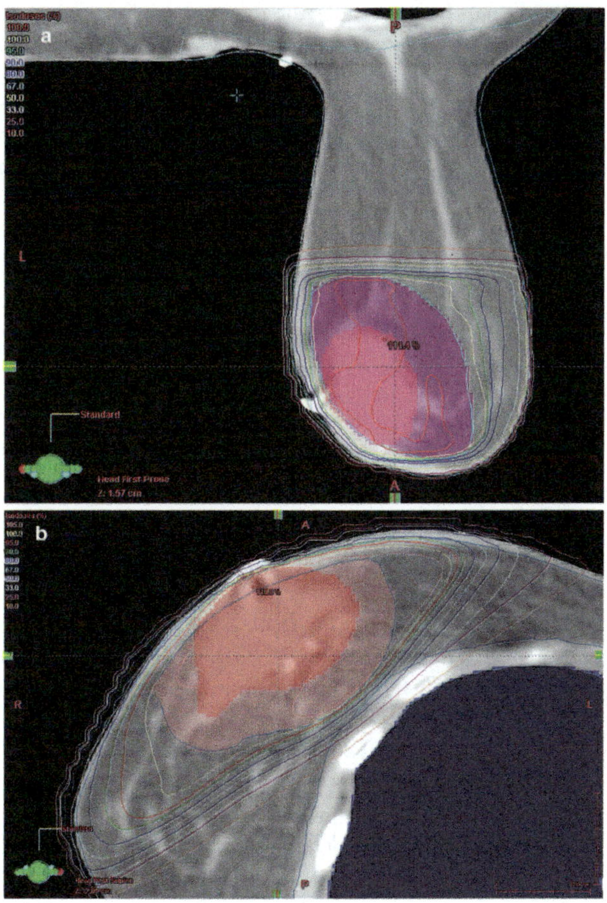

Fig. 10.1 (**a**, **b**) A patient with cancer in the right breast positioned in both the prone (**a**) and supine (**b**) positions. When prone, the cavity breast away from the chest wall by gravity, allowing treatment of the breast using opposed tangent fields and maximal sparing of the lungs

was based on the patient's preference since there was no significant difference in lung sparing between the supine and prone positions.

Among the 200 left breast cancer patients, the prone position was optimal in 85 % (170/200), with lung volume reduced by a mean of 93 cc (SD 72, range 9–334 cc) and heart volume reduced on average by 11 cc (SD 23, range 0–220 cc). However, in 15 % of left breast patients, the best position to reduce the volume of the heart in the treatment field was supine, reducing on average by 6 cc (SD 8, range 0–41 cc). Prone positioning was more likely to be the optimal choice regardless of breast size. Among patients with A/B cup size (<750 cc breast volume), 83 % were better treated prone (125/151). For C cup (>750 cc and <1500 cc) and D cup (>1500 cc) patients, the prone position was optimal in 96 % (168/175) and 99 % (73/74), respectively.

Sparing of the heart and lung tissue is particularly significant, given evidence from the Early Breast Cancer Trialists' Collaborative Group (EBCTCG) demonstrates that traditional radiotherapy, delivered with the patient in the supine position, increases both cardiac morbidity and the incidence of lung cancer [8]. Moreover, recent data indicates that as the mean heart dose increases, there is a dose-dependent rise in the risk of ischemic heart disease [9]. This adverse effect is present within 5 years after radiotherapy and persists up to 30 years after undergoing treatment.

Additionally, positioning patients prone considerably reduces the breast tissue motion associated both with cardiac systole and respiration [10]. Using CINE imaging to capture patient positioning during treatment, over 4,000 EPID images were evaluated for motion for ten patients treated with 15 fractions. In the prone position, intrafraction movement was limited to a mean value of 0.13 cm, with a 95 % confidence interval of 0.12–0.15 cm [11]. Morrow et al. [12] obtained similar results for women in the prone position as did Becker et al. [13] using 4D-CT analysis. Both authors showed reduced motion in the prone position compared to the supine position.

10.2.2 Algorithms for Predicting the Optimal Position: Supine versus Prone

A secondary objective of NYU 05–181 was the development of an algorithm to predict optimal positioning for treatment. In this trial, the supine position was superior in 15 % of left breast patients. A two-step process was employed to review 198 of the 200 left breast patients [14]. First, patients were divided into two groups based on their in-field heart volume in the prone position. The prone position was designated the preferred treatment position for patients with in-field heart volume < or = 0.1 cc (n = 149). Forty-nine patients with in-field heart volume >0.1 cc were further classified using a weighted support vector machine (SVM) that maximized specificity while preserving sensitivity. Three geometric features, (1) heart orientation about the right-to-left axis, (2) the distance between the heart and tumor, and (3) volume of lung within the treatment field, were also determined to provide the best accuracy. Using this two-stage process, only 9.6 % of patients required a second CT scan in the supine position to confirm their optimal position (Fig. 10.2).

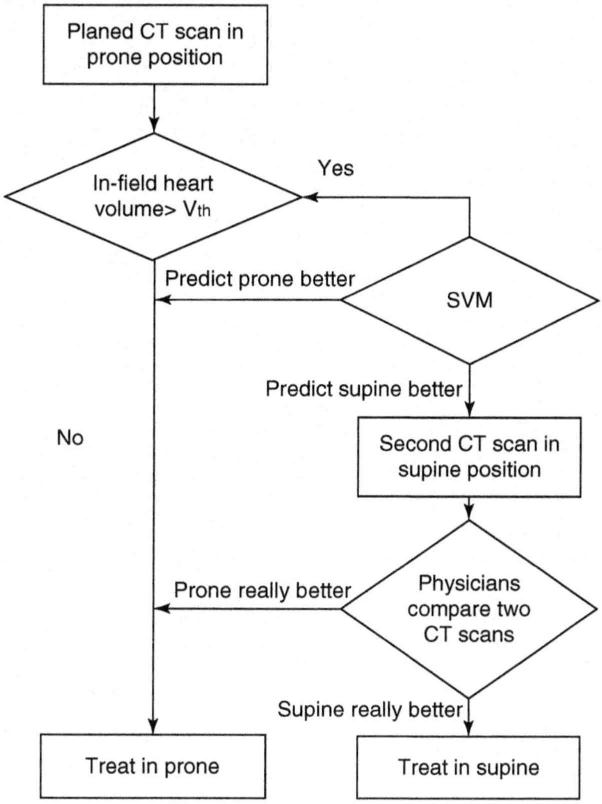

Fig. 10.2 Flow chart of two-step classification process for left breast cancer patients. Vth (0.1 cc) is a threshold volume to initially distinguish patients who may be optimally treated in the supine position

10.3 The Evolution of Prone Breast Board Design

A prone setup requires adequate support and immobilization for planning and treatment.

To this aim, multiple sequential solutions were tested ranging from basic Styrofoam cutouts to engineered modifications of the treatment couch [15]. Commonly, commercially available "breast boards" are used, and their design has evolved over time with the twofold goal of optimizing daily reproducibility/immobilization and patient comfort.

An initial model constructed at the University of Southern California featured a wooden platform with its distal end extending over the edge of the treatment couch to enable full couch rotation (Fig. 10.3b). At the level of the breast, there were removable concentric inserts to accommodate different breast sizes. A contralateral insert was placed to close the opening; then the patient was positioned so that the target breast was centered in the ipsilateral opening. This design was only suitable for partial breast treatment because part of the breast was superior to the wooden platform. Also, the patients' arms were kept adjacent to the breast so the ipsilateral arm would have been within the treatment field.

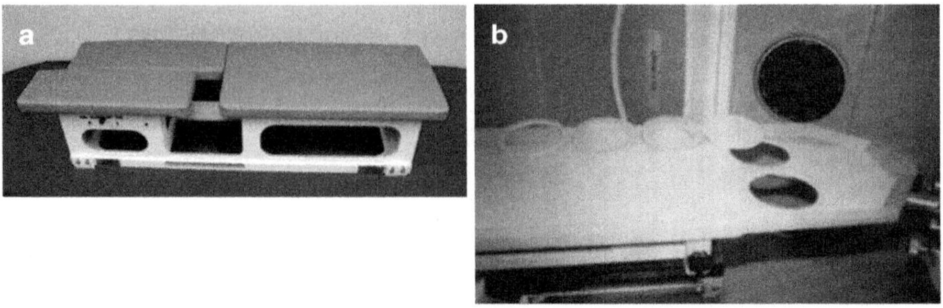

Fig. 10.3 (**a, b**) Prone breast devices developed at MSKCC (**a**) and the University of Southern California (**b**)

Fig. 10.4 Prone breast device developed at NYU. Tangential fields were possible because sidebars were absent. The prone board does not extend over the distal end of the treatment couch. To enhance patient comfort, the arms were raised above the head, and a thin, soft cushion was placed on top of the prone board

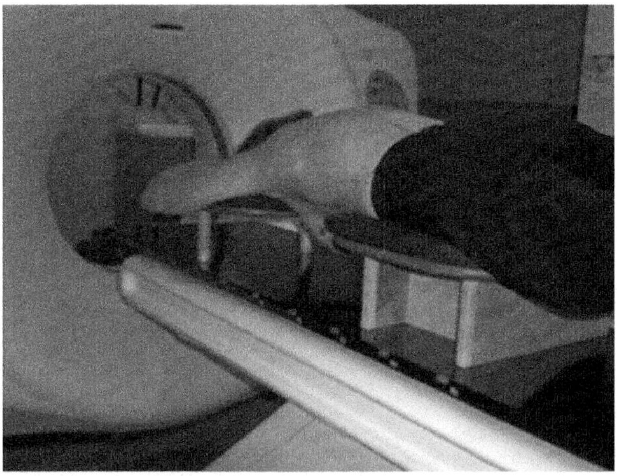

An earlier model from Memorial Sloan-Kettering Cancer Center featured an opening through which the index breast hung (Fig. 10.3a). The size of the opening was adjusted via a sliding insert. The patient's arm was placed at the patient's side or above their head. In addition, a wedge was placed under the contralateral chest to rotate the patient toward the treated breast.

At NYU, the USC model was modified to eliminate the sidebars and to position the patient with their arms up (Fig. 10.4). Although this design improved patient comfort, the wooden board was extremely heavy and difficult to maneuver.

The next version of the NYU prone board aimed to simplify board transport while enhancing patient comfort. It consisted of two 12.5 cm thick Styrofoam lined superiorly with a 2-inch thick memory foam (Fig. 10.5). The board consisted of three elements, connected by VELCRO and modifiable to create an opening on the side of the index breast. The lightweight materials expedited prone board assembly and removal from the treatment couch. In addition, the memory foam enabled reproducibility of the treatment setup since the same degree of compression would be applied by the patient's weight during each radiation therapy session.

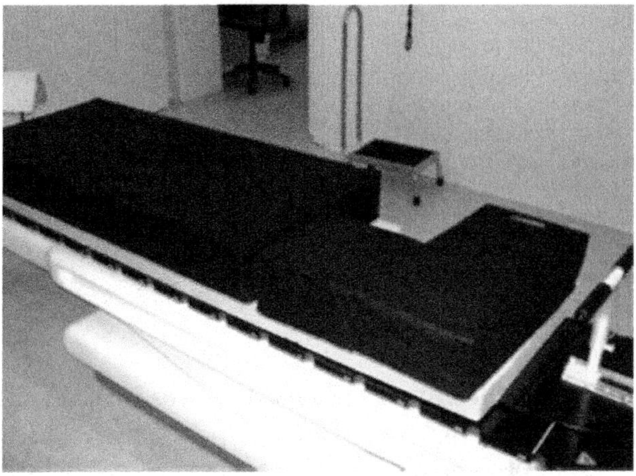

Fig. 10.5 Next-generation prone breast device developed at NYU. A 2-inch thick memory foam layer was placed on top of 12.5 inches of Styrofoam wrapped in a washable vinyl cover

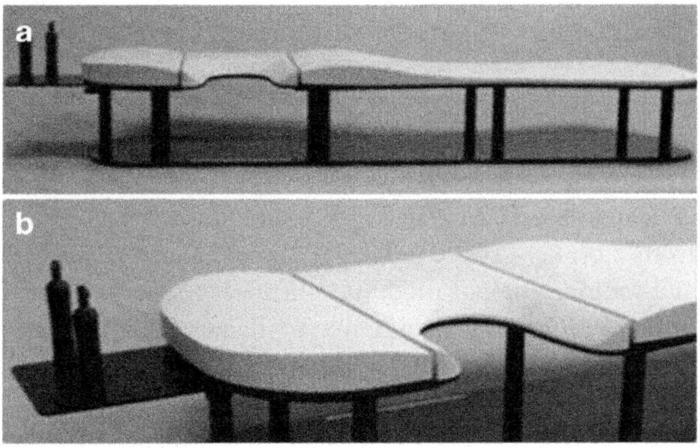

Fig. 10.6 (**a**) The ClearVue™ System (Orbital Therapy): carbon fiber plate and board, soft cover for patient comfort. (**b**) The central segment can be removed and reoriented to accommodate left or right breast patients

However, this model could not be indexed to the treatment couch, and there were no holding bars to maintain the patient's arms and hands in the same position. Verifying accurate positioning using lasers and imaging at regular intervals was essential.

The NYU experience, in part, informed the development of modern-day commercially available devices for prone breast irradiation. The ClearVue™ model (Fig. 10.6a, b) is a lightweight device made of carbon fiber and designed to rest on top of the treatment couch. It provides good access to the breast and visibility for accurate setup. The soft cushion is ergonomically designed for patient comfort. Varian's unit, the Access360™ (Fig. 10.7), functions as an extension of the treatment couch. It is also built of carbon fiber with a soft cushion top. In addition, the supraclavicular region can be visualized before treatment, to ensure exact positioning, via an uncovered section located at the cranial end of the mesh. One limitation is that large-angle superior-oblique fields are not possible since they would cause gantry collision with the arms of the patient.

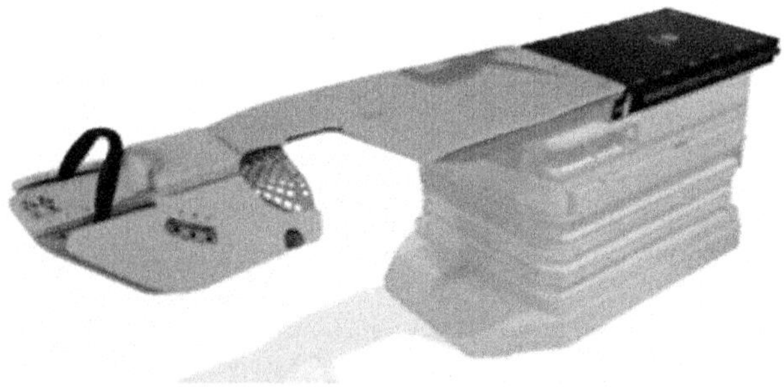

Fig. 10.7 The Access360™ (Varian Medical Systems): built of carbon fiber mesh, with a soft cushion on top. It attaches to the cranial end of the treatment couch. Supraclavicular treatment is possible through an uncovered section of the mesh

10.4 Selection of a Dose Fractionation Scheme for Postoperative Prone Hypofractionated Radiation Therapy

The adoption of hypofractionated regimens for breast irradiation has gradually increased over the past decade. Compared to the traditional 6-week course of 30 treatments, hypofractionated regimens offer both time and cost savings for patients and practitioners. Moreover, there is no apparent difference in clinical efficacy, toxicity, or cosmetic outcome.

Randomized trials in hypofractionated breast irradiation have used doses ranging from 2.66 Gy [16] to 3.3 Gy [17] per fraction. At NYU, we used a tumor α/β of 4 and radiobiological modeling of the biologically effective dose (BED) to design a hypofractionated schedule that replicates tumor control, early and late toxicity rates of 46–50 Gy to the whole breast, and a sequential tumor bed boost of 10–14 Gy. The choice of an α/β of 4 for tumor control is consistent with estimates from RMH/GO3 trial [17] and UK START trials [18, 19] that used a tumor control α/β of 4 and 4.6, respectively (Table 10.1). Based on the linear/quadratic formula, we estimated a prescription dose of 40.5 Gy to the whole breast in 15 fractions (2.7 Gy per fraction) and a concomitant boost of 0.5 Gy to the postoperative tumor bed plus margin for a total of 48 Gy, to achieve biological equivalence to a standard fractionation regiment of 6 weeks, sequentially to the breast and tumor bed.

10.5 Prone Breast Intensity-Modulated Radiation Therapy: 5-Year Results of NYU 03–30 and 05–181

Both the EORTC [20] and Lyon [21] boost trials demonstrated a reduction in the local failure rate with the addition of a 10–16 Gy tumor bed boost to traditional regimens of 50 Gy whole breast irradiation. In initial randomized trials of whole breast hypofractionated radiation therapy, between 43 and 75 % of patients received a tumor bed boost. However, most of these studies delivered the boost sequentially. There is a paucity of data regarding the incorporation of concomitant tumor bed

Table 10.1 Comparison of hypofractionated trial regimens

Trial	Hypofractionated whole breast dose	Tumor bed boost dose	α/β for tumor control
RMH/GO3	39 or 42.9 Gy in 13 fractions	14 Gy in 7 fractions	4
START A	39 or 41.6 Gy in 13 fractions	10 Gy in 5 fractions	4.6
START B	40 Gy in 15 fractions	10 Gy in 5 fractions	4.6
NYU 03–30 and 05-181	40.5 Gy in 15 fractions	7.5 Gy in 15 fractions	4

boost in hypofractionated schedules. At NYU, we designed trials to examine the combination of hypofractionation and a concomitant tumor bed boost.

The first prospective trial, NYU 03–30, was a phase I/II feasibility study of hypofractionated prone whole breast IMRT with a concomitant tumor bed boost. Eligible patients were pre- or postmenopausal women with stage I–II biopsy-proven invasive breast cancer status postlumpectomy with at least 1 mm negative margins. All patients with tumors >5 mm underwent sentinel node and/or axillary lymph node staging. Patients were excluded if more than 8 weeks separated their primary therapy (surgery or chemotherapy) and the start of radiation therapy. A minimum of 2 weeks between the last dose of chemotherapy and the start of radiation therapy was also required for patients who received adjuvant chemotherapy. Systemic therapy was prescribed at the discretion of the medical oncologist.

NYU 05–181, a prospective trial to determine optimal treatment positioning (see Sect. 10.2.1), enrolled patients with similar features. In addition, women with ductal carcinoma in situ (DCIS) were eligible, but sentinel node/axillary lymph node staging was not required for DCIS patients. Women with three or fewer lymph nodes involved by cancer were eligible for both trials. Exclusion criteria included previous radiation therapy to the ipsilateral breast, active connective tissue disorders, or a prior or concurrent malignancy (with the exception of squamous or basal cell skin cancer) unless the patient had been disease-free for more than 5 years.

For both trials, all patients underwent computed tomography (CT) simulation. The planning target volume for the breast (PTV1) was defined as the contoured ipsilateral whole breast (CTV1) reduced by 5 mm in all directions to account for the build-up region at the skin interface and penumbra effects along the posterior, superior, and inferior borders. The lumpectomy cavity (CTV2) with a 1 cm uniform margin defined the concomitant boost volume (PTV2). Delineation of the lumpectomy cavity was guided by all available clinical and radiographic data, including preoperative imaging such as screening/diagnostic mammogram, wire localization or MRI, the seroma cavity on the planning CT, surgical clips placed at the time of surgery, and the lumpectomy scar.

Using multiple beam arrangements, the index breast was treated to 40.5 Gy in 15 fractions at 2.7 Gy per fraction daily, Monday through Friday, over a 3-week interval. During each treatment a concomitant boost of 0.5 Gy was delivered to the tumor bed (total dose to PTV2, 48 Gy). A plane connecting the midline to the anterior surface of the latissimus dorsi muscle on CT defined the posterior edge of the field.

This technique ensured full coverage of the PTV1 regardless of prone or supine positioning. The boost was integrated directly into the IMRT optimization and treatment to intentionally produce a heterogeneous dose distribution within the breast and achieve a higher dose within the PTV2. The optimization and calculations were performed using Helios/Eclipse software. Normal tissue constraints stipulated that no more than 5 % of the heart volume receive >18 Gy and no more than 10 % of the ipsilateral lung receive >20 Gy.

10.5.1 NYU 03–30 and 05–181 Study Population Demographics

Between September 2003 and August 2009, a total of 490 women were enrolled in both the NYU 03–30 and 05–181 trials. The median age of at the time of consent was 56 (range 28–94 years old). Four hundred and four patients had invasive carcinoma (82 %), and 86 patients had DCIS (18 %). Among the 404 patients with invasive cancer, the average tumor size was 12.96 mm. Eighty-three percent of the combined cohort had T1 tumors, and the remaining 17 % had T2 tumors. Stage I was the most prevalent accounting for 72 % of patients, and 25 % had stage IIA cancer. Most patients were node negative (85 %). Eighty-two percent of the women had estrogen receptor-positive disease, and 61 % had progesterone receptor-positive disease. Only 9 % had HER2/Neu-positive invasive disease. Systemic chemotherapy was given to 37 % of patients with invasive disease, and 39 % received antihormonal therapy.

10.5.2 Results: Locoregional Control and Survival

After a median follow-up of 4 years, seven patients (1.4 %) had a locoregional recurrence resulting in a 98.6 % local control rate. Four of the seven recurrences were within the lumpectomy bed, and one was located elsewhere in the breast. The remaining two recurrences were in the ipsilateral supraclavicular and infraclavicular lymph nodes. In addition, 4 patients developed contralateral disease, half were invasive carcinoma, and half were DCIS. Five other patients developed distant metastases. There were 15 deaths with five attributed to breast cancer for a 4-year overall survival rate of 97 %.

We also reported a 5-year update on the 404 women with invasive disease who had participated in NYU 03–30 and 05–181 [22]. At a median follow-up of 60 months, 8 patients had developed an ipsilateral breast recurrence, and 3 patients developed regional recurrence. The number of contralateral breast cancer cases and patients who developed distant metastases were 4 and 5 patients, respectively. Four of the five patients who developed distant disease had stage IIA disease. Fifteen patients died for a 5-year cumulative survival rate of 98.72 %; however, only five patients died of breast cancer.

10.5.3 NYU 03–30 and 05–181 Results: Toxicities

Toxicity was assessed after completion of treatment at 1, 3, 6, and 12 months and then annually to assess long-term sequelae. Acute effects were graded using the Radiation Therapy Oncology Group toxicity criteria, and late effects were categorized using the Late Effects on Normal Tissues/Subjective, Objective, Management, and Analytic criteria (LENT/SOMA). Late toxicities were determined by the treating radiation oncologist or the nurse practitioner. Patients rated their overall cosmesis as excellent, good, fair, or poor at each yearly visit. The most common side effects were as follows: grade 1 pigmentation change, 19 %; grade 1 breast fibrosis, 19 %; grade 1 breast retraction, 5 %; and grade 1 breast telangiectasia, 14 %. Telangiectasia was the most frequent grade 3 toxicity and occurred in 1 % of patients (6 of 404). Less than 6 % of patients experienced grade 2 breast fibrosis, breast retraction, breast edema, or arm lymphedema. Similarly, less than 1 % of patients developed any grade 3 treatment-related toxicity.

Three hundred and seventy-seven women agreed to self-assess their cosmetic result, and the majority (82 %) rated their cosmetic outcome as excellent/good. Although 16 % deemed their cosmesis fair, it is important to note that the majority attributed their cosmetic outcome to the initial surgery, and dissatisfaction with the surgical results was recorded in the medical record prior to initiation of radiotherapy.

Therefore, our trial suggests that concomitant boost during hypofractionated breast irradiation is both feasible and efficacious with acceptable cosmetic results.

10.6 Preliminary Results of WBI Using Two Different Tumor Bed Boost Strategies: NYU Protocol 09–0030

Based on the success of the prone hypofractionated concomitant boost trials, we next tested two different strategies for delivering a lumpectomy bed boost. Radiobiological principles suggest that a weekly boost may be advantageous. In most radiation therapy departments, there is a treatment break for 72 h over the weekend. Tumor repopulation during this interval may diminish the biologic effectiveness of the dose delivered on Friday. Irradiating the tumor bed with a larger dose on Friday could potentially mitigate the detrimental effects of the weekend-long treatment break.

We designed a phase III randomized study to test two different boost arms. The first arm consisted of whole breast radiotherapy with a concomitant boost over the course of 3 weeks that had been evaluated in the studies NYU 03–30 and NYU 05–181. Using an α/β ratio of 4, the BED for this regimen of 3.2 Gy × 15 fractions was 86 Gy_4. For the second arm, we selected a treatment schedule that most closely approximated the BED of the concomitant boost arm. The weekly boost arm consisted of delivering 2.7 Gy five times per week (Monday to Friday) during

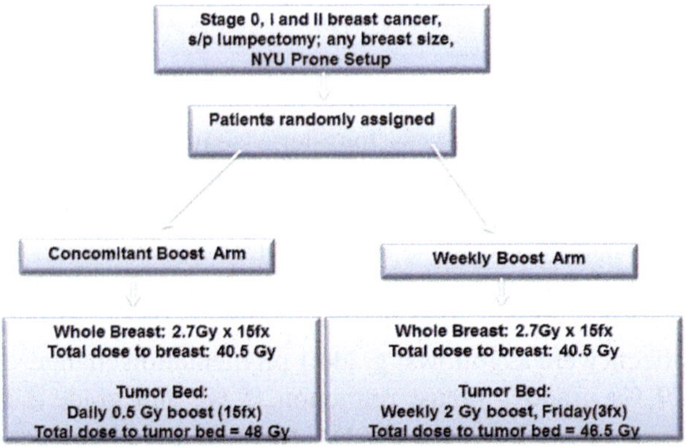

Fig. 10.8 Schema of NYU 09–0030

the 3 weeks (i.e., 2.7 Gy × 15 fractions). On each of the three Fridays, an additional 2 Gy was delivered to the tumor bed in addition to the 2.7 Gy whole breast dose such that the tumor bed received 4.7 Gy on each of the three Fridays (Fig. 10.8). The BED of this regimen was 85 Gy_4 to the tumor bed. Assuming a rate of 10 % grade 2 or greater acute toxicity on the concomitant boost arm, we hypothesized that the proportion of patients with grade 2 or greater acute toxicity on the weekly boost arm would be no more than 15 %. Acute toxicity was defined as occurring within 60 days of the start of radiotherapy.

For this trial, all patients underwent computed tomography (CT) simulation. The planning target volume for the breast (PTV1) was defined as the contoured ipsilateral whole breast (CTV1) reduced by 5 mm in all directions to account for the build-up region at the skin interface and penumbra effects along the posterior, superior, and inferior borders. The lumpectomy cavity (CTV2) with a 1 cm uniform margin defined the concomitant or weekly boost volume (PTV2).

10.6.1 NYU 09–0030 Study Population Demographics

Between 2009 and 2012, 400 women with stage 0–II breast cancer were enrolled on the clinical trial with 202 on the daily boost arm (Arm 1) and 198 on the weekly boost arm (Arm 2). The eligibility criteria were similar to those for the NYU 03–30 and NYU 05–181 studies. The mean age of patients at the time of consent was 56. The majority of patients had T1 tumors (111 on Arm 1 and 130 on Arm 2) with a mean tumor size of 1.5 cm. Estrogen receptor positivity was present in over 80 % of patients' tumors (84.2 % on Arm 1 and 79.3 % on Arm 2), and over 70 % of patients had progesterone receptor-positive disease (73.8 % on Arm 1 and 74.7 % on Arm 2). HER2/Neu overexpression was detected in 9.5 % of patients' tumors. Approximately 12 % of patients on either arm had node-positive disease (11.9 % on Arm 1 and 12.6 % on Arm 2), and 29.8 % received chemotherapy (59 patients on Arm 1 and 60 patients on Arm 2). Nearly half of the patient cohort (48.8 %) received antihormonal therapy. Almost all patients were treated in the prone position with the exception of 4 patients.

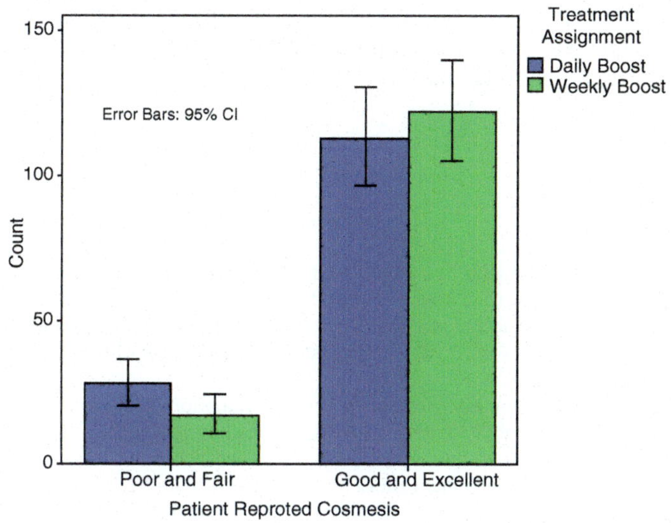

Fig. 10.9 Patient-reported cosmetic outcome according to treatment arm on the NYU 09–0030 trial

10.6.2 NYU 09–0030 Preliminary Results

At 5 years of follow-up, there was no difference in recurrence-free survival between the two arms. Fewer than 10 % of patients experienced grade 2 or higher acute toxicities (21 patients on Arm 1 and 16 patients on Arm 2). The most common side effects were as follows: grade 1 erythema, 83 %; grade 1 breast edema, 24.3 %; grade 1 fibrosis, 8.2 %; and grade 1 retraction/atrophy, 9.5 %. There were no statistically significant differences in the toxicity rates between the two arms. Of 280 women who evaluated their cosmetic result, 84 % rated their outcome as excellent/good (113 on Arm 1 and 122 on Arm 2, Fig. 10.9). These initial results suggest that a weekly tumor bed boost is a viable alternative to daily concomitant boost as it is not associated with a higher rate of acute toxicity, poor cosmetic outcome, or worse recurrence-free survival rate than daily concomitant boost.

10.7 Conclusions

The theoretical advantages of combining prone positioning and hypofractionated radiation therapy were clinically confirmed in multiple prospective clinical trials completed at NYU. Our experience has demonstrated that prone hypofractionated radiation therapy produces acceptable clinical and cosmetic results. Moreover, prone positioning significantly reduces the irradiated heart and lung volume and has a direct impact on the future risk of ischemic heart disease and lung cancer.

Additional follow-up is needed to ensure that the long-term toxicities and clinical outcomes remain comparable to traditional treatments that employ supine positioning and longer treatment schedules.

References

1. Jozsef G, Luxton G, Formenti SC. Application of radiosurgery principles to a target in the breast: a dosimetric study. Med Phys. 2000;27(5):1005–10.
2. Formenti SC, et al. Prone accelerated partial breast irradiation after breast-conserving surgery: preliminary clinical results and dose-volume histogram analysis. Int J Radiat Oncol Biol Phys. 2004;60(2):493–504.
3. Cross MA, Elson HR, Aron BS. Breast conservation radiation therapy technique for women with large breasts. Int J Radiat Oncol Biol Phys. 1989;17(1):199–203.
4. Bentel GC, Marks LB. A simple device to position large/flaccid breasts during tangential breast irradiation. Int J Radiat Oncol Biol Phys. 1994;29(4):879–82.
5. Grann A, Mccormick B, Chabner ES, Gollamudi SV, Schupak KD, Mychalczak BR, Heerdt AS, Merchant TE, Hunt MA. Prone breast radiotherapy in early- stage breast cancer: a preliminary analysis. Int J Radiat Oncol Biol Phys. 2000;47(2):319–25.
6. Formenti SC, et al. Phase I-II trial of prone accelerated intensity modulated radiation therapy to the breast to optimally spare normal tissue. J Clin Oncol. 2007;25(16):2236–42.
7. Formenti S, et al. Results of NYU 05–181: a prospective trial to determine optimal position (prone versus supine) for breast radiotherapy. Int J Radiat Oncol Biol Phys. 2009;75(3):S203–4.
8. Clarke M, et al. Effects of radiotherapy and of differences in the extent of surgery for early breast cancer on local recurrence and 15-year survival: an overview of the randomised trials. Lancet. 2005;366(9503):2087–106.
9. Darby SC, et al. Risk of ischemic heart disease in women after radiotherapy for breast cancer. N Engl J Med. 2013;368(11):987–98.
10. el-Fallah AI, Plantec MB, Ferrara KW. Ultrasonic measurement of breast tissue motion and the implications for velocity estimation. Ultrasound Med Biol. 1997;23(7):1047–57.
11. DeWyngaert JK, Mitchella JD, Alonso-Basanta M, Formenti SC. Intrafraction organ motion in breast radiation therapy: a comparison of prone versus supine patient positioning. Int J Radiat Oncol Biol Phys. 2006;66(3):S177–8.
12. Morrow NV, et al. Intra- and interfractional variations for prone breast irradiation: an indication for image-guided radiotherapy. Int J Radiat Oncol Biol Phys. 2007;69(3):910–7.
13. Becker SJ, Patela RR, Mackie TR. Accelerated partial breast irradiation with helical tomotherapy: prone or supine setup? Int J Radiat Oncol Biol Phys. 2006;66(3):S230.
14. Zhao X, et al. A support vector machine (SVM) or predicting preferred treatment position in radiotherapy of patients with breast cancer. Med Phys. 2010;37(10):5341–50.
15. Huppert N, et al. The role of a prone setup in breast radiation therapy. Front Oncol. 2011;1:31.
16. Whelan TJ, Pignol JP, Levine MN, et al. Long-term results of hypofractionated radiation therapy for breast cancer. N Engl J Med. 2010;362(6):513–20.
17. Owen JR, et al. Effect of radiotherapy fraction size on tumour control in patients with early-stage breast cancer after local excision: long-term results of a randomized trial. Lancet Oncol. 2006;7(6):467–71.
18. START Trialists' Group. The UK Standardization of Breast Radiotherapy (START) trial B of radiotherapy hypofractionation for treatment of early breast cancer: a randomized trial. Lancet. 2008;371(9618):1098–107.
19. START Trialists' Group. The UK Standardization of Breast Radiotherapy (START) trial A of radiotherapy hypofractionation for treatment of early breast cancer: a randomized trial. Lancet Oncol. 2008;9(4):331–41.

20. Bartelink H, et al. Impact of a higher radiation dose on local control and survival in breast-conserving therapy of early breast cancer: 10-year results of the randomized boost versus no boost EORTC 22881–10882 trial. J Clin Oncol. 2007;25(22):3259–65.
21. Romestaing P, et al. Role of a 10-Gy boost in the conservative treatment of early breast cancer: results of a randomized clinical trial in Lyon, France. J Clin Oncol. 1997;15(3):963–8.
22. Osa EO, et al. Prone breast intensity modulated radiation therapy: 5-year results. Int J Radiat Oncol Biol Phys. 2014;89(4):899–906.

Chapter 11
The Canadian Experience with Hypofractionation

Julie Arsenault and Timothy Whelan

Contents

J. Arsenault
Department of Radiation Oncology, Juravinski Cancer Centre,
699 Concession Street, 3rd Floor, Hamilton ON L8V 5C2, Canada
e-mail: jarsenau@hhsc.ca

T. Whelan (✉)
Department of Oncology, McMaster University & Juravinski Cancer Centre,
699 Concession Street, Rm. 4-204, Hamilton ON L8V 5C2, Canada
e-mail: twhelan@hhsc.ca; evansdi@hhsc.ca

D.W. Arthur et al. (eds.), *Short Course Breast Radiotherapy: A Comprehensive Review of Hypofractionation, Partial Breast, and Intra-Operative Irradiation*,
DOI 10.1007/978-3-319-24388-7_11

11.1 Introduction

The majority of women with early breast cancer are now treated with breast-conserving surgery. Randomized trials have demonstrated that whole-breast irradiation (WBI) following breast-conserving surgery reduces the risk of local recurrence and prevents the need for mastectomy [1–4]. More recently the Early Breast Cancer Trialists' Collaborative Group meta-analysis demonstrated that WBI also reduces breast cancer mortality [5].

The majority of trials that evaluated the role of WBI following breast-conserving surgery used conventional fractionation of 50 Gy in 25 daily fractions over a period of 5 weeks with or without a boost to the primary site for 1–1½ weeks [1–3]. Despite the benefits of this approach, it is estimated that a significant proportion of women do not receive WBI following breast-conserving surgery, in part because of the inconvenience and cost of having to come for daily treatments for 5–6 weeks [6]. Over the years, there have been ongoing efforts to reduce treatment morbidity and treatment time in order to improve the overall experience for patients.

Early reports suggested that using larger doses of radiation per fraction (hypofractionated radiotherapy) over a shorter overall duration might be as safe and effective as standard fractionation radiotherapy [7–10]. Hypofractionated radiotherapy has the advantage of being more convenient for patients and less resource intensive. These early studies led to the evaluation of hypofractionated WBI in randomized controlled trials. In the UK, two trials of WBI following breast-conserving surgery were performed: START A which compared 50 Gy in 25 fractions over 5 weeks to 41.6 Gy or 39 Gy in 13 fractions over 5 weeks and START B which compared 50 Gy in 25 fractions over 5 weeks to 40 Gy in 15 fractions over 3 weeks [11, 12]. The results of these trials led to the adoption of hypofractionation for the treatment of women requiring WBI following breast-conserving surgery in the UK. A similar comparison of WBI schedules after breast-conserving surgery was conducted in Canada.

11.2 The Canadian Hypofractionation Trial

The Ontario Clinical Oncology Group (OCOG) randomized controlled trial was conducted to assess the non-inferiority of hypofractionated WBI compared to standard fractionation [13]. Patients were accrued from 1993 to 1996. Following breast-conserving surgery and axillary node dissection, women with node-negative breast cancer were randomized to WBI of 50 Gy in 25 daily fractions over a period of 35 days or accelerated hypofractionated WBI of 42.5 Gy in 16 daily fractions over a period of 22 days. Women were excluded if they had positive resection margins, tumors larger than 5 cm, or breast width of more than 25 cm. Radiation was delivered Monday through Friday using tangential fields and 4–6 MV photons.

One thousand two hundred and thirty-four women were enrolled in the study; 612 were randomized to standard WBI and 622 were randomized to hypofractionation. At 5 years, the risk of local recurrence was 3.2 % in the standard arm compared to 2.8 % in the hypofractionated arm (absolute difference 0.4 percentage points; 95 % CI, −1.5 to 2.4) [13]. There was no difference in overall survival or disease-free survival between groups. The EORTC Cosmetic Rating System (excellent, good, fair, or poor) was used to report cosmetic outcome. At 5 years, only 22.6 % of patients in the standard arm and 23.2 % of patients in the hypofractionated arm had fair or poor cosmetic outcome (absolute difference –0.6 percentage points; 95 % CI, –6.5 to 5.5) [13].

At 10 years, these findings persisted with a risk of local recurrence of 6.7 % for standard irradiation and 6.2 % for hypofractionation (absolute difference 0.5 percentage points; 95 % CI, –2.5 to 3.5) [14]. A subgroup analysis confirmed that the effect was similar irrespective of patient age, tumor size, estrogen receptor status, and the use of systemic therapy. While a subgroup analysis did suggest that hypofractionation was less effective for patients with high-grade tumors, a subsequent evaluation using central review did not confirm this finding [14, 15]. The overall survival was 84.4 % for women treated with standard WBI and 84.6 % with hypofractionation. Radiation-related toxicity was also similar between groups. There was no grade 4 skin toxicity, and grade 3 toxicity was observed in 4 % or less of patients. 28.7 % of patients who received standard fractionation and 30.2 % of women who received hypofractionation had a fair or poor cosmetic outcome (absolute difference −1.5 percentage points; 95 % CI, –9.8 to 6.9) [14]. These data confirmed that hypofractionation was non-inferior to standard fractionation for women requiring WBI following breast-conserving surgery.

11.3 Patient Selection

Since the OCOG trial, women treated with breast-conserving surgery with node-negative or node-positive breast cancer (where regional nodal irradiation is not being considered) are candidates for hypofractionation [14]. For women with large breast size where a uniform dose distribution (within ± 7 % of the prescribed dose) cannot be achieved, or for women with breast implants, conventional fractionation of 50–50.4 Gy in 25–28 fractions may be a preferred alternative.

11.4 Physics and Techniques

This section describes the approaches at our own institution, the Juravinski Cancer Centre (JCC) in Hamilton, Ontario. Some variations of this may occur at other institutions. The approach used for WBI is similar for hypofractionation and conventional fractionation.

11.4.1 Simulation

Patients undergo CT simulation in the supine position on a standard breast board. In rare instances, for patients with large pendulous breasts, an Aquaplast breast mold may help mobilize the breast onto the chest wall, but is associated with an increased skin reaction. Other institutions have evaluated the role of the prone technique, in particular for lesions that are located away from the chest wall [16–20]. This technique reduces the skin dose and in some instances may also help to reduce the dose of radiation to the underlying structures such as the heart and lung. It has been associated with some inconsistency in day-to-day setup [21].

11.4.2 Deep Inspiration Breath Hold

For patients treated with WBI, various techniques have been evaluated to minimize the dose of radiation to the heart and avoid late cardiac toxicity. At the JCC, voluntary deep inspiration breath hold (vDIBH) is used. The technique is used for the majority of left-sided breast cancers. Additionally, patients with right-sided breast cancer may gain some benefit depending on the size and location of the heart.

For this approach, patients are instructed to hold their breath following a deep inspiration. In this process, the chest expands, moving the heart farther away from the chest wall. In vDIBH, an external surrogate is placed on the patient's abdomen, which moves with breathing and captures the breathing pattern at the time of simulation and treatment. In rare instances where vDIBH cannot be performed, a heart shield may be inserted to reduce the heart dose to acceptable limits, provided it does not shield the seroma planning target volume (PTV).

11.4.3 Treatment Plan and Treatment Delivery

A tangential beam arrangement is used to treat the entire breast with two parallel-opposed beams. In order to optimize dose homogeneity throughout the breast, wedges and segmentation (field within field technique) are used. Radiotherapy is delivered using megavoltage photons, with energies ranging from 6 to 18 MV. Higher-energy photon utilization is minimized to avoid the skin-sparing effect.

A dose-volume histogram is constructed to evaluate the target coverage and dose to organs at risk. The lung and heart doses are kept as low as possible. As a guide, the ipsilateral lung V20 is kept below 13–15 %. For right-sided breast cancer, the dose to 5 % of the heart is kept to <5 % of the dose and ideally <100 cGy mean heart dose. For left-sided disease, the dose to 5 % of the heart is kept to <10 % of the dose and ideally <200 cGy mean heart dose.

For treatment verification, portal images are obtained on the first day of treatment and repeated as necessary until the treatment position is satisfactory and reproducible. They may be repeated as desired and especially if setup issues arise during treatment.

11.4.4 Boost Irradiation

The use of boost irradiation to the tumor bed following WBI has been shown to decrease the risk of local recurrence [22–24]. At our institution, we normally give boost irradiation after hypofractionated WBI to patients at higher risk of local recurrence such as women age < 50, or those with high grade disease, or close or positive margins.

Although boost irradiation was not incorporated in the Canadian hypofractionation trial, it was used in the START A and B trials and did not affect the overall results of these studies. In addition, other recent studies support that hypofractionated WBI plus sequential boost treatment is well tolerated with minimal morbidity. The Canadian Randomized Trial of Accelerated Partial Breast Irradiation (RAPID) compared accelerated partial-breast irradiation to WBI. In the control arm of the study ($n = 1065$ patients), 82 % of patients received hypofractionation, and of these, 21 % received additional low-dose boost irradiation (10 Gy in 4–5 fractions). In an exploratory analysis the use of boost irradiation was not associated with increased adverse cosmesis at 3 years compared to no boost irradiation (15.5 % (15/97) vs. 16.7 % (74/442), $p = 0.88$) [25]. MD Anderson reported the early results of their study comparing standard WBI of 50 Gy in 25 fractions followed by a boost of 10–14 Gy in 5–7 fractions to hypofractionated WBI of 42.5 Gy in 16 fractions followed by a boost of 10–12.5 Gy in 4–5 fractions [26]. Two hundred and eighty seven patients were enrolled, 149 to standard fractionation and 138 to hypofractionation. Rates of acute grade ≥2 toxicity were significantly lower for patients treated with hypofractionation [26]. These data and our own clinical experience suggest that boost irradiation of 10–12.5 Gy in 4–5 fractions following hypofractionation is well tolerated. Longer follow-up is required to fully assess late treatment morbidity.

11.5 Special Indications

11.5.1 Ductal Carcinoma In Situ

The Canadian hypofractionation trial did not include patients with DCIS, but did include patients with microinvasive disease and patients with an extensive DCIS component as long as the resection margins were clear. Extrapolating from the original hypofractionation trials, hypofractionation has been used for the treatment of

DCIS following breast-conserving surgery in a number of studies. For example, a multicenter retrospective review of 440 DCIS cases treated with breast-conserving surgery followed by hypofractionated WBI delivered to a dose of 42.5 Gy in 16 daily fractions was conducted in the province of Quebec. Of these cases, 125 patients (28 %) received a sequential tumor bed boost of 10 Gy in four fractions. At 5 years, the local recurrence-free survival was 97 %. Although longer follow-up is needed, the authors concluded that hypofractionated WBI to a dose of 42.5 Gy in 16 fractions provides good local control following breast-conserving surgery for DCIS [27]. Similarly, a retrospective review of DCIS cases in Ontario was conducted using the Ontario Cancer Registry (OCR) between January 1994 and December 2003 [28]. Of 1609 women, 971 were treated with conventional WBI and 638 with hypofractionated WBI. At a median follow-up of 9.2 years, LR-free survival was 89 % for hypofractionation compared to 86 % for conventional fractionation ($p=0.03$) [28]. Finally, a retrospective review of 266 patients with DCIS treated with breast-conserving surgery and adjuvant WBI was conducted in Toronto, Ontario. Of the 266 women, 162 (61 %) received hypofractionated WBI (42.4 Gy in 16 fractions or 40 Gy in 16 fractions plus a boost of 12.5 Gy) [29]. At 4 years, the risk of recurrence was comparable between groups (7 % with hypofractionation and 6 % with conventional fractionation, $p=0.9$) [29]. Based on these limited data, we do use hypofractionation for patients with DCIS who are treated with WBI.

11.5.2 High-Grade Disease

Although most patients in hypofractionation trials had low-risk invasive disease, an important minority had high-risk disease (age < 50, tumor size > 2 cm, and high grade or estrogen receptor negative). An unplanned subgroup analysis from the Canadian trial suggested that hypofractionation was less effective for patients with high-grade tumors [14]. A reanalysis with central review did not confirm these findings [15], and a meta-analysis of the UK START trials was unable to show a detrimental effect of hypofractionation for high-grade disease [11, 12, 30, 31]. Based on these results, patients with high-grade tumors are treated with hypofractionation. In such instances, radiation oncologists may wish to consider additional boost irradiation.

11.5.3 Post-chemotherapy

In the Canadian trial, 11 % of patients received chemotherapy, primarily cyclophosphamide, methotrexate, and 5-fluorouracil, and 42 % received tamoxifen [14]. In the START A and B trials, 36 % and 20 % of patients received chemotherapy, respectively, and an anthracycline-based regimen was used in the majority (70 % and 59 %, respectively) [11, 12]. Tamoxifen was used in 79 % and 87 % of patients, respectively [11, 12]. As a result, patients treated with chemotherapy or hormonal therapy are routinely treated with hypofractionation. As per routine practice, chemotherapy is delivered prior to WBI, and hormonal therapy may be delivered concurrently or following WBI.

11.5.4 Regional Nodal Irradiation

Despite extensive experience supporting the use of hypofractionation for WBI there is less evidence supporting its use for regional nodal irradiation. Hypofractionation was used in the original British Columbia trial of postmastectomy radiotherapy where the dose to the regional nodes was 35 Gy in 16 daily fractions. While lymphedema was increased from 3.2 to 9.1 % with the use of regional nodal irradiation, no cases of brachial plexopathy were reported [32].

In a retrospective study from the Royal Marsden Hospital, 449 patients treated with locoregional radiotherapy received mean doses to the brachial plexus of 46 Gy in 15 fractions or 54 Gy in 27–30 fractions. Brachial plexopathy was observed in 5.9 % and 1.0 % of patients, respectively ($p=0.09$) [33]. Although the majority of patients were treated with older techniques with risk of overlapping fields, there remains some concern for increased morbidity when hypofractionation is used for regional nodal irradiation without adequate reduction of the total dose.

In START A, one case of brachial plexopathy was observed when 41.6 Gy in 13 fractions was used ($n=99$) [11]. No cases of brachial plexopathy were observed with 39 Gy in 13 fractions or 40 Gy in 15 fractions as used in the START A and B trials, but small numbers of patients were treated ($n=179$) [11, 12]. Radiation oncologists may wish to wait for more data on longer follow-up before using hypofractionation for regional therapy. In rare occasions in older women, we have used hypofractionation for regional nodal irradiation, but the total dose had been reduced to 38–40 Gy in 16 fractions.

11.6 Biomarkers and Hypofractionation

Biomarkers can help predict disease prognosis and response to treatment. In breast cancer, there is evidence to support the use of biomarkers to predict the risk of distant recurrence and response to systemic therapy [34–36]. Data on the ability of biomarkers to predict local recurrence and response to radiotherapy has been more limited. Recently, a better understanding of breast cancer molecular subtypes has led to their evaluation with respect to local recurrence and response to radiation [37, 38].

In the OCOG hypofractionation trial, tumor blocks were collected to evaluate the ability of tumor grade, intrinsic subtype, and hypoxia to predict response to hypofractionated WBI following breast-conserving surgery. The primary outcome was local recurrence (LR). Blocks were available for 989 of 1234 patients enrolled in the trial. Pathology was reviewed centrally (including grade), and tumors were classified by molecular subtype using immunohistochemistry for a six biomarker profile (ER, PR, HER-2, Ki67, CK5/6, and EGFR). Tumor hypoxia was also assessed using immunohistochemistry for HIF-1alpha, CAIX, or GLUT-1 [15].

Of 989 patients included in this cohort, 63 had a LR at a median follow-up of 12 years. In a multivariate Cox model, molecular subtype was the only factor significantly associated with LR. At 10 years, Luminal A and basal-like tumors had a better prognosis with a LR-free survival of 95.5 %. Luminal B tumors had a LR-free survival of 92.1 %, and HER2-enriched tumors had a LR-free survival of 83.1 %. The HER2-enriched subtype had the worst prognosis (HR 5.87, 95 % CI 2.38–14.48, $p<0.001$). There was no interaction between molecular subtype and treatment schedule suggesting that molecular subtype did not predict response to hypofractionation. Hypoxia markers were associated with more aggressive disease (such as high grade); however, they were not associated with a higher rate of LR [15].

11.7 Health Services Implications

In Ontario, a population-based retrospective cohort study was conducted to assess the WBI fractionation pattern of care before and after the presentation and publication of the OCOG fractionation study [39]. A total of 41,747 women treated with breast-conserving therapy between 1984 and 2008 were included in the analysis. Radiation was given most often in 16 or 25 fractions, and 16 % of patients received boost irradiation. A Poisson regression analysis was conducted to identify factors that may affect the use of shorter WBI fractionation. Older patients and those living farther from the cancer center were more likely to be treated with hypofractionation [39]. There were large differences in the use of hypofractionation between centers, ranging from 31.5 to 90.8 % [39].

Hypofractionation had been used in Ontario prior to the hypofractionation trial. When the OCOG fractionation study results were presented at the ASCO Annual Meeting in 2000, there was an increase in the use of hypofractionation from 48 to 68 %. Although an overall increase in the use of hypofractionation in Ontario was observed, important variations in practices persisted between centers at the end of the study period [39].

Similar studies on the health services implications of hypofractionated WBI have been published in the USA, suggesting that the uptake of hypofractionation is even lower. Bekelman et al. conducted a retrospective, observational cohort study of the uptake and cost of post-lumpectomy hypofractionated vs. conventional WBI in the USA between 2008 and 2013 [40]. Patients were included in one of two cohorts: the "hypofractionation-endorsed cohort" ($n=8924$), which included patients ≥ 50 years of age without nodal involvement or chemotherapy, and the "hypofractionation-permitted cohort" ($n=6719$), which included patients <50 years of age or those with nodal involvement or chemotherapy. Study endpoints included the use of hypofractionation and standard fractionation, as well as total and radiotherapy-related costs and patient out-of-pocket expenses. During the study period, the use of hypofractionated WBI in the hypofractionation-endorsed cohort increased from 10.6 to 34.8 % compared to 8.1 to 21.2 % in the hypofractionation-permitted cohort [40]. There was a statistically significant reduction in adjusted mean total health-care expenditures per patient in the first year after diagnosis with the use of hypofractionation compared to conventional fractionation, with savings of 9.1 % (95 % CI, 5.3–12.8) in the hypofractionation-endorsed cohort and 11.8 % (95 % CI, 7.6–15.8) in the hypofractionation-permitted cohort. Radiotherapy-related costs were also significantly lower with hypofractionation (mean difference of $4338 for the hypofractionation-endorsed cohort and $4785 for the hypofractionation-permitted cohort, $p < 0.001$). Patient out-of-pocket expenses were not significantly different between groups [40].

Similarly, Wang et al. conducted a retrospective study of breast cancer patients in the National Cancer Data Base from 2004 to 2011 to assess the relationship between patient, hospital, and cancer characteristics and the adoption of shorter radiation schedules [41]. Of 113,267 women eligible for hypofractionated WBI, 11.7 % were treated with hypofractionation and 88.3 % with conventional fractionation. Logistic regression was used to identify predictors of the use of hypofractionation. Patients treated at academic institutions, as well as older patients and patients residing farther from the cancer center, were more likely to be treated with hypofractionation. Disease characteristics suggestive of more aggressive pathology, such as large tumor size, poor differentiation, and ER-negative disease, were associated with a lower likelihood of treatment with hypofractionation [41].

In an effort to explore this variability further, a study of patients registered by the Michigan Radiation Oncology Quality Consortium (MROQC) between 2011 and 2013 was conducted [42]. The purpose of the study was to determine the variability in use of hypofractionated WBI at the physician and practice levels compared to the variability attributed to patient characteristics. Data were collected from 13 centers, including six academic centers, and 43 treating physicians. Of 913 patients with T1-2, N0 breast cancer treated with breast-conserving surgery and WBI, 283 (31 %) were treated with hypofractionated WBI. Patient characteristics used in the multilevel model included body mass index (BMI), separation, laterality, age, chemotherapy use, estrogen receptor status, use of hormonal therapy, and distance from the treatment facility. The use of hypofractionated WBI varied from 2 to 80 % between facilities. The variability in use of hypofractionation was mostly attributed to the practice (51 %) vs. the provider (21 %) and patient characteristics (28 %). Patients were more likely to receive hypofractionated WBI if they were older (≥50 years), if they had a smaller body habitus (separation < 25 cm), and if they did not receive chemotherapy [42].

These results support an overall increase in the use of hypofractionation since the publication of the hypofractionated WBI trials [11–13]. However, significant variations in practice persist, and many patients appropriate for shorter radiation regimens are still receiving conventional fractionation WBI. Further studies evaluating the factors that may contribute to an individual physician's treatment decisions would be beneficial. Hypofractionated WBI is more convenient for patients, is less expensive, and has the potential to improve the availability and use of radiation treatments for breast cancer patients.

When two therapies are found to be equally effective, as is the case for hypofractionated and standard WBI, it would make sense that the treatment recommendation would consist of the one with improved convenience and cost. As part of a Choosing Wisely campaign, the American Society for Radiation Oncology (ASTRO) created a list of five interventions that should be discussed between physicians and patients before their use [43]. This was done in an effort to provide high-quality patient care and reduce cost. An online survey of multiple ASTRO committees and disease site resource panels identified 34 potential items. A working group was then created to score the items and conduct a literature review for each of the items, and a top five list was created. The first of the five items was that WBI following breast-conserving surgery in women age ≥ 50 with early-stage disease should not be initiated without discussion of shorter radiation schedules [43]. The authors highlight that in select low-risk patients, hypofractionation provides similar results to conventional fractionation, improves efficiency, and reduces health-care cost.

11.8 Conclusion

Hypofractionated WBI is associated with low rates of LR and limited toxicity after breast-conserving surgery when compared to conventional fractionation WBI. Data suggests that hypofractionation can be used safely with boost irradiation and systemic chemotherapy. Additionally, comparable local control has been reported for patients with DCIS and high-grade disease.

In addition to being more convenient for patients, hypofractionation is associated with cost-savings. Despite that, the use of hypofractionation continues to be quite variable throughout Canada and the USA. Further work will be required to assess the additional factors that influence physician decisions regarding the use of hypofractionation.

References

1. Fisher B, Anderson S, Bryant J, et al. Twenty-year follow-up of a randomized trial comparing total mastectomy, lumpectomy, and lumpectomy plus irradiation for the treatment of invasive breast cancer. N Engl J Med. 2002;347:1233–41.
2. Veronesi U, Luini A, Del Vecchio M, et al. Radiotherapy after breast-preserving surgery in women with localized cancer of the breast. N Engl J Med. 1993;328:1587–91.
3. Forrest AP, Stewart HJ, Everington D, et al. Randomised controlled trial of conservation therapy for breast cancer: 6-year analysis of the Scottish trial. Lancet. 1996;348:708–13.
4. Clark RM, Whelan T, Levine M, et al. Randomized clinical trial of breast irradiation following lumpectomy and axillary dissection for node-negative breast cancer: an update. J Natl Cancer Inst. 1996;88:1659–64.

5. Early Breast Cancer Trialists' Collaborative Group (EBCTCG), Darby S, McGale P, et al. Effect of radiotherapy after breast-conserving surgery on 10-year recurrence and 15-year breast cancer death: meta-analysis of individual patient data for 10,801 women in 17 randomized trials. Lancet. 2011;378(9804):1707–16.
6. Virnig B, Habermann E, Al-Raie W, et al. Increased use of breast-conserving surgery: preferred treatment or failure to provide adequate local therapy? Breast Cancer Res Treat. 2007;106(Suppl 1):S188. abstract.
7. Fowler JF. The linear-quadratic formula and progress in fractionated radiotherapy. Br J Radiol. 1989;62:679–94.
8. Ash DV, Benson EA, Sainsbury JR, Round C, Head C. Seven-year follow-up on 334 patients treated by breast conserving surgery and short course radical post-operative radiotherapy: a report of the Yorkshire Breast Cancer Group. Clin Oncol (R Coll Radiol). 1995;7:93–6.
9. Olivotto IA, Weir LM, Kim-Sing C, et al. Late cosmetic results of short fractionation for breast conservation. Radiother Oncol. 1996;41:7–13.
10. Shelley W, Brundage M, Hayter C, Paszat L, Zhou S, Mackillop W. A shorter fractionation schedule for postlumpectomy breast cancer patients. Int J Radiat Oncol Biol Phys. 2000;47: 1219–28.
11. START Trialists' Group, Bentzen SM, Agrawal RK, et al. The UK Standardisation of Breast Radiotherapy (START) Trial A of radiotherapy hypofractionation for treatment of early breast cancer: a randomised trial. Lancet Oncol. 2008;9:331–41.
12. START Trialists' Group, Bentzen SM, Agrawal RK, et al. The UK Standardisation of Breast Radiotherapy (START) Trial B of radiotherapy hypofractionation for treatment of early breast cancer: a randomised trial. Lancet. 2008;371:1098–107.
13. Whelan T, MacKenzie R, Julian J, et al. Randomized trial of breast irradiation schedules after lumpectomy for women with lymph node-negative breast cancer. J Natl Cancer Inst. 2002;94:1143–50.
14. Whelan T, Pignol JP, Levine MN, et al. Long-term results of hypofractionated radiation therapy for breast cancer. N Engl J Med. 2010;362:513–20.
15. Bane A, Whelan T, Pond GR, et al. Tumor factors predictive of response to hypofractionated radiotherapy in a randomized trial following breast conserving therapy. Ann Oncol. 2014;25: 992–8.
16. Mulliez T, Veldeman L, van Greveling A, et al. Hypofractionated whole breast irradiation for patients with large breasts: a randomized trial comparing prone and supine position. Radiother Oncol. 2013;108(2):203–8.
17. Formenti S, DeWyngaert JK, Jozsef G, Goldberg JD. Prone vs supine positioning for breast cancer radiotherapy. JAMA. 2012;308(9):861–3.
18. Lymberis SC, Lymberis SC, deWyngaert JK, Parhar P, et al. Prospective assessment of optimal individual position (prone versus supine) for breast radiotherapy: volumetric and dosimetric correlations in 100 patients. Int J Radiat Oncol Biol Phys. 2012;84(4):902–9.
19. Formenti SC, Gidea-Addeo D, Goldberg JD, et al. Phase I-II trial of prone accelerated intensity modulated radiation therapy to the breast to optimally spare normal tissue. J Clin Oncol. 2007;25:2236–42.
20. Formenti SC, Hsu H, Fenton-Kerimian M, et al. Prone accelerated partial breast irradiation after breast-conserving surgery: five year results of 100 patients. Int J Radiat Oncol Biol Phys. 2012;84(3):606–11.
21. Kirby AM, Evans PM, Helyer SJ, Donovan EM, Convery HM, Yarnold JR. A randomised trial of supine versus prone breast radiotherapy (SuPr study): comparing set-up errors and respiratory motion. Radiother Oncol. 2011;100(2):221–6.
22. Bartelink H, Horiot JC, Poortmans P, et al. Impact of a higher radiation dose on local control and survival in breast-conserving therapy of early breast cancer: 10- year results of the randomized boost ver- sus no boost EORTC 22881–10822 trial. J Clin Oncol. 2007;25:3259–65.
23. Romestaing P, Lehingue Y, Carrie C, et al. Role of a 10-Gy boost in the conservative treatment of early breast cancer: results of a randomized trial in Lyon, France. J Clin Oncol. 1997;15: 963–8.

24. Poortmans PM, Collette L, Horiot JC, et al. Impact of the boost dose of 10 Gy versus 26 Gy in patients with early stage breast cancer after a microscopically incomplete lumpectomy: 10-year results of the randomised EORTC boost trial. Radiother Oncol. 2009;90:80–5.
25. Olivotto I, Whelan TJ, Parpia S, et al. Interim cosmetic and toxicity results from RAPID: a randomized trial of accelerated partial breast irradiation using three-dimensional conformal external bream radiation therapy. J Clin Oncol. 2013;31(32):4038–45.
26. Shaitelman SF, Buchholz TA, Hunt KK, et al. Hypofractionated whole breast irradiation results in less acute toxicity and improved quality of life at 6 months compared to conventionally fractionated whole breast irradiation: results of a randomized trial, ASTRO Annual Meeting. Abstract LBA3. Presented September 14, 2014.
27. Hathout L, Hijal T, Théberge V, et al. Hypofractionated radiation therapy for breast ductal carcinoma in situ. Int J Radiat Oncol Biol Phys. 2013;87(5):1058–63.
28. Lalani N, Paszat L, Sutradhar R, et al. Long-term outcomes of hypofractionation versus conventional radiation therapy after breast-conserving surgery for ductal carcinoma in situ of the breast. Int J Radiation Oncol Biol Phys. 2014;90(5):1017–24.
29. Williamson D, Dinniwell R, Fung S, Pintilie M, Done SJ, Fyles AW, et al. Local control with conventional and hypofractionated adjuvant radiotherapy after breast-conserving surgery for ductal carcinoma in situ. Radiother Oncol. 2010;95(3):317–20.
30. Haviland J, Owen JR, Dewar JA, et al. The UK Standardisation of Breast Radiotherapy (START) trials of radiotherapy hypofractionation for the treatment of early breast cancer: 10-year follow-up results of two randomised controlled trials. Lancet Oncol. 2013;14:1089–94.
31. Haviland J, Yarnold JR, Bentzen SM. Hypofractionated radiotherapy for breast cancer. N Engl J Med. 2010;362(19):1843.
32. Ragaz J, Olivotto IA, Spinelli JJ, et al. Locoregional radiation therapy in patients with high-risk breast cancer receiving adjuvant chemotherapy: 20-year results of the British Columbia randomized trial. J Natl Cancer Inst. 2005;97(2):116–26.
33. Powell S, Cooke J, Parsons C. Radiation-induced brachial plexus injury: follow-up of two different fractionation schedules. Radiother Oncol. 1990;18:213–20.
34. Paik S, Shak S, Tank G, et al. A multigene assay to predict recurrence of tamoxifen-treated, node-negative breast cancer. N Engl J Med. 2004;351:2817–26.
35. Paik S, Tang G, Shak S, et al. Gene expression and benefit of chemotherapy in women with node-negative, estrogen receptor-positive breast cancer. J Clin Oncol. 2006;24:3726–34.
36. Parker J, Mullins M, Cheang MC, et al. Supervised risk predictor of breast cancer based on intrinsic subtypes. J Clin Oncol. 2009;27:1160–7.
37. Nguyen PL, Taghian AG, Katz MS, et al. Breast cancer subtype approximated by estrogen receptor, progesterone receptor, and HER-2 is associated with local and distant recurrence after breast-conserving therapy. J Clin Oncol. 2008;26:2373–8.
38. Voduc KD, Cheang MC, Tyldesley S, Gelmon K, Nielsen TO, Kennecke H. Breast cancer subtypes and the risk of local and regional relapse. J Clin Oncol. 2010;28:1684–97.
39. Ashworth A, Kong W, Whelan T, Mackillop WJ. A Population-based study of the fractionation of postlumpectomy breast radiation schedules. Int J Radiation Oncol Biol Phys. 2013;86(1): 51–7.
40. Bekelman J, Sylwestrzak G, Barron J, et al. Uptake and costs of hypofractionated vs conventional whole breast irradiation after breast conserving surgery in the United States, 2008–2013. JAMA. doi:10.1001/jama.2014.16616.
41. Wang EH, Mougalian SS, Soulos PR, et al. Adoption of hypofractionated whole-breast irradiation for early-stage breast cancer: a national cancer data base analysis. Int J Radiation Oncol Biol Phys. 2014;90(5):993–1000.
42. Jagsi R, Griffith KA, Heimburger D, et al. Choosing wisely? Patterns and correlates of the use of hypofractionated whole-breast radiation therapy in the state of Michigan. Int J Radiation Oncol Biol Phys. 2014;90(5):1010–6.
43. Hahn C, Kavanagh B, Bhatnagar A, et al. Choosing wisely: the American Society for radiation oncology's top 5 list. Pract Radiat Oncol. 2014;4:349–55.

Chapter 12
United Kingdom Experience: Clinical Trial Evolution, Techniques, Data, and Toxicity

John Yarnold and Navita Somaiah

Contents

12.1 The START Trials

Late-reacting normal tissues are more sensitive to fraction size than most cancers (i.e., low α/ß ratio 0.5–6 Gy) and are relatively spared by fractions ≤2.0 Gy [1]. UK interest in breast cancer hypofractionation was stimulated by a 1984 publication by the Canadian radiation biologist, Bruce Douglas, who first suggested breast cancer might be different [2]. He estimated a value of 4–5 Gy for the α/β of locally advanced and recurrent breast cancer based on a reanalysis of clinical dose-response data first published by the South African radiation oncologist, Lionel Cohen [3]. This estimate represented an early clinical application of the linear-quadratic model, and it

J. Yarnold (✉) • N. Somaiah
Division of Radiotherapy and Imaging, Institute of Cancer Research & Royal Marsden NHS Foundation Trust, London, UK
e-mail: john.yarnold@icr.ac.uk

D.W. Arthur et al. (eds.), *Short Course Breast Radiotherapy: A Comprehensive Review of Hypofractionation, Partial Breast, and Intra-Operative Irradiation*,
DOI 10.1007/978-3-319-24388-7_12

was immediately put to the test in the UK Royal Marsden Hospital/Gloucestershire Oncology Centre (START-pilot) trial, 1986–1998 [4, 5]. The UK Standardisation of Breast Radiotherapy Trial A (START-A) trial, 1998–2003, was based on the results of this pilot trial [4–7]. At the same time, the START-B trial tested a commonly-used schedule in the UK, 40.0 Gy in 15 fractions over 3 weeks, against 50.0 Gy in 25 fractions in the same population of patients, whose characteristics are summarized in Table 12.1.

The START-pilot and START-A trials each incorporated two dose levels of a 13-fraction regimen controlling for overall treatment time (5 weeks) by treating on alternate days (Mon, Wed, Fri, Tue, Thu, etc.). The choice of 13 fractions was purely practical, allowing two patients prescribed 13 fractions to share the same appointment time on the same treatment machine. Fraction sizes iso-effective with the control schedule of 50.0 Gy in 25 fractions were estimated using α/β values judged to represent the upper and lower limits of sensitivity for the dose-limiting late-reacting normal tissues. The upper test dose (13×3.3 Gy) used in the START-pilot trial assumed $\alpha/\beta = 6.0$ Gy, and the lower test dose (13×3.0 Gy) assumed $\alpha/\beta = 1.8$ Gy. Based on the results of these comparisons in the START-pilot, which suggested an α/β of around 3 Gy for late adverse effects, 13×3.2 Gy replaced 13×3.3 Gy in the START-A trial. This regimen was predicted to be iso-effective with 50.0 Gy in 25 fractions assuming $\alpha/\beta = 3.2$ Gy. The lower test dose (13×3.0 Gy) remained unchanged. By controlling treatment time across all groups, and assuming linearity between test dose levels, the study design aimed to allow direct estimates of α/β for adverse effects and tumor control, by interpolation if necessary.

The primary end point of the START-pilot trial was late adverse effects, but that of the START-A trial was tumor control, see Tables 12.2 and 12.3. Based on a

Table 12.1 Patient and treatment characteristics of UK randomized trials of adjuvant breast hypofractionated radiotherapy

	START-pilot [4, 8]	START-A [6]	START-B [9]	FAST [10]
Years accrual	1986–1998	1998–2002	1999–2001	2004–2007
Total number of patients	1410	2236	2215	915
Standard arm (Gy/fr/weeks)	50/25/5	50/25/5	50/25/5	50/25/5
Test arm A (Gy/fr/weeks)	42.9/13/5	41.5/13/5	40.0/15/5	30/5/5
Test arm B (Gy/fr/weeks)	39/13/5	39/13/5	n/a	28.5/5/5
Mean age (years)	54.5	57.2	57.4	62.5
Node + (%)	32.7	28.8	22.8	0
Mastectomy (%)	0	15	8	0
Tumor ≥ T2 (%)	42.5[a]	48.6[b]	35.9[b]	17.8[b]
Boost (%)	74.5	60.6	42.6	0
Chemotherapy (%)	13.9	35.5	22.2	0
Regional radiotherapy (%)	20.6	14.2	7.3	0

[a]Clinical T stage
[b]Pathological stage

Table 12.2 Rates of local tumor relapse in UK hypofractionation trials in early breast cancer

Trial	Randomization (Gy/fraction)	Percent 3-yr local relapse	Percent 5-yr local relapse (95 % CI)	Percent 10-yr local relapse (95 % CI)
START-pilot [4, 8]	50.0/25		7.9 (5.4–10.4)	12.1 (8.8–15.5)
	42.9/13		7.1 (4.6–9.5)	9.6 (6.7–12.6)
	39.0/13		9.1 (6.4–11.7)	14.8 (11.2–18.3)
START-A [6, 7]	50.0/25		3.4 (2.3–5.1)	6.7 (4.9–9.2)
	41.6/13		3.1 (2.0–4.7)	5.6 (4.1–7.8)
	39.0/13		4.4 (3.1–6.2)	8.1 (6.1–10.7)
START-B [7, 9]	50.0/25		3.3 (2.4–4.6)	5.2 (3.9–6.9)
	40.0/15		1.9 (1.2–3.0)	3.8 (2.7–5.2)
FAST [10]	50.0/25	0.7		
	30.0/5	0		
	28.5/5	0		

Table 12.3 Clinically assessed moderate or marked late adverse effects in UK hypofractionation trials for patients treated by breast conservation surgery

Trial	Randomization (Gy/fractions)	Percent breast shrinkage at 10 yr (95 % CI)
START-pilot [4]	50.0/25	63.8
	42.9/13	74.4
	39.0/13	58.0
START-A [7]	50.0/25	34.2 (29.8–39.2)
	41.6/13	31.4 (27.2–36.0)
	39.0/13	30.0 (25.7–34.8)
START-B [9]	50.0/25	31.2 (27.9–34.9)
	40.0/15	26.2 (23.1–29.6)
FAST [11]	50.0/25	*9.5 (6.5–13.7)*[a]
	30.0/5	*17.3 (13.3–22.3)*[a]
	28.5/5	*11.1 (7.9–15.6)*[a]

[a]3-year rates for *any* late adverse effect

combined total of 278 local-regional tumor relapses in both trials at 10 years follow up, the adjusted α/β value for tumor control was 3.5 Gy (95 % CI 1.2–5.7), compared to 3.5 Gy (95 % CI 0.7–6.4) for clinically assessed breast shrinkage and 4.7 Gy (95 % CI 2.4–7.0) for breast induration. The results were, therefore, consistent with the hypothesis that a 13-fraction regimen delivered over 5 weeks could be as safe and effective as 50.0 Gy in 25 fractions in the adjuvant breast cancer setting.

Whereas the 13-fraction schedules offer high explanatory power, they are not convenient in the routine clinical setting. The START-B trial, although weak in explanatory power, was designed to test a 3-week schedule delivering 40.0 Gy in 15 fractions of 2.67 Gy, a regimen designed by Ralston Paterson at the Christie

Hospital, Manchester, with a long history of prior use in the UK [12]. The START-B trial recorded lower 10-year rates of clinically assessed breast shrinkage (hazard ratio, HR=0.83; 95 % CI, 0.66–1.04; p=0.06) and of breast induration (HR=0.81; 95 % CI, 0.64–1.03; p=0.084) after 15 fractions of 2.67 Gy, relationships confirmed by prospective patient self-reported 5-year assessments of a range of adverse effects (see Fig. 12.1) [9, 13]. Assuming α/β=3 Gy for late adverse effects, 40.0 Gy in 15 fractions is equivalent to 45.5 Gy in 2.0 Gy fractions. In other words, 40.0 Gy in 15 fractions is gentler on late-reacting normal tissues than 50.0 Gy in 25 fractions, the hazard ratio (HR) of 0.83 implying 17 fewer moderate/marked adverse effects among every 100 women treated with this schedule. Although there were only 95 local-regional tumor relapses in START-B, the HR for this end point was 0.77 (95 % CI, 0.51–1.16), consistent with non-inferiority for local-regional relapse after the 15-fraction regimen. The residual imprecision indicated by the upper and lower 95 % CI limits for the absolute difference between 40.0 Gy in 15 fractions and the control schedule in START-B suggests that local-regional tumor relapse is unlikely (≤2.5 %) to be more than 1 % higher, and perhaps 1 % or 2 % lower, than after 50.0 Gy in 25 fractions. The START-B schedule of 40.0 Gy in 15 fractions was adopted as the UK standard of care in 2009 for women prescribed adjuvant radiotherapy for early breast cancer [14]. In the most recent nationwide audit, conducted during a 2-week period in November 2011, 88 % of all dose prescriptions for women with early breast cancer in the UK used this schedule (Imogen Locke, personal communication).

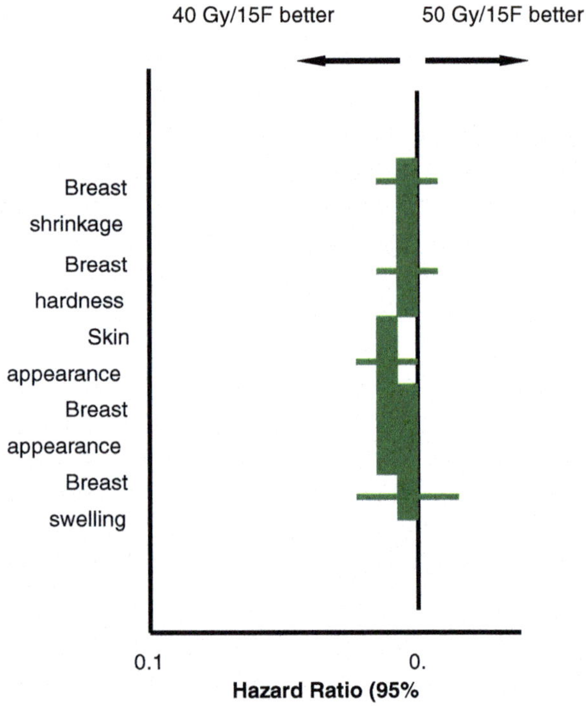

Fig. 12.1 Patient self-assessments of late adverse effects after breast conservation surgery in the START-B trial [9]

12.2 Are There Residual Concerns?

12.2.1 Length of Follow-Up

Adverse effects of radiotherapy evolve over decades, and an important question is whether the HR for dose-limiting adverse effects in experimental and control groups at relatively early time points are reliable indicators for the same adverse effects at much later time points. Comparisons of HR at 5 and 10 years for a range of adverse effects scored in the START trials are consistent with the predictive value of the 5-year time point. In fact, the 10-year relationships between treatment groups are established by year 3 and suggest that 10-year data are mature enough to base treatment decisions on [7]. This conclusion is not restricted to hypofractionation. The EORTC 22881–10882 trial confirmed that the relative risk of induration 14 years after randomization to breast boost dose versus no boost dose after 50 Gy in 25 fractions of whole breast radiotherapy could be accurately quantified within 5 years of treatment [15].

12.2.2 Patient and Tumor Subgroups

The patient and tumor characteristics of the three START trials are representative of patients with early breast cancer treated in the UK before 2004, with the exception that mastectomy patients are underrepresented (see Tables 12.1 and 12.4). There is no suggestion of any difference in treatment effects on tumor control for any of the subgroups recorded in the START trials, including patients with high grade disease (see Fig. 12.2).

Table 12.4 Patient and treatment characteristics in the UK START-pilot, START–A, and START-B trials (N=5861)

	Number patients (%)
Age <50 years	1389 (24)
Age ≥50 years	4472 (76)
Breast conserving	5348 (91)
Mastectomy	513 (9)
pN-	4318 (74)
pN+	1421 (24)
Grade 1	1213 (21)
Grade 2	2398 (41)
Grade 3	1272 (22)
No cytotoxics	4346 (74)
Cytotoxics	1480 (25)

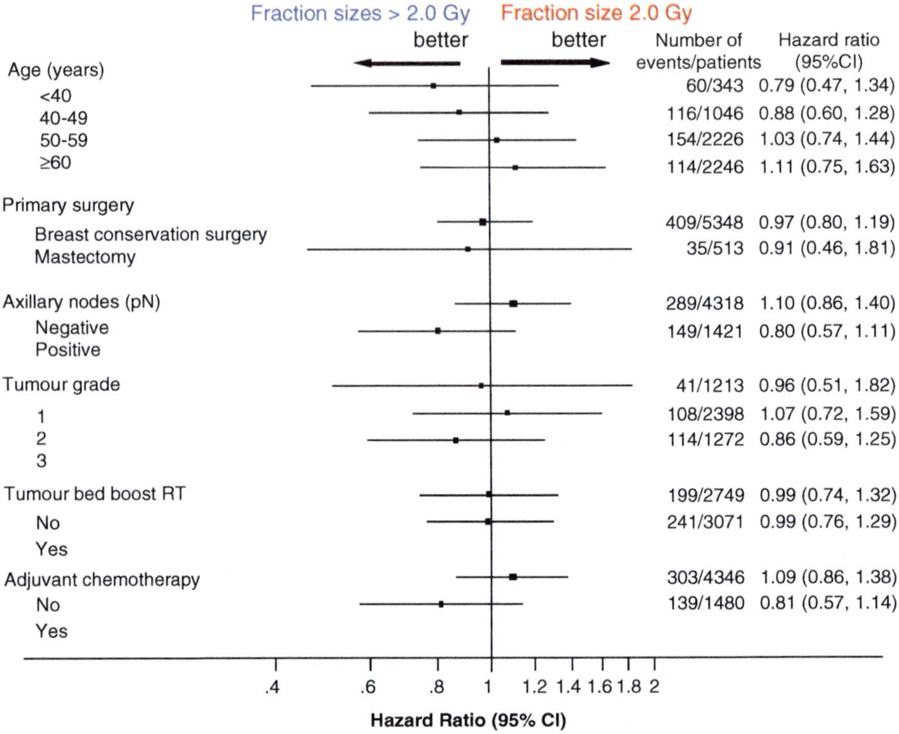

Fig. 12.2 Meta-analysis of tumor control in START-pilot, START-A, and START-B trials [7]

12.2.3 Cardiac and Lung Toxicity

A common concern relates to heart damage. There are no data relating to the fractionation sensitivity of this organ, but we suggest this concern is misdirected. Given the sensitivity of heart to conventionally fractionated radiotherapy, and the absence of a lower dose threshold for radiation-induced heart disease, the priority should be to protect this organ whatever fractionation regimen is used [16]. Even if cardiac protection is incomplete, the equivalent total dose delivered to the heart by 40 Gy in 15 fractions is lower than after 50 Gy in 25 fractions for a range of assumed fractionation sensitivities (see Table 12.5) [17]. Fractionation issues are also less relevant where the lung is concerned, since lung tolerance within the treatment volume is exceeded whichever dose regimen is used. As for the heart, a priority is to minimize lung volume, whatever dose prescription is used.

Table 12.5 Equivalent total doses in 2.0 Gy fractions delivered by currently used hypofractionated regimens, assuming different values of α/β [17]

	Equivalent dose in 2.0 Gy fractions		
α/β value	50 Gy/25 Fr	42.5 Gy/16 Fr	40 Gy/15 Fr
3.0 Gy	50.0	48.5	45.5
1.5 Gy	50.0	51.0	48.0

Table 12.6 "Double trouble" is always important but "triple trouble" has minimal implications for hypofractionation [20]

	Total equivalent dose (Gy) if α/β = 3 Gy, and you use fractions of:		
Breast dose inhomogeneity	2 Gy	4 Gy	6 Gy
100 %	50.0 ↓	50.0	50.0
105 %	53.6 → "double trouble"	54.0 →	54.3 "triple trouble"

12.2.4 *"Triple Trouble" and Large-Breasted Patients*

Double trouble was a term coined by Withers to describe the impact of unplanned dose inhomogeneities ("hotspots") when 2.0 Gy fractions are prescribed to the 100 % isodose [18]. Due to the mathematical form of the linear-quadratic dose-effect relationship, hotspots are penalized more severely in a hypofractionated treatment, so-called triple trouble [19]. In practice, triple trouble is of no clinical significance if hotspots are limited in volume, and dose gradients are restricted to between 95 and 107 % of the reference isodose (see Table 12.6). This should reassure those reluctant to prescribe hypofractionation in large-breasted women, who would otherwise gain from the reduced rates of moist desquamation and consequential late effects (telangiectasia and induration in the inframammary fold).

12.2.5 *Postmastectomy Radiotherapy*

A common question is whether it is safe to prescribe hypofractionation after removal of the breast, in the light of the underrepresentation of this population in the START trials. However, favorable patient-reported outcomes in the 513 women entered into the START trials postmastectomy suggest this is safe (see Tables 12.4 and 12.7 for data from 232 women in START-A trial) [13]. Patients prescribed 40 Gy in 15 fractions are expected to develop lower rates of long-term cutaneous atrophy and

Table 12.7 Patient-reported outcomes for breast conservation and mastectomy patients enrolled in START-A trial [13]

	Type of primary surgery	
	Breast-conserving surgery ($n=848$)	Mastectomy ($n=232$)
Change in skin appearance since radiotherapy		
50 Gy	1	1
41.6 Gy	0.92 (0.68–1.25)	0.53 (0.28–0.99)
39 Gy	0.63 (0.45–0.88)	0.64 (0.34–1.17)
Skin problems on or in area of affected breast		
50 Gy	1	1
41.6 Gy	1.02 (0.70–1.50)	0.90 (0.39–2.10)
39 Gy	0.87 (0.58–1.30)	1.07 (0.48–2.38)
Pain in area of affected breast		
50 Gy	1	1
41.6 Gy	1.29 (0.92–1.82)	0.82 (0.42–1.61)
39 Gy	1.01 (0.70–1.45)	0.87 (0.45–1.69)

symptoms referable to the rib cage than after 50 Gy in 25 fractions. The same considerations apply to women irradiated pre- or post-breast reconstruction, for whom the lower dose intensity of the 15-fraction regimen in terms of risk of adverse effects ought to be particularly appropriate, but who were poorly represented in the START trials conducted 1998–2003.

12.2.6 Lymphatic Radiotherapy

After irradiation of the axilla and/or supraclavicular fossa in over 400 patients within hypofractionated arms of the RMH/GOC, START-A, and START-B trials, there was no increase in reports of brachial plexopathy at a median follow-up of ≥6 years [4–7, 9]. A single case of mild brachial plexopathy in START-A after 41.6 Gy in 13 fractions presented in a patient with hereditary polydactyly (accessory thumb) who had no other radiation sequelae, consistent with a tissue-specific sensitivity syndrome. Whatever reasonable value of α/β, 40 Gy in 15 fraction regimen is gentler on the normal tissues, including brachial plexus, than 50 Gy in 25 fractions, being equivalent to 47 Gy in 2 Gy fractions if $\alpha/\beta=2$ Gy or 49 Gy in 2 Gy fractions if $\alpha/\beta=1$ Gy. In conclusion, if radiotherapy centers are confident in safety of their techniques when prescribing 50 Gy in 25 fractions, they can expect a reduced risk of late adverse effects after 40 Gy in 15 fractions under the same conditions.

12.2.7 Inoperable Breast Cancer

There is no randomized evidence testing hypofractionation in patients with macroscopic disease, where fractionation sensitivity might be modified, in either direction, by differences including tumor kinetics and hypoxia. However, the data published by Lionel Cohen in 1952 and used by Bruce Douglas to estimate an α/β value in the range 4–5 Gy were derived from women with locally recurrent and inoperable breast cancer. There are also retrospective data from France reporting outcome of 5 once-weekly fractions of 6.5 Gy fractions to the whole breast in 115 patients undergoing primary radiotherapy for nonmetastatic breast cancer (reference point unspecified) followed in 101/115 women by 1–3 tumor bed boost doses of 6.5 Gy [21]. Late effects, most commonly induration, were classified as grade 1 in 19 cases, grade 2 in 21 cases, and grade 3 in 6 patients at a median of 41 months. In our institution, high-dose palliation using once-weekly fractions of 6.0 Gy are prescribed in frail patients with inoperable disease in the breast/chest wall, for whom the weekly visits are relatively non-tiring and associated with much less moist desquamation than the equivalent regimen delivered using 2.0 Gy fractions. Assuming $\alpha/\beta = 3$ Gy for late adverse effects, 36 Gy in 6 fractions of 6.0 Gy delivers the equivalent to 65 Gy in 2.0 Gy equivalents, corresponding to 11 Gy in 2.0 Gy equivalents per fraction, a dose intensity appropriate for partial breast/chest wall volumes restricted to clinical disease.

12.3 Hypofractionation and Dose Intensity Modulation

Simple field-in-field techniques, intensity-modulated radiotherapy (IMRT), 3D conformal RT, and rotational techniques can exploit hypofractionation for dose intensity modulation. The most common application is simultaneous integrated boost (SIB) to the tumor bed during whole breast radiotherapy, which modulates fraction size rather than fraction number. The UK IMPORT HIGH trial, ($N = 2650$), applies IMRT and image-guided radiotherapy to modulate fraction size across the breast in women requiring a tumor bed boost in addition to adjuvant whole breast radiotherapy (see Fig. 12.3) [22]. The tumor excision cavity must be marked with titanium clips, and whole breast, tumor bed, and organs at risk must be outlined prior to randomization. The control group receives 40 Gy in 15 fractions to the whole breast followed by 16 Gy in 8 fractions to the tumor bed using megavoltage X-rays. Given very low risks of local tumor relapse beyond the index quadrant, the test groups are prescribed a 10 % reduction in total dose to the whole breast (36 Gy in 15 fractions of 2.4 Gy). The SIB delivers 48 Gy in 15 fractions of 3.2 Gy in test group 1 compared to 53 Gy in 15 fractions of 3.5 Gy in test group 2. Assuming an α/β ratio of

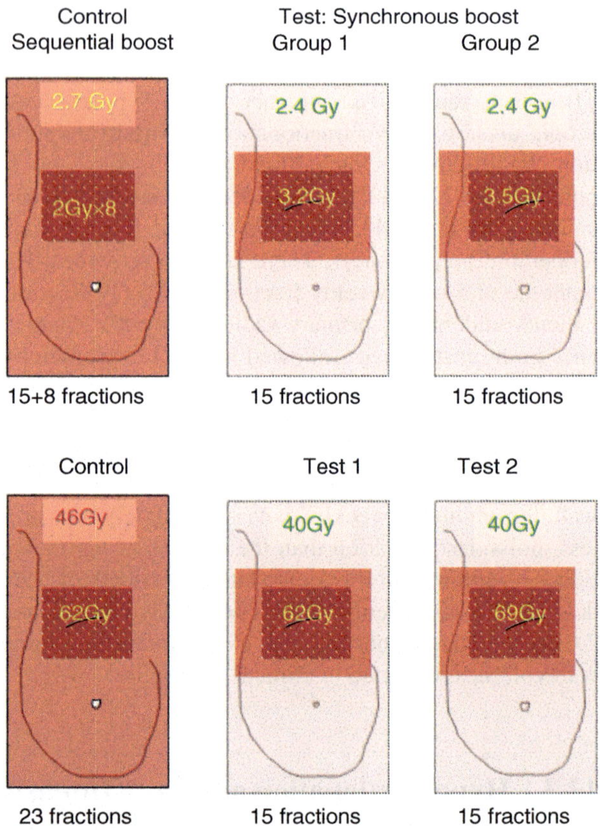

Fig. 12.3 UK IMPORT HIGH trial (N=2568): upper schema shows dose prescriptions; lower schema shows dose intensities in 2.0 Gy equivalents compared to standard fractionation, assuming $\alpha/\beta = 3$ Gy

3.0 Gy, the total tumor bed doses delivered to the control, test 1 and test 2 groups, are 62, 62, and 69 Gy in 2 Gy equivalents, respectively.

The modest dose reduction to whole breast in both test groups is equivalent to a reduction from 46 Gy in 2 Gy fractions (control) to 40 Gy in 2 Gy fractions (test 1 and 2), assuming $\alpha/\beta = 3$ Gy. This is expected to reduce late adverse effects referable to the breast and chest wall in both test groups. Given very low rates of local relapse outside the index quadrant, the inferior HR for local control in this large volume (HR approximately 0.5 instead of 0.3) is expected to have only a marginal impact on local control rates. Overall, adverse event rates are expected to be significantly lower in test group 1 compared to control, considering that the same 62 Gy equivalent total dose is delivered to the tumor bed volume in both test 1 and control groups. On average, integral total doses (function of dose × volume) to test 2 and control groups are comparable, dose being moved from the whole breast into the tumor bed volumes. Patient-reported outcomes will be needed to help define how to redistribute dose intensity in order to gain the optimal balance of local cancer control and adverse effects.

12.4 What Are the Limits of Whole Breast/Chest Wall Hypofractionation?

Fifteen fractions are unlikely to represent the useful limits of hypofractionation for whole breast radiotherapy. Following the 5-year analysis of the START trials in 2008, UK trialists designed a randomized trial (FAST Trial, $N=915$) testing late adverse effects of two dose levels of a 5-fraction regimen delivered once-weekly [10]. Five fractions of 5.7 Gy or 6.0 Gy were predicted to be equivalent to 25 fractions of 2.0 Gy, assuming values for $\alpha/\beta=3.0$ Gy or 4.0 Gy, respectively, since based on early and late human skin responses, the linear-quadratic model appears to perform reliably over this range of radiation fraction sizes. Three-year rates of physician-assessed moderate/marked adverse effects in the breast were 17.3 % (13.3–22.3 %, $p<0.001$) for 30 Gy and 11.1 % (7.9–15.6 %, $p=0.18$) for 28.5 Gy compared with 9.5 % (6.5–13.7 %) after 50 Gy (see Table 12.3). Change in photographic breast appearance, the primary end point, gave an estimate of α/β of 2.6 Gy (95 % CI 1.4–3.7). Although consistent with the estimates generated by the START trials, it is possible that markedly lower rates of moist desquamation and associated consequential late effects in the hypofractionated schedules slightly reduce the α/β estimate for "true" late adverse effects. At a median follow-up in survivors of 37.3 months, only two local tumor relapses have been recorded.

After the UK switched to 40.0 Gy in 15 fractions in 2009, this schedule became the reference schedule, not only for the IMPORT HIGH trial but also for the FAST-Forward trial evaluating a 5-fraction regimen of whole breast radiotherapy delivered in 1 week. Assuming $\alpha/\beta=3$ Gy for dose-limiting adverse effects, 27.0 Gy in 5 fractions of 5.4 Gy (test group 1) were predicted to be equivalent to 40.0 Gy in 15 fractions (45.5 Gy in 2.0 Gy equivalents under the same assumption of α/β). As in earlier trials, a second test group tested 26.0 Gy in 5 fractions of 5.2 Gy, equivalent to 42.6 Gy in 2.0 Gy equivalents under the same assumption and 48.0 Gy in 2.0 Gy equivalents if $\alpha/\beta=2.5$ Gy (see Table 12.8). Recruiting between November 2011 and March 2014, 4000 patients prescribed radiotherapy to the whole breast or postmastectomy chest wall are currently in follow-up, with local control as primary end point. An extension to this trial using the same randomized treatment options is opening in 2015 to assess arm swelling as primary end point in 600 patients prescribed lymphatic radiotherapy.

In conclusion, a 15-fraction regimen of local-regional radiotherapy has been standard of care in the UK since 2009 for women treated by breast-conserving

Table 12.8 Equivalent total doses in 2.0 Gy fractions of regimens being tested in the UK FAST Forward trial ($N=4000$) under different assumptions of α/β

	Equivalent total dose (Gy) in 2.0 Gy fractions		
Regimen	α/ß = 3.0	α/ß = 2.0	α/ß = 1.5
40Gy/15 F/3 W	45.5	46.7	47.6
27 Gy/5 F/1 W	45.5	50.0	53.2
26 Gy/5 F/1 W	43.0	46.8	49.8

surgery or mastectomy for early breast cancer. Initial uncertainties relating to selected patient and tumor subgroups have been resolved for the majority of radiation oncologists by dialogue and acceptance of national guidelines. Hypofractionation lends itself to dose intensity modulation using synchronous boost techniques, which are currently under test in a randomized trial. Finally, the FAST-Forward trial evaluates a 5-fraction schedule of local-regional radiotherapy delivered in 1 week, a regimen that approaches the limits of whole breast hypofractionation.

References

1. Thames HD, et al. Fractionation parameters for human tissues and tumors. Int J Radiat Biol. 1989;56(5):701–10.
2. Douglas BG, Castro JR. Novel fractionation schemes and high linear energy transfer. Prog Exp Tumor Res. 1984;28:152–65.
3. Cohen L. Radiotherapy in breast cancer I. The dose-time relationship theoretical considerations. Br J Radiol. 1952;25(300):636–42.
4. Yarnold J, et al. Fractionation sensitivity and dose response of late adverse effects in the breast after radiotherapy for early breast cancer: long-term results of a randomised trial. Radiother Oncol. 2005;75(1):9–17.
5. Owen JR, et al. Effect of radiotherapy fraction size on tumour control in patients with early-stage breast cancer after local tumour excision: long-term results of a randomised trial. Lancet Oncol. 2006;7(6):467–71.
6. Bentzen SM, et al. The UK Standardisation of Breast Radiotherapy (START) Trial A of radiotherapy hypofractionation for treatment of early breast cancer: a randomised trial. Lancet Oncol. 2008;9(4):331–41.
7. Haviland JS, et al. The UK Standardisation of Breast Radiotherapy (START) trials of radiotherapy hypofractionation for treatment of early breast cancer: 10-year follow-up results of two randomised controlled trials. Lancet Oncol. 2013;14(11):1086–94.
8. Owen JR, et al. Fractionation sensitivity of breast cancer: results of a randomised trial. Eur J Onc Suppl. 2003;1:S9.
9. Bentzen SM, et al. The UK Standardisation of Breast Radiotherapy (START) Trial B of radiotherapy hypofractionation for treatment of early breast cancer: a randomised trial. Lancet. 2008;371(9618):1098–107.
10. Agrawal RK, et al. First results of the randomised UK FAST Trial of radiotherapy hypofractionation for treatment of early breast cancer (CRUKE/04/015). Radiother Oncol. 2011;100(1):93–100.
11. FAST Trialists Group, Agrawal RK, Alhasso A, Barrett-Lee PJ, Bliss JM, Bliss P, Bloomfield D, Bowen J, Brunt AM, Donovan E, Emson M, Goodman A, Harnett A, Haviland JS, Kaggwa R, Morden JP, Robinson A, Simmons S, Stewart A, Sydenham MA, Syndikus I, Tremlett J, Tsang Y, Wheatley D, Venables K, Yarnold JR. First results of the randomised UK FAST Trial of radiotherapy hypofractionation for treatment of early breast cancer (CRUKE/04/015). Radiother Oncol. 2011;100(1):93–100.
12. Paterson R. In: Paterson R, editor. The treatment of malignant disease by radium and x-rays. 1st ed. London: Edward Arnold;1948. p. 622.
13. Hopwood P, et al. Comparison of patient-reported breast, arm, and shoulder symptoms and body image after radiotherapy for early breast cancer: 5-year follow-up in the randomised Standardisation of Breast Radiotherapy (START) trials. Lancet Oncol. 2010;11(3):231–40.
14. Harnett A, et al. Diagnosis and treatment of early breast cancer, including locally advanced disease--summary of NICE guidance. BMJ. 2009;338:b438.

15. Collette S, et al. Predictors of the risk of fibrosis at 10 years after breast conserving therapy for early breast cancer: a study based on the EORTC Trial 22881–10882 'boost versus no boost'. Eur J Cancer. 2008;44(17):2587–99.
16. Darby SC, et al. Risk of ischemic heart disease in women after radiotherapy for breast cancer. N Engl J Med. 2013;368(11):987–98.
17. Appelt AL, Vogelius IR, Bentzen SM. Modern hypofractionation schedules for tangential whole breast irradiation decrease the fraction size-corrected dose to the heart. Clin Oncol (R Coll Radiol). 2013;25(3):147–52.
18. Withers HR. Biologic basis of radiation therapy. In: Perez CA, Brady LW, editors. Principles and practice of radiation oncology. Philadelphia: J.B. Lippincott Co; 1992. p. 64–96.
19. Jones B, et al. The role of biologically effective dose (BED) in clinical oncology. Clin Oncol (R Coll Radiol). 2001;13(2):71–81.
20. Yarnold J, et al. Hypofractionated whole-breast radiotherapy for women with early breast cancer: myths and realities. Int J Radiat Oncol Biol Phys. 2011;79(1):1–9.
21. Courdi A, et al. Long-term results of hypofractionated radiotherapy and hormonal therapy without surgery for breast cancer in elderly patients. Radiother Oncol. 2006;79(2):156–61.
22. Coles C, Yarnold J. The IMPORT trials are launched (September 2006). Clin Oncol (R Coll Radiol). 2006;18(8):587–90.

Part III
Accelerated Partial Breast Irradiation

Chapter 13
Patient Selection for Accelerated Partial Breast Irradiation (APBI)

Laurie W. Cuttino

Contents

13.1 Introduction

The concept of irradiating only a portion of the affected breast dates back to the 1980s, when breast conservation was proven in multiple trials to be equivalent to mastectomy. One of the first investigations of accelerated partial breast irradiation (APBI) was undertaken at Guy's Hospital in the United Kingdom. The investigators hoped that a simplification of breast radiotherapy might allow more women to undergo breast conservation as well as possibly improve cosmetic outcome and allow for more rapid delivery of chemotherapy [1]. A low-dose-rate iridium implant was used to treat the area surrounding the lumpectomy cavity. Unfortunately, the incidence of local recurrence was significantly higher than expected, leading some to conclude that APBI was inferior to whole-breast irradiation (WBI). Investigators at the Christie Hospital published a similarly discouraging experience using electrons to treat the area around the lumpectomy cavity [2]. The suboptimal results in these original investigations of APBI were, in part, largely due to a lack of rigorous

L.W. Cuttino, MD
Department of Radiation Oncology, Virginia Commonwealth University Health System, 401 College Street, Box 980058, Richmond, VA 23298-0058, USA
e-mail: lcuttino@mcvh-vcu.edu

D.W. Arthur et al. (eds.), *Short Course Breast Radiotherapy: A Comprehensive Review of Hypofractionation, Partial Breast, and Intra-Operative Irradiation*, DOI 10.1007/978-3-319-24388-7_13

selection criteria. These trials included patients with large, clinically palpable tumors and lacked thorough review of surgical margins or lymph node status. Implants were performed at the time of surgery, with two-dimensional techniques and no assurance that the appropriate target was covered by the prescription dose.

In the United States, APBI was initially investigated using interstitial brachytherapy at William Beaumont Hospital (WBH) and at the Ochsner Clinic. Investigators at WBH used stringent inclusion and exclusion criteria for patients offered partial breast irradiation as part of institutional Phase II trials. Patients were required to be >40 years old, with invasive ductal carcinoma (IDC), surgical margins >2 mm, and axillary lymph node dissection of levels I and II with <3 nodes positive, no extensive intraductal component (EIC), and no residual microcalcifications on post-lumpectomy mammogram. A complete summary of the inclusion and exclusion criteria for the original WBH trials using interstitial brachytherapy is presented in Table 13.1. When balloon-based brachytherapy was introduced several years later, WBH conducted another institutional trial and developed updated selection criteria based on the evolution of breast cancer management, including the use of sentinel lymph node biopsy. Patients were required to be >40 years old, with either IDC or ductal carcinoma in situ (DCIS), tumor size <3.0 cm, surgical margin >2 mm, and lymph node assessment (for invasive histology only) with <3 nodes positive. Patient selection criteria for balloon-based APBI at WBH are presented in Table 13.2. Long-term outcomes using these criteria are excellent [3].

13.2 Society Patient Selection Guidelines

The American Brachytherapy Society (ABS) first published patient selection guidelines in 2003. Soon to follow were guidelines from the American Society of Breast Surgeons (ASBrS) [4]. Both were conservative in nature and based on the data and knowledge of breast cancer patterns of failure known at that time. Since then,

Table 13.1 Initial patient selection guidelines at William Beaumont Hospital (interstitial brachytherapy)

Inclusion	Exclusion
Invasive ductal carcinoma	Infiltrating lobular carcinoma
Surgical margins >2 mm	Skin involvement
ALND of levels I and II with <3 LN positive	Significant areas of LCIS
No extensive intraductal component	Pure DCIS
No residual microcalcifications on post-lumpectomy mammogram	Diffuse suspicious microcalcifications on initial mammogram (exceeding >3 cm or involving >1 quadrant)
Age >40 years	Paget's disease
Breast was technically suitable for interstitial implant	

ALND axillary lymph node dissection, *LCIS* lobular carcinoma in situ, *DCIS* ductal carcinoma in situ

Table 13.2 Initial patient selection guidelines at William Beaumont Hospital (balloon brachytherapy)

Inclusion	Exclusion
IDC or pure DCIS Tumor size ≤3.0 Surgical margin ≥2 mm Nodal assessment for invasive carcinoma Age >40 0–3 positive lymph nodes	Applicator-to-skin distance less than 5 mm

IDC infiltrating ductal carcinoma, *DCIS* ductal carcinoma in situ

Table 13.3 Patient selection guidelines from ABS [5] and ASBrS [4]

ABS	ASBrS
Age >50 IDC, ILC, and DCIS Size <3 cm No tumor on ink Node negative No LVSI	Age >45 (IDC), > 50 (DCIS) Histology: IDC, DCIS Size <3 cm Negative microscopic margins Node negative

IDC infiltrating ductal carcinoma, *ILC* infiltrating lobular carcinoma, *DCIS* ductal carcinoma in situ, *LVSI* lymphovascular space invasion

guidelines from both societies have been recently updated and are presented in Table 13.3 [4, 6].

In 2008, the American Society of Radiation Oncology (ASTRO) convened a Task Force of experts in the field of breast cancer to develop a consensus statement regarding patient selection criteria and best practices for the use of APBI outside the context of a clinical trial. The primary purpose was "to identify a subset of patients with a very low risk of clinically occult disease remote from the lumpectomy cavity." Recommendations were based on the results of a systematic literature review and were supplemented by the expert opinions of the Task Force members. The Task Force proposed three patient groups: a "suitable" group, for whom APBI outside of a clinical trial is acceptable; a "cautionary" group, for whom caution and concern should be applied when considering APBI outside of a clinical trial; and an "unsuitable" group, for whom APBI outside of a clinical trial is not generally considered warranted. The proposed selection criteria for the "suitable" group were derived from the inclusion criteria and characteristics of patients enrolled in prospective single-arm studies with a minimum of 4 years' follow-up. The "cautionary" group included those patients for whom the Task Force expressed uncertainty regarding the appropriateness of APBI, although at least some patients in this group had been included in single-arm prospective trials. The "unsuitable" group included those patients for whom there was very limited evidence from clinical trials to support the use of APBI [5]. The ASTRO consensus statement recommendations for APBI are summarized in Table 13.4.

Shortly after the publication of the ASTRO recommendations, the Groupe Européen de Curiethérapie-European Society for Therapeutic Radiology and

Table 13.4 ASTRO consensus statement guidelines [7]

Factor	"Suitable"	"Cautionary"	"Unsuitable"
Age	60 years old	50–59	<50
BRCA 1 or 2 mutation	Not present	–	Present
Tumor size	≤2 cm	>2 cm, ≤3 cm	>3 cm
Tumor stage	T1	T0 or T2	T3 or T4
Margin status	Negative by ≥2 mm	Close (<2 mm)	Positive
Grade	Any	–	–
LVSI	No	Limited/focal	Yes
ER status	Positive	Negative	–
Multicentricity	Unicentric only	–	Present
Multifocality	Clinically unifocal with total size ≤2 cm	Clinically unifocal with total size 2.1–3.0 cm	Multiple foci >3 cm apart
Histology	Invasive ductal or other favorable subtype	Invasive lobular	
Pure DCIS	Not allowed	≤3 cm	If >3 cm
EIC	Not allowed	≤3 cm	If >3 cm
Associated LCIS	Allowed	–	–
Nodal stage	pN0 (i^-, i^+)	–	pN1, pN2, pN3
Nodal surgery	SLNB or ALND	–	None performed
Neoadjuvant therapy	Not allowed	–	If used

BRCA breast cancer susceptibility gene, *LVSI* lymphovascular space invasion, *DCIS* ductal carcinoma in situ, *EIC* extensive intraductal component, *LCIS* lobular carcinoma in situ, i^- immunostain negative, i^+ immunostain positive, *SLNB* sentinel lymph node biopsy, *ALND* axillary lymph node dissection

Oncology (GEC-ESTRO) breast cancer working group developed guidelines for patient selection [7]. Like ASTRO, GEC-ESTRO divides patients into three groups: low risk, intermediate risk, and high risk. Unlike other society recommendations, however, the use of APBI off-protocol is only advised for the low-risk group. Treatment as part of a clinical trial is recommended for the intermediate-risk group. APBI is not recommended at all for patients in the high-risk group, even if they are participating in a clinical trial. GEC-ESTRO guidelines are summarized in Table 13.5.

Thus, four societies have published guidelines on patient selection for APBI. None of these sets of recommendations is identical, nor do they represent the patient population originally investigated by the institutions which pioneered the technique. Practitioners of APBI in the United States were presented with a significant challenge when the ASTRO recommendations were published in 2009. These recommendations placed patients, particularly younger patients and those with in situ histology, into the "cautionary" or even "unsuitable" categories, when these same patients had been treated for over a decade under the original ABS and ASBrS guidelines. It is difficult to synthesize an understanding of appropriate patient selection from the current, largely divergent, society recommendations. The three societies based in the United States agree only that ideal candidates have infiltrating

Table 13.5 GEC-ESTRO patient selection guidelines [8]

Low risk	Intermediate risk	High risk
Age ≥50 Margins ≥2 mm Negative nodes Unicentric, unifocal disease Tumor ≤3 cm No EIC, invasive lobular histology, or LVSI	Age 41–49 Margins <2 mm ≤3 nodes positive	Age ≤40 Positive margins ≥4 nodes positive or unknown axillary status Multicentric disease Tumor size >3 cm LVSI or EIC present

EIC extensive intraductal component, *LVSI* lymphovascular space invasion

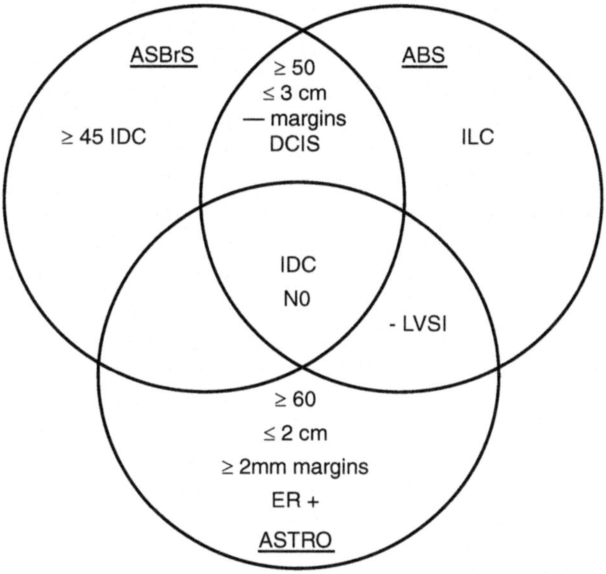

Fig. 13.1 Comparison of guidelines from US Societies

ductal carcinoma with negative lymph nodes. All other factors differ among the guidelines. A diagram demonstrating the intersection of these three society guidelines and diagraming agreement and disagreement is presented in Fig. 13.1. The only factors deemed clearly unsuitable for treatment with APBI according to both ASTRO and GEC-ESTRO are tumor size >3 cm and positive surgical margins. A diagram demonstrating the discordance of what is felt to be unsuitable by the largest professional societies is shown in Fig. 13.2.

13.3 Predictive Value of Society Patient Selection Guidelines

Although each society has developed a different set of selection guidelines, it is safe to say that each shared a common goal: to identify patients at high risk for failure after APBI. When published the ability of these guidelines to predict local

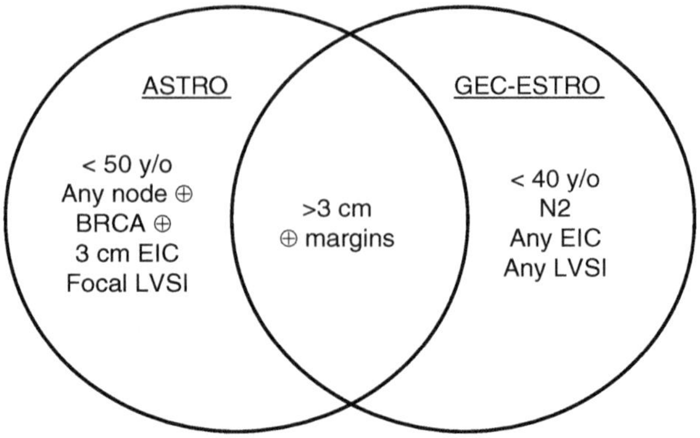

Fig. 13.2 ASTRO vs. GEC-ESTRO "unsuitable" factors

recurrence was questioned. Multiple investigators subsequently applied the ASTRO guidelines to their APBI datasets [3, 8–10]. To date, only one of these analyses has demonstrated an increased IBTR for either the "cautionary" or "unsuitable" groups. In fact, the only publication demonstrating any association between ASTRO group and outcome is a retrospective of patients treated with intraoperative radiotherapy with electrons (ELIOT) at the European Institute of Oncology [11]. All the 1,822 cases except for 25 could be classified according to ASTRO consensus statement: 294 patients met the criteria for inclusion into the suitable group, 691 patients into the cautionary group, and 812 patients into the unsuitable group. The 5-year rate of ipsilateral breast recurrence for suitable, cautionary, and unsuitable groups were 1.5, 4.4, and 8.8 %, respectively ($p=0.0003$). This analysis included a disproportionately high percentage of patients with unsuitable characteristics as well as employing a different definition of estrogen receptor status from other series. In addition, intraoperative electron therapy differs significantly from other APBI techniques in target definition and delivery and is not widely used outside Italy. Thus, this analysis has limited relevance when considering if the ASTRO groups are truly predictive of recurrence after APBI.

More recently, a pooled analysis of patients treated at WBH and on the ASBrS MammoSite Registry trial was performed, demonstrating no association between ASTRO group and recurrence [10]. APBI was used to treat 2127 cases of early-stage breast cancer (WBH, $n=678$; ASBrS, $n=1449$). Three forms of APBI were used at WBH (interstitial, $n=221$; balloon-based, n=255; or 3-dimensional conformal radiation therapy, $n=206$), whereas all Registry Trial patients received balloon-based brachytherapy. Patients were divided according to the ASTRO consensus statement into "suitable" ($n=661$, 36.5 %), "cautionary" ($n=850$, 46.9 %), and "unsuitable" ($n=302$, 16.7 %) categories. Tumor characteristics and clinical outcomes were analyzed according to risk group. The median follow-up time was 60.6 months. The WBH cohort had more node-positive disease (6.9 % vs. 2.6 %, $P<.01$) and cautionary patients (49.5 % vs. 41.8 %, $P=.06$). The 5-year actuarial ipsilateral breast tumor recurrence (IBTR), regional nodal failure (RNF), and distant metastasis (DM) for the

Table 13.6 Association between recurrence and ASTRO risk group

Series	*n*	Median f/u (years)	IBTR suitable (%)	IBTR cautionary (%)	IBTR unsuitable (%)	Conclusion
WBH [3]	199	10.7	4.4	7.4	2.1	No difference
Wisconsin [8]	322	5.0	1.6	4.8	6.6	Trend, not significant
ASBrS trial [9]	1025	4.5	2.6	5.4	5.3	No difference
ASBrS/WBH [10]	2127	5.0	2.5	3.3	4.6	No significant difference, trend towards increased IBTR in unsuitable due to elsewhere failures and new primaries
ELIOT [11]	1797	NR	1.5	4.4	8.8	Significant association

WBH William Beaumont Hospital, *ASBrS* American Society of Breast Surgeons MammoSite Registry Trial, *ELIOT* European Institute of Oncology intraoperative electron therapy

whole cohort were 2.8, 0.6, 1.6 %. The rate of IBTR was not statistically higher between suitable (2.5 %), cautionary (3.3 %), and unsuitable (4.6 %) patients ($P=.20$). The nonsignificant increase in IBTR for the cautionary and unsuitable categories was due to increased elsewhere failures and new primaries ($P=.04$), not tumor bed recurrence ($P=.93$), leading the authors to conclude that the current ASTRO consensus statement guidelines did not adequately differentiate patients at an increased risk of IBTR or tumor bed failure in the largest patient cohort analyzed to date. A summary of the analyses of recurrence according to ASTRO group is summarized in Table 13.6.

13.4 Evidence-Based Risk Factors for Recurrence

If the ASTRO consensus statement risk groups do not predict for an increased risk of local failure after APBI, which factors have been shown to be related to IBTR? Young age, large tumor size, close or positive margins, LVSI, estrogen receptor (ER) negative disease, lobular histology, DCIS, EIC, and positive nodes are all considered to be either cautionary/intermediate-risk or unsuitable/high-risk features according to the various society recommendations. These same features, however, have been demonstrated to be associated with increased risk of local failure after standard whole-breast irradiation [12–14]. Multiple analyses of APBI datasets have been performed in attempt to determine if certain factors are associated with an increased risk IBTR [3, 8, 10, 15, 16]. A summary of the published series investigating the association between various factors and IBTR after APBI is presented in Table 13.7. The recent pooled analysis of patients treated at WBH and on the ASBrS

MammoSite trial demonstrated that young age (<50 years vs. >50 years) and ER negative disease were associated with increased risk of IBTR after APBI. No other factors (including ASTRO risk group) were significantly associated.

Investigators at the Medical University of South Carolina (MUSC) found that patients with involved lymph nodes were more likely to experience local failure [15]. Again, it should be noted that patients with these risk factors are also more likely to fail locally after standard whole-breast irradiation. Both the groups at WBH and MUSC have published matched-pair analyses of patients treated at these institutions with APBI and WBI and have found that the risk factors for recurrence

Table 13.7 Predictors of local recurrence after APBI

Series	*n*	f/u (years)	Factor	OR	*p* value	Not associated
ASBrS/WBH [10]	2127	5.1	Age <50 ER neg	2.02 2.71	0.04 <0.01	Tumor size Margin status Nodal status Tumor grade ASTRO group
MUSC [15]	183	3.8	Positive nodes	6.39	0.02	Age ER neg HER-2 status LVSI EIC DCIS Margin status
WBH [3]	199	10.7	none	–	–	Age <50 Tumor size Lobular histology EIC Tumor grade ER neg Margin status Nodal status
Bryn Mawr [16]	109	3.0	None	–	–	ER neg (trend but not significant) Age Tumor size Close margins LVSI Lobular histology
Wisconsin [8]	322	5.0	ER neg Lobular histology	NR NR	0.002 0.004	Univariate only. Multivariate analysis did NOT identify any features associated with IBTR given small number of events

WBH William Beaumont Hospital, *ASBrS* American Society of Breast Surgeons MammoSite, *ER* neg estrogen receptor negative, *MUSC* Medical University of South Carolina, *LVSI* lymphovascular space invasion, *EIC* extensive intraductal component, *DCIS* ductal carcinoma in situ, *IBTR* ipsilateral breast tumor recurrence after APBI were the same as those for recurrence after WBI and that patients with these factors did not have improved outcomes after WBI [3, 15]. Thus, of all the "high-" risk factors identified by the various societies, only young age (<50 years), ER negative disease, and involved lymph nodes have actually been shown by data to be associated with increased risk of IBTR after APBI. Since these same factors are also associated with increased local failure after WBI, they may be associated with higher risk of local failure after *any* form of breast-conserving therapy, regardless of radiotherapy technique.

13.5 Conclusion

With appropriate patient selection, long-term data for patients treated with accelerated partial breast irradiation (APBI) demonstrates excellent outcomes and low risk of local recurrence [17–19]. In the United States, the most widely used guidelines are those developed by ASTRO and published in 2009. The authors of the original consensus statement deserve recognition for their extraordinary work in developing the initial guidelines for the application of this technique based on the data available at the time. The data, however, have grown in tremendously volume and matured in follow-up in the 8 years since the consensus panel met. A second expert panel has been organized to incorporate the more recent analyses of risk factors for IBTR after APBI. Revised and updated ASTRO guidelines are expected to be published by the end of 2015. Until long-term data from randomized trials is available, debate will continue over the ideal patient population to treat with APBI. While the presently available guidelines are imperfect, they were created to ensure conservative patient management and safety. It is suggested that these guidelines should be followed by practitioners until replaced with more current recommendations.

References

1. Fentiman IS, Poole C, Tong D, et al. Inadequacy of iridium implant as sole radiation treatment for operable breast cancer. Eur J Cancer. 1996;32A:608–11.
2. Ribeiro GG, Magee B, Swindell R, Harris M, Banerjee SS. The Christie Hospital breast conservation trial: an update at 8 years from inception. Clin Oncol (R Coll Radiol). 1993;5:278–83.
3. Shah C, Antonucci JV, Wilkinson JB, et al. Twelve-year clinical outcomes and patterns of failure with accelerated partial breast irradiation versus whole-breast irradiation: results of a matched-pair analysis. Radiother Oncol. 2011;100:210–4.
4. The American Society of Breast Surgeons consensus statement for accelerated partial breast irradiation. https://www.breastsurgeons.org/statements/PDF_Statements/APBI.pdf
5. Smith BD, Arthur DW, Buchholz TA, et al. Accelerated partial breast irradiation consensus statement from the American Society for Radiation Oncology (ASTRO). Int J Radiat Oncol Biol Phys. 2009;74:987–1001.

6. Shah C, Vicini F, Wazer DE, Arthur D, Patel RR. The American Brachytherapy Society consensus statement for accelerated partial breast irradiation. Brachytherapy. 2013;12:267–77.
7. Polgar C, Van Limbergen E, Potter R, et al. Patient selection for accelerated partial-breast irradiation (APBI) after breast-conserving surgery: recommendations of the Groupe Europeen de Curietherapie-European Society for Therapeutic Radiology and Oncology (GEC-ESTRO) breast cancer working group based on clinical evidence (2009). Radiother Oncol. 2010;94:264–73.
8. McHaffie DR, Patel RR, Adkison JB, Das RK, Geye HM, Cannon GM. Outcomes after accelerated partial breast irradiation in patients with ASTRO consensus statement cautionary features. Int J Radiat Oncol Biol Phys. 2011;81:46–51.
9. Shaitelman SF, Vicini FA, Beitsch P, Haffty B, Keisch M, Lyden M. Five-year outcome of patients classified using the American Society for Radiation Oncology consensus statement guidelines for the application of accelerated partial breast irradiation: an analysis of patients treated on the American Society of Breast Surgeons MammoSite Registry Trial. Cancer. 2010;116:4677–85.
10. Wilkinson JB, Beitsch PD, Shah C, et al. Evaluation of current consensus statement recommendations for accelerated partial breast irradiation: a pooled analysis of William Beaumont Hospital and American Society of Breast Surgeon MammoSite Registry Trial Data. Int J Radiat Oncol Biol Phys. 2013;85:1179–85.
11. Leonardi MC, Maisonneuve P, Mastropasqua MG, et al. How do the ASTRO consensus statement guidelines for the application of accelerated partial breast irradiation fit intraoperative radiotherapy? A retrospective analysis of patients treated at the European Institute of Oncology. Int J Radiat Oncol Biol Phys. 2012;83:806–13.
12. Goldstein NS, Kestin L, Vicini F. Factors associated with ipsilateral breast failure and distant metastases in patients with invasive breast carcinoma treated with breast-conserving therapy. A clinicopathologic study of 607 neoplasms from 583 patients. Am J Clin Pathol. 2003;120:500–27.
13. Nguyen PL, Taghian AG, Katz MS, et al. Breast cancer subtype approximated by estrogen receptor, progesterone receptor, and HER-2 is associated with local and distant recurrence after breast-conserving therapy. J Clin Oncol. 2008;26:2373–8.
14. Werkhoven E, Hart G, Tinteren H, et al. Nomogram to predict ipsilateral breast relapse based on pathology review from the EORTC 22881–10882 boost versus no boost trial. Radiother Oncol. 2011;100:101–7.
15. Zauls AJ, Watkins JM, Wahlquist AE, et al. Outcomes in women treated with MammoSite brachytherapy or whole breast irradiation stratified by ASTRO Accelerated Partial Breast Irradiation Consensus Statement Groups. Int J Radiat Oncol Biol Phys. 2012;82:21–9.
16. Stull TS, Catherine Goodwin M, Gracely EJ, et al. A single-institution review of accelerated partial breast irradiation in patients considered "cautionary" by the American Society for Radiation Oncology. Ann Surg Oncol. 2012;19:553–9.
17. Polgar C, Fodor J, Major T, Sulyok Z, Kasler M. Breast-conserving therapy with partial or whole breast irradiation: ten-year results of the Budapest randomized trial. Radiother Oncol. 2013;108:197–202.
18. Shah C, Badiyan S, Ben Wilkinson J, et al. Treatment efficacy with accelerated partial breast irradiation (APBI): final analysis of the American Society of Breast Surgeons MammoSite((R)) breast brachytherapy registry trial. Ann Surg Oncol. 2013;20:3279–85.
19. Strnad V, Hildebrandt G, Potter R, et al. Accelerated partial breast irradiation: 5-year results of the German-Austrian multicenter phase II trial using interstitial multicatheter brachytherapy alone after breast-conserving surgery. Int J Radiat Oncol Biol Phys. 2011;80:17–24.

Chapter 14
Physics of APBI

Dorin A. Todor

Contents

14.1 Introduction

APBI (accelerated partial-breast irradiation) treatments can be delivered using external beam or brachytherapy techniques. Interstitial brachytherapy using LDR (low-dose rate) Ir-192 seeds was historically the first modality used for APBI and consequently has the longest follow-up. More recently, external beam treatment has been used, either as photon, proton beams, or highly collimated electron beams, the latest being more often associated with intraoperative techniques relatively popular in Europe. New brachytherapy sources have been developed, including a miniature low-energy (~50 kV) electronic brachytherapy source and existent sources (e.g., Pd-103) commonly used as permanent seed implants for PBI, i.e., prostate cancer [25, 29, 31]. However, more commonly, APBI brachytherapy is associated with HDR (high-dose rate) treatment using Ir-192. The relatively high-energy source (~380 keV) at the tip of a thin wire is placed, using a computer-controlled afterloader device, in precisely specified positions for time intervals determined during

D.A. Todor
Department of Radiation Oncology, School of Medicine, Virginia Commonwealth University, 401 College St, PO Box 980058, Richmond, VA 23298, USA
e-mail: dorin.todor@vcuhealth.org

D.W. Arthur et al. (eds.), *Short Course Breast Radiotherapy: A Comprehensive Review of Hypofractionation, Partial Breast, and Intra-Operative Irradiation*,
DOI 10.1007/978-3-319-24388-7_14

the planning phase. Given the fact that the treatment is delivered very fast compared with the average half-time of cellular repair processes, one can establish equivalence between multiple sources loaded simultaneously (LDR) and one source, as is the basis for the HDR paradigm. During treatment, the single HDR source is successively placed in specified positions along applicators, called dwell positions, for specified amounts of time called dwell times. Thus, after combining a well-determined target, a specified applicator, and a given strength of an Ir-192 source, an HDR treatment plan is generated through specifying dwell positions and their associated dwell times. The highly radioactive source cannot be placed in direct contact with tissues, and therefore, various devices or "applicators" are used to both contain and to guide the source in the desired positions.

The first technique developed for APBI was multicatheter interstitial brachytherapy (see Chap. 15). With this approach, the treatment time is reduced from the traditionally 5 weeks to 5–8 days with the potential of reducing it further. The technique was initially used to deliver a tumor bed boost after whole-breast irradiation, and it has been a prominent APBI technique in North America and Europe. Catheters are placed through the breast tissue surrounding the lumpectomy cavity typically at 1–1.5-cm intervals, the number of catheters being determined by the size and shape of the target. The configuration of the catheters is guided by the understanding of brachytherapy dosimetry. Initially, the target volume was defined as the lumpectomy cavity plus a 2-cm margin, except where these target dimensions were limited by the extent of breast tissue (i.e., the chest wall and skin). At the initiation of mulitcatheter APBI, the catheter placement was guided by fluoroscopy (with surgical clips placed to mark the lumpectomy cavity), while the planning was based on orthogonal radiographs, so no true PTV was actually employed.

Even though from a technical perspective an interstitial implant is the most flexible technique, it does require specialized training and considerable experience. In an effort to make APBI more accessible, a number of devices were created with the goal of reducing the level of invasiveness, making the technique simpler and more reproducible [2, 9]. Essentially, there are two categories of devices: balloon-based devices (MammoSite, Contura MLB, and MammoSite ML) and strut-based devices (SAVI, ClearPath). The MammoSite was historically the first intracavitary balloon-based device available for breast brachytherapy. Of interest, this device was in fact following in the footsteps and on the basis of another balloon device used for brain brachytherapy: GliaSite RTS – a balloon filled with liquid I-125 [18].

In 2003, investigators at the William Beaumont Hospital [3, 36] developed and described the first and probably most used EBRT APBI technique, three-dimensional-conformal radiotherapy (3D-CRT). This technique was created as an option to invasive procedures and adopted for use as one of the allowed treatment modalities for patients randomized to APBI in the National Surgical Adjuvant Breast and Bowel Project B-39/Radiation Therapy Oncology group (NSABP/RTOG) 0413 phase III trial [37]. Further improvements in dose homogeneity, OARs sparing and deliver efficiency were obtained in techniques developed since 2003, using photon beams alone, combinations of photons and electrons, protons in conjunction with various setup, and imaging and motion (breathing) control techniques.

14.2 Radiation Sources for Breast HDR

Iridium has long been the workhorse of HDR brachytherapy. Its history starts with iridium having been used with brachytherapy in 1958 as seeds by Ulrich Henschke and then, from the early 1960s, mainly as wires [4]. Andrassy, in a debate on the best HDR isotope, sets up the history when pointing out the fact that sometimes it is forgotten that there was a time when most afterloaders used Cobalt-60: "In the 1950–1960s, when the production of isotopes by neutron activation became feasible, Co-60 complemented Cs-137 as the standard nuclide in radiation therapy. Its application has been studied in many countries all over the world, and broad clinical experience in teletherapy, as well as in brachytherapy has been gained. All in all, several hundred HDR afterloader units equipped with Co-60-sources have been utilized in clinics ever since, the majority of them for gynecological applications. The technical development of sources with higher specific activity was the starting point for HDR remote afterloading. Clinical data and dose delivery concepts to achieve equivalent outcomes in Low Dose Rate (LDR) and HDR-applications had been worked out using Co-60 sources. In the 1970s, the manufacture of miniaturized Ir-192 sources shifted market preference to this nuclide. Smaller size and source diameter allowed new application modalities, e.g., interstitial therapy, as well as dose optimization due to stepping source technology. At the same time, the extrapolation of experience obtained from traditional brachytherapy nuclides to Ir-192 was based on the similarity of physical dose distributions" [1]. The dominance of iridium–192 as an HDR source is based on several factors: the first of which is that it has a reasonable long half-life (73.81 days), so a typical source exchange occurs approximately every 2 months. Two additional technical advantages include that this isotope has a relatively low average energy (~.38 Mev, with a range from 0.136 to 1.062 MeV) and a half value layer of ~ 0.3 cm Pb, so it is relatively easily shielded. Nevertheless, the lead shielding for a room designated solely for brachytherapy can be expensive. The second advantage is its high specific activity (450 Ci/g), allowing the construction of high activity sources (10 Ci) of small diameter (0.6–1.1 mm). 192Ir is produced from enriched 191Ir targets (37 % natural abundance) in a reactor by the (n, γ) reaction, creating HDR 192Ir sources (typically 1-mm diameter by 3.5-mm length cylinders) with activities exceeding 4.4 TBq. HDR 192Ir sources are encapsulated in a thin titanium or stainless steel capsule and laser welded to the end of a flexible wire. Electrons from β-decay are absorbed by the core and the capsule.

As a novel approach to brachytherapy, the Xoft Axxent source is an electronic microminiature X-ray tube [31]. Despite a small diameter of the X-ray tube – 2.25 mm – the need for a flexible cooling catheter makes the HV catheter 5.4 mm, large enough to make its use impossible in most if not all applicators designed for Ir-192. The electronic source generates a 50-kV photon spectrum in a roughly spherical distribution. The depth dose characteristics of this source were designed to roughly mimic HDR 192Ir; however, there are important differences. The lower photon energy of this source results in greater attenuation. Unlike HDR 192Ir, electronic brachytherapy (EBT) does not require a shielded vault. This reduces costs and allows for portability of the system, which can lead to greater access for patients particularly in more remote locations or non-shielded operating and treatment rooms. There are also dosimetric implications of a lower-energy spectrum that results in more rapid dose falloff with depth in tissue. With a standard dose prescription at 1 cm from the balloon surface, the dose to structures proximal to this point is higher with EBTEBT as compared to that of an Ir192 source, and the dose to structures beyond this point is lower. Dickler et al. evaluated the dosimetric differences between Xoft and MammoSite [12]. They showed that the dose to the lung and heart was significantly lower with EBT; lung V30 of 1.1 % vs. 3.7 % and heart V5 of 9.4 % vs. 59.2 % for EBT and iridium-based brachytherapy (IBB) respectively. The dose to nontarget breast was also lower: breast V50 of 13 % vs. 19.8 %, respectively. However, the volume of dose hotspots was significantly higher with EBT. The V150, V200, and V300 were 59.4 % vs. 41.8 %, 32 % vs. 11.3 %, and 6.7 % vs. 0.4 %, respectively. Another consideration for EBT is that the relative biological effectiveness (RBE) for low-energy photons is higher and on the order of 1.2–2, depending on energy and depth. This has currently not been taken into account in the prescribed dose for EBT, which uses the same prescription of 34.0 Gy in 10 fractions as used with IBB using HDR 192Ir. Electronic sources do not fall under existent regulatory scrutiny of radioactive sources. ASTRO Emerging Technology Committee issued a report on electronic brachytherapy providing a descriptive overview of the technologies, current and future projected applications, comparison of competing technologies, potential impact, and potential safety issues [23].

169Ytterbium has been discussed for a long time as a possible alternate HDR source, and a number of papers that describe the advantages of Yb-169 compared with Ir-192, including for a balloon device [20], have been published. Yb-169 emits photons with energies ranging from 50 to 308 keV (average energy 93 keV) and decays with a half-life of 32 days. While the use and management of a radioactive source with a shorter half-life is clearly a disadvantage, the lower average energy clearly would require significantly less shielding than iridium. In the dosimetric balloon study, the plans using 169Ytterbium source result in less volume receiving doses of 150 and 200 % of the prescription, a greater homogeneity (DHI) and lower maximum dose [20].

14.3 Spectrum of APBI External Beam Radiation Treatment (EBRT)

The generic category of "external beam" APBI treatment contains numerous techniques. There are many advantages over the brachytherapy techniques, most obvious advantages being the noninvasiveness of the treatment and the widespread availability as most radiation therapy centers already perform 3D-CRT for other cancers and the staff is familiar with the technical demands and quality assurance issues [34]. Historically, the first and probably most used technique was 3D-CRT, developed and initially described by investigators at the William Beaumont Hospital [3, 36]. This technique uses three to five tangentially positioned noncoplanar beams. This technique was adopted for use as one of the allowed treatment modalities for patients randomized to APBI in the National Surgical Adjuvant Breast and Bowel Project B-39/Radiation Therapy Oncology group (NSABP/RTOG) 0413 phase III trial [37]. The prescription dose used for NSABP/RTOG protocol is 3.85 Gy twice daily (separated by at least 6 h) to a total dose of 38.5 Gy delivered within 1 week [10].

A combination of photons and en face electrons was proposed in order to create a simpler approach similar to the standard tangents with the patient in supine position [33]. In their study, a three-field technique consisting of 6 MV or 10 MV opposed conformal "mini"-tangential photons and en face electrons was employed on 70 % of the patients. The average contribution of the electron field was 20 %. For some patients with large breast size or deep seroma location, an en face photon field or multiple additional fields were thought to be needed to achieve acceptable PTV dose coverage.

While the simplicity of these approaches made them very popular, the desire to improve dose inhomogeneity in the target leads to the use of IMRT techniques. Another advantage of IMRT is the reduction in volume of high-dose irradiation to normal breast tissue and dose reduction to organs at risk (OAR): the heart and ipsilateral lung. The outcome and toxicity of IMRT-based methods is somewhat controversial, with some investigators reporting very low acute toxicity compared with WBI, while others, using APBI in conjunction with active breathing control, reported unacceptable cosmesis [14, 16]. A version of IMRT, tomotherapy, combines a helical intensity-modulated delivery (the couch moves continuously through the bore of a gantry simultaneously with the rotation of gantry-mounted LINAC) with the integrated image-guided system and thus can be described as computed axial tomography-guided IMRT [17]. The potential of tomotherapy for APBI treatments is, to a large extent, as in all EBRT modalities, dependent on the visibility of lumpectomy cavity and its position relative to the chest wall [21]. VMAT (volumetric-modulated arc therapy) and IMAT (intensity-modulated arc therapy) techniques were developed to preserve the idea of the continuously rotating gantry but expanding the narrow beam used for delivery in tomotherapy to a volumetric one. With the use of dynamic multi-leaf collimation and changing the field shape continuously as the gantry rotates around the patient, this EBRT technology claims similar advantages to tomotherapy: efficient delivery, dose conformity, dose homogeneity, and sparing of OARs [41, 42].

More recently, proton beam-based treatment has been explored. In theory, proton beams have a low entrance dose and a region of uniform high dose and a sharp falloff. This leads to homogeneous, conformal dose distributions and significant OARs sparing. For breast treatment, one can argue that proton therapy would produce a lower integral dose to the body; however, the production of secondary neutrons could significantly reduce this advantage. Passive scattering proton beam (PSPB), a technique in which the proton beam is spread out laterally and longitudinally, was shown to reduce dose to OARs (normal breast tissue, lungs, and heart) compared to 3D-CRT but has the disadvantage of delivering close to 100 % of the prescription dose to the skin for each beam [33]. Intensity-modulated proton therapy (IMPT) was investigated as a modality that had the potential to decrease the skin dose [38]. In a dosimetric study in which two plans were created for each of the 11 patients studied – one using two tangential beams and the other plan used one tangential beam and one en face beam – the authors concluded that IMPT is sensitive to delivery uncertainties (intrafractional motion including respiratory motion and interfractional motion, including setup uncertainties): "With the better and better understanding of IMPT uncertainties and advanced techniques to limit its uncertainties, IMPT may have real advantages over PSPB. At the current state of the art, however, PSPB appears as good as, if not better than, IMPT dosimetrically and more robust" [38].

It is interesting to note that while the usual argument against brachytherapy is that it is too "...dependent on the skill and training of radiation oncologist", the simplicity of delivery of brachytherapy treatments is often replaced by a very long list of issues affecting correct and reproducible delivery of EBRT. This list includes the necessity of special (and uncomfortable) immobilization devices, setup errors and uncertainties, the need for image-guided methods (electronic portal imaging devices (EPID), implanted fiducial markers with in-room megavoltage (MV) or kilovoltage (kV) X-rays, in-room CT or cone beam CT, optical or video 3D surface imaging), organ motion, and the need for motion management (implemented as active breathing control (ABC) or moderate deep inspiration breath hold (DIBH)). Adding to all the uncertainties related to proton treatments is the fact that most treatments are prescribed using the Cobalt Gray Equivalent (CGE) accounting for the higher relative biologic effectiveness (1.1 at mid-spread-out Bragg peak, but ranging from 0.7 to 1.6) of protons compared with photons [22]. While for many years studies concentrated on measurements of the relative biological effectiveness (RBE) of the energetic particles for end points like cell killing, it was recently shown that "densely ionizing radiation elicits signaling pathways quite distinct from those involved in the cell and tissue response to photons" [13], thus making the "effect-matching" of photon and proton treatments even more difficult.

14.4 Target Delineation in APBI

The rationale behind the reduced target volume in APBI, compared with WBI (whole-breast irradiation), stems from data on clinical patterns of failure (recurrences) of early-stage breast cancer patients treated with lumpectomy followed by WBI. Through the development of APBI using various delivery modalities and devices, the target definition also evolved. The general construct for the PTV involves outlining the tumor bed (equivalent terms are also lumpectomy cavity, excision cavity, cavity, etc.) or its surrogates (e.g., balloon surface, STRUT surrogate) as GTV and then applying a certain margin to create a CTV (clinical target volume) and another margin to create a PTV (planning target volume). While the

PTV in general is bound by the breast, it is not unusual for the PTV used for evaluation (PTV_EVAL) to be bound by pectoralis muscle, chest wall, and/or a 5-mm layer from the skin surface. Due to the fact that one does not need to account for motion and setup errors in brachytherapy (CTV equal PTV), PTV volumes in EBRT are significantly larger than in brachytherapy.

In balloon-based methods, the uncertainty of delineating the lumpectomy cavity is removed and replaced by the much more reliable delineation of the balloon surface. Of course, the implicit assumption is that the balloon is correctly placed in the center of lumpectomy cavity and inflated balloon stretches the tissue isotropically. For an increased visibility on CT images and automatic delineation, a small quantity of iodine-based contrast is used in the water. A PTV_EVAL is created using a 1.0-cm expansion from the balloon surface for CTV but limited by the first 5 mm of skin and the chest wall. A one centimeter expansion is used in the case of balloon-based brachytherapy devices due to stretching of the tissue surrounding the lumpectomy cavity. If air or fluid is retained within the lumpectomy cavity after inflation of the applicator's balloon, the displacement of the tissue away from the applicator's surface must be accounted for. The air/fluid trapped should be contoured separately on each CT slice and a total volume should be calculated to determine the percentage of the PTV_EVAL that is displaced. This percent displacement must be limited so that:

$$(\%\text{PTV\_EVAL coverage}) - \left[(\text{vol. trapped air} / \text{vol PTV\_EVAL}) \times 100\right] =\geq 90\%$$

The PTV_EVAL originated as a structure used to *evaluate* an existent plan for PBI under the NSABP B39-RTOG0314 clinical trial. The simple idea was that since the external beam (EB) RT dose calculation algorithms were unreliable close to interfaces (i.e., the skin) and since the trial was supposed to compare brachytherapy and external beam treatments, creating a structure that would remove the 5 mm of skin seemed almost normal. The pectoralis muscle, chest wall, and ribs were deemed "nontarget" tissues and also removed from the PTV.

While the PTV, as a 1-cm margin from the balloon surface, would almost always be symmetrical (unless the balloon would be less than 1 cm away from the skin), the PTV_EVAL, by being limited by the 5-mm skin structure and the chest wall and pectoralis, would be, in most cases, asymmetric relative to the central balloon axis (and implicitly its central lumen). In the single-lumen MammoSite era, there was nothing one could do to customize the coverage for an asymmetric PTV_EVAL, whether the PTV would be "whole" – as in the case of a balloon placed deep in the breast – or modified (see Fig. 14.1), the dose distribution created was invariably a radially symmetrical shape. So even though there were no two explicit structures, one for planning and one for evaluation (as that was the case, for example, in EBRT), there was in fact an implicit planning structure simply because the device could only create a radially symmetrical dose distribution. With the introduction of multiple treatment lumens, which have the potential to create a dose distribution truly conformal to the PTV_EVAL, the question whether PTV_EVAL is in fact a planning

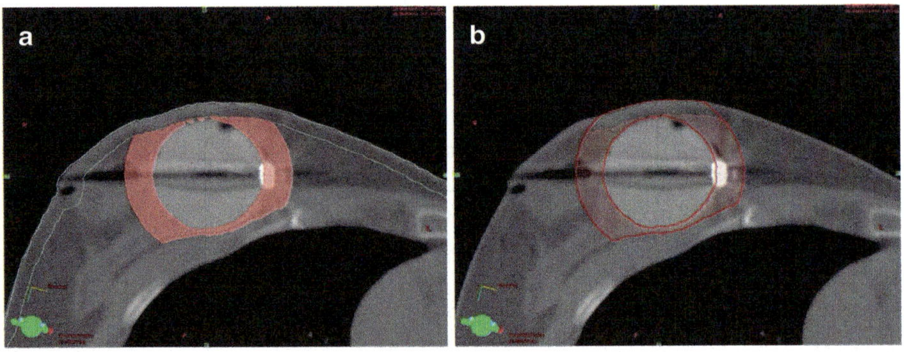

Fig. 14.1 (**a**) A “classic” (NSABP-B49/RTOG 0413) PTV_EVAL. (**b**) A “novel” PTV_EVAL containing the 5 mm of skin normally removed

structure, an evaluation structure, or both should be revisited. The answer is far from being of just academic interest and more likely has important implications for how the new devices are being used. In the strut-based devices, issues are similar except that the surrogate for cavity, which for balloon is obvious and easy to delineate, becomes less obvious, namely, a pseudo-surface encompassed by the struts.

In EBRT methods, the extent of the margins for creating CTV and PTV is different depending on cavity size and surgical closure techniques, patient position (supine vs. prone), institution, setup methods and breathing motion management, and delivery method (3D-CRT, IMRT, VMAT, tomotherapy, etc.). In a study comparing four different EBRT techniques, the PTV was defined by adding different margins depending on the directional safety margin status of each lumpectomy cavity (i.e., medial, lateral, superior, inferior, and deep margins measured from the tumor front after the examination of the surgical specimen: 2, 1.5, and 1 cm for resection margins <1 cm, 1–2 cm, and >2 cm, respectively) [19]. These unequal margins typically lead to smaller PTV volumes than most clinical other trials. By comparison, the guidelines for PTV delineation in the EBRT arm of NSABP B-39/ RTOG 0413 are as follows: “The CTV will be defined by uniformly expanding the excision cavity volume by 15 mm. However, the CTV will be limited to 5 mm from the skin surface and by the posterior breast tissue extent (chest wall and pectoralis muscles are not to be included). The PTV, defined as a uniform 10-mm expansion of the CTV, will provide a margin around the CTV to compensate for the variability of treatment set-up and motion of the breast with breathing. The PTV is saved and is used to generate the beam aperture with an additional margin to take penumbra into account. Since a substantial part of the PTV often extends outside the patient (especially for superficial cavities), the PTV is then copied to a PTV_EVAL, which is edited. This PTV_EVAL is limited to exclude the part outside the ipsilateral breast and the first 5 mm of tissue under the skin (in order to remove most of the buildup region for the DVH analysis) and excluding (if applicable) the PTV expansion beyond the posterior extent of breast tissue (chest wall, pectoralis muscles and lung). This PTV_EVAL is the structure used for DVH constraints and analysis.”

14.5 Fundamentals of Brachytherapy Physics

The physics of breast brachytherapy is in no way different from the physics of brachytherapy in general. In fact, while essential in our understanding of dose delivered to target tissues, physics is one component in a long list of "ingredients" necessary for a successful brachytherapy treatment. Without the claim that this is an exhaustive one, here is a comprehensive list of such ingredients:

1. One or more radiation sources with calibration traceable to a standards laboratory
2. Understanding of the radiation emitted by the sources and the effects of encapsulation, wires, etc.
3. Dosimetric system/model for the computation of dose distribution and treatment time
4. Understanding and good geometrical and material description of applicators
5. Accurate positioning of sources
6. Accurate timing of source placement
7. Accurate description of tissues (composition and mass energy absorption coefficients)
8. Accurate description of radiation biological effects in the targeted tissues as well as "normal" tissues

In August 2012, a report of the High Energy Brachytherapy Source Dosimetry (HEBD) Working Group published its "Recommendations of the American Association of Physicists in Medicine (AAPM) and the European Society for Radiotherapy and Oncology (ESTRO) on dose calculations for high-energy (average energy higher than 50 keV) photon-emitting brachytherapy sources was presented, including the physical characteristics of specific 192Ir, 137Cs, and 60Co source models" as well as consensus datasets for commercially available high-energy photon sources.

Without getting into the details of the dose computation formalism and radiation source descriptions within this formalism, all of which are well described in literature, we will address physics issues directly related to balloon brachytherapy. In general, four factors influence the single-source dose distribution for photon-emitting sources:

- Distance (inverse-square law)
- Absorption and scattering in the source core and encapsulation
- Photon attenuation and
- Scattering in the surrounding medium

The inverse-square law is the best known and is strictly a geometric consequence of any isotropic source emitting photons in a 3D space. It assumes no attenuation or scattering of photons by the medium. Of the four factors influencing the dose distribution, the inverse-square law is by far the most important. For a pure isotropic point source, the dose will decrease by a factor of 100 between the distances of 0.5 and 5 cm. The influence of the remaining factors over the same distance range rarely exceeds a factor of 2 or 3. The tissue surrounding the source affects the dose distribution in two competing ways: dose is reduced by the attenuation of primary photons and at the same time is increased by the scattered photons. Photons are being emitted in all directions from the source and are interacting with the tissue by means of Compton scattering and photoelectric absorption. Thus, each volume element of tissue is effectively radiating scattered photons in all directions, many of which contribute to the dose at the point of interest.

One can see that up to distances of about 5 cm, the attenuation of primary photons and the buildup of dose from scattered photons are compensating each other, leading to an almost "pure" inverse-square distance law (Fig. 14.2). At larger distances, seldom of interest for clinical purposes, attenuation wins, and the falloff is faster. Compton scattering, which dominates photon absorption and scattering above 100 keV, depends mainly on electron density (electrons/g) of the medium, which is nearly constant for all biologic materials. Thus, for Ir-192 HDR brachytherapy, tissue composition is largely irrelevant and water as medium is a very good approximation, validating the use of TG-43 formalism in most clinical applications. The only limitation of TG-43 is assuming that medium is infinite and thus scatter contribution is always in full. In the "evolution of brachytherapy treatment planning," the authors examined the sensitivity of common treatment sites to dosimetric limitations of the current dose computation formalism (TG-43) [30]. They concluded that, for breast HDR, significant differences between planned and delivered dose are likely to occur due to one factor only: scattering. In breast, relatively close to the radiation source and applicators are two interfaces: one between breast and air and the other between the breast tissue and the lung. As a result, a part of the contribution from scatter will be lost, and likely the planned dose will be an overestimation of the dose actually delivered. It is interesting to note that this is also applicator dependent. In interstitial implants, the source is in the immediate proximity of the tissue; thus, dose is delivered largely by primary photons, and thus, the

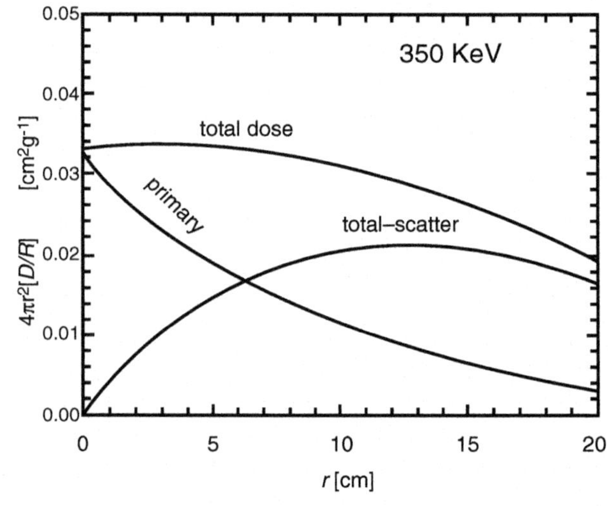

Fig. 14.2 Contributions of primary and scattered photons to total absorbed dose at the photon energies of 350 keV. The dose distributions are multiplied by the distance squared and normalized to the primary photon energy (From Carlsson and Ahnesjö [12])

missing scatter will impact very little the difference between planned and delivered dose (typically 2–3 %). A direct comparison of TG-43-based dose calculations to MC simulations in the CT-based geometries of 18 multicatheter breast patients taking into account four tissue types was included in a study introducing an analytical scatter correction technique [26]. Average results, reported in terms of dose-volume statistics for the PTV, skin, lung, and heart, verified the magnitude of the TG-43 dose overestimation (i.e., 2.6±0.6 % for PTV D_{90}, 4.7±1.2 %, 5.3±0.9 %, 2.1±3.7 % for the skin, lung, and heart $D_{0.1\text{cm}^3}$, respectively).

In balloon brachytherapy, the tissue is a few cm away (can be as many as 3–4 cm) from the source, making the scatter a more important component of dose. Thus, the missing scatter due to the breast tissue-air interface can bring the difference between planned and delivered dose to 10–15 %.

The SAVI device poses even more significant problems, given that the device itself is not filled with water, but air [28]. Without taking into account any uncertainty that may arise in a clinical scenario in which the delivered dose may be perturbed by proximity to the skin/air interface or near the lung, the dose discrepancy between TG-43 and MC calculated dose, strictly due to the air cavity of the SAVI device, was found to be of the order of 8–9 % for the largest device available (10 struts).

14.6 CT Planning and Dose Optimization

Before discussing about dose optimization, one needs to stress the importance of optimal placement. In the case of multicatheter brachytherapy, implant orientation is based on the size, shape, and location of the intended target while also considering patient comfort and location of potential punctate scarring from catheter entrance and exit. The number of catheters and planes needed is governed by the target geometry and brachytherapy principles. In regard to intracavitary devices, there are many constraints on how a device is to be implanted including patient's anatomy, patient convenience, and cavity location. However, in addition, optimal placement of an intracavitary device must take into account the particularities of the device and the way dose distribution is created. The principles of device orientation apply to all intracavitary devices and are exemplified with the following Contura MLB case (Fig. 14.3). One can see that the asymmetry of the PTV_EVAL can be bounded by two lines (in yellow) in two of the orthogonal views. Ideally, the central lumen would be oriented along the bisector (upper left panel), and catheters 1 and 3 would also be positioned along the bisector (lower panel right). The entry direction of the device is dictated by the shape of the cavity and by the length of the tissue that needs to be traversed to reach the cavity. However, there is no reason not to rotate the device, once inserted, so that it is in optimal position. If catheters 1–3 are along the bisector, and catheters 2–4 are oriented along the shorter "axis" of PTV_EVAL, the optimizer would very likely weigh heavily on 1–3 in order to create an elongated dose distribution and would use very little catheters 2 and 4. In a less than optimal

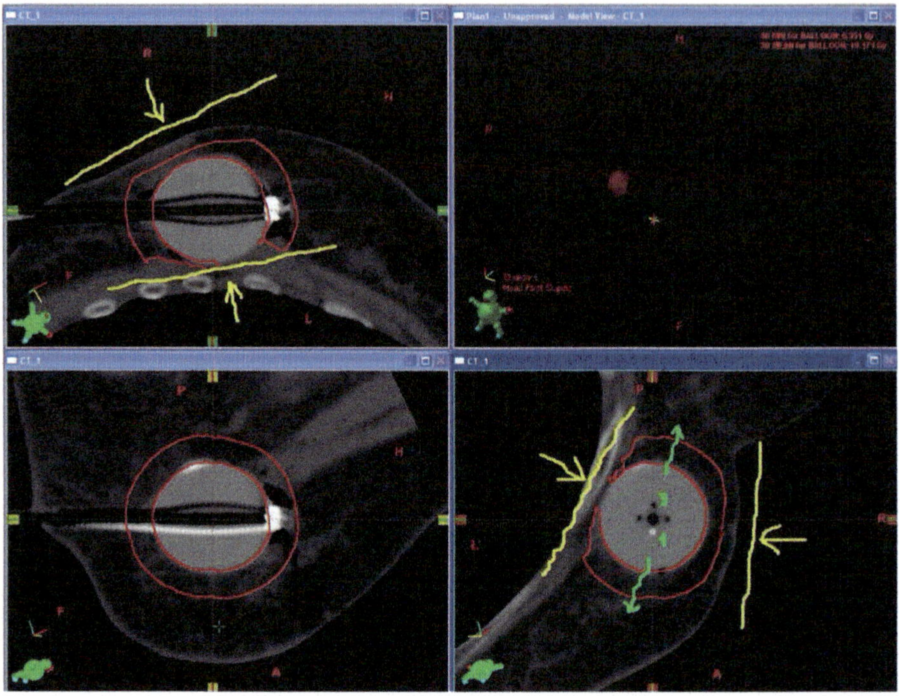

Fig. 14.3 Orthogonal views of a Contura multilumen plan. In *yellow* are shown the "bounding" planes of the PTV_EVAL

position, the optimizer would likely distribute dwell times in all catheters, thus leading to a more spherical, less conformal dose distribution.

A preliminary CT scan can be used for rotating the balloon in the optimal position. For the final treatment planning CT, the patient should be in a position reproduced in each of the treatments. Every particular aspect (arm, wedges used to rotate the patient, etc.) should be recorded and reproduced in each of the treatment positions. The CT should start at or above the mandible and extend several cm below the inframammary fold (including the entire lung). A CT scan thickness of $\leq$5 mm, preferably 2–3 mm, should be employed. The following structures will be contoured: the gross target volume (GTV), the clinical target volume (CTV), the planning target volume (PTV), and the PTV_EVAL trapped air and/or fluid and ipsilateral breast. The chin, shoulders, and entire ipsilateral breast should be included in the scan. The target and normal tissue structures must be outlined on all CT slices.

In a multicatheter implant, the GTV is represented through a combination of residual seroma cavity, postoperative changes, and, if present, surgically placed clips. In the case of intracavitary device-based brachytherapy, the contour of the balloon or the pseudo-surface encompassed by the struts becomes a surrogate

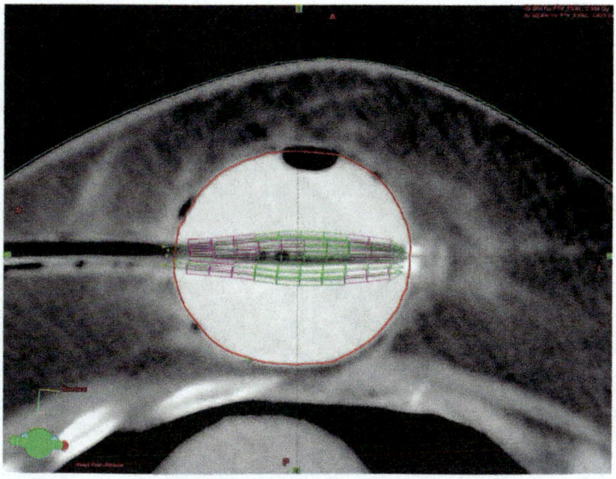

Fig. 14.4 Outline of a multilumen balloon after automatic segmentation. Also shown are the applicators

definition of the lumpectomy cavity (GTV). The balloon can be outlined (segmented) automatically, based on an increased CT number, compared with adjacent tissue (Fig. 14.4). This can be easily achieved using a few milliliters of an iodine based diluted in the water or saline used to inflate the balloon. The PTV_EVAL is created by uniformly expanding by 1 cm. The structure is limited to 5 mm from the skin surface and the chest wall and pectoralis.

Very important for planning is an avoidance structure. The pseudo-structure is obtained by expanding the PTV_EVAL by 3–4 mm and then subtracting the PTV_EVAL itself, resulting in a thin rim surrounding the PTV_EVAL (Fig. 14.5). Additional constraints can be imposed on this structure, together with the ones already described for the PTV_EVAL.

The next step is defining the geometry of the applicators. Identifying and delineating each numbered catheter in a multicatheter implant with the treatment planning system is time-consuming but critically important. For the balloon-based devices, a rigid relative geometry of the treatment lumens (e.g., Contura MLB, MammoSite ML) allows the importing of the applicator from a template library, dramatically reducing the time needed to outline the applicators and at the same time insuring a perfect and reproducible definition of the applicators even on less than optimal quality images. Once applicators are delineated, one defines the dwell positions by specifying, for each catheter, lumen or strut, a starting dwell position, a dwell increment – typically 5 mm, but it can be any value greater than 1 mm, system dependent – and an ending dwell position.

While there are many ways of creating a dose distribution, among them, manual and geometrical optimization, the only "true" optimization is the so-called volume or DVH-based optimization. Each of the structures that will be subjected to dose-

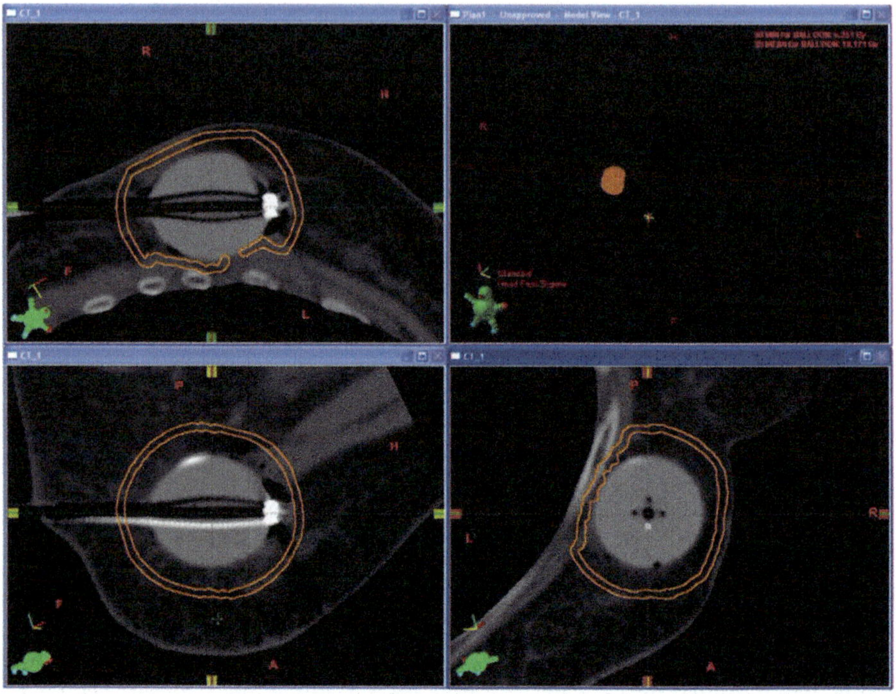

Fig. 14.5 The avoidance structure (a *thin ring* around PTV_EVAL) is shown here

volume constraints are sampled in a number of points, typically hundreds to a few thousands, depending on the volume. The reason for doing this is that in order to speed up the optimization process, one can choose to calculate dose in a much smaller number of points than the total number of dose voxels that the structure inherently has, based on the resolution of the dose matrix. While upper and lower constraints are placed on the dose-volume histogram for the target PTV_EVAL, the avoidance structure placed outside the target is the one limiting higher than prescription dose "spilling" into the normal tissue and thus driving the dose conformance. Good structures and good constraints will produce optimal plans. If one needs to manually "tweak" an already optimized plan, it is very likely that either the optimizer is not performing adequately (might be too sensitive and easily "captured" by local minima) or the set of constraints does not adequately or completely reflect the goals for the plan.

During "volume optimization," dose-volume constraints are placed on the histograms for PTV_EVAL and the avoidance structure (an example with typical constraints is shown in Fig. 14.6). Depending on the shape of the PTV_EVAL, one can limit the volume of the avoidance structure receiving prescription dose to a few percentage (1–10 %), thus increasing the "conformality" of the dose to the PTV_EVAL.

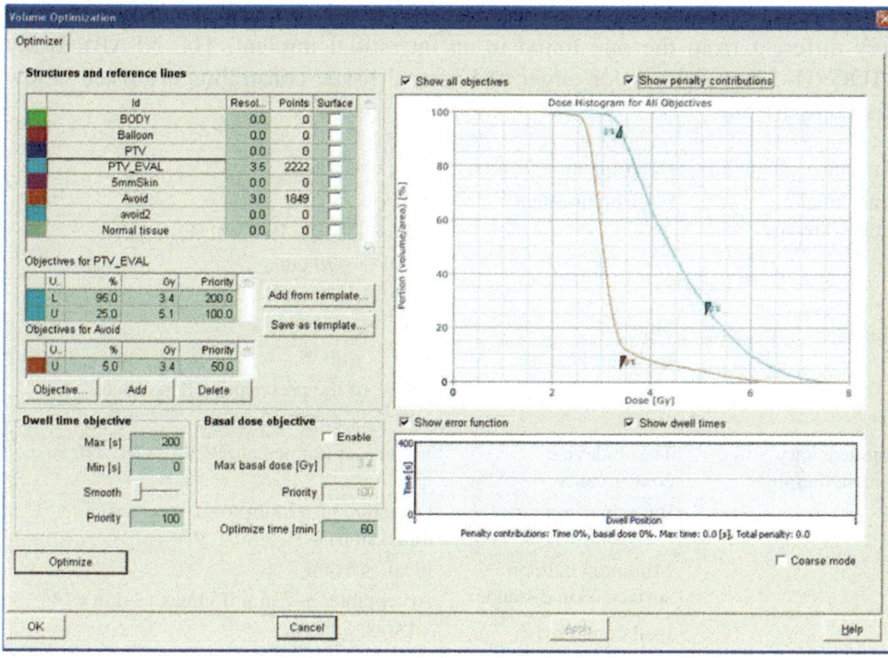

Fig. 14.6 Typical DVH optimization parameters for PTV_EVAL and the avoidance structure are shown

14.7 Dosimetry in Brachytherapy: Outcome Measures and Toxicity Analysis

Data about toxicity and dosimetric limits associated with various side effects originated after studying interstitial implants, historically the first APBI modality. A manuscript by Wazer et al. analyzed variables associated with late toxicity long-term cosmetic outcome after high-dose-rate interstitial brachytherapy [39]. They found that "suboptimal cosmetic outcome was significantly associated with the number of source dwell positions, V150, and V200 and inversely associated with DHI (0.77 vs. 0.73; p_0.05). The risk of Grade 1/2 skin toxicity was significantly associated with V150 and V200 and inversely associated with DHI (0.77 vs. 0.71; p_ 0.009). The risk of Grade 0/1 vs. Grade 2–4 subcutaneous toxicity was significantly associated only with a lower value of DHI (0.77 vs. 0.73; p_ 0.02). To further explore factors that might contribute to the risk of fat necrosis (symptomatic or asymptomatic), a separate analysis showed that only dose hotspots as reflected in V150 and V200 were significantly associated with elevated risk." It is interesting that while DHI proved to be a very strong indicator of late skin toxicity and late subcutaneous toxicity, its use in balloon brachytherapy completely disappeared. A probable explanation is in the fact that while most balloons can only achieve a DHI of about 0.7, the type of dose inhomogeneity in the target tissue around a balloon is very different from the one found in an interstitial implant. The NSABP B-39/ RTOG 04–13 guidelines for target and normal tissue constraints are listed below (for comparison):

Treatment technique	Determination factors	Dose constraints
Interstitial brachytherapy	Dose homogeneity	DHI ≥0.75
		DHI=(1–V150 %/V100 %)
		V150 % ≤70 cm^3
		V200 % ≤20 cm^3
	Skin	Skin Dmax <100 %
	Ipsilateral breast	V50 % ≤60 %
	Target	>90 % of the prescription dose covers
		>90 % of the PTV_EVAL
Intracavitary brachytherapy	Tissue-device conformance	Volume of trapped air/PTV_EVAL <10 %
	Balloon symmetry	Deviation of <2 mm from expected dimensions
	Minimum balloon surface–skin distance	Ideal: ≤7 mm
		Acceptable: 5–7 mm if Dmax to skin <145 %
	Ipsilateral breast	V150% ≤50 cm^3
		V200% ≤10 cm^3
		V50% <60 %
	Target	>90 % of the prescription dose covers >90 % of the PTV_EVAL (after accounting for volume of trapped air)

In later trials (e.g., multi-institutional phase IV Contura registry trial), dosimetry parameters were improved as the dosimetric coverage was increased to V95 >=95 %, while the max skin dose was decreased to 125%PD and max dose to the proximal rib, previously unconstrained, was set to no more than 145 %. In a comparison between multicatheter implants, Contura multilumen balloon and MammoSite single lumen, the multicatheter implants were found to have the lowest skin and chest wall dose, but between the two balloons, Contura was found to have the lowest skin and rib dose: 82 %PD and 82 %, respectively, vs. 94 %PD and 105 % for MammoSite [11]. A recent study of patterns of failure, patient selection, and dosimetric correlates for late toxicity after APBI using MammoSite balloon brachytherapy [35] established an even lower limit for max skin dose: "skin dose >100 % significantly predicted for the development of telangiectasia (50 % vs. 14 %, $p<.0001$)," "rediscovering" the initial constraint set for multicatheter implants. Despite reports on late chest wall toxicity after MammoSite breast brachytherapy [6] describing "fractures occurred in ribs with V (37) Gy and V (44) Gy each well below 33 %," no clear threshold were detected. In the first analysis of the American Society of Breast Surgeons MammoSite breast brachytherapy registry trial [32], excellent results were noted, and they compared favorably with other forms of APBI with similar follow-up. The toxicity rates with single-lumen brachytherapy-based APBI were low with fewer than 10 % of patients developing infections, 13 % symptomatic seromas, and 2.5 % fat necrosis, numbers comparable with WBI outcomes.

14.8 Dose Calculation Formalism: Effects of Contrast and Air

In 1995, the American Association of Physicists in Medicine (AAPM) Task Group No. 43 published a clinical protocol on dosimetry for interstitial brachytherapy sources, known as the "TG-43 formalism," and provided reference dosimetry datasets for commercially available 192Ir, 125I, and 103Pd sources.

While AAPM has reviewed and published reference-quality dosimetry datasets for low-energy brachytherapy sources in a number of reports (TG-43, TG-43U1, and TG-43U1S1), no similar effort has been attempted by AAPM or the European Society for Radiotherapy and Oncology (ESTRO) for high-energy sources. To fill this void, the AAPM Brachytherapy Subcommittee (BTSC) formed the High-Energy Brachytherapy Source Dosimetry (HEBD) Working Group to focus on photon-emitting brachytherapy sources with average energy higher than 50 keV. The report [24] reviewed published dosimetry for commonly used for high-energy 192Ir, 137Cs, and 60Co sources, critically reviewed the TG-43U1 formalism and developed a complete consensus dataset to support clinical planning for each source model.

New advances of dose calculation algorithms using sophisticated model-based dose calculations (MBDC) have been recently introduced for brachytherapy treatment planning systems (TPS). While TG-43 models a single source in an effectively infinite water phantom, MBDC model sources, applicators, patient heterogeneities, interfaces, and boundaries.

Two commercially available systems, the BrachyVision Acuros (BV-Acuros) (Varian, Palo Alto, CA) and the Oncentra Advanced Collapsed Cone Engine (ACE) (Elekta, Netherlands) MBDCs. BV-Acuros is a grid-based Boltzmann solver (GBBS) that deterministically solves the linear Boltzmann transport equation. Oncentra ACE is a collapsed cone convolution (CCC) algorithm which has been developed specifically for performing dose calculations for brachytherapy.

AAPM issued a report of a Task Group 186 [5] on the topic of model-based calculation formalism beyond TG-43. In conclusion, it was stated that "…it is important to acknowledge that the bulk of clinical brachytherapy dosimetry experience is with radiation transport and energy deposition in water, with dose to water reported (as calculated under the TG-43 approach). Hence, for the time being the recommendation that TG-43 calculations be performed in parallel with model-based dose calculations is crucial. Only in this way will the radiation therapy community become familiar with dose differences, including the impact on prescription dose and doses to points, organs and regions of interest."

For the breast irradiation with Ir-192, the most important factor impacting TG-43 dose calculation is the lack of complete scatter around the implant, leading to an overestimate of the skin dose (and to a smaller extent, target coverage). The magnitude of this overestimation was addressed by a number of investigators [15, 27] using multiple methods (TLD measurements, Monte Carlo simulations, etc.). The effects were found to be dependent on the balloon diameter, with up to 9.8 % for a 4 cm balloon and 13.2 % for a 6 cm balloon with no tissue beyond the prescription distance at the breast-skin interface. Smaller magnitude effects were noted on the breast-lung interface, with 6.7 and 9.6 % differences for the small and large balloon diameters, respectively.

Also studied intensively were the effects of contrast in the balloons and that of air pockets. While mixing radiopaque iodine-based contrast with water or saline helps visualizing the balloon contour, an increased absorption and attenuation can lead to a dose reduction if only a TG-43 calculation is performed (as opposed to a heterogeneity-corrected calculation). In a study [15], concentrations ranging from 5 to 25 % by volume of iodine-based radiopaque solution were simulated in balloons with diameters between 4 and 6 cm. The dose rate reduction at the typical prescription line of 1 cm away from the balloon surface ranged from - 0.8 % for the smallest balloon diameter and contrast concentration to a maximum of – 5.7 % for the largest balloon diameter and contrast concentration, relative to a water-filled balloon. Limiting the contrast concentration to 10 % would insure less than 3 % reduction in the prescription dose, regardless of balloon diameter. In terms of air pockets effects, the dose near the balloon surface may be increased by 0.5 % per cm^3 of air [8]. Monte Carlo simulation suggests that the interface effect (enhanced dose near surface) is primarily due to Compton electrons of short range (<0.5 mm).

Some of the issues regarding inhomogeneity and boundaries are exacerbated by the use of low-energy source like Xoft Axxent. In a study comparing TG-186-based calculations with TG-43 for balloon applicators [40], based on a prescription dose of 34 Gy, the average D90 to PTV was reduced by between ~4 and ~40 %, depending on the scoring method (dose to water (Dw, m) and dose to medium (Dm, m)), compared to the TG-43 result. Max skin dose was also reduced by 10–15 % due to the absence of backscatter not accounted for in TG-43. The final conclusion of the study was that "tissue heterogeneities, applicator, and patient geometries demonstrate the need for a more robust dose calculation method for low-energy brachytherapy sources."

14.9 Conclusions

Accelerated partial-breast irradiation is a new technology that provides faster, more convenient treatment after breast conserving. Of all the APBI modalities, intracavitary brachytherapy is probably the technique at the confluence of an important number of desirable features. Given the single entry catheter, as opposed to multiple catheters in interstitial implants, it is probably the easiest to tolerate for patients.

Relying on the device as a GTV surrogate instead of the delineation of an uncertain lumpectomy cavity, together with the use of library plans, makes planning an easy task. While our dose computation formalisms are evolving, we do have a reasonable good understanding of the dosimetric factors which play a role in good outcomes of the treatment. Long-term follow-up and guidelines like those outlined in RTOG 0413/ NSABP B-39 national phase III trial will hopefully demonstrate the long-term effectiveness and safety of this method for selected patients with early breast cancer.

References

1. Andrassy M, Niatetsky Y, Perez-Calatayud J. Controversies. Co-60 versus Ir-192 in HDR brachytherapy: scientific and technological comparison. Rev Fis Med. 2012;13(2):125–30.
2. Arthur DW, Koo D, Zwicker RD, Tong S, Bear HD, Kaplan BJ, et al. Partial breast brachytherapy after lumpectomy: low-dose-rate and high-dose-rate experience. Int J Radiat Oncol Biol Phys. 2003;56:681–9.
3. Baglan KL, Sharpe MB, Jaffray D, et al. Accelerated partial breast irradiation using 3D conformal radiation therapy (3D-CRT). Int J Radiat Oncol Biol Phys. 2003;55(2):302–11.
4. Baltas D, Sakelliou L, Zamboglou N. The physics of modern brachytherapy for oncology. New York: Taylor & Francis; 2007.
5. Beaulieu L, Carlsson Tedgren A, Carrier JF, Davis SD, Mourtada F, Rivard MJ, Thomson RM, Verhaegen F, Wareing TA, Williamson JF. Report of the task group 186 on model-based dose calculation methods in brachytherapy beyond the TG-43 formalism: current status and recommendations for clinical implementation. Med Phys. 2012;39(10):6208–36.
6. Brashears JH, Dragun AE, Jenrette JM. Late chest wall toxicity after MammoSite breast brachytherapy. Brachytherapy. 2009;8(1):19–25.
7. Carlsson AK, Ahnesjö A. The collapsed cone superposition algorithm applied to scatter dose calculations in brachytherapy. Med Phys. 2000;27(10):2320–32.
8. Cheng CW, Mitra R, Li XA, Das IJ. Dose perturbations due to contrast medium and air in mammosite treatment: an experimental and Monte Carlo study. Med Phys. 2005;32(7): 2279–87.
9. Cuttino LW, Todor D, Arthur DW. CT-guided multi-catheter insertion technique for partial breast brachytherapy: reliable target coverage and dose homogeneity. Brachytherapy. 2005;4(1):10–7.
10. Cuttino LW, Todor D, Pacyna L, Lin PS, Arthur DW. Three-dimensional conformal external beam radiotherapy (3D-CRT) for accelerated partial breast irradiation (APBI): what is the correct prescription dose? Am J Clin Oncol. 2006;29(5):474–8.
11. Cuttino LW, Todor D, Rosu M, Arthur DW. Skin and chest wall dose with multi-catheter and MammoSite breast brachytherapy: Implications for late toxicity. Brachytherapy. 2009;8(2):223–6.
12. Dickler A, Kirk MC, Coon A, Bernard D, Zusag T, Rotmensch J, Wazer DE. A dosimetric comparison of Xoft Axxent Electronic Brachytherapy and iridium-192 high-dose-rate brachytherapy in the treatment of endometrial cancer. Brachytherapy. 2008;7(4):351–4.
13. Durante M. New challenges in high-energy particle radiobiology. Br J Radiol. 2014;87(1035):20130626.
14. Jagsi R, Ben-David MA, Moran JM, et al. Unacceptable cosmesis in a protocol investigating intensity-modulated radiotherapy with active breathing control for accelerated partial-breast irradiation. Int J Radiat Oncol Biol Phys. 2010;76(1):71–8.
15. Kassas B, Mourtada F, Horton JL, Lane RG. Contrast effects on dosimetry of a partial breast irradiation system. Med Phys. 2004;31(7):1976–9.

16. Livi L, Buonamici FB, Simontacchi G, et al. Accelerated partial breast irradiation with IMRT: new technical approach and interim analysis of acute toxicity in a phase III randomized clinical trial. Int J Radiat Oncol Biol Phys. 2010;77(2):509–15.
17. Mackie TR, Holmes T, Swerdloff S, et al. Tomotherapy: a new concept for the delivery of dynamic conformal radiotherapy. Med Phys. 1993;20(6):1709–19.
18. Monroe JI, Dempsey JF, Dorton JA, Mutic S, Stubbs JB, Markman J, Williamson JF. Experimental validation of dose calculation algorithms for the GliaSite RTS, a novel 125I liquid-filled balloon brachytherapy applicator. Med Phys. 2001;28(1):73–85.
19. Moon SH, Shin KH, Kim TH, et al. Dosimetric comparison of four different external beam partial breast irradiation techniques: three-dimensional conformal radiotherapy, intensity modulated radiotherapy, helical tomotherapy, and proton beam therapy. Radiother Oncol. 2009;90(1):66–73.
20. Munro JJ, Medich DC. Dosimetric comparison of three radiation sources used in balloon-based breast. Brachytherapy. 2007;6:80–81.
21. Oliver M, Chen J, Wong E, Van Dyk J, Perera F. A treatment planning study comparing whole breast radiation therapy against conformal, IMRT and tomotherapy for accelerated partial breast irradiation. Radiother Oncol. 2007;82(3):317–23.
22. Paganetti H, Niemierko A, Ancukiewicz M, Gerweck LE, Goitein M, Loeffler JS, Suit HD. Relative biological effectiveness (RBE) values for proton beam therapy. Int J Radiat Oncol Biol Phys. 2002;53(2):407–21.
23. Park CC, Yom SS, Podgorsak MB, Harris E, Price Jr RA, Bevan A, Pouliot J, Konski AA, Wallner PE, Electronic Brachytherapy Working Group. American Society for Therapeutic Radiology and Oncology (ASTRO) Emerging Technology Committee report on electronic brachytherapy. Int J Radiat Oncol Biol Phys. 2010;76(4):963–72.
24. Perez-Calatayud J, Ballester F, Das RK, Dewerd LA, Ibbott GS, Meigooni AS, Ouhib Z, Rivard MJ, Sloboda RS, Williamson JF. Dose calculation for photon-emitting brachytherapy sources with average energy higher than 50 keV: report of the AAPM and ESTRO. Med Phys. 2012;39(5):2904–29.
25. Pignol JP, Keller B, Rakovitch E, Sankreacha R, Easton H, Que W. First report of a permanent breast 103Pd seed implant as adjuvant radiation treatment for early-stage breast cancer. Int J Radiat Oncol Biol Phys. 2006;64(1):176–81.
26. Poon E, Verhaegen F. Development of a scatter correction technique and its application to HDR 192Ir multicatheter breast brachytherapy. Med Phys. 2009;36:3703–13.
27. Raffi JA, Davis SD, Hammer CG, Micka JA, Kunugi KA, Musgrove JE, Winston Jr JW, Ricci-Ott TJ, DeWerd LA. Determination of exit skin dose for 192Ir intracavitary accelerated partial breast irradiation with thermoluminescent dosimeters. Med Phys. 2010;37(6):2693–702.
28. Richardson SL, Pino R. Dosimetric effects of an air cavity for the SAVI partial breast irradiation applicator. Med Phys. 2010;37(8):3919–26.
29. Rivard MJ, Davis SD, DeWerd LA, Rusch TW, Axelrod S. Calculated and measured brachytherapy dosimetry parameters in water for the Xoft Axxent x-ray source: an electronic brachytherapy source. Med Phys. 2006;33:4020–32.
30. Rivard MJ, Venselaar JL, Beaulieu L. The evolution of brachytherapy treatment planning. Med Phys. 2009;36(6):2136–53.
31. Rusch TW, Davis SD, DeWerd LA, Burnside RR, Axelrod S, Rivard MJ. Characterization of a new miniature x-ray source for electronic brachytherapy. Med Phys. 2004;31:1807.
32. Shah C, Badiyan S, Ben Wilkinson J, Vicini F, Beitsch P, Keisch M, Arthur D, Lyden M. Treatment efficacy with accelerated partial breast irradiation (APBI): final analysis of the American Society of Breast Surgeons MammoSite(®) breast brachytherapy registry trial. Ann Surg Oncol. 2013;20(10):3279–85.
33. Taghian AG, Kozak KR, Katz A, Adams J, Lu HM, Powell SN, et al. Accelerated partial breast irradiation using proton beams: initial dosimetric experience. Int J Radiat Oncol Biol Phys. 2006;65:1404–10.
34. Todor D, Becker S, Orton CG. Point/counterpoint. Brachytherapy is better than external beam therapy for partial breast irradiation. Med Phys. 2013;40(8):080601.

35. Vargo JA, Verma V, Kim H, Kalash R, Heron DE, Johnson R, Beriwal S. Extended (5-year) outcomes of accelerated partial breast irradiation using MammoSite balloon brachytherapy: patterns of failure, patient selection, and dosimetric correlates for late toxicity. Int J Radiat Oncol Biol Phys. 2014;88(2):285–91.
36. Vicini FA, Remouchamps V, Wallace M, et al. Ongoing clinical experience utilizing 3D conformal external beam radiotherapy to deliver partial-breast irradiation in patients with early-stage breast cancer treated with breast-conserving therapy. Int J Radiat Oncol Biol Phys. 2003;57(5):1247–53.
37. Vicini F, Winter K, Straube W, et al. A phase I/II trial to evaluate three dimensional conformal radiation therapy confined to the region of the lumpectomy cavity for Stage I/II breast carcinoma: initial report of feasibility and reproducibility of Radiation Therapy Oncology Group (RTOG) Study 0319. Int J Radiat Oncol Biol Phys. 2005;63(5):1531–7.
38. Wang X, Zhang X, Li X, Amos RA, Shaitelman SF, Hoffman K, Howell R, Salehpour M, Zhang SX, Sun TL, Smith B, Tereffe W, Perkins GH, Buchholz TA, Strom EA, Woodward WA. Accelerated partial-breast irradiation using intensity-modulated proton radiotherapy: do uncertainties outweigh potential benefits? Br J Radiol. 2013;86(1029):20130176.
39. Wazer DE, Kaufman S, Cuttino L, DiPetrillo T, Arthur DW. Accelerated partial breast irradiation: an analysis of variables associated with late toxicity and long-term cosmetic outcome after high-dose-rate interstitial brachytherapy. Int J Radiat Oncol Biol Phys. 2006;64(2):489–95.
40. White SA, Landry G, Fonseca GP, Holt R, Rusch T, Beaulieu L, Verhaegen F, Reniers B. Comparison of TG-43 and TG-186 in breast irradiation using a low energy electronic brachytherapy source. Med Phys. 2014;41(6):061701.
41. Yu CX. Intensity-modulated arc therapy with dynamic multileaf collimation: an alternative to tomotherapy. Phys Med Biol. 1995;40(9):1435–49.
42. Yu CX, Li XA, Ma L, et al. Clinical implementation of intensity modulated arc therapy. Int J Radiat Oncol Biol Phys. 2002;53(2):453–63.

Chapter 15
Overview of Outcomes with Accelerated Partial Breast Irradiation

Chirag Shah, Shireen Parsai, Rupesh Kotecha, Rahul Tendulkar, and Frank A. Vicini

Contents

15.1 Introduction

Historically, randomized trials and meta-analyses have demonstrated the benefits on local control, and breast cancer mortality with adjuvant whole breast irradiation (WBI) following breast-conserving surgery (BCS) [1–4]. However, review of patterns of failure in patients undergoing breast-conserving therapy has demonstrated that the majority of local recurrences occur within close proximity to the lumpectomy cavity [5]. Accelerated partial breast irradiation (APBI), which is based on the concept of radiotherapy to the area surrounding the lumpectomy cavity, has emerged as a treatment option for women with early-stage breast cancer over the past several decades. By limiting the volume of normal tissue treated, APBI has the potential for reduced toxicity, but also improved patient convenience as treatment is completed in 1 week or less [6, 7]. This directly addresses the underutilization of breast-conserving therapy and offers a solution to the large number of patients who fail to complete the 5–6-week course of adjuvant external beam WBI due to social and economic considerations [8].

C. Shah, MD (✉) • S. Parsai • R. Kotecha • R. Tendulkar
Department of Radiation Oncology, Cleveland Clinic, Taussig Cancer Institute, Cleveland, USA
e-mail: csshah27@hotmail.com

F.A. Vicini
Michigan Healthcare Professionals/21st Century Oncology, Farmington Hills, USA

D.W. Arthur et al. (eds.), *Short Course Breast Radiotherapy: A Comprehensive Review of Hypofractionation, Partial Breast, and Intra-Operative Irradiation*, DOI 10.1007/978-3-319-24388-7_15

As technology has improved over time, APBI has similarly evolved and now incorporates multiple treatment techniques and options. The initial APBI technique was a multicatheter interstitial brachytherapy implant that used a high-dose-rate (HDR), low-dose-rate (LDR), or pulsed-dose-rate (PDR) technique and represents the most mature APBI data available at this time. Subsequently, less technically complex brachytherapy techniques have been developed including a single-lumen applicator with further innovations leading to the development of multi-lumen and strut-based applicators. These newer devices allow for increased dosimetric flexibility, a known limitation with single-lumen applicators [9, 10]. Finally, for those patients wishing to limit further invasive procedures, external beam radiotherapy techniques have been developed including 3-dimensional conformal radiotherapy (3D-CRT), intensity-modulated radiation therapy (IMRT), and proton therapy. This chapter will present outcomes with each APBI technique with a focus on randomized data as well as prospective, single institution, and retrospective series.

15.2 Interstitial Brachytherapy

Interstitial brachytherapy, as noted above, represents the initial technique developed to deliver APBI and has been utilized as a boost or as monotherapy. While more mature treatment data and clinical outcomes for patients treated with early forms of the technique are available in the literature, these studies were limited by technique differences compared to current practice, a lack of modern imaging, inconsistent patient selection criteria, and less rigid quality assurance procedures [11, 13]. Therefore, this section will primarily focus on modern interstitial APBI.

Data from the National Institute of Oncology in Hungary represents the most robust and mature data available for modern interstitial APBI. The initial prospective study of 45 patients accrued between 1996 and 1998. All patients received HDR interstitial implants, and eligibility criteria limited included early-stage breast cancer patients with tumors less than 2 cm, negative margins, pathologically negative lymph nodes (micrometastases allowed), and low-grade disease. With a median follow-up of 133 months, the 12-year rate of ipsilateral breast tumor recurrence (IBTR) was 9.3 % with a corresponding cause-specific survival (CSS) of 91.1 %. Rates of toxicity remained low with a majority of patients (77.8 %) reporting a excellent/good cosmesis and only one reported case of grade 3 fibrosis (2.2 %) [14]. The results of this prospective study prompted the initiation of a subsequent randomized trial in which 258 women were randomized to receive WBI or partial breast irradiation (PBI). Partial breast irradiation in this trial was primarily delivered with HDR multicatheter brachytherapy ($n=88$) to a dose of 36.4 Gy delivered in 7 fractions, while a subset of patients received a limited electron field PBI ($n=40$) to a dose of 50 Gy in 25 fractions. Ten-year outcomes for this study reported no statistically significant differences in the rates of local recurrence between patients treated with WBI and PBI (5.1 % vs. 5.9 %) as well as equivalent rates of disease-free survival (DFS), CSS, and overall survival (OS). It is important to note that although clinical outcomes between the groups were similar, patients treated with PBI were found to have higher rates of excellent/good cosmetic outcomes compared to those treated with WBI (81 % vs. 63 %, $p<0.01$) [15].

The Radiation Therapy Oncology Group (RTOG) protocol 9517 was a phase II trial designed to evaluate multicatheter interstitial APBI. Of the 99 patients enrolled in this study, 66 patients received HDR brachytherapy (34 Gy in 10 twice-daily fractions within 5 days) and 33 patients received LDR brachytherapy (45 Gy in 3.5–5 days). At 5 years, the rates of IBTR remained low at 3 % and 6 % for the HDR and LDR cohorts, respectively. The reported grade 3 toxicity rate across all patients was 13 % with the majority of toxicity due to skin dimpling (37 %), fibrosis (45 %), telangiectasias (45 %), and symptomatic fat necrosis (15 %). Seventy-five percent of patients were satisfied with their treatment, and 66 % reported a excellent/good cosmetic outcome following treatment [16, 17]. In order to compare outcomes with WBI, a matched pair analysis was performed at William Beaumont Hospital in which 199 patients treated with HDR interstitial APBI were matched to 199 patients treated with WBI based on age, tumor size, nodal status, estrogen receptor status, and hormonal therapy. At 12 years, no significant differences in clinical outcomes (local recurrence, regional recurrence, DFS, CSS, OS) were noted between the two cohorts with the exception of reduced distant metastases with APBI [18]. A similar analysis was performed at Washington University in which 202 interstitial APBI patients were matched with 94 WBI patients with no difference in local control noted between the groups with greater than 5 years of follow-up. It is important to note that in this study, the interstitial APBI cohort of patients was found to have a 17.6 % rate of fat necrosis and 10.1 % rate of symptomatic fat necrosis with 95 % of patients having a excellent/good cosmesis at 3 years [19–21].

A phase I/II protocol from Harvard evaluated 50 patients with LDR interstitial APBI on a dose-escalation protocol. With greater than 11 years of follow-up, the local recurrence rate was 15 % with 67 % of patients reporting excellent/good cosmesis. Toxicity profiles were elevated with 54 % of patients having moderate/severe fibrosis and 9 and 13 % of patients having grade 3 or 4 skin/subcutaneous toxicity, respectively [22]. Another phase II trial from a multicenter collaboration in Germany and Austria enrolled 274 patients with low-risk breast cancer, tumors less than 3 cm in size resected with negative surgical margins. Patients received APBI with PDR ($n=175$) or HDR ($n=99$). At 5 years, the rate of IBTR was 2.9 % with a 0.4 % rate of grade 3 or higher toxicity with PDR and 2.2 % with HDR. Acute toxicity was seen in 6.6 % of patients, and 90 % of patients had excellent/good cosmesis [23]. A summary of data with interstitial APBI is presented in Table 15.1 [14–29].

A closed phase III multicenter (GEC-ESTRO, NCT00402519) trial evaluated HDR/PDR interstitial APBI and randomized patients to either standard WBI (50 Gy/25 fractions) with a boost (10 Gy/5 fractions) or interstitial APBI with a primary end point of local control. Inclusion criteria for this trial include women 40 years and older with stage 0–II breast cancer with tumors $\leq$3 cm, node negative (except DCIS), and clear resection margins at least 2 mm in any direction. Results from this study are anticipated in the next few years.

Table 15.1 Outcomes with interstitial APBI

Series; year published	Patients (*n*)	Median follow-up (months)	Technique	Complications/cosmesis	Local control
Hungarian; 2010	45	133	HDR	2.2 % Grade 3 fibrosis, no grade 3 telangiectasia, 2.2 % fat necrosis, 77.8 % excellent/good cosmesis	12-year LR 9.3 %
Hungarian randomized; 2013	258 (128 PBI, 88 brachytherapy)	124	HDR/electrons	81 % excellent/good cosmesis	10-year LR 5.1 % (no significant difference)
RTOG 9517; 2008/2014	99	73	HDR (66)/LDR (33)	13 % grade 3 toxicity, 45 % fibrosis, 15 % fat necrosis, 66 % excellent/good cosmesis	5-year LR 3 %/6 % (HDR/LDR)
William Beaumont Hospital; 2011	199	127	HDR		No difference in 12-year LR (3.8 % vs. 5.0 %)
Washington University; 2012	202	60	HDR	17.6 % rate of fat necrosis, 10.1 % rate of symptomatic fat necrosis, 95 % excellent/good cosmesis	5-year LC 97 %; no difference in local control with matched whole breast cohort
Harvard University; 2012	50	133	LDR	9 %/13 % grade 3/4 toxicity, 54 % moderate/severe fibrosis, 34 % telangiectasia, 35 % fat necrosis, 67 % excellent/good cosmesis	12-year LC 15 %
Germany/Austria; 2011	274	63	PDR (175)/HDR (99)	0.4 %/2.2 % grade 3 or greater with PDR/HDR, 90 % excellent/good cosmesis	5-year LR 2.9 %

Series; year published	Patients (n)	Median follow-up (months)	Technique	Complications/cosmesis	Local control
Ochsner Clinic; 2000	51	75	LDR/HDR	8 % grade 3 or 4 toxicity; comparable outcomes, toxicity, cosmesis compared to WBI	75-month 2 % LR
Florence; 1995	115	50	LDR (Ir-192)		5-year LR 6 %
University of Kansas; 2001	24	47	HDR	100 % excellent/good cosmesis	No LR
Tufts; 2007	32		HDR	27.3 % fat necrosis, 89 % excellent cosmesis	5-year LR 6.1 %
University of Wisconsin; 2008	247	48	HDR	93 % excellent/good cosmesis	5-year LR 2.2 %
Virginia Commonwealth University; 2003	44	42	LDR (11)/HDR (31)	79.6 %/90 % excellent/good cosmesis with LDR/HDR	No LR
Orebro Medical Centre; 2009	50	86	PDR	12 % fat necrosis, 56 % excellent/good cosmesis	7-year LC 96 %

15.3 Applicator-Based Brachytherapy

Applicator-based brachytherapy began with the FDA approval of the MammoSite single-lumen applicator. This technology allowed for the delivery of APBI without the technical complexity or requirements of multicatheter brachytherapy. The initial study evaluated 70 patients, 43 of whom completed treatment to a dose of 34 Gy in 10 fractions over 1 week. With a median follow-up of 5.5 years, no patients developed a local recurrence, and the procedure was well tolerated, with an infection rate of 9.3 % and a seroma formation rate of 32.6 % (12 % symptomatic). Excellent/good cosmesis was observed in 83 % of treated patients with a skin spacing >7 mm associated with reduced rates of telangiectasia and retraction as well as improved cosmetic outcomes. Also, seroma formation was found to be associated with an open placement technique [31]. Similar findings were noted in a preliminary analysis from William Beaumont Hospital of 80 patients. Three-year rates of local recurrence were 2.9 % with 88 % of patients reporting a excellent/good cosmesis; however, lower rates of cosmesis were noted with spacing less than 7 mm and in patients receiving chemotherapy. The toxicity profile was comparable with a 10 % rate of symptomatic seroma, 8.8 % rate of fat necrosis, and an 11.3 % rate of infection [32].

The largest series with applicator-based brachytherapy to date comes from the American Society of Breast Surgeons (ASBS) MammoSite Registry. Between 2002 and 2004, 1,449 patients with early-stage breast cancer were prospectively enrolled and treated using a single-lumen applicator. With a median follow-up of 63 months, the 5-year rate of IBTR was 3.8 %, with estrogen receptor negativity and larger tumor size associated with IBTR. At 60, 72, and 84 months, the rates of excellent/good cosmesis were 91.3 %, 90.5 %, and 90.6 % with a 2.5 % rate of fat necrosis and a 9.6 % rate of infection. Final toxicity analysis demonstrated that the rate of any complication was 24.2 % at 1 year and 38.5 % at any time, whereas for noninfectious complications, the rates were 14.8 % and 28.9 %, respectively. Symptomatic seromas were seen in 13 % of cases. These rates were comparable to the toxicity and infection rates observed in patients treated with standard and hypofractionated external beam radiation therapy [32, 33]. Similar findings were noted in a multi-institutional analysis of 483 patients treated with a single-lumen applicator between 2000 and 2004. Though follow-up was short at 24 months, there was 1.2 % local failure rate and a 91 % rate of excellent/good cosmesis. The rate of infection was 9 % (4.8 % with closed technique) with infection impacting overall cosmetic outcome. A skin spacing of less than 6 mm was associated with increased risk of acute skin reaction and subsequent development of telangiectasias [34]. Similar results have been noted from multiple single institution series, which are presented in Table 15.2 [30–46].

In order to improve dosimetric outcomes and enhance the ability to sculpt dose in order to achieve increased target coverage while reducing dose to normal tissue structures (e.g., skin, chest wall, and normal breast tissue), multi-lumen

Table 15.2 Outcomes with applicator-based APBI

Series; year published	Patients (*n*)	Follow-up (months)	Technique	Complications/cosmesis	Local control
MammoSite FDA; 2007	43	65	Single lumen	32.6 % seroma, 12 % symptomatic seromas, 9.3 % infections, 83.3 % excellent/good cosmesis	5-year LR 0 %
William Beaumont Hospital; 2007	80	22	Single lumen	10 % symptomatic seromas, 11.3 % infections, 8.8 % fat necrosis, 88 % excellent/good cosmesis	3-year LR 2.9 %
MammoSite Registry; 2013	1,449	63	Single lumen	13.4 % symptomatic seromas, 9.6 % infections, 13.0 % telangiectasia, 2.5 % fat necrosis, 91.3 % excellent/good cosmesis	5-year LR 3.8 %
Multi-institutional (United States); 2008	483	24	Single lumen	9 % infections, 91 % excellent/good cosmesis	2-year LR 1.2 %
Contura Phase 4; 2014	342	36	Multi-lumen	4.4 % symptomatic seroma, 8.5 % infection, 88 % excellent/good cosmesis	3-year LR 2.2 %
University of California, San Diego; 2009/2011	30/100	12/21	Strut applicator	No symptomatic seroma, fat necrosis/2 cases of symptomatic seroma, 1.9 % fat necrosis	1 % LR (reported in 2011)
St. Vincent's; 2004	31	11	Single lumen	7 % grade 3 moist desquamation, 16 % infections, 86 % excellent/good cosmesis	
Tufts; 2004/2006	28/38	12/17	Single lumen	11 % grade 2–4 fibrosis/76 % seroma rate	
Multi-institutional (Europe); 2006	23	20	Single lumen	3 cases of rupture, 39 % seroma, 26 % telangiectasia, 56 % hyperpigmentation, 91 % erythema	
Rush; 2007	70	26	Single lumen		Crude local failure rate 5.7 %
Magee-Women's Hospital; 2009	92	24	Single lumen	Higher rate of seroma with open placement (79 %), skin spacing associated with cosmesis	

(continued)

Table 15.2 (continued)

Series; year published	Patients (*n*)	Follow-up (months)	Technique	Complications/cosmesis	Local control
University of South Carolina; 2010	111	46	Single lumen	90 % excellent/good cosmesis	4-year ipsilateral breast control 5 %
The Breast Center, Georgia; 2012	46	36	Multi-lumen	4.3 % persistent seroma, no grade III toxicity, 2.2 % telangiectasia, 97 % excellent/good cosmesis	2 % LR,

applicators were subsequently developed. Dosimetric studies validated an improved skin and rib dose as well as the ability to treat cases with skin spacing less than 7 mm, capitalizing on the ability of the technique to modulate dose [9, 10, 42]. A multi-institutional analysis demonstrated that similar acute toxicities were noted for multi-lumen applicators even with close skin and rib parameters as compared to single-lumen techniques with greater spacing [42]. Long-term results from a multi-institutional series of 342 patients treated with a multi-lumen device demonstrated a 2.2 % recurrence rate at 3 years with 88 % excellent/good cosmesis. Infection was seen in 8.5 % of patients and a symptomatic seroma rate of 4.4 %, with improved outcomes seen in high-volume centers [43]. Similarly, strut-based devices have been developed to improve upon the initial applicators. A preliminary experience in 30 patients using this technique demonstrated improved target coverage and no symptomatic seromas or fat necrosis at 1 year even with limited skin spacing, which was subsequently confirmed in a update of 100 patients [45, 46].

Two population-based studies evaluated toxicity outcomes with brachytherapy-based APBI. Smith et al. evaluated 92,735 women 67 years or older with invasive breast cancer diagnosed between 2003 and 2007. A total of 85,783 received whole breast irradiation and 6,952 received brachytherapy. The study found that rates of subsequent mastectomy were higher with brachytherapy as were rates of infectious and noninfectious complications with no difference in survival noted [47]. Similar findings were noted in smaller Medicare analysis from Presley et al. [48]. These studies have significant limitations including short follow-up (median 3 years for Smith et al., minimum 1 year of follow-up for Presley et al.), a lack of patient/pathologic data, limited patient population (67 years or older), a failure to evaluate toxicities that are higher with WBI (e.g., pulmonary, cardiac), and a use of older data prior to the utilization of multi-lumen applicators. Also, they were claims-based analysis, which would allow for a contralateral mastectomy to be scored as a treatment-related mastectomy and have methodology with significant limitations as noted by Chen et al. and Kuske et al. [49, 50]. These retrospective data also conflict with level I evidence from randomized and prospective studies that have shown excellent clinical outcomes and low toxicity rates.

15.4 External Beam Techniques

External beam APBI was evaluated in early trials; however, these studies did not utilize modern radiotherapy techniques and were found to have higher rates of local recurrence [51, 52]. Over the past two decades more modern techniques have been developed using 3D-CRT and IMRT [53, 54]. The appeal of external beam APBI is the ability to deliver accelerated courses of radiotherapy without additional invasive procedures. Nonetheless, the trade-off has traditionally been an increase in normal breast tissue irradiated and, therefore, the potential for increased treatment-related toxicity.

The RAPID trial was a randomized trial comparing hypofractionated/standard fractionated WBI (42.5 Gy/16 fractions or 50 Gy/25 fractions ± boost) with 3D-CRT APBI (38.5 Gy/10 fractions). From 2006 to 2011, the trial enrolled 2,135 women with tumors less than 3 cm following breast-conserving surgery. With a median follow-up of 36 months, 3D-CRT APBI was associated with higher rates of adverse cosmesis (29 % vs. 17 %) as well as higher rates of grade 1 or 2 toxicity with no difference in the rate of grade 3 toxicity [55]. RTOG 0319 was a phase II trial that evaluated 3D-CRT APBI in patients with stage I/II (less than 3 cm) breast cancer following partial mastectomy with 52 patients enrolled and treated to a dose of 38.5 Gy in 10 fractions. At a median follow-up of 5.3 years, 64 % of patients had excellent/good cosmesis, a decrease from the 82 % observed at 1 year. Grade 3 toxicity remained rare at 5.8 % with 37 % of patients having grade 1 toxicity and 50 % experiencing grade 2 toxicity [56]. Similar results were seen in smaller series from the University of Michigan and Tufts University; Liss et al. reported a series of 34 patients treated with IMRT with a median follow-up of 5 years. In this series, 73.3 % of patients had excellent/good cosmesis with 3.3 % rate of grade 2 fibrosis and an overall 97 % local control rate [57, 58].

One of the largest single institution series with 3D-CRT APBI comes from William Beaumont Hospital. Using the aforementioned technique, 205 patients were treated between 2000 and 2011. With a median follow-up of 4.8 years, the 5-year rates of IBTR, CSS, and OS were 0 %, 99T, and 92 %, respectively. Eighty-one percent of patients reported a excellent/good cosmesis with a 7.5 % rate of grade 3 fibrosis and 7.6 % rate of telangiectasias (no other grade 3 toxicities noted) [59]. Similarly, a series of 100 patients from New York University, treated with 3D-CRT using a prone technique, found a 5-year local recurrence rate of 1 % with 89 % of patients having excellent/good cosmesis and minimal grade 3 toxicities [60]. Furthermore, due to concerns regarding the potential for toxicity based on the studies noted above, an interim analysis of the NSABP B-39 trial was performed, and in patients treated with the 3D-CRT technique, a 3 % rate of grade 3 or greater fibrosis was observed [61].

One technique that offers the potential to reduce toxicity with external beam APBI is intensity-modulated radiation therapy (IMRT). One of the largest single institution series using this technique comes from the Rocky Mountain Cancer Center. With a median follow-up of 53 months, there was a 0.7 % rate of IBTR with

Table 15.3 Outcomes with external beam APBI

Series; year published	Patients (*n*)	Follow-up (months)	Technique	Complications/cosmesis	Local control
RAPID; 2013	2,135	36	3D-CRT	3D-CRT associated with higher rates of adverse cosmesis and grade 1/2 toxicity	
RTOG 0319; 2013	52	63	3D-CRT	5.8 % grade 2 toxicity, 3.3 % grade 2 fibrosis, 64 % excellent/good cosmesis	6 % LR
University of Michigan; 2014	34	60	IMRT	3.3 % grade 2 fibrosis, 73.3 % excellent/good cosmesis	3 % LR
Tufts; 2013	80	32	3D-CRT	7.5 % grade 3/4 fibrosis, 11 % fat necrosis, 81 % excellent/good cosmesis	
William Beaumont Hospital; 2013	192	56	3D-CRT	7.5 % grade 3 fibrosis, 7.6 % telangiectasias, 81 % excellent/good cosmesis	5 year LR 0 %
NYU; 2012	100	64	3D-CRT-prone	Grade 3 toxicity 2 %, 89 % excellent/good cosmesis	5-year LR 1 %
NSABP B-39/ RTOG 0413; 2011	1,367	37	3D-CRT	3 % grade 3 or greater fibrosis, 89 % excellent/ good cosmesis	
Rocky Mountain; 2013	136	53	IMRT	3.6 % telangiectasia, 88.2 % excellent/good cosmesis	4-year LR 0.7 %
University of Florence; 2015	520	60	IMRT	0 % grade 3 toxicity, 95.1 % excellent/good cosmesis	No difference in IBTR or overall survival with APBI at 5 years
Massachusetts General Hospital; 2014	98	82	Protons	More common skin toxicities, 62 % excellent/good cosmesis	7-year LR 11 %
Loma Linda; 2014	100	60	Protons	No grade 3 acute skin toxicity, 90 % excellent/ good cosmesis	5-year ipsilateral breast tumor recurrence-free survival 97 %
Christie; 1996	708	96	Electron		8-year LR 25 %
United Kingdom; 2005	174	96	Multiple		8-year LR 12 %

Table 15.3 (continued)

Series; year published	Patients (n)	Follow-up (months)	Technique	Complications/cosmesis	Local control
Canadian multi-institutional; 2011	104	36	3D-CRT	1 grade 3 toxicity, 82 % excellent/good cosmesis	1 local recurrence
Seoul National University; 2013	30	59	Protons	Excellent/good cosmesis 69 %	No LR
Massachusetts General Hospital; 2014	19	82	Protons	7-year excellent/good cosmesis 62 %, increased toxicity with protons	7-year local recurrence 11 %

100 % and 97 % CSS and OS, respectively. Eighty-eight percent of patients rated their cosmesis excellent/good with a 3.6 % rate of telangiectasias and two rib fractures noted [62]. Similarly, a randomized study from the University of Florence compared IMRT APBI with WBI in 520 women. With 5-year follow-up, no difference in IBTR (1.5 % vs. 1.4 %, $p=0.86$) or overall survival was noted. Acute grade 3 toxicity was observed in 6.5 % of patients with WBI and 0 % with APBI, whereas excellent cosmesis was noted in 95.1 % of APBI patients and 89.6 % of WBI patients [63].

Another APBI technique is proton therapy. Dosimetric data was promising; however, initial studies demonstrated high rates of acute skin toxicity with 79 % of patients having moderate/severe skin changes and 22 % experiencing severe moist desquamation. An update of the Massachusetts General Hospital experience of 98 patients found that at 7 years, 62 % of patients had excellent/good cosmesis (as compared with 95 % for photons) with increased rates of telangiectasias, pigmentation changes, and late skin toxicity [64–66]. More recent studies including an update of the Loma Linda trial have demonstrated improvement in outcomes with refinement of the technique and with 5-year follow-up demonstrated no grade 3 or greater acute skin toxicity and 90 % of patients experiencing excellent/good cosmesis [67]. A summary of studies evaluating external APBI with the various different techniques is presented in Table 15.3 [55–69].

15.5 Conclusions

With increasing availability of recurrence and toxicity data with long-term follow-up, APBI continues to gain traction as rates of recurrence are low and toxicity is comparable or improved as compared to WBI. Interstitial APBI, representing the technique with the longest follow-up, has demonstrated equivalent outcomes compared with WBI based on data from a randomized trial as well as prospective studies, matched pair analyses, and retrospective reviews. Furthermore, toxicity rates with this technique remain low with long-term follow-up beyond 10 years. Applicator-based APBI allows for a greater number of patients to have access to APBI due to the reduced technical complexity of the technique as compared with multicatheter interstitial APBI. Over the past decade, there has been an evolution in applicators from single-lumen to multi-lumen and strut devices, which correspondingly has led to improved dosimetric outcomes. While data with long-term follow-up is limited, toxicity data with the multi-lumen approach is promising at this time. Finally, external beam APBI offers the promise of a noninvasive APBI approach. Despite recent data suggesting higher toxicity rates with 3D-CRT, new techniques including IMRT and improved image guidance may address some of the differences between external beam APBI and brachytherapy and allow for comparable toxicity profiles in the years to come.

In the next several years, outcomes from randomized trials including the NSABP B-39/RTOG 0413 and GEC-ESTRO trial will provide clinicians with further clinical data upon which to make treatment decisions regarding adjuvant radiotherapy. Further, with increased data comes the ability to risk stratify patients and tailor local therapy to a patient's specific clinical and pathologic features as well as tumor genetics.

References

1. Fisher B, Anderson S, Bryant J, et al. Twenty-year follow-up of a randomized trial comparing total mastectomy, lumpectomy, and lumpectomy plus irradiation for the treatment of invasive breast cancer. N Engl J Med. 2002;347:1233–41.
2. Veronesi U, Cascinelli N, Mariani L, et al. Twenty-year follow-up of a randomized study comparing breast-conserving surgery with radical mastectomy for early breast cancer. N Engl J Med. 2002;347:1227–32.
3. Litiere S, Werutsky G, Fentiman IS, et al. Breast conserving therapy versus mastectomy for stage I-II breast cancer: 20 year follow-up of the EORTC 10801 phase 3 randomised trial. Lancet Oncol. 2012;13:412–9.
4. Darby S, McGale P, Correa C, et al. Effect of radiotherapy after breast-conserving surgery on 10-year recurrence and 15-year breast cancer death: meta-analysis of individual patient data for 10,801 women in 17 randomised trials. Lancet. 2011;378:1707–16.
5. Gage I, Recht A, Gelman R, et al. Long-term outcome following breast-conserving surgery and radiation therapy. Int J Radiat Oncol Biol Phys. 1995;33:245–51.
6. Wilkinson JB, Martinez AA, Chen PY, et al. Four-year results using balloon-based brachytherapy to deliver accelerated partial breast irradiation with a 2-day dose fractionation schedule. Brachytherapy. 2012;11:97–104.
7. Swanson TA, Vicini FA. Overview of accelerated partial breast irradiation. Curr Oncol Rep. 2008;10:54–60.
8. White A, Richardson LC, Krontiras H, et al. Socioeconomic disparities in breast cancer treatment among older women. J Women Health. 2014;23:335–41.
9. Brown S, McLaughlin M, Pope DK, et al. A dosimetric comparison of the multilumen balloon breast brachytherapy catheter vs. the single-lumen MammoSite balloon device in patients treated with accelerated partial breast irradiation at a single institution. Brachytherapy. 2011;10:68–73.
10. Gurdalli S, Kuske RR, Quiet CA, et al. Dosimetric performance of Strut-Adjusted Volume Implant: a new single-entry multicatheter breast brachytherapy applicator. Brachytherapy. 2011;10:128–35.

11. Poti Z, Nemeskeri C, Fekeshazy A, et al. Partial breast irradiation with interstitial 60CO brachytherapy results in frequent grade 3 or 4 toxicity. Evidence based on a 12-year follow up of 70 patients. Int J Radiat Oncol Biol Phys. 2004;5:1022–33.
12. Fentiman IS, Deshmane V, Tong D, et al. Caesium (137) implant as sole radiation therapy for operable breast cancer: a phase II trial. Radiother Oncol. 2004;71:281–5.
13. Cionini L, Marzano S, Pacini P, et al. Iridium implant of the surgical bed as the sole radiotherapeutic treatment after conservative surgery for breast cancer. Radiother Oncol. 1995;35:S1.
14. Polgar C, Major T, Fodor J, et al. Accelerated partial breast irradiation using high-dose-rate interstitial brachytherapy: 12-year update of a prospective clinical study. Radiother Oncol. 2010;94:274–9.
15. Polgar C, Fodor J, Major T, et al. Breast-conserving therapy with partial or whole breast irradiation: ten-year results of the Budapest randomized trial. Radiother Oncol. 2013;108:197–202.
16. Arthur DW, Winter K, Kuske RR, et al. A Phase II trial of brachytherapy alone after lumpectomy for select breast cancer: tumor control and survival outcomes of RTOG 95–17. Int J Radiat Oncol Biol Phys. 2008;72:467–73.
17. Rabinovitch R, Winter K, Kuske R, et al. RTOG 95–17, a Phase II trial to evaluate brachytherapy as the sole method of radiation therapy for Stage I and II breast carcinoma- year 5 toxicity and cosmesis. Brachytherapy. 2014;13:17–22.
18. Shah C, Antonucci JV, Wilkinson JB, et al. Twelve-year clinical outcomes and patterns of failure with accelerated partial breast irradiation versus whole-breast irradiation: results of a matched-pair analysis. Radiother Oncol. 2011;100:210–4.
19. Ferraro DJ, Garsa AA, Dewees TA, et al. Comparison of accelerated partial breast irradiation via multicatheter interstitial brachytherapy versus whole breast radiation. Radiat Oncol. 2012;7:53.
20. Garsa AA, Ferraro DJ, Dewees T, et al. Analysis of fat necrosis after adjuvant high-dose-rate interstitial brachytherapy for early stage breast cancer. Brachytherapy. 2013;12:99–106.
21. Garsa AA, Ferraro DJ, DeWees T, et al. Cosmetic analysis following breast-conserving surgery and adjuvant high-dose-rate interstitial brachytherapy for early-stage breast cancer: a prospective clinical study. Int J Radiat Oncol Biol Phys. 2013;85(4):965–70.
22. Hattangadi JA, Powell SN, MacDonald SM, et al. Accelerated partial breast irradiation with low-dose-rate interstitial implant brachytherapy after wide local excision: 12-year outcomes from a prospective trial. Int J Radiat Oncol Biol Phys. 2012;83:791–800.
23. Strnad V, Hildebrandt G, Potter R, et al. Accelerated partial breast irradiation: 5-year results of the German-Austrian multicenter phase II trial using interstitial multicatheter brachytherapy alone after breast-conserving surgery. Int J Radiat Oncol Biol Phys. 2011;80:17–24.
24. Ott OJ, Hildebrandt G, Potter R, et al. Accelerated partial breast irradiation with multi-catheter brachytherapy: local control, side effects, and cosmetic outcomes for 274 patients. Results of the German-Austrian multi-centre trial. Radiother Oncol. 2007;82:281–6.
25. King TA, Bolton JS, Kuske RR, et al. Long-term results of wide-field brachytherapy as the sole method of radiation therapy after segmental mastectomy for T(is,1,2) breast cancer. Am J Surg. 2000;180:299–304.
26. Krishnan L, Jewell WR, Tawfik OW, et al. Breast conservation therapy with tumor bed irradiation alone in a selected group of patients with Stage I breast cancer. Breast J. 2001;7:91–6.
27. Patel RR, Christensen ME, Hodge CW, et al. Clinical outcome analysis in "high-risk" versus "low-risk" patients eligible for national surgical adjuvant breast and bowel B-39/radiation therapy oncology group 0413: five-year results. Int J Radiat Oncol Biol Phys. 2008;70:970–3.
28. Arthur D, Koo D, Zwicker RD, et al. Partial breast brachytherapy after lumpectomy: low-dose-rate and high-dose-rate experience. Int J Radiat Oncol Biol Phys. 2003;56:681–9.
29. Johansson B, Karlsson L, Liljegren G, et al. Pulsed dose rate brachytherapy as the sole adjuvant radiotherapy after breast-conserving surgery of T1-2 breast cancer: first long time results from a clinical study. Radiother Oncol. 2009;90:30–5.

30. Benitez PR, Keisch ME, Vicini F, et al. Five-year results: the initial clinical trial of MammoSite balloon brachytherapy for partial breast irradiation in early-stage breast cancer. Am J Surg. 2007;194:456–62.
31. Chao KK, Vicini FA, Wallace M, et al. Analysis of treatment efficacy, cosmesis, and toxicity using the MammoSite breast brachytherapy catheter to deliver accelerated partial-breast irradiation: the William Beaumont Hospital experience. Int J Radiat Oncol Biol Phys. 2007;69:32–40.
32. Shah C, Badiyan S, Ben Wilkinson J, et al. Treatment efficacy with accelerated partial breast irradiation (APBI): final analysis of the American Society of Breast Surgeons MammoSite breast brachytherapy trial. Ann Surg Oncol. 2013;20:3279–85.
33. Shah C, Khwaja S, Badiyan S, et al. Brachytherapy-based partial breast irradiation is associated with low rates of complications and excellent cosmesis. Brachytherapy. 2013;12:278–84.
34. Cuttino LW, Keisch M, Jenrette JM, et al. Multi-institutional experience using the MammoSite radiation therapy system in the treatment of early-stage breast cancer: 2-year results. Int J Radiat Oncol Biol Phys. 2008;71:107–14.
35. Chen S, Dickler A, Kirk M, et al. Patterns of failure after MammoSite brachytherapy partial breast irradiation: a detailed analysis. Int J Radiat Oncol Biol Phys. 2007;69:25–31.
36. Harper JL, Watkins JM, Zauls AJ, et al. Six-year experience: long-term disease control outcomes for partial breast irradiation using MammoSite balloon brachytherapy. Am J Surg. 2010;199:204–9.
37. Haley M, Beriwal S, Heron DE, et al. MammoSite accelerated partial breast irradiation: a single-institution outcomes analysis with 2 years of followup. Brachytherapy. 2009;8:9–13.
38. Shah NM, Tenenholz T, Arthur D. MammoSite and interstitial brachytherapy for accelerated partial breast irradiation: factors that affect toxicity and cosmesis. Cancer. 2004;101:727–34.
39. Evans SB, Kaufman SA, Price LL, et al. Persistent seroma after intraoperative placement of MammoSite for accelerated partial breast irradiation: incidence, pathologic anatomy, and contributing factors. Int J Radiat Oncol Biol Phys. 2006;65:333–9.
40. Richards GM, Berson AM, Rescigno J, et al. Acute toxicity of high-dose-rate intracavitary brachytherapy with the MammoSite applicator in patients with early-stage breast cancer. Ann Surg Oncol. 2004;11:739–46.
41. Niehoff P, Polgar C, Ostertag H, et al. Clinical experience with MammoSite radiation therapy system for brachytherapy of breast cancer: results from an international phase II trial. Radiother Oncol. 2006;79:316–20.
42. Shah C, Ghilezan M, Arthur D, et al. Initial clinical experience with multilumen brachytherapy catheters for accelerated partial breast irradiation. Brachytherapy. 2012;11:369–73.
43. Cuttino LW, Arthur DW, Vicini F, et al. Long-term results from the Contura Multi-Lumen balloon breast brachytherapy catheter phase 4 registry trial. Int J Radiat Oncol Biol Phys. 2014;90:1025–9.
44. Israel PZ, Robbins A, Shroff P, et al. Three-year clinical outcome using the Contura multilumen balloon breast brachytherapy catheter to deliver accelerated partial breast irradiation (APBI): improving radiation standards for the optimal application of APBI. Brachytherapy. 2012;11:316–21.
45. Yashar CM, Blair S, Wallace A, et al. Initial clinical experience with strut-adjusted volume implant brachytherapy applicator for accelerated partial breast irradiation. Brachytherapy. 2009;8:367–72.
46. Yashar CM, Scanderberg D, Kuske R, et al. Initial clinical experience with the strut-adjusted volume implant (SAVI) breast brachytherapy device for accelerated partial-breast irradiation (APBI): first 100 patients with more than 1 year follow-up. Int J Radiat Oncol Biol Phys. 2011;80:765–70.
47. Smith GL, Xu Y, Buchholz TA, et al. Association between treatment with brachytherapy vs whole-breast irradiation and subsequent mastectomy, complications, and survival among older women with invasive breast cancer. JAMA. 2012;307:1827–37.

48. Presley CJ, Soulos PR, Herrin J, et al. Patterns of use and short-term complications of breast brachytherapy in the national medicare population from 2008–2009. J Clin Oncol. 2012;30:4302–7.
49. Chen PY. Accelerated partial breast irradiation: keeping guidelines in step with evolving data. Int J Radiat Oncol Biol Phys. 2014;88:263–5.
50. Kuske RR, Young SS. Breast brachytherapy versus whole-breast irradiation: reported differences may be statistically significant but clinically trivial. Int J Radiat Oncol Biol Phys. 2014;88:266–8.
51. Magee B, Swindell R, Harris M, et al. Prognostic factors for breast recurrence after conservative breast surgery and radiotherapy: results from a randomized trial. Radiother Oncol. 1996;39:223–7.
52. Dodwell DJ, Dyker K, Brown J, et al. A randomised study of whole-breast vs tumour-bed irradiation after local excision and axillary dissection for early breast cancers. Clin Oncol. 2005;17:618–22.
53. Baglan KL, Sharpe MB, Jaffray D, et al. Accelerated partial breast irradiation using 3D conformal radiation therapy (3D-CRT). Int J Radiat Oncol Biol Phys. 2003;55:302–11.
54. Formenti SC, Truong MT, Goldberg JD, et al. Prone accelerated partial breast irradiation after breast-conserving surgery: preliminary clinical results and dose-volume histogram analysis. Int J Radiat Oncol Biol Phys. 2004;60:493–504.
55. Olivotto IA, Whelan TJ, Parpia S, et al. Interim cosmetic and toxicity results from RAPID: a randomized trial of accelerated partial breast irradiation using three-dimensional conformal external beam radiation therapy. J Clin Oncol. 2013;31:4038–35.
56. Chafe S, Moughan J, McCormick B, et al. Late toxicity and patient self-assessment of breast appearance/satisfaction on RTOG 0319: a phase 2 trial of 3-dimensional conformal radiation therapy-accelerated partial breast irradiation following lumpectomy for stages I and II breast cancer. Int J Radiat Oncol Biol Phys. 2013;86:854–9.
57. Liss AL, Ben-David MA, Jagsi R, et al. Decline of cosmetic outcomes follow accelerated partial breast irradiation using intensity modulated radiation therapy: results of a single-institution prospective clinical trial. Int J Radiat Oncol Biol Phys. 2014;89:96–102.
58. Leonard KL, Hepel JT, Hiatt JR, et al. The effect of dose-volume parameters and interfraction interval on cosmetic outcome and toxicity after 3-dimensional conformal accelerated partial breast irradiation. Int J Radiat Oncol Biol Phys. 2013;85:623–9.
59. Shah C, Wilkinson JB, Lanni T, et al. Five-year outcomes and toxicities using 3-dimensional conformal external beam radiation therapy to deliver accelerated partial breast irradiation. Clin Breast Cancer. 2013;13:206–11.
60. Formenti SC, Hsu H, Fenton-Kerimian M, et al. Prone accelerated partial irradiation after breast-conserving surgery: five-year results of 100 patients. Int J Radiat Oncol Biol Phys. 2012;84:606–11.
61. Julian TB, Constantino JP, Vicini FA, et al. Early toxicity results with 3D conformal external beam (CEBT) from the NSABP B-39/RTOG 0413 accelerated partial breast irradiation (APBI) trial. Presented at the 2011 American Society of Clinical Oncology annual meeting, 4–8 June 2011, Chicago.
62. Lei RY, Leonard CE, Howell KT, et al. Four-year clinical update from a prospective trial of accelerated partial breast intensity-modulated radiotherapy (APBIMRT). Breast Cancer Res Treat. 2013;140:119–33.
63. Livi L, Meattini I, Marrazzo L, et al. Accelerated partial breast irradiation using intensity-modulated radiotherapy versus whole breast irradiation: 5-year survival analysis of a phase 3 randomised controlled trial. Eur J Cancer. 2015;51:451–63.
64. Taghian AG, Kozak KR, Katz A, et al. Accelerated partial breast irradiation using proton beams: initial dosimetric experience. Int J Radiat Oncol Biol Phys. 2006;65:1404–10.
65. Kozak RR, Smith BL, Adams J, et al. Accelerated partial- breast irradiation using proton beams: initial clinical experience. Int J Radiat Oncol Biol Phys. 2006;66:691–8.

66. Galland-Girodet S, Pashtan I, MacDonald SM, et al. Long-term cosmetic outcomes and toxicities of proton therapy compared with photon-based-3-dimensional conformal accelerated partial-breast irradiation: a phase 1 trial. Int J Radiat Oncol Biol Phys. 2014;90:493–500.
67. Bush DA, Do S, Lum S, et al. Partial breast radiation therapy with proton beam: 5-year results with cosmetic outcomes. Int J Radiat Oncol Biol Phys. 2014;90:501–5.
68. Berrang TS, Olivotto I, Kim DH, et al. Three-year outcomes of a Canadian multicenter study of accelerated partial breast irradiation using conformal radiation therapy. Int Radiat Oncol Biol Phys. 2011;81:1220–7.
69. Chang JH, Lee NK, Kim JY, et al. Phase II trial of proton beam accelerated partial breast irradiation in breast cancer. Radiother Oncol. 2013;108:209–14.

Chapter 16
The Evolution of Brachytherapy Techniques and the Current Arizona Approach

Robert R. Kuske

Contents

16.1 Introduction: A 24-Year Historical Perspective on Accelerated Partial Breast Irradiation

Dr. Bernard Aron, former chairman of radiation oncology at the University of Cincinnati, insisted that his residents learn brachytherapy techniques. "Brachytherapy is a tool that every complete radiation oncologist needs to have in his/her toolbox" [1]. In addition to the easier and simpler intracavitary brachytherapy that is commonly employed for gynecologic malignancies such as cervical and endometrial carcinoma, he encouraged his trainees to use interstitial brachytherapy for head and neck cancers, soft tissue sarcomas, and breast conservation boost. Later, he would admit that he did not give primary breast brachytherapy much thought because of

R.R. Kuske, MD, FAACE
Virginia G. Piper Cancer Center, Radiation Oncology, Arizona Breast Cancer Specialists and Center for Cancer Care, Scottsdale, AZ, USA
e-mail: rkuske@breastmd.com

D.W. Arthur et al. (eds.), *Short Course Breast Radiotherapy: A Comprehensive Review of Hypofractionation, Partial Breast, and Intra-Operative Irradiation*, DOI 10.1007/978-3-319-24388-7_16

the two negative trials from the United Kingdom, the Guy's and Christie Hospital trials [12]. At the current time, brachytherapy is not being taught in most radiation oncology residency programs, so there is danger that this useful means of delivering a tumoricidal dose of radiation could become a lost art.

In October 1991, a woman from Venezuela with a stage T2 N0 M0 ductal carcinoma of the right supra-areolar breast presented before the multidisciplinary Conference and Clinic at the Ochsner Clinic in New Orleans. Aware that there were alternatives to mastectomy and that there were no linear accelerators in her home country at the time within 8 hours of her home, she insisted that her physician consultants come up with an alternative to the standard 6.5 weeks of external beam breast irradiation.

The surgical oncologist at the Clinic, John Bolton, MD, suggested that we consider offering her wide-volume brachytherapy, similar to how we had been treating soft tissue sarcomas. He noted that the published local control rates with single plane implants covering the surgical bed with generous margins were excellent, allowing limb preservation [2]. Our soft tissue sarcoma brachytherapy results in New Orleans mirrored those published in this series. The low-dose rate brachytherapy was designed to deliver a radiation dose capable of sterilizing microscopic extensions of sarcoma beyond the surgical margin, which was microscopically clear. An inherently hotter central dose inside the peripheral envelope offers a built-in boost dose to the surface area at greatest risk for tumor cells after surgical excision.

An added benefit particularly attractive to this patient: since the treatment is delivered with low-dose rate iridium seeds within plastic catheters imbedded directly within the tissues that harbored the malignancy, a tumoricidal dose could be given much more quickly, in 3–5 days instead of the conventional 6–7 weeks of external beam whole breast irradiation.

Since the margins were not evaluated in Venezuela, Dr. Bolton took her back to surgery for a reexcision in New Orleans, and an axillary dissection for staging was also planned. In the operating room, with the wound open and exposed, multiple brachytherapy catheters were inserted, with 1.2 cm between each catheter within a plane and approximately 2.5 cm between the two planes, superficial and deep. The goal was to bracket the lumpectomy cavity between two planes of catheters and extend them peripherally 2 cm beyond the surgical edge in all directions, except superficial and deep where the skin and pectoralis major fascia provide anatomic limits to coverage.

The prescription dose was 45 Gy in 3 1/2 days with low-dose rate (LDR) seeds but with the antiquated 2-dimensional non-CT single slice treatment planning of that day. The seeds were loaded 1 cm deep to the skin entry and exit sites on both the proximal and distal sides of the implant, so that a seed was not at the skin surface creating a pockmark and/or telangiectasia. This is in contrast to modern 3-dimensional treatment planning, where the seed positions in the z-plane are placed from each edge of the target volume, rather than skin to skin. The seed strength was 1 millicurie per seed, and the dose was delivered in 3 days as an inpatient with shielding and radiation precautions. On day 4, the patient was on a plane back to Venezuela, her family, and her business. Photos of her breast immediately after catheter removal and at the time of her 10-year follow-up are shown in Fig. 16.1.

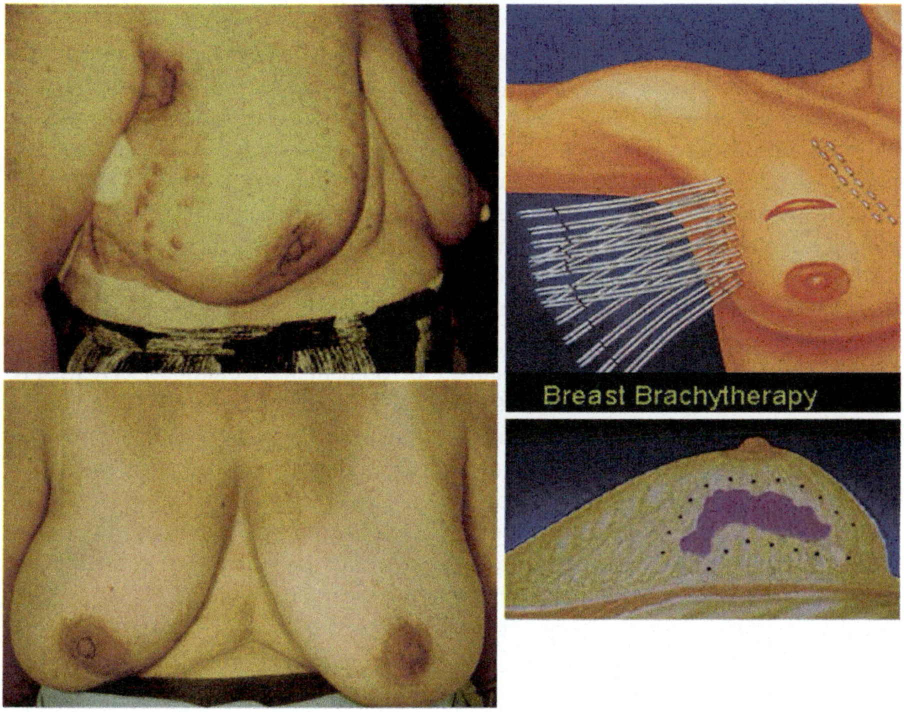

Fig. 16.1 The first APBI patient in the modern era: freehand catheter insertion with the wound open at the time of reexcision and axillary dissection

The breast team at the Ochsner Clinic was encouraged by the results in this patient, the first patient treated with early stage (T2 N0) breast cancer, negative surgical margins, and wide-volume breast brachytherapy alone in the modern era. Her breast maintained its softness over time, in contrast to the woody induration seen with brachytherapy as a boost. The cosmetic outcome was excellent.

We submitted a phase II trial to the Institutional Review Board (IRB). Initially, 23 patients were to be treated by interstitial brachytherapy, followed by a 2-year hiatus to evaluate acute and subacute toxicity and cosmesis. The study then extended after the 2-year break to 163 patients after a favorable review of the initial data. Selection criteria included pathologic tumor size ≤4 cm, excision with negative margins (no ink on tumor), and negative nodes or 1–3 positive without extracapsular extension. There were no age restrictions, DCIS and lobular histologies were allowed as long as the pathologic extent was ≤4 cm, and an extensive intraductal component to an invasive cancer was allowed. We treated women with low- and high-dose rate (HDR) brachytherapy in alternating blocks of 10 patients each to avoid selection bias. The HDR dose (32 Gy in 8 fractions over 4 days or 34 Gy in 10 fractions over 5 days) was independently calculated by pre-eminent biologists/physicists to be similar to the LDR regimen for tumor control probability (TCP) and late tissue effects (LTE). The 32 Gy dose focused on TCP, while the 34 Gy dose favored LTE.

The published results for the first 50 patients were presented as a matched pair analysis comparing select brachytherapy patients to whole breast irradiation patients treated by the same selection criteria, the same physicians, with similar stage, age, and follow-up intervals [3]. Tumor control, toxicity, and cosmesis were similar between the matched pairs. There was no significant difference between low- and high-dose rate results, so the subsequent study extension was primarily HDR.

HDR was also favored because the dose was delivered over ~10–15 min with the patient staying in precisely the same supine position in which she was planned. LDR patients, on the other hand, were sitting in chairs reading, eating, brushing their teeth, etc., and the catheter positions in the breast changed, sometimes dramatically, by posture.

After IRB review, the trial was extended to 163 patients, including 19 DCIS, 116 invasive ductal, 7 invasive ductal with EIC, 11 lobular, 6 tubular, and 4 mucinous histologies. Twenty-four patients were node positive. Overall, 71 % of the patients were treated with HDR brachytherapy. Five patients (3 %) had breast, 4 nodal (2.5 %), and 7 distant (4.3 %) recurrence at a median follow-up of 65 months [4].

The New Orleans excellent outcomes were mirrored by the William Beaumont Hospital [5], providing impetus toward Radiation Therapy Oncology Group (RTOG) Trial 95–17. It was important to discover that quality brachytherapy could be executed at institutions remote from experienced expert centers of excellence. RTOG 95–17 is the first cooperative group phase II trial of partial breast irradiation. This trial accrued 100 patients (99 eligible) from 10 institutions. The one patient deemed ineligible by RTOG had sentinel lymph node biopsy only, and the protocol was written before the sentinel node era.

It should be remembered that this trial was written in 1994, so there were no CT-based 3-dimensional treatment plans and the brachytherapy was primitive compared to modern standards. Dosimetry was planned from orthogonal films with dummy seed strands placed within the catheters. In the z-plane, the dose was delivered from skin to skin, in contrast to proximal-to-distal target volume coverage performed today. The implants tended to be one or two planes rather than current volume implants.

Despite this low-technology brachytherapy and inclusion of radiation oncology centers without the experience of the original pioneers, the results were quite impressive. At over 12 years follow-up, the ipsilateral breast recurrence rate is 4.1 % actuarial at 5 years and 6.2 % at 10 years. There were only 3 regional nodal failures (3.1 %) despite over 20 % of patients being initially node positive [6, 7].

Research in accelerated partial breast irradiation is blossoming, with more than a dozen international randomized trials ongoing or finished, registry trials with large numbers of patients, and numerous single institution publications. Investigation in APBI has been a model for how medicine should evolve, from a single patient giving us the concept, to prospective IRB-approved single institution trials at two hospitals, to a national phase II cooperative group trial, to multiple international phase III trials.

Soon, we will have direct comparisons between conventional 6-week whole breast irradiation and 5-day partial breast irradiation. The NSABP B-39/RTOG 0413 North American randomized trial with 4214 enrolled patients completed accrual in April 2013. Results should be forthcoming in the next couple of years, with considerable statistical power. The European phase III randomited trid of 1,184 patients treated between 2004–9 with 6 weeks of whole breast in radiation vs. interstitial brachy therapy APBT will be presented at the annual meeting of the American Society of Theropetic Radiology and oncology in october, 2015.

16.2 A New Hypothesis and a Potential Paradigm Shift

There has been a 119-year tradition of treating the entire breast in all breast cancers, no matter how small, with no or minimal regional spread, or how favorable the biology. Sir William Halstead proposed the original hypothesis that the entire organ needed to be treated and all possible extensions of the malignancy, including nodal regions. This concept withstood the test of time, at least until a few decades ago.

In the early 1980s, the Halstead hypothesis was challenged but only to the extent that comprehensive breast irradiation rather than the scalpel could treat the entire breast.

Attempts at partial breast surgery without whole breast irradiation were failures, with local recurrence rates in the range of 30–40 % [8].

A principle of radiation oncology is: When treating large volumes or entire organs, a lower-dose per fraction improves tolerance by decreasing the late effects (e.g., fibrosis, microvascular damage, telangiectasia, and necrosis) of irradiation. In consideration of the goal of optimizing cosmetic outcome in the treatment of early stage breast cancer with breast-preserving approaches, the original pioneers of breast conservation therapy chose to treat the ipsilateral breast with relatively low daily doses of irradiation in the range of 180–200 cGy per fraction. The whole breast was treated to 4500–5000 cGy, followed usually by a boost to the excision site plus a margin to 6000–6600 cGy over 6–7 weeks.

The breast team at the Ochsner Clinic in New Orleans hypothesized in 1991 that:

1. In select breast cancers, true biologically significant multicentricity is rare, and more recent improvements in breast imaging (e.g., breast MRI) and pathology (e.g., meticulous margin assessment of an oriented lumpectomy specimen) may further reduce the risk of disconnected multi-quadrant disease.
2. Virtually extending the surgical margins by eliminating contiguous breast cancer extensions beyond the surgical edge with focused dose-intense radiation might lower the true local recurrence rate.
3. Since the radiation source is immediately in the vicinity of the tissue at risk, brachytherapy can be given in a shorter time period, accelerating the treatment time, potentially making breast conservation radiotherapy more accessible to eligible women.
4. As a result of the physics of brachytherapy, the dose falls off rapidly away from the source dwell positions, decreasing normal tissue exposure to radiation, potentially preventing sequelae to the heart, lung, chest wall, skin, lymphatic, and uninvolved breast irradiation.

5. The shorter overall treatment duration allows all the local therapy for breast cancer to be given upfront, with systemic therapy to follow without delay, potentially maximizing local and systemic control of the malignancy.
6. Partial breast irradiation may allow more options for salvage therapy in the event of local relapse.
7. Should plastic surgery be required in the future, the avoidance of whole breast irradiation may contribute to lower complication rates.

APBI represents a potential paradigm shift. The existing paradigm assumes that the entire breast needs to be treated by either surgery or limited surgery followed by whole breast irradiation. APBI introduces the concept that in appropriately selected breast cancers, only the affected portion of the breast needs to be treated. Since the treatment volume is limited, the treatment can be dramatically shortened from 6 weeks to 4–5 days.

16.3 The Target Volume

In the year 1991, we chose our target volume based upon published pathological and clinical analysis of the extent of breast cancer beyond the primary tumor. We also evaluated where sites of recurrence were found after breast-conserving surgery, with or without whole breast irradiation. We decided to embark upon initial clinical trials treating 2 cm beyond the surgical edge, unless the skin or pectoralis fascia intervened. Because the lumpectomy specimen is not always oriented, and we feared inaccuracy, we made the decision to treat 2 cm beyond the cavity edge without consideration for where the original tumor was located within the lumpectomy specimen. With improvements in imaging and 3-dimensional computer reconstructions, future research may map the original tumor within the postoperative breast and choose a margin that could be eccentric relative to the cavity.

Seven years after interstitial brachytherapy trials were initiated, the balloon intracavitary catheter was introduced. This new single-channel brachytherapy device sparked considerable discussion and thoughtful analysis about whether 1 cm might be sufficient in carefully selected patients. Some comfort in a tighter 1 cm margin was offered by the concept of tissue compression by the expanded balloon. An analysis by Vicini [9] put forth a hypothesis that 1 cm margin may be sufficient in carefully selected patients.

Currently, the choice of appropriate margin of irradiation is hotly debated and may vary with the age of the patient and the aggressiveness of the tumor. It is clear that 0 cm, or no radiation at all, results in unacceptably high local breast recurrence rates in the range of 30–40 % even with negative surgical margins [8]. The local recurrence rates with treating an additional 2 cm with interstitial brachytherapy are 4 % at 7 years in the New Orleans prospective clinical trials and 4 % at 5 years and 6 % at 10 years on the RTOG 95–17 multi-institutional prospective cooperative group phase II trial. Local recurrence rates with the balloon intracavitary catheter have proven acceptable. The balloon data has shorter follow-up intervals than the interstitial brachytherapy series, but in the next few years, 10-year outcomes should be available, and it is anticipated that results seen with balloon brachytherapy will match favorably with the results with interstitial brachytherapy.

For the phase III trial, considerable thought and discussion went into choosing the ultimate criteria of treating 1.5 cm beyond the lumpectomy cavity edge for interstitial brachytherapy, 1.0 cm for balloon and later strut-based intracavitary brachytherapy, and 1.5 cm plus 1.0 cm planning target volume (PTV) margin for the 3-D conformal option on this study. Based on the knowledge that the expanded balloon stretches and compresses the surrounding breast tissue when inflated, it was understood that a larger volume of actual tissue would be treated than what a 1 cm target volume represented. Therefore, the decision to use a 1 cm target volume for intracavitary treatment was made to better approximate a 1.5 cm target expansion as used in the alternative 2 treatment techniques. With 3-D conformal PBI (3-D-CRT), breathing motion and set-up uncertainty needed to be accounted for and therefore a 1 cm (total 2.5 cm) PTV was added to the 1.5 cm target. We have subsequently noted that the percentage of the ipsilateral breast covered by the 3D-CRT technique exceeds 50 % when the lumpectomy cavities are large.

The research in the field of PBI is currently very active, so it is anticipated that determination of the appropriate radiation margin around the excision cavity will be clearer in the future. Perhaps the margin will vary from patient to patient in the future, depending on tumor biology, patient characteristics, and the original tumor location. As seen in specimen radiographs, the tumor is frequently eccentrically located within a specimen, with a generous margin on one side and a close margin on another. It is conceivable that the radiation margin in the future may vary geometrically, based upon accurate and reliable pathological determination of surgical margin width in 3-dimensions.

16.4 Brachytherapy Techniques

16.4.1 Open Freehand Interstitial Catheter Insertion

Open freehand technique depends upon the skill of the brachytherapist to insert catheters or needles in an array that both covers the target volume and provides a spacing that will ensure a homogeneous dose distribution. It was the original method of breast brachytherapy, used by Geoffrey Keynes from England in the 1920s as the original breast conservation therapy [10]. With newer image-guided template techniques, freehand catheter insertion is now reserved for very small breasts or to supplement cold spots found upon evaluating template insertions or single entry devices.

At the time of a lumpectomy or reexcision, the radiation oncologist goes to the operating room with the surgeon. With the skin incision open, the extent of the surgical excision can be determined by probing the cavity with an index finger.

A sterile marker pen delineates the edges of the cavity onto the skin surface by lifting up the probing finger along the edges of the surgery and making a mark. A single, double, or rarely triple plane implant is then designed by marking the planned needle entry and exit sites on the skin (Fig. 16.1).

Keep in mind that brachytherapy catheter insertion at the time of surgery can be problematic because the pathology report will not be available for 2–3 days after surgery and catheter insertion. Documenting surgical margins and nodal status is essential before delivering the first brachytherapy dose! One must be prepared to pull the catheters or use them as a boost only. Patients should be forewarned of this possibility before the procedure. For this reason, most experienced brachytherapists now prefer image-guided insertions as a separate procedure 2–6 weeks after breast-conserving surgery and sentinel node mapping.

A single plane implant is indicated if the thickness of the tissue to be covered is 1.0 cm or less. This typically is the case for very medial lesions near the parasternal breast tissue or in very small breasts or in augmented breasts (see my other chapter). It is appropriate to design a single plane implant for one side of the target volume where it is thin and broaden it out into two planes (in a "Y" pattern) where the breast becomes thicker, such as under the nipple. A double plane is necessary if the tissue thickness is greater than 1.0 cm but less than 2.5 cm. A third plane is added when the target tissue exceeds or equals 2.5 cm.

The spacing between needles within a plane varies with the size of the implant. Smaller volumes require closer spacing, and larger volumes should be covered with wider spacing. For example, when using a single plane implant, the needle spacing typically is 1.0–1.2 cm. For double plane implants, the spacing is 1.2–1.5 cm. For multiplane implants with 3 or more planes (routine with modern volume implants), the separation between planes is 1.5–2 cm, and intercatheter separation within each plane is usually 1.5 cm. Closer catheters in volume implants result in an extraordinary total number or catheters, and are not necessary.

In high-risk superficial areas such as directly under the lumpectomy scar, smoother dose distributions are desirable. To avoid scalloping in of the dose under the skin, extra catheters should be added 0.7–1.0 cm deep to the surface between your original superficial catheters. By adding these extra catheters, called the "gauntlet under the skin," you can feather the dose under the skin by varying the dwell times without overdosing the skin surface and running the late risk of telangiectasia.

General principles of freehand technique include: (1) when in doubt about coverage, add an extra catheter in the OR, because you can always pull it or not use it if the dose distribution is acceptable without it, but it is harder (but not impossible!) to add it later after the patient has awoken; (2) catheter entry and exit locations should be selected at least 1 cm away from the target volume, or a source dwell will need to be in the skin, guaranteeing a telangiectatic spot; (3) ideally, the needles are perfectly straight and parallel to each other; (4) at the ends of the implant, placing an extra catheter in between the two planes will prevent bowing in of the isodose curves; and (5) crossing needles in a perpendicular orientation near the catheter entry and exit sites can be helpful in preventing a dipping-in of the dose at these

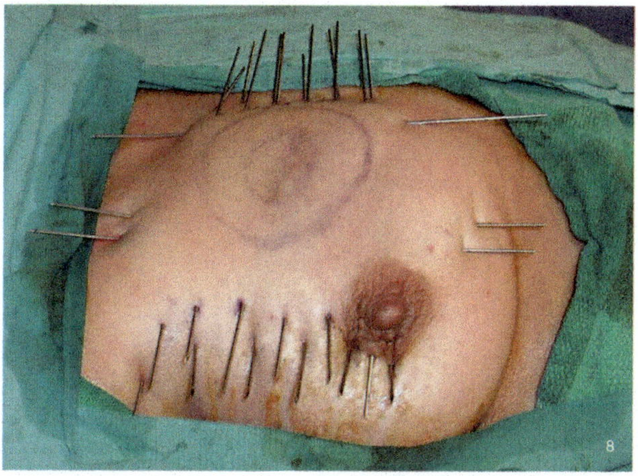

Fig. 16.2 When the target volume is close to the entry site of your needle, crossing needles can prevent scalloping in of the dose under the skin, so you do not need to load the radioactive source close to the skin surface

ends of the target volume. One or two catheters placed 1 cm below the skin surface along the original catheter entry/exit sites will prevent a scalloping in of the dose at the ends of a line source (Fig. 16.2).

Clearly, freehand techniques require skill and experience from the brachytherapist. For this reason, as well as for the pathology report issue described above, this technique is less commonly used than the other image-guided techniques shown in this chapter. This technique is still occasionally used with augmentation mammoplasty at the time of the lumpectomy with the wound open. The silicone surface can be seen as you guide each needle across the target volume. Direct visualization is helpful to avoid augmentation implant puncture and subsequent rupture. Because the peripheral edges of the target volume are not visible through the open wound at the right and left sides, it is much safer to have intraoperative ultrasound in order to avoid puncture. Alternatively, "pinch-view" catheter insertion with the template and CT guidance provides the safest and most reliable technique in augmented women [13].

16.4.2 Ultrasound-Guided Supine Catheter Insertion

Ultrasound can be very helpful in guiding needle insertion in a closed lumpectomy cavity. The junction between water (seroma) and breast tissue (fat) is clearly seen for the first 5–7 weeks after lumpectomy, unless for the surgeon sutures the cavity shut such as oncoplastic lumpectomies. In the presence of a seroma, the surgical excision cavity is readily seen by ultrasound. Using real-time ultrasound, it is feasible to guide each brachytherapy needle millimeter by millimeter across the breast at a chosen depth (Fig. 16.3a, b). The deep plane is inserted either along the surface

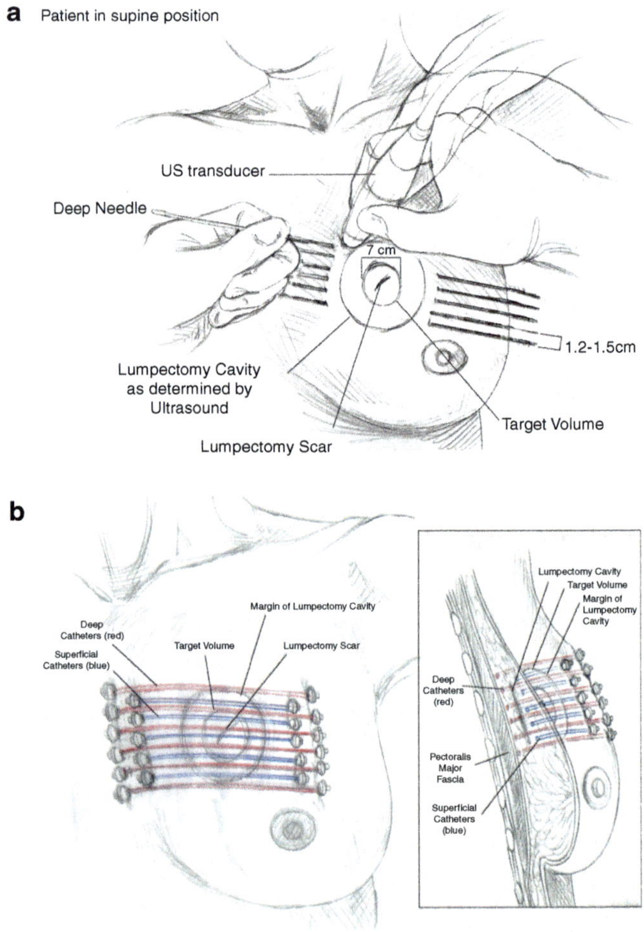

Fig. 16.3 (**a**) Ultrasound-guided brachytherapy with the left hand holding the transducer and the right hand the needle. (**b**) Watching the US monitor, while also checking the needles to be parallel, needle insertion is guided millimeter by millimeter across the breast tissue

of the pectoralis major muscle or 5 mm deep to the lumpectomy cavity. The superficial plane is inserted at a depth of 0.75–1.0 cm from the skin surface. A middle plane is added when the separation between the two planes, easily measured by the ultrasound device, exceeds 2.5–3 cm or at the ends of the implant to prevent bowing in of the isodose curves as described above.

Choose needles that are easily seen by the ultrasound transducer. The challenge is to make each needle go straight and parallel to the others while looking at the ultrasound monitor for proper depth. Some brachytherapists will have a diagnostic radiologist present to hold the transducer and monitor depth and target volume coverage, while others will use their dominant hand for needle insertion and the other hand to hold the transducer (Fig. 16.3a).

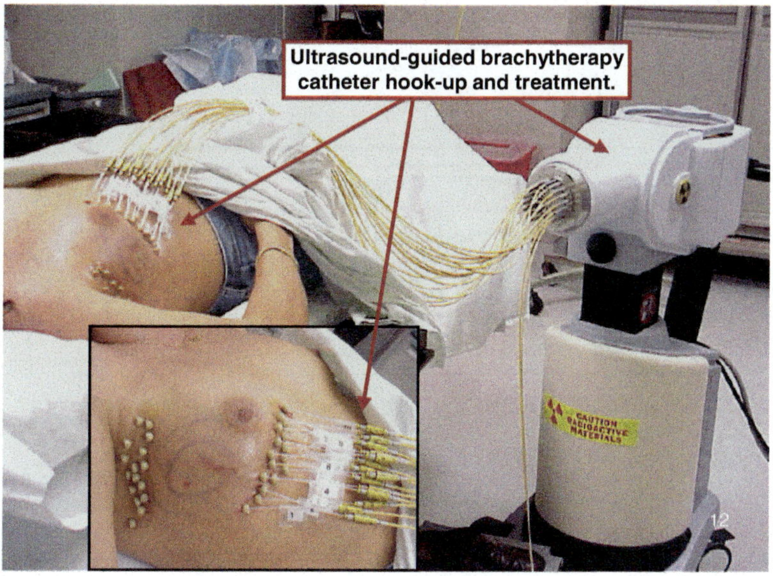

Fig. 16.4 Breast catheters are connected to yellow transfer tubes that are attached to the high-dose rate remote afterloader, which positions the iridium-192 source at precise locations inside the breast to deliver the prescribed dose

This technique is also skill dependent, since it is still a freehand technique without a template to ensure a geometrical array of catheters across the target volume. It can be done under local anesthesia with analgesia or under conscious sedation. Unless you are performing the implant at the time of axillary or breast surgery, general anesthesia is not required. In the presence of augmentation, keep in mind that a 25- or 27-gauge local anesthetic needle is more risky to pierce the augmentation implant than a 19-gauge brachytherapy needle, and they are more difficult to see on ultrasound.

Ultrasound catheter insertion in the supine position usually requires fewer catheters than the template-guided insertions below, because the breast flattens out in the supine position and there is no compression to elongate the lumpectomy cavity and subsequent target volume. This fact makes connection to the HDR iridium-192 remote afterloading machine easier (Fig. 16.4).

16.4.3 Image-Guided Prone Catheter Insertion with a Special Breast Template

This technique in the prone position on a stereotactic core needle breast biopsy table was described in the first edition of this textbook. Since then, we have abandoned this technique, so it will not be described herein. The prone method of

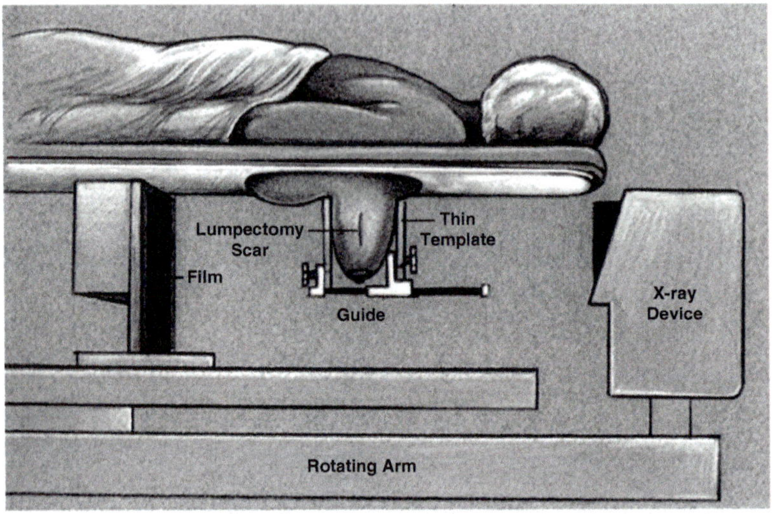

Fig. 16.5 1998 development of the prone technique on the stereotactic breast biopsy table with nonionic contrast in the cavity and a template to guide catheter insertion

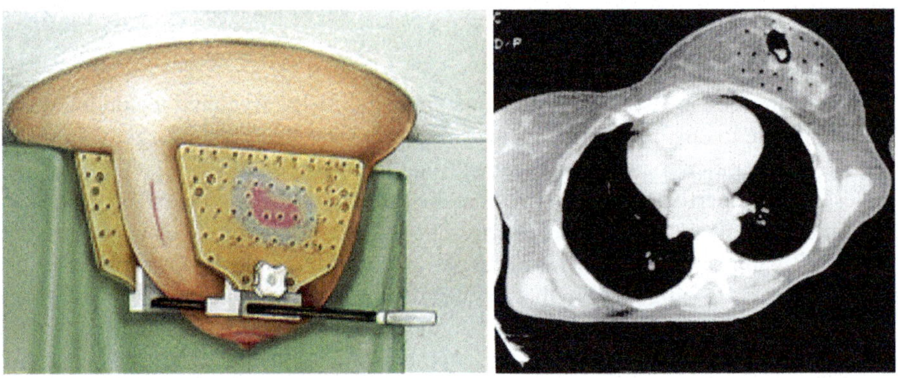

Fig. 16.6 Typical CT of the breast after brachytherapy. Note the excellent deep coverage along the pectoralis fascia and the 2 cm margin around the lumpectomy cavity

catheter insertion was advantageous because it was reproducible and guaranteed 3-dimensional coverage of the target volume. Gravity pulls the breast away from the chest wall, facilitating catheter insertion without fear of a pneumothorax (Figs. 16.5 and 16.6). But mammographic visualization of the lumpectomy cavity usually requires contrast injection, and the core biopsy tables are not generally available to radiation oncologists or surgeons, so we now prefer CT-guided brachytherapy catheter insertion. CT scanners are now available in almost all radiation oncology departments, making this procedure potentially available to centers all over the USA.

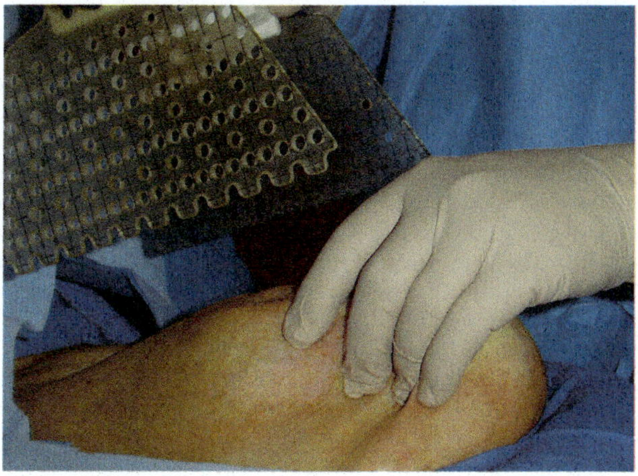

Fig. 16.7 In the supine CT-guided technique with the special template, the breast is grasped and pulled up and away from the chest wall while the two plates are squeezed to apply moderate compression

16.4.4 CT-Guided Supine Catheter Insertion with a Special Breast Template

The procedure can be performed on the radiation oncologist's own time on his or her own treatment planning CT scanner. Furthermore, the patient rests in a supine position, usually with her arm comfortably at her side, much more comfortable than being prone for a 1–2 h procedure (Table 16.1).

A typical procedure would go as follows: The patient or a nurse applies topical lidocaine cream (Emla) to the involved breast one to two hours before the start time. One hour before start time, the patient takes 60 mg Nucynta and 5 mg Valium. An optional extra step, that could be helpful, is to perform breast ultrasound to identify the seroma and map it out prior to the procedure. Using a straw to make an impression on the patient's skin, the projection of the cavity edge onto the skin can be mapped. This step can be helpful in facilitating accurate positioning of the template around the cavity and choosing template orientation. In 90+% of cases, the cavity is readily seen on CT, and contrast is not necessary. In these cases, proceed directly to the CT scanner without the next step.

If the cavity is old and not readily seen on CT, or the breast is dense, nonionic contrast injection into the cavity can help define the target. This procedure can be done by the radiation oncologist, but a diagnostic radiologist can provide this service. An ultrasound-compatible needle enters the skin at least 2 cm away from the seroma, to avoid leakage of contrast later, after small amount of local anesthetic has been injected to raise a skin wheal and along the planned path of the needle. The needle is positioned in the middle of the seroma using ultrasound guidance, and approximately 80 % of the seroma fluid is aspirated into a syringe. This decreases the target volume. Then 3 cc nonionic contrast and 2 cc air are injected directly into the cavity. The needle is withdrawn.

Table 16.1 Advantages of supine CT image-guided needle/catheter insertion

1. The lumpectomy cavity is frequently readily discernable by CT. If the breast is dense or the cavity is old, just 3 cc nonionic contrast (e.g., Omnipaque) can be injected directly into the lumpectomy cavity along with 2 cc air using ultrasound guidance. This extra step highlights the seroma as well as the crevices and outpouchings of the lumpectomy cavity
2. By manually lifting the breast off the chest wall while attaching a special template with pre-drilled holes, deep coverage to the pectoralis muscle can be achieved
3. Using modern CT-based 3-dimensional treatment planning software available in most radiation oncology departments, the rendered image of the breast can be viewed with the template attached. The view can be rotated on the computer until the front and back template holes are perfectly aligned
4. Once the cavity is contoured on each CT slice, the target volume is grown, using widely available computer software, by 1.5–2 cm. The holes necessary to cover the target volume are readily apparent in the "beam's eye view," or rather a needle's eye view. Reliable and reproducible coverage of the target volume by an array of thin plastic catheters is assured
5. Any margin around the lumpectomy cavity can be chosen (e.g., 1, 1.5, 2.0, 2.5 cm, etc.), and theoretically one could have broader coverage on one side of the cavity, where the margin is perhaps tighter and a smaller margin on the other side where the surgical margin is generous
6. The procedure can be performed totally under local anesthesia without conscious sedation, much safer and less expensive
7. The resultant catheter distribution is a volume implant, rather than one or two planes, allowing much more flexibility for dosimetry and coverage of odd cavity shapes
8. Assuming the template is attached in the same way, a radiation oncologist in a different state, or even a resident in training, would perform exactly the same implant as a very experienced brachytherapist would

The patient is taken to the radiation oncology CT scanner. The table is draped in sterile fashion. The patient's breast is prepped with Betadine or a similar solution. The lumpectomy site is palpated and correlated with the straw marks on the skin outlining the cavity. Tincture of benzoin, Mastisol, or the equivalent is applied to the skin before the template is attached to prevent slippage. Breast brachytherapy templates are commercially available from both Elekta and Varian Corporations. The template is positioned on the breast so that the surgical scar is between the two plates and visible to the physician. The surgical scar should not be up against one of the plates because you want the catheters to be parallel to the skin under the lumpectomy scar, not perpendicular, for dosimetry reasons.

The breast is vigorously lifted up and off the chest wall as the template is attached with moderate compression. The base of the template is positioned tightly up against the chest wall while the breast is being lifted so adequate deep coverage is guaranteed (Fig. 16.7). Immediately, to prevent template slippage, three CT-compatible needles are inserted around the lumpectomy site in a triangle to anchor the template (Fig. 16.8). These marker needles will also provide fiducial markers to facilitate orientation on CT and the treatment planning renderings. A 27-gauge needle is used to inject 0.5 % buffered lidocaine with epinephrine under the skin at each entry site (Fig. 16.9). A 25-gauge needle is used to inject deeper 0.1 % buffered lidocaine with epinephrine along the planned pathway of each brachytherapy needle (Fig. 16.10). We use Lactated Ringer's solution to dilute the local anesthetic, as it causes less

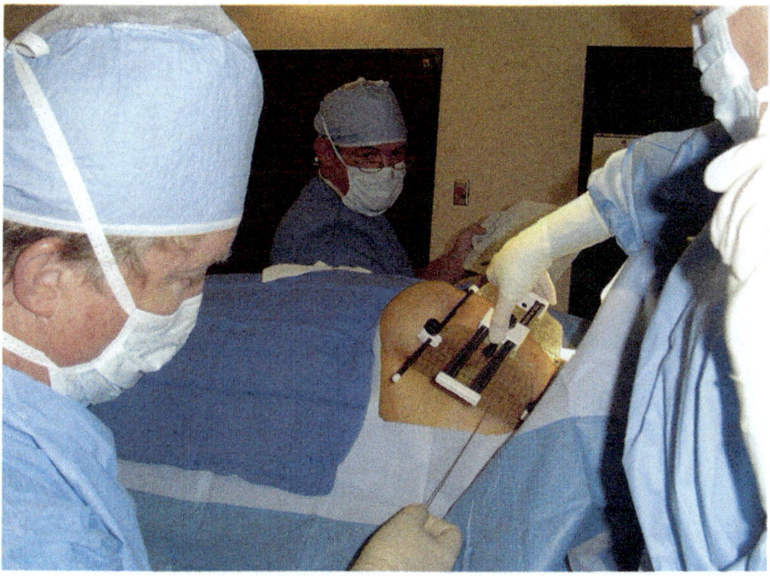

Fig. 16.8 With the nurse stabilizing the template so that it does not slip, the first of 3 anchoring needle are inserted, which also provide fiducial markers of 3 coordinate holes for subsequent 3-d planning

Fig. 16.9 Half % buffered "skin wheal" lidocaine with epinephrine is injected into the skin at each entry and exit site, and 0.1 % "tumescent" is injected deep into the parenchyma of the breast along the future path of each needle

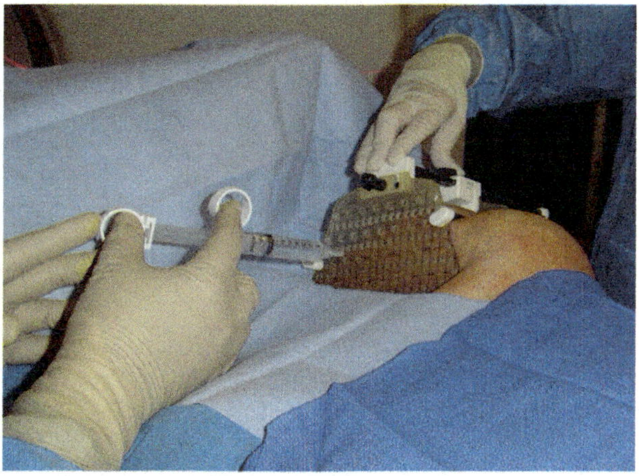

stinging than normal saline when injected into tissue. The template is covered with a sterile drape or towel, and a CT of the breast is obtained (Fig. 16.11). The images are electronically transferred to the treatment planning computer.

The CT images are reviewed on the treatment planning software, and the dosimetrist or medical physicist contours the lumpectomy cavity under supervision of the radiation oncologist who is sterile gloved and gowned (Fig. 16.12). The planning treatment volume (PTV) represents a 1.5–2 cm growth of the cavity and is

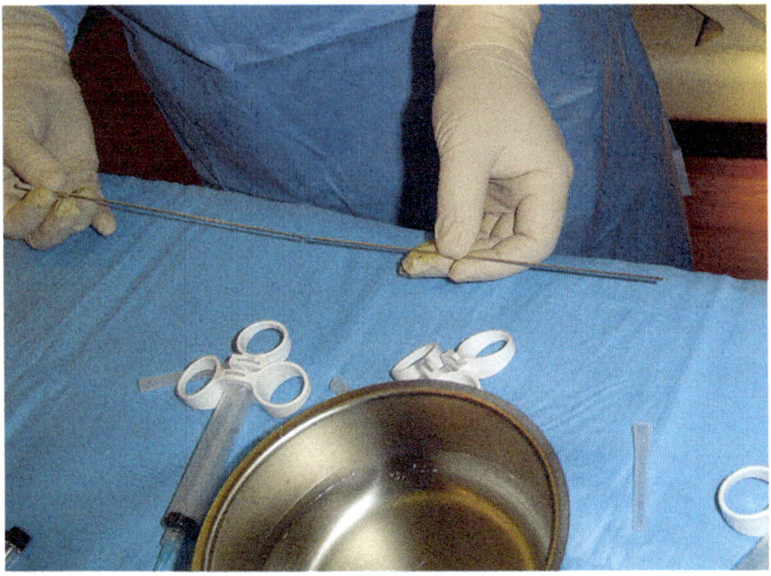

Fig. 16.10 Each hollow needle has a sharp-point removable central trocar for ease of insertion

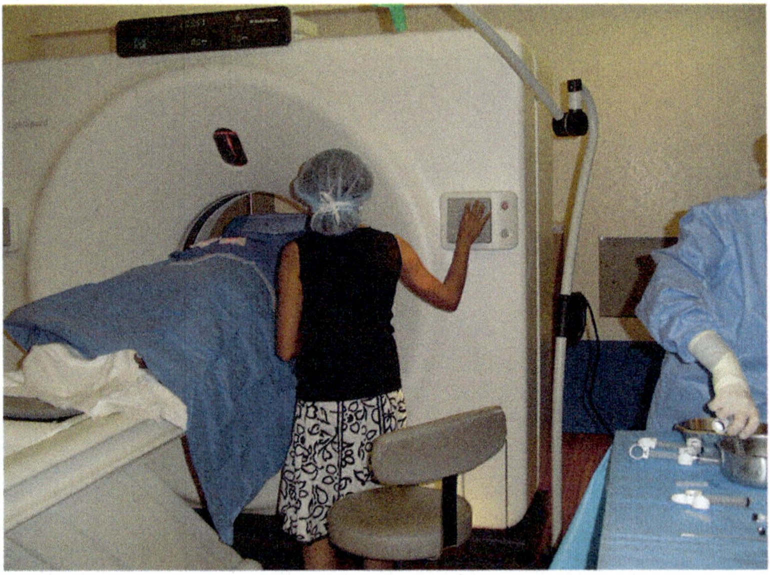

Fig. 16.11 A CT is obtained with the template and 3 needles in place

automatically generated by the computer. Using coordinate C12 (Elekta template) as a centering location, the front and back template holes are aligned. The lumpectomy cavity and PTV are transparently displayed on a "beam's eye view" with the

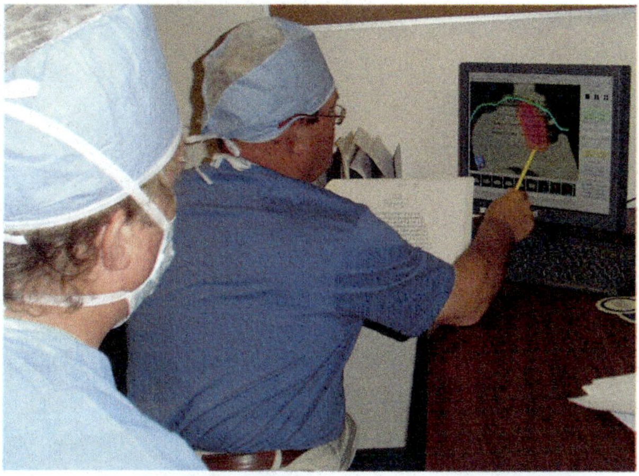

Fig. 16.12 The dosimetrist contours the lumpectomy cavity with supervision by the physician

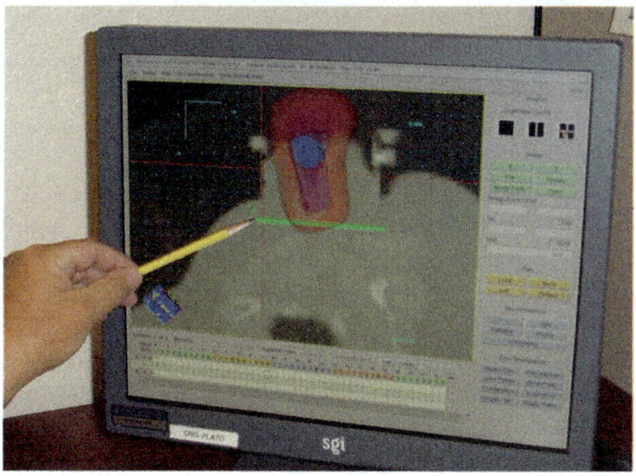

Fig. 16.13 The computer displays a 3-d rendition of the cavity and PTV, with the perspective rotated until the front and back template holes are perfectly aligned

holes of the front and back templates aligned (Fig. 16.13). The coordinates of template holes required to cover the PTV are then evident, and the computer rendering is printed out. A rule of thumb for any template catheter insertion method is to add a catheter beyond the PTV if the closest hole is inside the PTV. If the template hole is at the edge of the PTV, no additional catheter is necessary.

The radiation oncologist returns to the CT suite. Half-strength buffered local anesthetic is injected just under the skin surface to raise a skin wheal, and more dilute tumescent local anesthetic with epinephrine is injected directly down the planned holes of insertion for a relatively painless and bloodless procedure. Allow at least 5 min from local anesthetic injection to brachytherapy catheter insertion for total pain relief, and be sure to inject the skin wheal local on front and back sides of the template at chosen coordinates to eliminate needle entry and exit pain. A thick guiding template is attached to the thin front template, making sure that the needles are parallel and straight (Fig. 16.14).

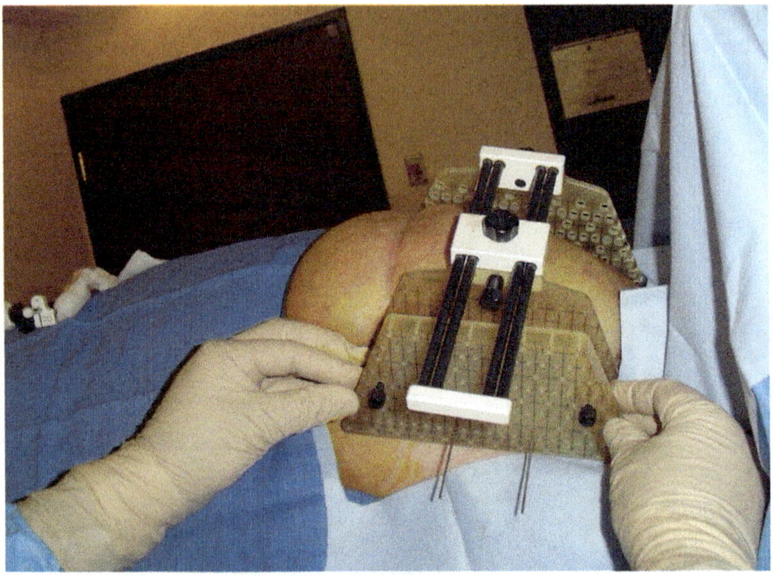

Fig. 16.14 After all needed coordinates for target coverage are determined and each pathway is locally anesthetized, the *thick guiding template* is attached to the front thin template

Since moderate compression is applied by the template, the cavity is somewhat spread out and elongated, causing the use of many more catheters than is usually seen with the old style one or two plane implants. An average of 20 catheters is inserted with this procedure.

This technique provides real-time documentation of coverage of the target volume and allows immediate adjustments or additional catheters. Deep coverage can be improved by an additional row of deep "sub-A" needles using CT guidance (Figs. 16.15 and 16.16), with you or your nurse lifting the template up and away from the chest wall. By staying parallel to the previous needles and checking the desired additional depth on the CT scan, one can avoid pneumothorax. If in doubt, take a few CT images after the needles are partway through the breast. All needles are inserted with the same analgesia and tumescent local anesthetic procedure described above.

After the needles are in place, the template is disassembled and removed from the breast, except that the front thin template is left attached temporarily. Plastic Comfort ® catheters (Elekta, Veneendal, NE) are then inserted inside the distal end of each needle and pulled until the needle is out. Once all the Comfort catheters have replaced all metal needles, the front thin template will easily fall off. The catheters are then pulled the rest of the way through the breast until the distal hemispherical buttons touch the skin at the entry position (Figs. 16.17 and 16.18). A button is placed at the other end of each catheter and fixed to the catheter using a heat-flanging device, securing it in place, and the catheter is trimmed to the button.

At the end, it may be advisable to add a few closely spaced superficial (0.7–10 mm below surface) catheters flanking the lumpectomy scar, called the "gauntlet under the skin," ensuring good superficial coverage without the prescription isodose

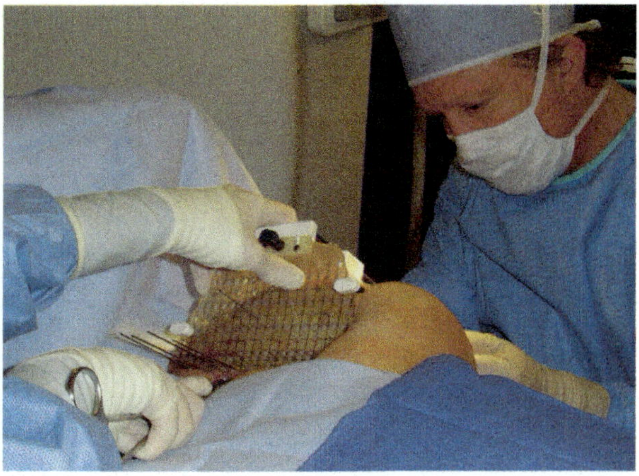

Fig. 16.15 For the deep A and (when needed) sub-A rows, the nurse uses O-ring forceps to compress the backside skin down so the needle tips exit rather than track under the skin

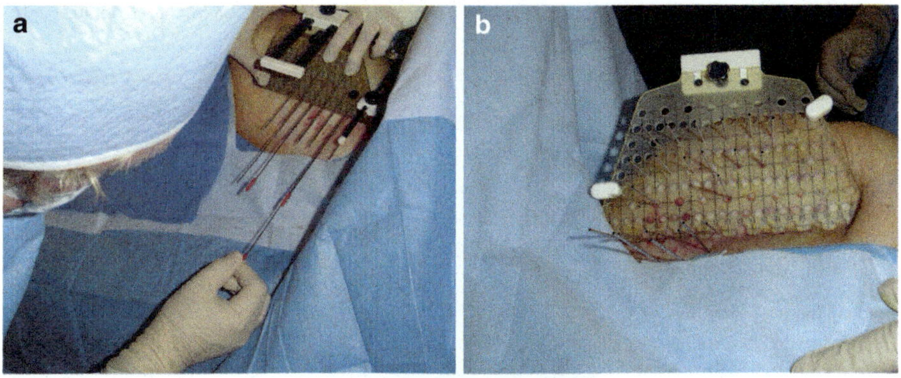

Fig. 16.16 (**a**) Deep catheters are planned beneath the template for adequate coverage of the PTV along the pectoralis muscle, and the dosimetrist/physicist has mapped a pathway that does not intersect with the pleura. The nurse and physician lift the template off the chest wall while the needles are inserted freehand. (**b**) On the backside template, the three deep sub-A needles are seen as they exit the skin. The backside template holes are wider since they provide no guidance and simply brace the other side of the breast

line going beyond the surface (Fig. 16.19). At the end of the procedure, the catheters do not protrude beyond the skin surface (Fig. 16.20), and connection to the HDR remote afterloader is easily accomplished (see Fig. 16.4).

Bacitracin ointment is applied at each entry/exit site, and a Surgi-Bra is used to hold ABD pads in place over the implant so no tape is necessary.

A treatment planning CT scan is obtained of the involved breast later that day or the next day, after any swelling as subsided. The lumpectomy cavity is contoured on each CT slice, and this volume is expanded the desired amount (usually 1.5–2 cm) on the computer as the PTV. Within each catheter, dwell times are selected at 0.5 cm intervals so that the prescription isodose line covers the PTV, with an acceptable (>0.75) dose homogeneity index. Treatment systems have dose optimization algorithms that facilitate PTV coverage, but it is important to make sure that none of the

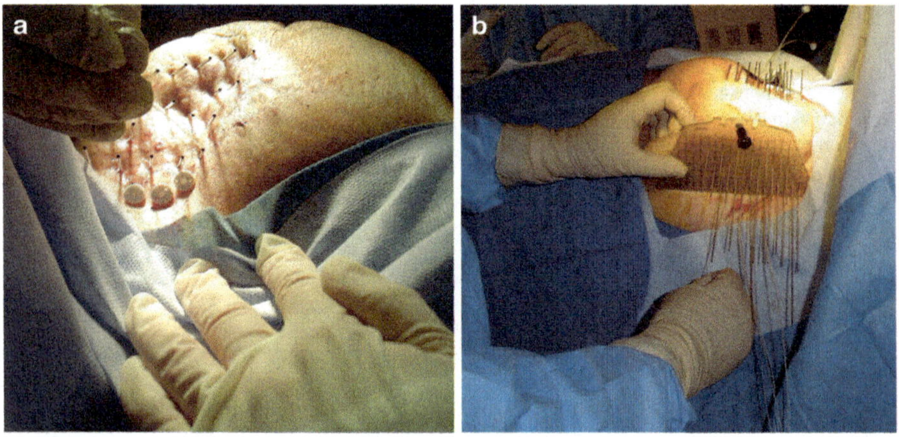

Fig. 16.17 (**a**) The thin portion of the plastic Comfort ® catheter is threaded through the backside end of the needle and (**b**) pulled through the other end until the thick portion hits the front template

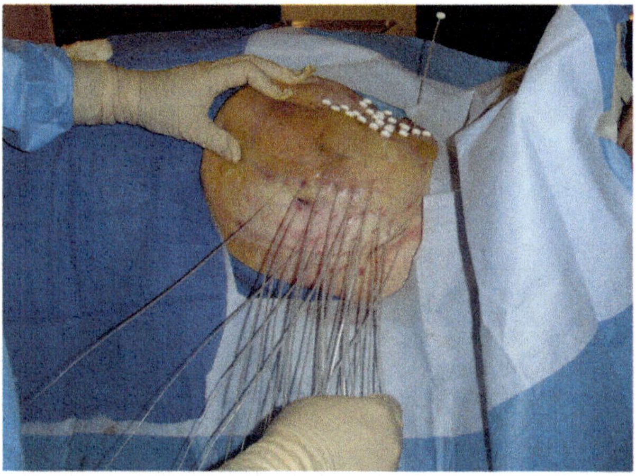

Fig. 16.18 The needle is then removed. After all needles are out, the front thin template falls off easily. The catheters are pulled until the back hemispherical button is flush with the skin

150 % isodose curves connect between one catheter and an adjacent one (i.e., contiguous V150s). We also ensure that the prescription line does not reach the skin surface.

16.4.5 Balloon Intracavitary Catheter Insertion

The MammoSite single lumen (SL) balloon can be inserted at the time of surgery or later as a separate procedure. In the first couple of years after the catheter became available, most of our MammoSite SL balloons were inserted at the time of surgery for the patient convenience of having everything done at once. Now, closed wound

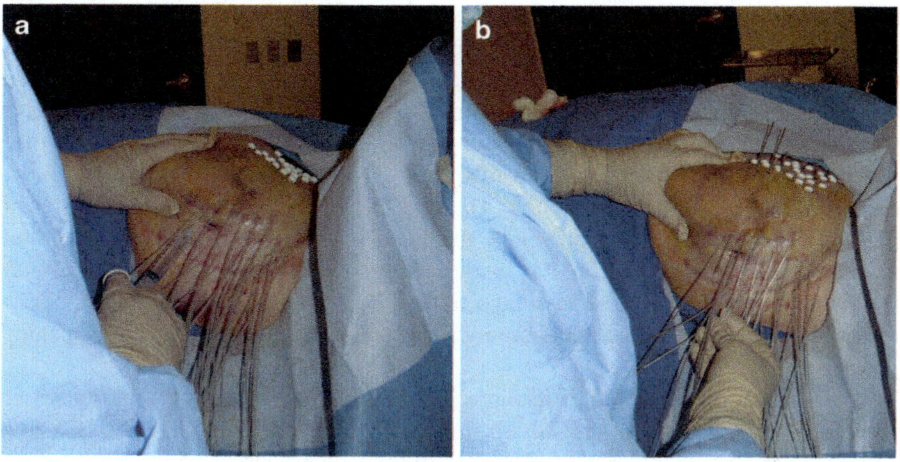

Fig. 16.19 (**a**) After the template is removed, the physicist/dosimetrist and MD survey the implant, deciding where extra (usually superficial) freehand needles may help cover potential cold spots. As before, skin and tumescent local anesthetic are injected through gaps in the target volume. (**b**) Needles are inserted freehand along the anesthetized path to fill potential cold spots and prevent scalloping in of dose underneath the lumpectomy scar

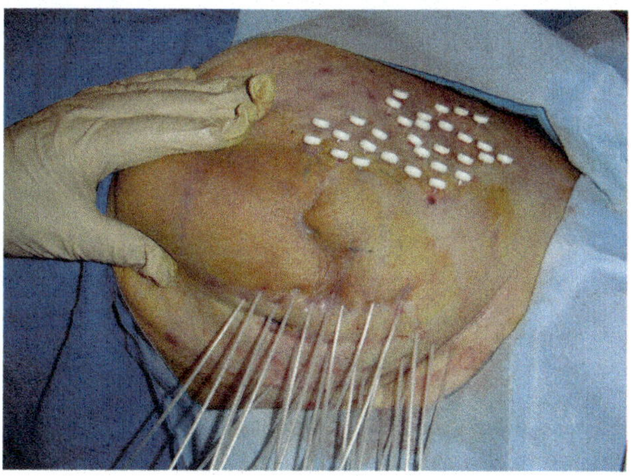

Fig. 16.20 The completed CT-guided multiplanar interstitial volume implant using the special template

catheter insertion is preferred because the pathology report is available confirming that the patient is indeed a candidate for APBI or the balloon. We can also perform a pre-implant ultrasound or CT to check the skin flap thickness and shape of the cavity, maximizing our success rate with balloon insertion. There are fewer aborted procedures, down from approximately 20 % with intraoperative insertion to 10 % with a closed wound. Finally, the sutured lumpectomy wound has fully healed and hemostasis has occurred, which further ensures the success of the balloon and provides a better cosmetic outcome.

We insert the MammoSite ML either with the scar-entry technique (SET) or the lateral trocar tunneling technique. The SET uses a #11 blade to reopen the lumpectomy scar approximately 0.75 cm using local anesthesia. The seroma is rarely more that 1–2 cm deep to the lumpectomy scar, making entry into the seroma easy. After the blade nick, a hemostat or Kelly clam is inserted under ultrasound guidance into the wound and gently opened, and this process repeated until you get a gush of seroma fluid emanating out the hole. Express all the seroma with the hemostat in place. Immediately upon removal of the hemostat, replace it with the deflated MammoSite catheter, checking its position using the ultrasound. Inflate the balloon while observing the ultrasound image. After the balloon is inflated, place Steri-Strips across the rest of the lumpectomy scar so that the wound does not propagate causing a dehiscence.

There are advantages and disadvantages of the SET technique. SET is an easier technique that avoids the large sharp threatening trocar. Since the ends of a line source are relatively colder, the anisotropy of the isodose curves helps pull the dose away from the skin, which is usually the most signicant problem with MammoSite SL, and the chest wall. An additional cosmetically detrimental scar on the breast is avoided.

The lateral trocar tunneling method is simpler if done at the time of lumpectomy or reexcision, but intraoperative insertions are plagued with the issues noted above. This procedure can be performed with a closed wound using ultrasound guidance. Since breast tissue tends to collapse around the longer lateral pathway, the large trocar is necessary to provide a path for the catheter into the lumpectomy cavity. This trocar results in a larger scar on the breast, typically 2 cm.

With either technique, good tissue conformance to the balloon surface must be checked. Separations of the breast tissue you wish to treat from the prescription isodose curve, by air gaps or seroma/hematoma fluid collections, are to be avoided.

16.4.6 SAVI or Contura Insertions

The SAVI is a "Strut Adjustable Volume Implant" device, designed to be a hybrid between interstitial brachytherapy with multiple catheters and the single-entry simplicity of the balloon catheter. SAVI consists of 6, 8, or 10 individual catheters that open after positioning within the lumpectomy cavity using a screwing mechanism (Fig. 16.21). When open, this device is more football shaped or elliptical than round. Air and seroma tend to enter the open central part of the device, allowing the struts to be in direct contact with the cavity walls. If the skin is less than 1.0 cm from the cavity, this device allows the dosimetrist to sculpt the dose away from the skin, protecting the skin from radiation overdosage. Similarly, the device can protect the chest wall, lung, and heart for left breast cancers.

The surgeon or the radiation oncologist can insert a SAVI. It is important to position the device along the long axis of the cavity, since the device is "football shaped," so pre-planning with ultrasound or CT is required. We contour the lumpectomy

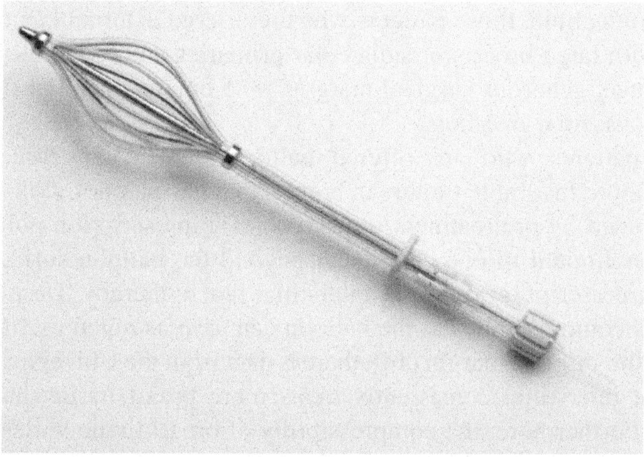

Fig. 16.21 The single-entry multicatheter SAVI device

cavity on each CT slice. The radiation physicist can perform 3-d planning, choosing the optimal entry site and angle in order to optimize SAVI positioning within the cavity. Obviously, real-time ultrasound may achieve the same result, but the two together maximize the chance for implant success.

The Contura is a balloon device that has off-set (by 5 mm) internal catheters that also permits the shaping of the prescription isodose line thus allowing reduction of the skin surface dose and rib dose. The insertion technique mirrors that of MammoSite balloon catheter insertion. One word of advice for both multilumen devices (SAVI and Contura): Quality Assurance prior to each treatment is mandatory to ensure that the device has not rotated, altering the desired dose profile.

16.5 Judgment: Selecting the Optimal Technique for a Particular Patient

The major decision trees are:

1. Whether to offer external beam PBI techniques or breast brachytherapy [11]
2. If you have decided that breast brachytherapy is preferable, do you select balloon intracavitary, SAVI, or interstitial breast brachytherapy techniques?

For issues and concerns highlighted in the summary section of this chapter, most of the author's patients will receive brachytherapy over external beam PBI. Please note that these are theoretical concerns, and more data will be required before one can apply these selection criteria uniformly. The NSABP/RTOG phase III trial allows the participant to select the APBI technique to be used; therefore, a selection bias will preclude meaningful data analysis comparing APBI techniques.

In the author's clinic, those patients who are offered external beam PBI are usually women with large breasts or subareolar primaries and favorable tumor factors such as older age, generous surgical margins >0.5 cm, and smaller tumors lacking EIC or lymphovascular invasion.

Similarly, patients who are offered balloon intracavitary brachytherapy or Contura have more favorable tumors in breasts that have a thick skin-cavity separation as determined by pretreatment ultrasound. The prescription point for the balloon catheter is limited to one centimeter beyond the balloon surface which is in contrast to the prescription point for interstitial brachytherapy. Despite claims that breast tissue is compressible and the balloon can treat as much as 1.6 cm of breast tissue beyond the surgical margin [14], there is data from the University of Wisconsin indicating that interstitial consistently treats more breast tissue than the balloon catheter [15]. Furthermore, the compressibility of breast tissue varies between premenopausal dense breasts and postmenopausal fatty breasts.

Because of the physics of balloon intracavitary brachytherapy, prescribing beyond 1 cm results in extraordinary high doses in the breast tissue touching the balloon, so this is strictly forbidden. Interstitial brachytherapy is only limited by the number of catheters inserted and is determined by geographic coverage. By its nature, interstitial brachytherapy can cover any size or shape cavity, so it is much more dose-controllable than the balloon catheter. As a result, most patients who cannot be treated by the balloon, for geometric reasons, can be treated with interstitial breast brachytherapy.

In all cases, a thorough discussion with the breast surgeon, preferably in a multidisciplinary breast oncology clinic/conference, is important. As a team, you must decide which selection criteria you will use when considering APBI and if the selection criteria will change based on the APBI technique used. You may decide, as we have, to offer interstitial brachytherapy to such higher-risk patients and balloon or 3-d techniques to the favorable patients with acceptable skin separations or 3-d locations.

The clinical judgment and decision-making offered above represents the experience and theoretical concerns of the author and his breast oncology team. Ongoing clinical trials should shed light in the future on appropriate selection criteria for each technique and indeed breast PBI in general.

16.6 Summary

This chapter has reviewed 6 techniques of covering the target volume with brachytherapy. Each has its advantages and disadvantages, and *a strong recommendation* is for the radiation oncology/surgical team to have many, if not all, techniques of delivering partial breast irradiation in their armamentarium. If a patient who is otherwise a candidate for partial breast irradiation is unable to receive it by one technique, it is far preferable to be able to take care of her by another technique than to resort back to 6 weeks of whole breast external beam radiotherapy. For phase III clinical trials, it is critically important to try to keep the patient on the selected arm of the study even if technical issues make one PBI technique problematic.

Intraoperative radiotherapy (IORT) is plagued by poor quality assurance. With both electron beam and soft x-rays (Intrabeam and Xoft), documentation that the target tissue receives the prescribed dose is inadequate. How much breast tissue is pulled into the electron cylinder? What about the breast tissue clinging to the undersurface of the skin that is retracted by skin-hooks and not within the cylinder? How reproducible is the IORT electron method from one surgeon to the next? For soft x-rays, when is treating only 2 mm of breast tissue enough? What if there is a small hematoma, seroma, or air pocket separating the device from the tissue by more than 2 mm? How does the radiation oncologist verify tissue conformance to the metal ball or balloon? And how do you proceed after the IORT is delivered if the pathology report reveals that the patient has positive surgical margins, or multiple metastatic lymph nodes, or unsuitable tumor biology for APBI?

There are theoretical reasons why brachytherapy may result in better outcomes than external beam PBI techniques, such as 3-d conformal or intensity-modulated radiotherapy. First, brachytherapy is prescribed to the periphery of the target volume, with all tissue inside this envelope receiving a significantly higher dose of radiation. We call this the inherent "boost" provided by the dose inhomogeneity that is part and parcel in brachytherapy. Indeed, the radiation dose immediately adjacent to a source dwell position within a catheter can be very high. The central higher radiation dose with brachytherapy can improve local control but also result in possible fat necrosis, fibrosis, telangiectasia, or other late effects of irradiation.

Second, the rapid fall-off of dose away from the catheter(s) should reduce the exposure of normal tissue to radiation. External beam PBI techniques can traverse significant amounts of normal tissue to get to the target, such as the thyroid gland, opposite breast, lung, heart, chest wall, uninvolved breast tissue, skin, or other organs that simply get in the way of the beam. Low doses of irradiation may be even more carcinogenic than therapeutic doses; so long-term effects must be watched for the next 10–25 years on these organs.

Third, the typically homogeneous dose distribution with external beam PBI has inspired the experts in the field to recommend higher prescribed doses than with brachytherapy, 385 cGy per fraction in contrast to 340 cGy per fraction of brachytherapy, for example. The net effect is higher total prescribed dose, higher dose per fraction, and more normal tissue exposure to radiation with external beam PBI techniques. Only the clinical trials will shed ultimate light on the impact these theoretical concerns will have on outcomes.

One issue that has not been resolved involves our current practice of uniformly treating a certain margin (1–2 cm) around the lumpectomy cavity, regardless of where the tumor is centered or where the pathologic margin is closest. When viewing specimen radiograms, it is rare that the lesion is centered within the excised tissue. Instead the visible lesion tends to be more commonly eccentrically located near one aspect of the specimen, with a large area of uninvolved fat or normal breast tissue at one end and the tumor approximating the edge on the other end. Ideally, one would want to generously treat the breast tissue adjacent to the close margin and minimize treatment to the breast tissue on the side that has generous surgical margins. Practically, however, contouring partial breast irradiation in this manner has technical challenges, and it is easier to simply treat all margins to a given distance.

The future of breast brachytherapy is promising, with many techniques for accomplishing target volume coverage and more innovations to come as industry interest in this expanding technology blossoms. Meticulous attention to detail in selecting patients and covering the target volume is key to future success. Learning the above techniques is essential to serving your patients and participating in clinical trials. Avenues for learning these techniques include studying this textbook, visiting the clinics of experienced breast brachytherapists, formal schools offered by societies and equipment manufacturers, and of course building your own clinical experience.

References

1. Aron BS. Teaching of radiation oncology residents. University of Cincinnati College of Medicine. 1984.
2. Brennan MF, Hilaris B, Shiu MH, et al. Local recurrence in adult soft tissue sarcoma: a randomized trial of brachytherapy. Arch Surg. 1987;122:1289.
3. King TA, Bolton JS, Kuske RR, et al. Long-term results of wide-field brachytherapy as the sole method of radiation therapy after segmental mastectomy for T(is,1,2) breast cancer. Am J Surg. 2000;180:299–304.
4. Kuske RR, Boyer C, Bolton JS, et al. Long-term results of the Ochsner Clinic prospective phase II breast brachytherapy trial. San Antonio Breast Meeting, 2004.
5. Baglan KL, Martinez AA, Frazier RC, et al. The use of high-dose brachytherapy alone after lumpectomy in patients with early-stage breast cancer treated with breast-conserving therapy. Int J Radiat Oncol Biol Phys. 2001;50:1003–11.
6. Kuske RR, Winter K, Arthur D, et al. A phase II trial of brachytherapy alone following lumpectomy for stage I or II breast cancer: initial outcomes of RTOG 95–17. J Contemp Brachytherapy. 2014;6(2):231–235. doi:10.5114/jcb.2014.43779.
7. Arthur DW, Winter K, Kuske RR, et al. A phase II trial of brachytherapy alone after lumpectomy for select breast cancer: tumor control and survival outcomes of RTOG 95–17. Int J Radiat Oncol Biol Phys. 2008;72:467–73.
8. Morrow M, Harris JR. Local management of invasive breast cancer. In: Harris JR, Lippman ME, Morrow M, Osborne CK, editors. Diseases of the breast. 2nd ed. Lippincott Williams and Wilkins; 2000. p. 528. table 6.
9. Vicini FA, Baglan K, Kestin L, et al. The emerging role of brachytherapy in the management of patients with breast cancer. Semin Radiat Oncol. 2002;12:31–9.
10. Keynes G. Conservative treatment of cancer of the breast. BMJ. 1937;2:643.
11. Vicini FA, Remouchanps V, Wallace M, et al. Ongoing clinical experience utilizing 3D conformal external beam radiotherapy to deliver partial-breast irradiation in patients with early-stage breast cancer treated with breast-conserving therapy. Int J Radiat Oncol Biol Phys. 2003;57:1247–53.
12. Ribeiro GG, Dunn G, Swindell R, et al. Conservation of the breast using two different radiotherapy techniques: interim report of a clinical trial. Clin Oncol (R Coll Radiol). 1990;2:27–34.

13. Kuske RR. Breast brachytherapy in women with breast cancer in the presence of augmentation mammoplasty. Radiol Soc North Am. Presence of Augmentation. Int J Radiat Oncol Biol Phys. 2012;84:S87.
14. Edmundson GK, Vicini FA, Chen PY, et al. Dosimetric characteristics of the MammoSite RTS: a new breast brachytherapy applicator. Int J Radiat Oncol Biol Phys. 2002;52:1132–9.
15. Patel R, et al. Presented at the 3rd annual school of breast brachytherapy, Las Vegas; 2005.

Chapter 17
Intracavitary Brachytherapy: Techniques, Data, Toxicity

Rakesh R. Patel

Contents

17.1 Introduction

Studies evaluating accelerated partial breast irradiation (APBI) as an alternative adjuvant treatment after breast-conserving surgery for early-stage breast cancer have demonstrated excellent outcomes [1, 17, 18, 22]. The method with the longest-standing history and supporting outcome data for APBI is multicatheter interstitial brachytherapy. The advent of a single-channel intracavitary device, the MammoSite balloon, has allowed a more simple and reproducible approach and has in turn led to a significant increase in the number of patients treated with APBI. Second-generation APBI methods have been built upon on favorable clinical outcomes while overcoming certain limitations inherent in these techniques.

In this chapter, the design rationale, potential advantages, and published clinical data of each method are reviewed.

R.R. Patel
The Targeted Radiation Institute at VMOC,
5725 West Las Positas Blvd, Suite 100, Pleasanton, CA 94588, USA
e-mail: rpatel@vmoc.com; iupatel@yahoo.com

D.W. Arthur et al. (eds.), *Short Course Breast Radiotherapy: A Comprehensive Review of Hypofractionation, Partial Breast, and Intra-Operative Irradiation*,
DOI 10.1007/978-3-319-24388-7_17

17.2 First-Generation Brachytherapy

17.2.1 Multicatheter Interstitial

Interstitial multicatheter breast brachytherapy has been in clinical use for several decades and has significantly more mature outcome data than any other APBI method [10, 17, 22]. The APBI application of this approach arose from its initial use to administer a boost dose to the tumor bed region in addition to whole breast irradiation. During this outpatient procedure, typically 15–25 needles are placed through the breast tissue. The needles are spaced about 1 cm apart in multiple planes in order to cover the surgical cavity plus a 1- to 2-cm margin, correlating with the region at highest risk of harboring residual microscopic disease. Advancements in image-guidance measures such as CT, ultrasound, and stereotactic digital mammography have significantly improved the accuracy and reproducibility of this APBI method [3, 14]. Following the outpatient placement procedure, individualized treatment planning is performed, which specifies predetermined dwell times and the positions of the radioactive source within the multiple catheters. Importantly, in any catheter system, the presence of multiple lumens offers a significant potential advantage by allowing maximal adjustment of the specific dwell positions and dwell times of the HDR source, resulting in highly tailored isodose distributions. This, coupled with more advanced 3D CT-based dosimetry with automatic catheter reconstruction tools and inverse optimization methods, has further improved target volume delineation, planning target volume coverage, avoidance of nearby critical structures, and dose homogeneity [5]. The multiple catheter interstitial technique offers the greatest control and tailoring of radiation dose delivery to variations in lumpectomy cavity size, shape, or location within the breast.

The primary disadvantage of this approach is the technical challenge for physicians and invasiveness of multicatheter insertion, which has diminished the use and restricted the adoption of this APBI technique to relatively few academic centers. Although the development of image-guided implant techniques has reduced the learning curve and improved reproducibility, this approach does require additional time, skill, and specialized training. However, the inherent dosimetric capabilities proved instrumental in development of modern intracavitary devices currently in wide use.

17.2.2 Single-Lumen Intracavitary

In early 2002, the MammoSite (MS) Radiation Therapy System (HOLOGIC, Inc., Bedford, MA, USA) was developed to increase the availability of APBI by simplifying the breast brachytherapy procedure for physicians and patients alike [6]. The applicator system consists of a semiflexible catheter that is 6 mm in diameter and 15 cm long with an inflatable balloon attached to the distal end. It can be placed easily either intraoperatively or postoperatively using a single entry into the breast and is inflated symmetrically within the lumpectomy cavity. The spherical single-lumen balloons are currently available in 4- to 5-cm diameter and 5- to 6-cm diameter sizes. After inflation with saline, the balloon is evaluated via CT (computerized tomography) or ultrasound to assure proper geometry, symmetry, and conformance.

An electronic form of brachytherapy (EBT) was developed to allow APBI to be performed in a patient procedure room with minimal shielding. This device (Axxent®, Xoft, Inc., Sunnyvale, CA) uses a kilovoltage X-ray source to also deliver HDR radiation to the tumor bed through a similar-shaped balloon applicator. Although early, 1-year follow-up data from a multicenter study suggests control rates, cosmesis, and tolerability may be similar to other forms of breast brachytherapy [15].

For these intracavitary methods, the catheter shaft has a single lumen that permits the transport of an HDR source into the center of the balloon, affording only a few dwell positions and thus a much quicker and simpler treatment planning process with a high reproducibility of target coverage. This results in a significantly shorter learning curve than interstitial brachytherapy. Multiple studies have revealed excellent local control rates with acceptable toxicity profiles relative to interstitial brachytherapy [18, 21].

Its primary drawbacks include the relatively restricted flexibility of treatment planning after applicator placement. This limits its applicability to only select patients, contingent upon several factors: (1) good conformance between the balloon surface and breast tissue (minimal air gaps), (2) optimal location and geometry of the surgical cavity, and (3) appropriate skin-to-balloon distance. In the initial trial, 30 % of patients proved ineligible for brachytherapy due to these technical reasons [11].

17.3 Next Generation: Multicatheter Intracavitary Brachytherapy

17.3.1 Rationale

In an effort to merge the simplicity and reproducibility of the single-entry MammoSite balloon device with the customization and dose flexibility of the multicatheter interstitial technique, the next generation of intracavitary devices was born. These devices have key differences in applicator design, placement technique, treatment planning, and quality assurance measures. However, they share basic goals: (1) to provide optimal target volume coverage, (2) to minimize normal tissue dose/toxicity, and (3) to expand the number of patients that are eligible for APBI by overcoming previous technical limitations of tissue nonconformance, central lumen asymmetry, and reduced skin-to-balloon or chest wall distance.

An important consideration when modifying the current single-lumen balloon APBI method is the ability to shape the radiation dose away from the chest wall and skin surface. This was not possible when two-dimensional or plain film treatment planning was routinely performed due the difficulty in assessing the gradient of radiation dose to the skin via a dose–volume histogram. As a result, for single-lumen balloon, the skin-to-balloon distance (or skin bridge) measurement has been used as a simple method of estimating the likely maximum dose to the skin surface. The typical maximum skin doses are significantly higher with single-lumen balloon brachytherapy relative to interstitial multicatheter brachytherapy, where multiple dwell positions allow tailored dose modulation. This restricted the patient eligibility recommendation to a minimal skin bridge of 5–7 mm.

Several reports have demonstrated a correlation between balloon-to-skin spacing and acute and late skin toxicity. Nine institutions participated in a pooled analysis of data evaluating clinical experience of the MammoSite RTS for delivering accelerated partial breast irradiation. Between 2000 and 2004, 483 patients were treated and treatment parameters were analyzed to identify factors affecting outcome. A skin spacing of <6 mm increased the risk of severe acute skin reaction ($p=0.017$) and telangiectasia ($p=0.028$). Importantly, the use of multiple dwell positions reduced the risk of severe hyperpigmentation ($p=0.0278$), also suggesting that a reduction in the skin dose correlates with a reduction with skin toxicity [2]. Similarly, in cases where the applicator is close to the chest wall, the dose to the ribs, lung, and heart can be significant with the higher dose per fraction of APBI.

Compared with standard single-lumen balloon brachytherapy, potential improvements in dosimetric capabilities are significant. This includes reduced skin and chest wall dose (thereby eliminating the 5- to 7-mm skin bridge requirement) and improved target (PTV_EVAL) coverage. As a result, the planning parameters can be made more stringent in an effort to reduce acute and late toxicity (Table 17.1).

17.3.2 Advances in Treatment Planning Systems

Key improvements in treatment planning hardware and software that facilitate the planning process, including contouring, automated catheter reconstruction, optimization tools, and dose–volume histogram analyses, were instrumental in enabling adoption of more advanced brachytherapy devices. CT-based three-dimensional planning is paramount in order to achieve reliable target coverage with maximal normal tissue sparing for all multicatheter approaches [3, 5, 12, 13, 16, 20]. Although

Table 17.1 Dosimetric planning parameters

	Interstitial	Single lumen balloon	Multi-lumen balloon	Strut-based
D90	>90 %	>90 %	–	–
D95	–	–	>95 %	>95 %
V150	≤70 cc	≤50 cc	≤50 cc	≤50 cc
V200	≤20 cc	≤10 cc	≤10 cc	≤20 cc
D_{max} skin	≤100 %	≤145 %	≤125%	≤100 %

the devices have evolved significantly over the past two decades, the conventional regimen for most HDR APBI techniques remains a dose of 34 Gy delivered twice daily at least 6 h apart over a period of ten fractions in 1 week. Treatment planning consists of outlining the lumpectomy cavity, which may contain seroma fluid and/or air plus an expansion of 1 cm of breast tissue. For all intracavitary HDR APBI methods, the planning target volume (PTV) is defined as the expanded volume minus the lumpectomy cavity often defined by the device itself (Fig. 17.1).

Importantly, the added multichannel flexibility does require rigorous quality assurance with imaging typically recommended to be obtained prior to each fraction in order to verify the position and geometry of the applicator within the breast. This can be done via plain X-ray, CT scout, CT, or ultrasound and should be correlated with the relevant measurement at the time of initial treatment planning.

17.3.3 Surgical Technique

Intracavitary devices can be placed at the time of surgery or preferably during a separate procedure after surgical pathology is reviewed. In a multi-institutional report, the results of 1403 cases from 87 institutions were studied, and it was found that 44 % of the applicators were placed using an open technique at the time of lumpectomy, 41 % used an ultrasound-guided lateral incision, and 14 % used the scar entry technique. As the trial progressed, the proportion of patients undergoing an open placement declined. In this large registry trial, there were no differences

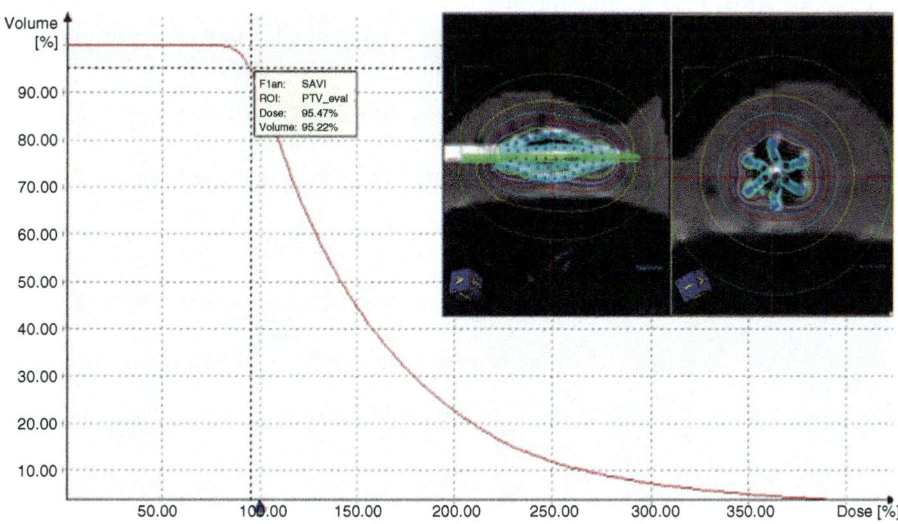

Fig. 17.1 Example of 3D treatment planning software, demonstrating dose optimization and dose–volume histogram analyses of a SAVI device using the Nucletron Oncentra Brachy planning system

among the three placement techniques in regard to skin distance, cavity conformance, or asymmetry, and no associations were found between placement technique and cosmetic outcome [25]. If the physician is not experienced with ultrasound-guided percutaneous methods, an alternative is to insert and leave a temporary balloon catheter indwelling at the time of lumpectomy surgery, which is then exchanged for the hybrid device.

17.4 Multi-lumen Balloons (MLB)

The MammoSite ML (*HOLOGIC, Inc., Bedford, MA, USA*) was introduced as a second-generation balloon brachytherapy method for more technically challenging cases. The polyurethane applicator includes three additional lumens parallel to the central channel. The size ranges from 3.5 to 5 cm diameter based on volume filling of 25–61 cc. This enables accommodating a range of lumpectomy bed sizes and allows some minor tailoring of the radiation dose cloud (Fig. 17.2).

A similar advancement in balloon technology was the Contura MLB radiation system (HOLOGIC, Inc., Bedford, MA, USA). The device has a polyethylene balloon at the end of a central shaft with four additional minimally displaced treatment catheters, all five of which can accommodate the HDR source. A key feature of the Contura device is a vacuum port on both ends of the balloon to remove fluid or air around the lumpectomy cavity, thereby improving the conformity of the target tissue to the balloon surface, leading to reproducible dose delivery and increased target volume coverage. This in turn increases the pool of patients that are technically eligible for APBI [19]. Unlike the non-balloon hybrid devices, the positions of the surrounding channels are not variable. They have a fixed 5-mm offset around the central channel. These channels provide additional source positions and thus allow

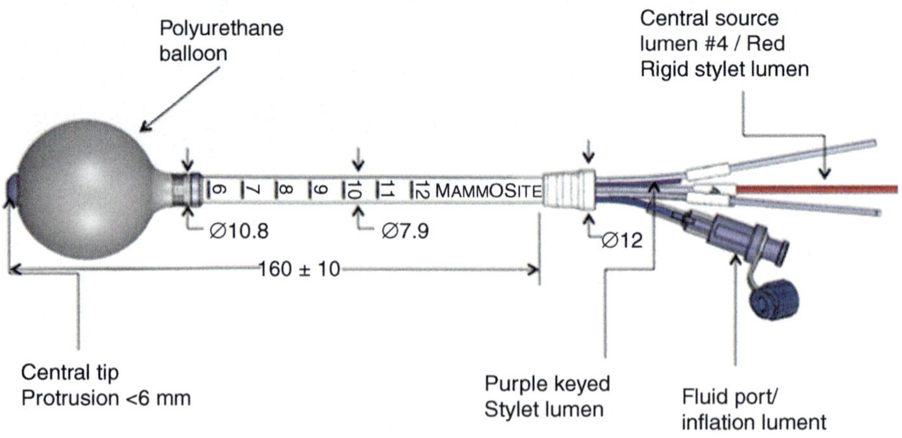

Fig. 17.2 MammoSite ML

increased dose flexibility compared to single-lumen devices. This can potentially lead to some increased sparing of normal tissues, including the heart, lung, chest wall, and skin (Fig. 17.3).

The improved dose modulation with MLB was shown in a dosimetric study in patients previously treated with the single-lumen MammoSite device. The MammoSite planning CT scans account for the additional lumens available in the MLB catheter. For balloons located between 10 and 5 mm from the skin, the MLB diminished the V_{150} to the breast by 20 % and reduced the chest wall dose by about 40 %. For balloons located ≤5 mm from the skin, the MLB device allowed the maximum dose to the skin to be less than 115 %, typically 30 % less than for a single-lumen balloon. Target volume coverage was also increased by 5–15 %. In addition, the additional dose flexibility may allow the treating physician to account for an asymmetric balloon implant with respect to the central channel, which was often a limitation of the single-lumen balloon method.

As expected, the clinical outcomes have demonstrated similar excellent locoregional control as first-generation methods given that the majority of patients have been prescribed the conventional 10 fraction regimen, twice daily over 5 days. One study with 46 patients published a 2 % (1 of 46 patients) local recurrence rate at 3

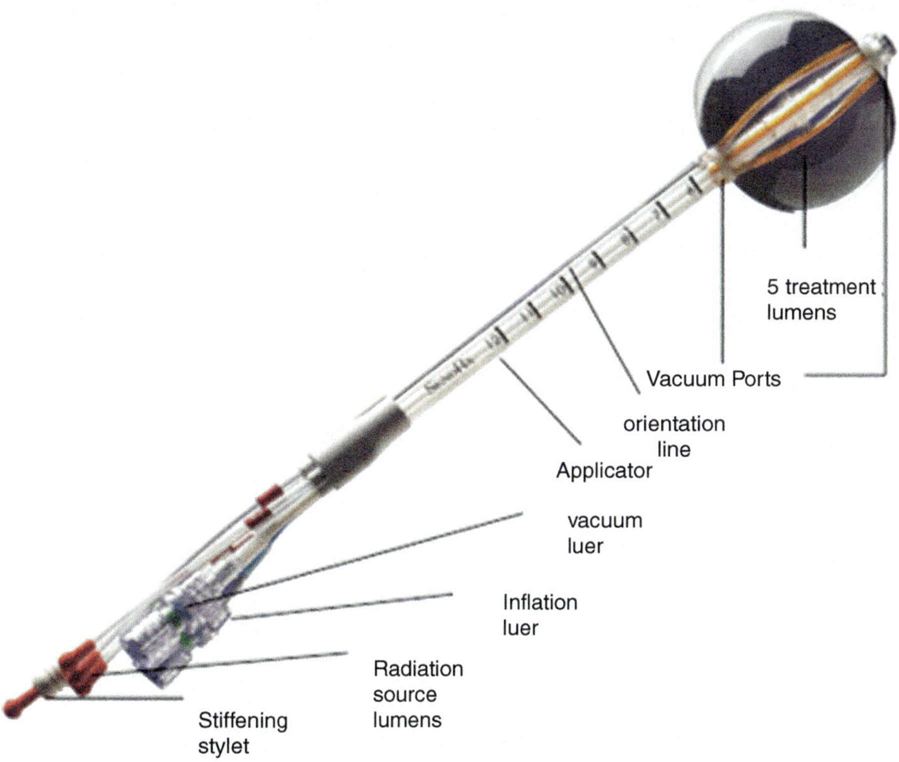

Fig. 17.3 Contura MLB

years. The median skin dose was 99.7 % of the prescribed dose and the PTV coverage was excellent (V95>98.8 %). No major toxicities were seen and the good/excellent cosmetic outcome was 97 % at 3 years [7].

A large multicenter registry trial comprised of 342 patients from 23 institutions was completed and also reported high local control rates with minimal acute or delayed toxicity. A total of ten patients had ipsilateral breast tumor recurrence (2.2 %) and the good/excellent cosmetic outcome was 88 % at a median follow-up of 3 years [4].

17.5 SAVI

The SAVI (strut adjusted volume implant) applicator (Cianna Medical, Aliso Viejo, CA, USA) was the first non-balloon hybrid device to reach the marketplace, and it also combines the dosimetric flexibility of multicatheter brachytherapy with the advantages of a single catheter entry into the breast. It is available in several sizes consisting of six, eight, or ten catheters that deploy into equal positions radially around a central strut. The device is inserted in collapsed form through a small skin incision. Once placed, it is then expanded to fit the lumpectomy cavity by rotating the hub of the device, which remains external to the patient's skin after deployment (Fig. 17.4).

With up to 11 total catheter lumens to accommodate the HDR source, the multiple peripheral struts of the SAVI enable radiation dose modulation in amounts customized for cavity characteristics, including proximity to the skin and chest wall, in contrast to the spherically symmetric distribution associated with balloon catheters, where radiation comes from a single point or line source. With the use of multiple dwell positions in each of the hollow struts, the flexibility in dose distribution can approach the conformality and distribution associated with multicatheter interstitial brachytherapy. This enhanced dose modulation capability has been shown in several studies. Gurdalli and colleagues found that, in 15 patients treated with the SAVI device, the skin doses were 10–13 % lower than published values for MammoSite, although the treatment plans were more complex than MammoSite plans, with an average number of dwell positions utilized of 106 [8].

The same group performed a dosimetric comparison of SAVI, Contura MLB, and MammoSite breast brachytherapy by inserting each of the applicators into a 5-cm diameter lumpectomy cavity in a human cadaver. The target volume coverage was excellent and similar for all three devices; however, given a 3-mm skin distance, the maximum skin doses differed significantly at 85, 142, and 182 % of the prescription dose for SAVI, MLB, and MS, respectively. This suggests that the dose modulation capability of the SAVI is the greatest of all the currently available HDR intracavitary devices and may have the least restrictions in terms of positioning of the cavity in relation to the skin surface (i.e., skin bridge) and chest wall [9].

Initial clinical experience was reported from a multicenter analysis of the first 100 patients treated with SAVI at a median follow-up of 21 months. This showed

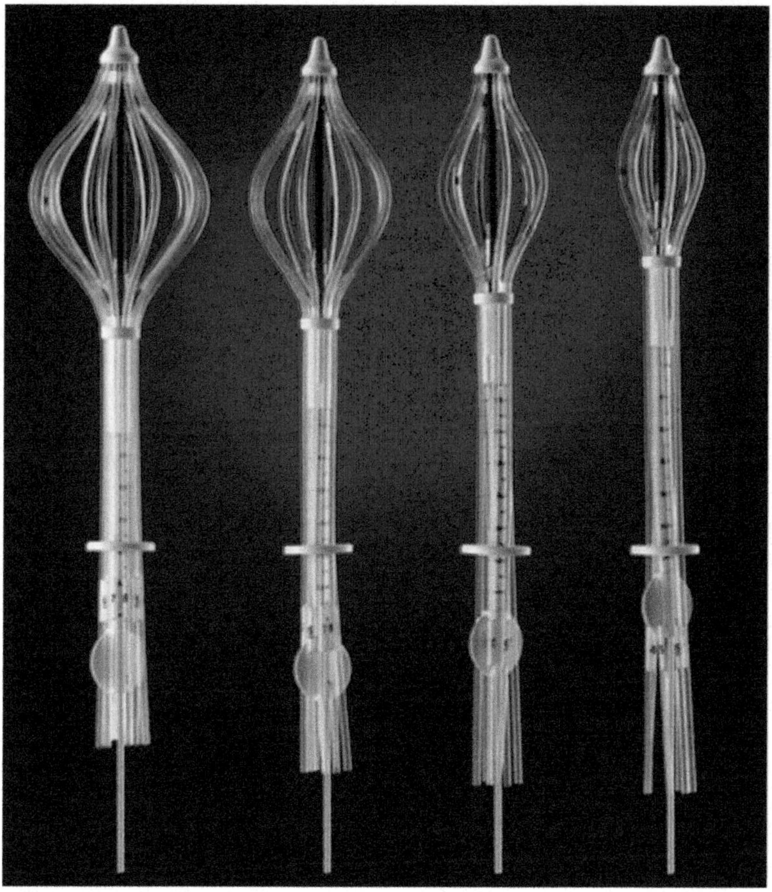

Fig. 17.4 SAVI

the local recurrence rate to be 1 % with favorable toxicity rates in terms of fibrosis, seroma, and telangiectasia. Furthermore, the study stratified patients by skin bridge and/or chest wall constraint and reported that up to 27 % of the patients would have not been potentially eligible for single-lumen balloon brachytherapy. The volumes receiving a specific higher % of the prescription dose (V150 and V200) were 27.8 and 14 cc, respectively [23]. These "hotspots" in the breast tend to be higher with the SAVI device since the struts housing the HDR source are approximating breast tissue similar to interstitial brachytherapy and unlike the MLB methods where the source is near the center in the internal lumens. Given that the toxicity tends to evolve over time, with the incidence of breast pain, fibrosis, and fat necrosis continuing to increase, longer-term data have been awaited to assess these toxicities. Several recent reports from the SAVI Collaborative Research Group (over 1000 patients from 14 institutions) have presented early and late toxicity rates that are low in incidence, low in grade, and favorable to other brachytherapy methods. The telangiectasia rate was 1.6 %, the symptomatic seroma rate was 3.2 %, and the fat necrosis rate was 0.5 % at 5 years [24].

17.6 Conclusion

Based on favorable clinical outcome data, accelerated partial breast irradiation is routinely offered as an alternative to conventional external beam whole breast irradiation following lumpectomy in select early-stage breast cancer patients. Development and integration of more advanced imaging and sophisticated 3D radiation treatment planning systems have spawned innovative multichannel intracavitary applicator systems capable of delivering higher-quality APBI. These approaches represent a new iteration of treatment technologies that seek to increase applicability to a broader group of patients, significantly improve ease of use for the physician, reduce normal tissue toxicity, and ultimately provide greater patient convenience without deteriorating existing breast cancer treatment outcomes.

References

1. Arthur DW, Morris MM, et al. Breast cancer: new radiation treatment options. Oncology (Williston Park). 2004;18(13):1621–9; discussion 1629–30, 1636–38.
2. Cuttino LW, Keisch M, et al. Multi-institutional experience using the mammosite radiation therapy system in the treatment of early-stage breast cancer: 2-year results. Int J Radiat Oncol Biol Phys. 2008;71(1):107–14.
3. Cuttino LW, Todor D, et al. CT-guided multi-catheter insertion technique for partial breast brachytherapy: reliable target coverage and dose homogeneity. Brachytherapy. 2005;4(1):10–7.
4. Cuttino LW, Arthur DW, et al. Long-term results from the Contura multilumen balloon breast brachytherapy catheter phase 4 registry trial. Int J Radiat Oncol Biol Phys. 2014;90(5):1025–9.
5. Das RK, Patel R, et al. 3D CT-based high-dose-rate breast brachytherapy implants: treatment planning and quality assurance. Int J Radiat Oncol Biol Phys. 2004;59(4):1224–8.
6. Edmundson GK, Vicini FA, et al. Dosimetric characteristics of the MammoSite RTS, a new breast brachytherapy applicator. Int J Radiat Oncol Biol Phys. 2002;52(4):1132–9.
7. Israel PZ, Robbins A, et al. Three-year clinical outcome using the Contura multilumen balloon breast brachytherapy catheter to deliver accelerated partial breast irradiation (APBI): improving radiation standards for the optimal application of APBI. Brachytherapy. 2012;11(4):316–21.
8. Gurdalli SK, Kuske R, et al. A dosimetric comparison of three different brachytherapy applicators for partial breast irradiation. Brachytherapy. 2008;7:143.
9. Gurdalli SK, Kuske R, et al. Dosimetric performance of SAVI: a new single-entry, multicatheter breast brachytherapy applicator. Brachytherapy. 2008;7:142–3.
10. Kamrava M, Kuske RR, et al. Outcomes of breast cancer patients treated with accelerated partial breast irradiation via multicatheter interstitial brachytherapy: the Pooled Registry of Multicatheter Interstitial Sites (PROMIS) Experience. Ann Surg Oncol. 2015. Epub ahead of print.

11. Keisch M, Vicini F, et al. Initial clinical experience with the MammoSite breast brachytherapy applicator in women with early-stage breast cancer treated with breast-conserving therapy. Int J Radiat Oncol Biol Phys. 2003;55(2):289–93.
12. Major T, Frohlich G, et al. Dosimetric experience with accelerated partial breast irradiation using image-guided interstitial brachytherapy. Radiother Oncol. 2007;90(1):48–55.
13. Ott OJ, Lotter M, et al. Accelerated partial-breast irradiation with interstitial implants: the clinical relevance of the calculation of skin doses. Strahlenther Onkol. 2007;183(8):426–31.
14. Patel RR, Das RK. Image-guided breast brachytherapy: an alternative to whole-breast radiotherapy. Lancet Oncol. 2006;7(5):407–15.
15. Patel RR, Beitsch PD, et al. Postsurgical treatment of early-stage breast cancer with electronic brachytherapy: outcomes and health-related quality of life at 1 year. Am J Clin Oncol. 2013;36(5):430–5.
16. Patel RR, Becker SJ, et al. A dosimetric comparison of accelerated partial breast irradiation techniques: multicatheter interstitial brachytherapy, three-dimensional conformal radiotherapy, and supine versus prone helical tomotherapy. Int J Radiat Oncol Biol Phys. 2007;68(3):935–42.
17. Polgár C, Fodor J, et al. Breast-conserving therapy with partial or whole breast irradiation: ten-year results of the Budapest randomized trial. Radiother Oncol. 2013;108(2):197–202.
18. Shah C, Badiyan S, et al. Treatment efficacy with accelerated partial breast irradiation (APBI): final analysis of the American Society of Breast Surgeons MammoSite(®) breast brachytherapy registry trial. Ann Surg Oncol. 2013;20(10):3279–85.
19. Tokita KM, Cuttino LW, et al. Optimal application of the Contura multilumen balloon breast brachytherapy catheter vacuum port to deliver accelerated partial breast irradiation. Brachytherapy. 2011;10(3):184–9.
20. Weed DW, Edmundson GK, et al. Accelerated partial breast irradiation: a dosimetric comparison of three different techniques. Brachytherapy. 2005;4(2):121–9.
21. Wilkinson JB, Beitsch PD, et al. Evaluation of current consensus statement recommendations for accelerated partial breast irradiation: a pooled analysis of William Beaumont Hospital and American Society of Breast Surgeon MammoSite Registry Trial Data. Int J Radiat Oncol Biol Phys. 2013;85(5):1179–85.
22. Wobb JL, Shah C et al. Brachytherapy-based accelerated partial breast irradiation provides equivalent 10-year outcomes to whole breast irradiation: a matched-pair analysis. Am J Clin Oncol. 2015. Epub ahead of print.
23. Yashar CM, Scanderbeg D, et al. Initial clinical experience with the Strut-Adjusted Volume Implant (SAVI) breast brachytherapy device for accelerated partial-breast irradiation (APBI): first 100 patients with more than 1 year of follow-up. Int J Radiat Oncol Biol Phys. 2011;80(3):765–70.
24. Yashar C, et al. Outcomes for APBI with strut-based brachytherapy: first 200 accrued patients (5-year report). Presentation at the 2014 annual meeting of the American Society for Radiation Oncology.
25. Zannis V, Beitsch P, et al. Descriptions and outcomes of insertion techniques of a breast brachytherapy balloon catheter in 1403 patients enrolled in the American Society of Breast Surgeons MammoSite breast brachytherapy registry trial. Am J Surg. 2005;190(4):530–8.

Chapter 18
External-Beam Accelerated Partial Breast Irradiation

Aaron Sabolch and Reshma Jagsi

Contents

As discussed elsewhere in this textbook, interest in accelerated partial breast irradiation (APBI) for the adjuvant treatment of breast cancer after breast-conserving surgery has grown substantially over the past two decades. This interest derives from the hope that targeting a smaller volume of breast tissue than that treated in traditional whole breast irradiation might allow for treatment to be completed more efficiently and with greater sparing of normal tissues. Such an approach might have similar efficacy to whole breast radiation in selected patients in whom radiation therapy to areas of the breast remote from the tumor bed might not be necessary.

Although early experience with APBI primarily involved brachytherapy techniques, more recent investigations have focused on external-beam techniques. In the current chapter, we will begin by discussing the motivation for developing external-beam techniques for APBI, early experiences in external-beam APBI technique development, recent data from clinical trials reporting early cosmetic outcomes in patients treated with external-beam APBI, and finally treatment planning considerations in this context.

A. Sabolch, MD
Department of Radiation Oncology, University of Michigan,
1500 E. Medical Center Drive, Ann Arbor, MI
e-mail: sabolch@med.umiche.du

R. Jagsi, MD, DPhil (✉)
Department of Radiation Oncology, University of Michigan,
1500 E. Medical Center Drive, UH-B2-C490, SPC5010, Ann Arbor, MI 48109, USA
e-mail: rjagsi@med.umich.edu

D.W. Arthur et al. (eds.), *Short Course Breast Radiotherapy: A Comprehensive Review of Hypofractionation, Partial Breast, and Intra-Operative Irradiation*,
DOI 10.1007/978-3-319-24388-7_18

18.1 Development of External-Beam Accelerated Partial Breast Irradiation

Although there are many potential advantages of brachytherapy for APBI, this approach relies heavily on physician expertise that may not universally be taught in training programs. Furthermore, brachytherapy may require an additional surgical procedure, potentially increasing the chances of a complication resultant from this invasive approach. In contrast, external-beam APBI, which has become more feasible owing to the development of sophisticated treatment planning systems, has the benefit of utilizing the standard linear accelerators that have become ubiquitous in radiation oncology practice. Additionally, by utilizing an external-beam approach analogous to that employed in other disease sites, the technique relies less on the surgical skill set and clinician expertise required by brachytherapy, making this approach more easily applied by all radiation oncologists.

Considerable research has been devoted to the development of external-beam APBI approaches. Such work has been particularly challenging because external-beam techniques involve the irradiation of a larger portion of the normal breast and greater dose homogeneity than with brachytherapy, and this has complicated the determination of appropriate dose and fractionation with this approach. Early randomized trials demonstrated concerning findings, both in terms of efficacy and toxicity, but subsequent investigations in numerous institutions have been more promising. This section reviews those studies.

Early in the history of the development of APBI, two randomized trials compared external-beam APBI versus whole breast radiotherapy [1–3]. The trial with the largest enrollment was performed at Christie Hospital in Manchester [1, 2]. Subjects were less than 70 years old, with tumors smaller than 4 cm. The axilla was required to be clinically negative, and margins after breast-conserving surgery needed to be macroscopically negative. Seven hundred eight women accrued to the trial. In the group randomized to APBI, an *en face*, 8–14 MeV electron beam was used to deliver 40–42.5 Gy in 8 fractions. The group receiving whole breast radiotherapy received 40 Gy in 15 fractions using tangential 4 MV photons. Additionally, this group also received a matched nodal treatment to 40 Gy in 15 fractions. Systemic therapy was not permitted. The median follow-up for the entire cohort was 65 months, and there were no differences in overall survival between the two groups. Six percent of those who received whole breast radiation experienced an isolated ipsilateral breast recurrence as a first event compared to 14 % of those in the APBI arm [2]. In addition to worse rates of disease control in the APBI arm, there were also worse complications. Marked telangiectasias were experienced by 33 % of the APBI arm versus 12 % of the whole breast arm. Likewise, marked fibrosis was seen in 14 % of the APBI group as compared to 5 % of those who underwent whole breast radiotherapy. Fat necrosis occurred in 5 % of the APBI arm but only 1 % of the control arm [2].

Another randomized trial that showed similarly cautionary results was performed at Leeds Hospital in Yorkshire [3]. This study enrolled women with pT1-2, N0-1 disease who had undergone lumpectomy as well as axillary lymph node dissection. Margins from the procedure were required to be macroscopically negative. Systemic therapy with cyclophosphamide, methotrexate, and fluorouracil, as well as tamoxifen, was frequently employed. In those randomized to partial breast irradiation, 55 Gy in 20 fractions was delivered via *en face* electrons or tangential photons. Whole breast radiotherapy consisted of tangential photon beams to 40 Gy in 15 fractions; this was followed by a boost to the tumor bed of 15 Gy in 5 fractions. A total of 174 women enrolled. After a median follow-up of 8 years, 24 % of those in the partial breast arm had a local-regional recurrence as opposed to only 9 % of those who underwent treatment of the whole breast. No cosmetic outcomes were described.

Although the results of the early British trials were concerning, more recent studies of external-beam APBI have utilized more stringent criteria for patient selection, modern planning techniques, and lower total dosages. Many of these studies have had more promising results, particularly with respect to efficacy and in some cases also cosmetic outcomes. For example, investigators at New York University pioneered the delivery of APBI with the patient in the prone position, such that the treated breast is free to fall beneath the table without obstruction [4, 5]. In a prospective study, these investigators included women with hormone receptor-positive tumors smaller than 2 cm and negative surgical margins. Those with nodal disease or an extensive intraductal component were excluded. The clinical target volume (CTV) was the lumpectomy cavity with a 2.7 cm margin to the planning target volume (PTV). Parallel-opposed mini-tangents were used to give 30 Gy in 5 fractions over 10 days. After 5 years of follow-up in 100 patients, local control was excellent at 99 %. Overall survival was excellent and no deaths from breast cancer were reported. Further, rates of cosmesis at 3 years – as judged by the patient on a 4-point scale – were excellent or good in 89 % of cases [4]. The use of such a scale – with scores of poor, fair, good, or excellent – was initially developed at Harvard, in a system in which the treated breast is compared to the contralateral side [6].

In contrast to the prone technique, investigators at William Beaumont Hospital focused on refining the use of external-beam APBI using supine positioning [7–10]. Initially, this technique was developed in a Phase I/II trial that enrolled 23 patients, all older than 50 years of age, with tumor size 3 cm or less, and at least 2 mm of negative margins following lumpectomy. The axilla was required to be pathologically negative. After CT simulation, a clinical target volume (CTV) was defined as the lumpectomy cavity plus 1–1.5 cm, with an additional 1 cm expansion to a planning target volume (PTV). Treatment planning consisted of three to seven non-coplanar photon beams in the most patients. The prescription dose was 34–38.5 Gy in 10, twice-daily fractions (extrapolated from doses used in studies with brachytherapy). Toxicity and cosmetic outcomes from this study showed good results in the majority of women. Subsequently, this technique was used in additional patients, and retrospective results from a total of 205 women were recently reported. After a median follow-up of almost 5 years, no local failures were reported, nor was there any death from breast cancer. Eighty-one percent of patients had excellent or good cosmesis [10].

Similar to the Beaumont experience, RTOG 0319 was a US cooperative group study that utilized 38 Gy in 10, twice-daily fractions in a Phase I/II feasibility trial, which enrolled 58 women [11, 12]. Entry criteria required tumors 3 cm or smaller, negative surgical margins, and three or fewer pathologically involved lymph nodes. Planning parameters were similar to those used in the Beaumont experience. However, unlike the single institution data reported above, the rate of in-breast recurrence was 6 % at a median follow of 4.5 years. Furthermore, when cosmesis was assessed by radiation oncologists, 26 % of women were judged to have unacceptable outcomes at 1 year, and this worsened to 42 % after 3 years of follow-up [12].

Investigators from Harvard reported on their initial dosimetric experience in a series of 61 patients with unicentric Stage I disease without evidence of involved margins, lymphovascular invasion, or an extensive intraductal component [13]. The majority of these patients were enrolled on a prospective Phase I/II protocol. After simulation in the supine position, the PTV was created by a 1.5–2.0 cm expansion of the tumor bed, edited back from skin surface, pectoralis, and chest wall. Most women were treated with 3DCRT to 32 Gy in 4 Gy fractions, delivered twice-daily over 4 days, though subsequent patients on the same protocol were treated to a total of 36 Gy. No formal normal tissue constraints were used, though efforts were made to reduce dose to the normal breast parenchyma to less than 50 % of the prescribed dose. Dose inhomogeneity was limited to less than 15 % of the prescription. The majority of patients were treated with a three-field technique of mixed mini-tangent photon beams and *en face* electrons. The median volume of ipsilateral breast receiving half the prescription dose was 52 %. The median dose inhomogeneity was 105 % though it exceeded 110 % in 11 % of patients [13].

A subsequent publication from the Harvard instigators has updated this series with 79 women treated with a median of follow-up of 83 months [14]. The authors reported cosmetic outcomes in these women – as evaluated by both the patient and the treating clinician on a 4-point scale. At 1 year following treatment, 93 % of patients rated their cosmesis as excellent or good, compared to 96 % at 7 years. Physicians rated 97 % of patients as having good or excellent cosmesis at 1 year, versus 94 % at 7 years [14]. A separate toxicity analysis also revealed that greater dose to the ipsilateral lung was associated with the development of pneumonitis; increases in the volumes receiving 20 Gy, 10 Gy, or 5 Gy were all found to be significantly correlated with such toxicity [15].

Canadian researchers have also reported their experience with 3DCRT APBI in a Phase II trial that enrolled women, age 40 or greater, with either invasive disease or DCIS [16]. Subjects were required to have tumors less than 3 cm in size, negative margins following lumpectomy, as well as an uninvolved axilla. Furthermore, the lumpectomy cavity was required to be 30 % or less of the ipsilateral breast volume. Patients were simulated in the supine position. The CTV was a 1.0–1.5 cm expansion of the lumpectomy cavity, excluding the chest wall and skin, and the PTV was a 1.0 cm expansion beyond this. The prescription was to deliver 35–38.5 in 10, twice-daily fractions. The primary dose constraints for the ipsilateral breast were to limit the volume receiving 95 % of the prescription to less than 25 % and to limit the volume receiving 50 % of the prescription to less than 50 %. Dose inhomogeneity was limited to 107 %. Cosmesis was assessed using the EORTC Cosmetic Rating System [17].

In total, 127 women enrolled on the trial, and 87 were available for evaluation after 3 years of follow-up. Eighty-seven percent of treatment plans met all dosimetric constraints. There was only a single local recurrence. Cosmesis was excellent or good in 85 % of patients 1 year after radiotherapy and in 82 % of patients at 3 years [16]. Longer follow-up has not yet been published.

More recently, a small randomized trial of 3DCRT APBI versus whole breast irradiation was reported by Spanish investigators [18]. Entry criteria required that subjects be age 60 or greater, with invasive disease, Grade 1 or 2, less than or equal to 3 cm in size. Women with positive or close margins less than 3 mm were not allowed on trial, nor were those with nodal involvement or an extensive intraductal component. CT simulation was performed in the supine position, and the PTV in the APBI arm was defined as the quadrant of the breast containing the lumpectomy cavity. Patients randomized to APBI received 37.5 Gy in 10, twice-daily fractions. Dose constraints were based upon those used in RTOG 0413/NSABP B-39 [19], and these are discussed in more detail later in this chapter. Patients randomized to whole breast radiotherapy received 48 Gy in 2 Gy daily fractions, followed by an optional 10 Gy boost. Cosmesis was assessed by patients as well as by physicians on a 4-point scale [6].

One hundred two women enrolled on the trial. For the APBI arm, the mean volume of the ipsilateral breast that received 50 % of the prescription dose was 52 %. After 5 years of follow-up, there were no local recurrences in either arm. Additionally, all patients in both arms rated their cosmesis as either excellent or good. However, 67 % of those in the standard radiotherapy arm rated themselves as having excellent cosmesis compared to 57 % in the APBI arm, though this difference was not significant (no p-value reported). Similarly, the final physician assessment of cosmesis found excellent or good cosmesis in 84 % of the control arm compared to 75 % of the APBI arm, though this difference was not significant (no p-value reported) [18].

In contrast to the 3DCRT approach, investigators from Colorado have published their experience with the use of intensity-modulated radiotherapy (IMRT) to deliver APBI [20–22]. This Phase II study enrolled women with either DCIS or T1N0M0 invasive disease, age 40 or older, with negative margins by at least 2 mm. Patients were simulated in the supine position. The CTV was defined as a 1–2 cm expansion of the lumpectomy cavity, edited to be at least 0.5 cm from the skin surface or chest wall, and the PTV was a 1 cm expansion beyond this. The prescription dose was 34–38.5 Gy in 10, twice-daily fractions. The volume of ipsilateral breast allowed to receive 50 % of the prescription was limited to 50 %. Following treatment, both patients and treating physicians graded cosmesis on a 4-point scale.

The study enrolled a total of 136 patients. IMRT plans utilized a median of 6 fields each. After a median follow-up of 53 months, the rate of local recurrence was 0.7 %. Patient-reported cosmesis was excellent or good in 98 % of cases at 1 year posttreatment, though this declined 91 % at 5 years. Likewise, physician-rated cosmesis fell from excellent or good in 98 % of cases at 1 year to 89 % at 5 years [20].

18.2 Growing Interest in Cosmetic Outcomes

As detailed above, cosmetic outcomes after external-beam APBI have varied considerably in different series. Single institution data from Tufts and the University of Michigan have raised further concerns about adverse cosmetic results with external-beam approaches and the dose-fractionation schedule that has become most commonly applied (38.5 Gy in 10, twice-daily fractions, as specified on the RTOG 0413/NSABP B39 randomized trial) [23–26].

At Tufts, 80 patients were treated with 3DCRT APBI, the results of which were retrospectively analyzed [25, 26]. The majority of women received therapy in the manner specified by RTOG 0413/NSABP B-39 [19]. Cosmesis was evaluated on a 4-point scale by the treating physician, and toxicity was assessed according to RTOG criteria. The median follow-up for all patients was 32 months. The mean age was 67 years, and the mean tumor size was 1.0 cm. At last follow-up, 19 % of patients had fair or poor cosmesis. Having an unacceptable cosmetic outcome was significantly correlated with the volume of the breast receiving 50, 80, and 100 % of the prescription dose, as well as with increasing maximum dose inhomogeneity. Not surprisingly given these high rates of poor cosmesis, patients also frequently experienced severe late toxicity: 8 % experienced Grade 3–4 subcutaneous fibrosis, and 11 % experienced fat necrosis [26].

Similar findings were reported from a Phase I/II trial of IMRT APBI conducted at the University of Michigan [23, 24]. This feasibility study enrolled women with either DCIS or Stage I disease, age 40 or greater, who had undergone excision with negative margins by at least 3 mm. There were several exclusion criteria, including the presence of lymphovascular invasion or an extensive intraductal component. CT simulation was in the supine position, and the PTV was defined as a 1.5 cm expansion of the lumpectomy cavity, edited such that it did not encroach within 0.5 cm of the skin surface. Treatment was delivered via beamlet IMRT with active breathing control to a total dose of 38.5 Gy in 10, twice-daily fractions. Dosimetric constraints were similar to that used on RTOG 0413/NSABP B-39 [19]. Cosmesis was assessed by the treating physician on a 4-point scale. Toxicity was assessed with the Common Terminology Criteria for Adverse Events (CTCAE) scale.

The study enrolled a total of 34 patients before being terminated early due to concerns of unacceptable cosmetic outcomes. Five-year results showed 97 % local control, though 27 % of patients had either fair or poor cosmesis. Further, cosmetic outcomes had continued to decline over the study's entire follow-up period. However, this did not correspond to a high rate of toxicity as measured on the standard CTCAE scale, as only 7 % of patients experienced any late Grade 3 toxicity, and no patient developed late Grade 3 fibrosis [23].

Of note, patients with unacceptable cosmesis were found to have a higher ratio of PTV volume to ipsilateral whole breast volume (WBV) than those with better cosmesis (18 % versus 13 %, $p=0.051$). Additionally, the authors found several dosimetric correlates of unacceptable cosmesis. Specifically, when compared to women with better outcomes, patients with fair/poor cosmesis had significantly higher portions of their WBV that received 20 %, 50 %, 80 %, and 100 % of the prescription dose [23, 24]. Since higher doses to normal tissue appeared to lead to worse cosmesis, the authors provisionally recommended limiting the portion of the WBV receiving 50 % of the prescription to less than 40 % of the volume [24]. Figure 18.1 demonstrates that the amount of dose delivered to normal breast tissue with external-beam techniques can vary substantially depending on approach and individual patient characteristics.

That increased dose to the breast may lead to worse outcomes is also supported by a recent Phase II dose escalation study [27]. This French study included women with pT1N0 disease. Patients underwent CT simulation in the supine position, and the PTV was defined as a 2.3–2.8 cm expansion of the lumpectomy cavity. There were two dosing schemas employed: 40 or 42 Gy in 10 fractions, twice daily, over 5 consecutive days delivered via mixed photon and electron plans. With both dose levels, only 50 % of the ipsilateral WBV was allowed to receive 50 % of the prescription. Toxicity was graded according to RTOG criteria. After enrolling a total of 48 patients, the trial was closed due to persistent Grade 3 fibrosis, telangiectasia, and breast pain in a patient at the 42 Gy dose level at 6 months after treatment. Overall, women in the 42 Gy group experienced higher rates of acute toxicity as well as worse and more frequent late toxicity than patients in the 40 Gy group. Detailed cosmetic outcomes were not reported [27].

The largest and most thorough analysis of cosmetic results with external-beam APBI to date is from the Randomized Trial of Accelerated Breast Irradiation (RAPID) [28]. This multicenter Canadian trial enrolled patients age 40 or older,

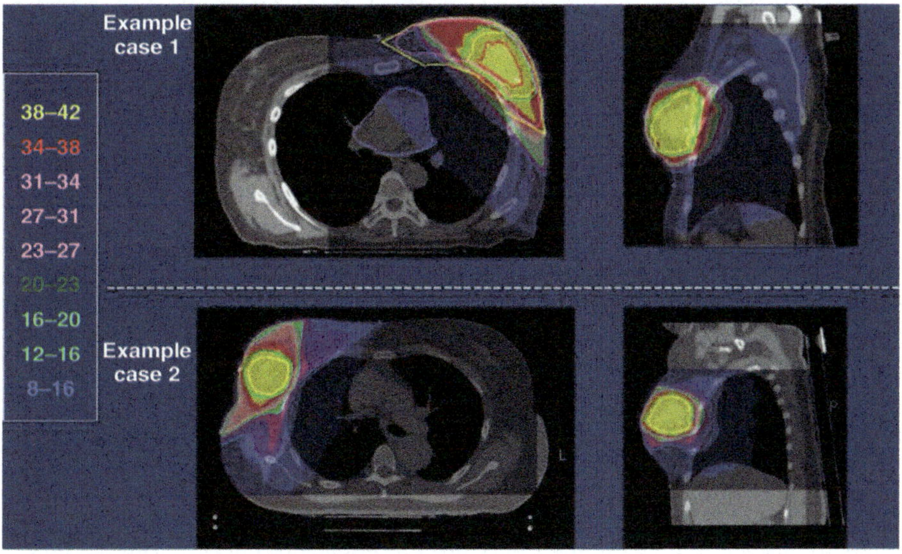

Fig. 18.1 Two different cases of external-beam APBI. These cases demonstrate how the proportion and volume of normal breast tissue receiving high radiation doses can vary from patient to patient (figure courtesy of Jagsi et al. 2010) [24]

with tumor 3 cm or less in size, negative surgical margins, and no axillary involvement. Women were randomized to whole breast irradiation – consisting of 42.5 Gy in 16 fractions or 50 Gy in 25 fractions with or without a boost to the lumpectomy cavity – versus external-beam APBI with 3–5 non-coplanar photon beams to a dose of 38.5 Gy delivered in 10, twice-daily fractions. For those in the APBI arm, the CTV was defined as a 1 cm expansion of the lumpectomy margin, with an additional 1 cm margin for PTV.

One of the strengths of this trial is its thorough assessment of cosmesis, which was evaluated by physicians, nurses, and patients themselves [28]. Two panels of physicians were blinded to treatment and examined digital photographs to rate cosmesis at 3 years posttreatment. Nurses utilized an EORTC tool specifically designed to evaluate breast cancer cosmesis [17], and patients used a validated questionnaire to report cosmetic outcomes [29, 30]. Finally, toxicity was recorded using CTCAE criteria.

The trial closed after enrolling 2135 subjects. After a median of 36 months follow-up, cosmetic outcomes were reported. Cosmesis was significantly worse in the APBI arm as compared to the whole breast radiotherapy arm. This effect persisted no matter which group judged cosmetic outcomes. Twenty-nine percent of APBI patients reported adverse cosmesis, compared to 18 % in the control arm ($p=0.0022$). Likewise, trained nurses found worse cosmesis in the APBI arm (29 % versus 17 %, $p<0.001$), as did physicians (35 % versus 17 %, $p=0.001$) [28].

Of note, these concerning rates of poor cosmesis did not correlate with CTCAE toxicity: Grade 3 or above toxicity was seen in only 1.4 % of the APBI arm. That cosmesis does not track well with CTCAE has been documented in other studies [12, 23, 24]. This raises the issue of whether the CTCAE tool is effective in capturing meaningful cosmetic information. Further, it emphasizes the need to develop more sophisticated measures of acute toxicity tailored to breast cancer treatment [31], in addition to tools specifically for evaluation of cosmesis.

Of additional concern, cosmetic results from RAPID continued to decline over the entire follow-up period [28]. For example, nurses rated 37 % of the APBI arm as having adverse cosmesis at 5 years, increased from 33 % at 3 years. Such a worsening of cosmesis over the course of time was also demonstrated by RTOG 0319 as well as the University of Michigan [12, 23].

Several authors have discussed the likely explanations for these poor cosmetic results [23, 28, 32]. To begin with, APBI delivered via external beam as opposed to brachytherapy may result in a higher integral dose to the breast [33]. In RAPID, the volume allowed to receive 95 % of the prescription dose was limited to less than 35 % of the total breast [28]. However, this still might be too great and speaks to the need for the development of better dosimetric constraints, as suggested by several investigations that have found a dose-volume relationship with cosmesis [23, 25, 26]. Additionally, evidence from clinical findings as well as biological modeling suggests that large fraction sizes may disproportionately impact cosmesis unless accompanied by a decrease in total dose [34, 35]. This might be especially relevant in cases of twice-daily treatments, when the normal breast parenchyma may not have sufficient time for repair [36].

In contrast to results from RAPID, investigators from the University of Florence recently reported encouraging cosmetic results from a randomized trial comparing external-beam APBI to whole breast irradiation [37, 38]. Women were eligible for enrollment if they were at least 40 years old with a tumor size of 2.5 cm or less. Of note, axillary nodal involvement was not among the exclusion criteria. Those randomized to receive whole breast irradiation received 50 Gy in 25 fractions, using tangential fields. This was followed by a boost of 10 Gy. Women in the APBI arm received 30 Gy in 5 fractions, delivered in a non-consecutive fashion over the course of 2 weeks. No twice-daily fractions were allowed. The CTV was a 1 cm expansion of the tumor bed, and the PTV was a 1 cm expansion beyond this. APBI was delivered using IMRT with 4 or 5 non-coplanar photon beams and a mean of 30 segments per plan.

In total 520 patients enrolled in the trial. After a median follow-up of 5 years, the rate of ipsilateral breast recurrence was 1.5 % in both arms [38]. Cosmetic outcomes were assessed in a non-blinded fashion by physicians using a 4-point scale [39]. Cosmesis was excellent in 95 % of those in the APBI arm compared to 90 % of those in the whole breast arm ($p=0.045$). Additionally, there were fewer instances of toxicity in those treated with APBI. Eighty percent of the APBI arm experienced no acute skin toxicity versus 34 % in the control arm ($p=0.0001$). As for late skin toxicity, 96 % of the APBI arm experienced no events, compared to 89 % of the whole breast group ($p=0.004$) [38].

There are several reasons why these cosmetic results may significantly differ from those reported by RAPID. First, RAPID included many more patients, and its cosmetic evaluation was both blinded and more thorough, as it was performed by physicians, nurses, and patients themselves. Nonetheless, this is unlikely to account for most of the differences in cosmesis. Rather, the treatment schedule employed by the Florence investigators, in which only a single fraction was given per day and without treatment on consecutive days, may have allowed for greater normal tissue recovery than possible with a twice-daily fractionation regimen. This explanation is consistent with the very low rates of toxicity experienced in the APBI arm. Furthermore, in contrast to the RAPID study, the investigators from Florence used an IMRT-based approach, which may have allowed greater dose homogeneity throughout the breast, as hot spots within the PTV were restricted to 105 % or less of the prescribed dose, and the volume of breast allowed to reach 15 Gy was less than 50 %. Of note, prior investigations that have reported poor outcomes with an IMRT-based approach have always been in the context of twice-daily treatments [23, 24]. Though the Florence results are promising, longer follow-up is needed to allow further maturation of the data, especially given how cosmetic outcomes following APBI have been shown to worsen with time [12, 23, 28].

It is hoped that ongoing concerns regarding cosmesis are addressed by RTOG 0413/NSABP B-39. This randomized Phase III trial of APBI versus whole breast radiation recently completed enrollment in 2013, after accruing 4311 patients. Three different treatment modalities were allowed for APBI (interstitial, intracavitary, and external beam), though most patients in the APBI arm were treated with the external-beam approach. Detailed cosmetic outcomes have not yet been reported.

Subjects on this trial have experienced low rates of CTCAE toxicity [40], but the findings of the studies reported above suggest that this may not necessarily correlate with cosmesis [23, 24, 28]. This study will also address issues of APBI's efficacy as well as the proper selection of patients, as it has enrolled many subjects who are younger than 50 years old, in addition to those with nodal disease, DCIS, or hormone receptor-negative tumors.

An additional trial that has recently closed but not yet reported efficacy or cosmetic outcomes is the IMPORT-LOW study, which was organized by the UK Medical Research Council. In this trial, women were randomized to partial breast irradiation of 40 Gy in 15 fractions delivered via IMRT or to whole breast radiotherapy consisting of 36 Gy to the entire breast along with a simultaneous integrated boost to the lumpectomy cavity to a total of 40 Gy, all given in 15 fractions. The trial has enrolled 2100 patients, and results have not yet been published.

18.3 Proton Therapy for Accelerated Partial Breast Irradiation

Although the aforementioned studies have used photons, electrons, or some combination thereof to deliver APBI, investigators have begun to examine treatment delivery with proton therapy. While proton therapy may potentially offer a dosimetric advantage in terms of both sparing normal tissue and also in reducing dose inhomogeneities [15, 41–44], there may be substantial skin dose, and clinical investigations have been heterogeneous and few, with mixed results [14, 45, 46].

Investigators from Loma Linda have reported their Phase II experience [42, 45]. This study enrolled women with invasive disease, 3 cm or less in size, without involved nodal disease, positive surgical margins, or an extensive intraductal component. Patients were simulated in the prone position, and the CTV was defined as 1 cm expansion of the lumpectomy cavity – edited back from skin and muscle – and the PTV was a 2 mm expansion beyond this. The prescription was 40 Gy in 10 daily fractions delivered over 2 weeks. Proton therapy plans generally involved 2–4 beams, all of which were treated daily. Normal tissue constraints were not reported. Cosmesis was graded by the patient and treating physician on a 4-point scale.

In total, 100 patients enrolled. After a median follow-up of 60 months, local control was 97 % within the ipsilateral breast. At last follow-up, over 90 % of patients and physicians rated cosmesis as good or excellent, and there was no worsening of cosmetic outcomes observed over time. Toxicity was low, as there were no grade 3 acute reactions, and late toxicity consisted primarily of mild telangiectasias [45].

Another Phase II study was reported by researchers from Korea [46]. Inclusion criteria specified that women must be at least 40 years old, with tumors 3 cm or less in size, without nodal disease or involved surgical margins. It did, however, allow patients with an extensive intraductal component. Patients were simulated in the supine position, and the PTV was created from the lumpectomy cavity using one of several different expansions, which varied by the width of the surgical margin: a 2 cm expansion was used for margins less than 1 cm, a 1.5 cm expansion for margins of 1–2 cm, and a 1 cm expansion for margins greater than 2 cm. The PTV was then edited such that it did not come within 3 mm of the skin surface nor was it allowed to enter into the chest wall. The prescription was 30 Gy, to be given in once-daily fractions over 5 consecutive days. Cosmetic results were evaluated by physicians on a 4-point scale, as well as by utilizing a system that measures vertical and lateral displacement of the nipple in comparison to that of the untreated breast [47].

The study enrolled a total of 30 patients, with almost 5 years of median follow-up. The first 15 patients accrued were treated via a single proton beam, whereas the final 15 patients were treated with 2 proton beams. There were no recurrences during the period of follow-up. Cosmesis was rated as excellent or good in approximately 80 % of patients at 2 months posttreatment, though this decreased to 69 % at 3 years. Nonetheless, the majority of those with fair or poor cosmesis were from the group treated with a single beam. Similarly, the single beam group experienced a significant amount of objective nipple displacement, though this effect was not exhibited by those treated with 2 beams [46].

Researchers from Harvard have also published their experience with proton therapy [14, 15, 41, 48]. The most recent report from this group describes the result of a Phase I study comparing proton therapy APBI versus APBI delivered with photons alone or a combination of photons and electrons [14]. Patients were required to have T1N0 tumors without involved surgical margins, lymphovascular invasion, or an extensive intraductal component. Patients underwent CT simulation in the supine position, and the PTV was created as a 1.5–2 cm expansion of the lumpectomy cavity. This was then edited back from the skin surface, pectoralis, and chest wall. The prescription dose was to 32 Gy, given in 8, twice-daily fractions over 4 consecutive days. For patients receiving proton therapy, 1–3 field plans were employed, though only a single field was treated for any given fraction. Patients who did not receive proton therapy were treated with 3DCRT APBI, typically with two tangential mini-tangent photon beams and an *en face* photon or electron beam. No formal dose constraints were utilized. Cosmesis was assessed on a 4-point scale by both patients and physicians.

The study enrolled a total of 19 patients who were treated with proton therapy and 79 who were treated with 3DCRT. After a median follow-up of 7 years, there were 3 local failures in the proton arm and 2 in the conventional arm ($p=0.2$). While there were no significant differences between the two groups in patient-reported cosmesis, this contrasted with physician-rated cosmesis, which was excellent or good in 62 % of those treated with protons as compared to 94 % of those treated with photons ($p=0.03$). Furthermore, late toxicities – most commonly consisting of telangiectasias and altered pigmentation – were significantly more frequent in the proton therapy group [14].

Given both the broad range of techniques used in these studies as well as the mixed cosmetic results, proton therapy APBI, like all other forms of APBI, is best still considered investigational. Physicians are strongly encouraged to utilize this approach only within the context of an appropriately designed clinical trial.

18.4 Planning Considerations

Given that external-beam APBI is still being actively investigated, physicians should enroll patients on clinical trials if at all possible. However, should a suitable patient desire treatment off protocol, we recommend that treatment adhere closely to the guidelines put forth in NSABP B-39 [19], which will be reviewed here, and consideration be given to even stricter dosimetric constraints where possible.

To begin, the patient should undergo standard CT simulation in the supine position, and the volume of the lumpectomy cavity should not exceed 30 % of the whole breast reference volume, for if it does, the patient is unsuitable for APBI. Of note, the ipsilateral whole breast reference volume is determined by measuring the volume encompassed by a standard tangential field arrangement, excluding any lung. See Fig. 18.2 for an example of the whole breast reference volume.

The CTV is then defined as a uniform 1.5 cm expansion of the lumpectomy cavity. It should encompass any surgical clips. However, this volume is limited such that it does not encroach within 0.5 cm of the skin surface, nor does it include any aspect of the pectoralis muscle or chest wall. See Fig. 18.3 for an example of CTV definition.

The PTV is defined as a 1.0 cm expansion of the CTV. This structure is used for generation of the beam apertures. However, for the purposes of dose-volume histogram (DVH) calculations and evaluation, an additional structure is created: PTV_EVAL. This structure is identical to the PTV except that it is not permitted to come within 0.5 cm of the skin surface, nor is it allowed to contain any pectoralis, chest wall, or lung. See Fig. 18.4a, b for examples of PTV and PTV_EVAL construction, respectively.

Planning should use three-dimensional conformal techniques to incorporate 3–5 non-coplanar beams, none of which should directly enter a critical organ at risk such as the heart, lung, or contralateral breast. The isocenter is usually placed in the center of the PTV. The prescription dose most typically administered in the USA is 38.5 Gy, delivered in 10, twice-daily fractions, with a minimum of 6 h between

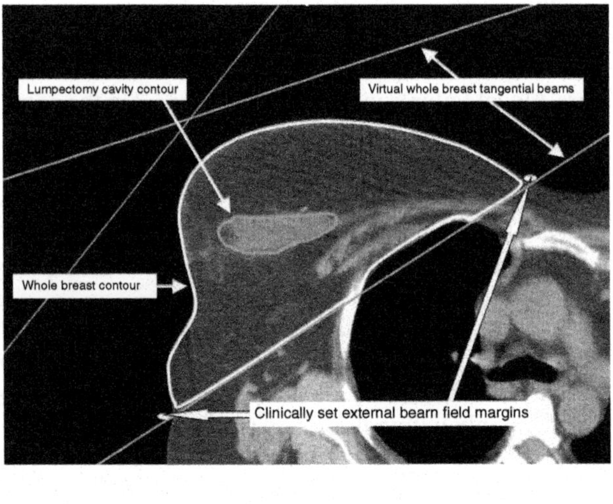

Fig. 18.2 Construction of a whole breast volume based upon the area defined by virtual tangential beams minus lung parenchyma (figure courtesy of RTOG 0413/ NSABP B-39) [19]

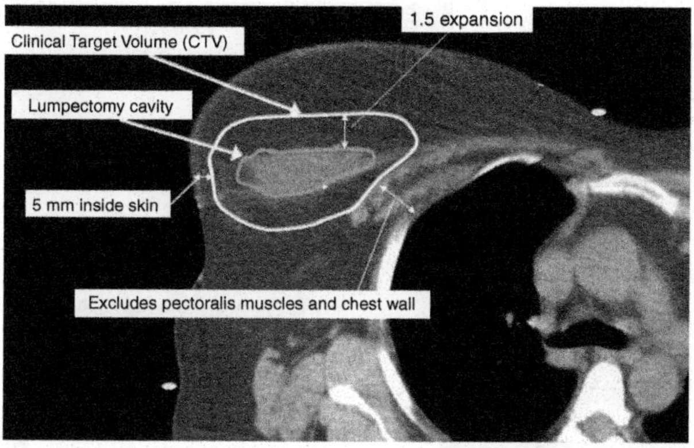

Fig. 18.3 The CTV is created by a 1.5 cm expansion of the lumpectomy cavity. It excludes any pectoralis muscle or chest wall. It is also limited to within 0.5 cm of the skin surface (figure courtesy of RTOG 0413/NSABP B-39) [19]

treatments. Treatment is usually completed over the course of 5 consecutive days. However, promising results from Florence as well as cautionary findings from RAPID and certain institutions should prompt further investigation of the optimal dose and fractionation schedule in this setting [23–26, 28, 38].

There are several normal tissue constraints of which the clinician should be aware. For the ipsilateral breast, NSABP B-39 guidelines suggest that less than 60 % of the whole breast reference volume should receive 50 % or more of the prescription dose (V50) [19]. However, given the cosmetic results and dosimetric correlates found by investigators at the University of Michigan, we would recommend that every effort be made to keep the V50 below 40 % [23, 24]. V100 should be kept less than 35 % and lower wherever possible.

The contralateral breast – contoured using the same technique as that used for the ipsilateral breast reference volume – should have a maximum point dose of less than 3 % of the prescription dose. V30 of the ipsilateral lung should be kept less than 15 %, while V5 of the contralateral lung should be less than 15 %. For right-sided tumors, V5 should be less than 5 % of the heart, though for left-sided lesions this constraint is relaxed to a V5 of less than 40 % of the heart. Finally, the thyroid should be allowed a maximum point dose of 3 % of the prescription.

Though these normal tissue constraints are an excellent starting point, it may be possible to accomplish an even lower dose to the ipsilateral whole breast reference volume than that required by NSABP B-39, and such a lower integral dose may improve cosmesis [23, 24, 26]. For instance, in the University of Michigan series, increasing V20, V50, V80, and V100 were significantly correlated with worse cosmetic outcomes, even when the NSABP B-39 dose constraints were met [23]. This emphasizes the importance of minimizing dose to the ipsilateral breast as much as possible.

It remains to be seen whether prospective studies will reveal better dosimetric constraints that will minimize the risk of poor cosmesis while still allowing adequate target coverage. In order to further this knowledge as well as provide the best

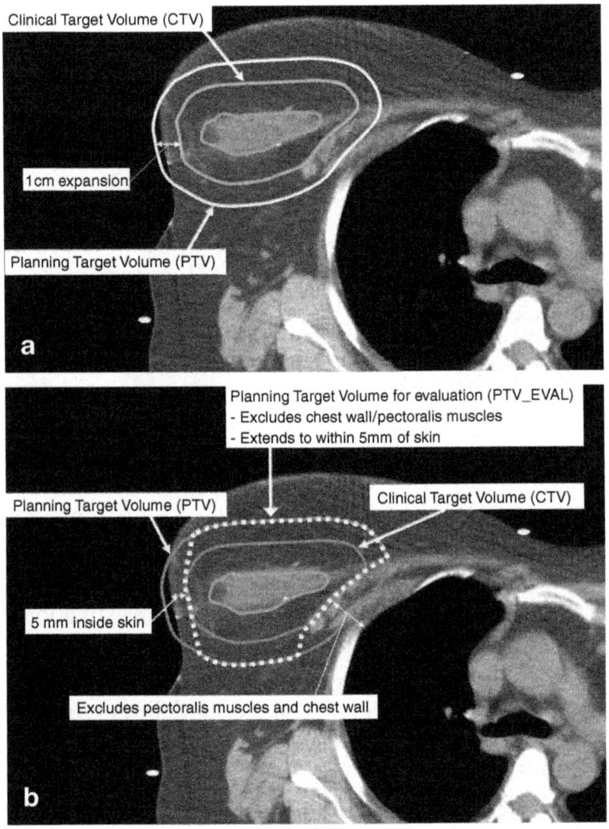

Fig. 18.4 (**a**) The PTV is defined as a 1.0 cm expansion of the CTV. This structure is used for generation of the beam apertures (figure courtesy of RTOG 0413/NSABP B-39) [19]. (**b**) For the purposes of DVH calculations and evaluation, an additional structure is created: PTV_EVAL. This structure is identical to the PTV except that it is not permitted to come within 0.5 cm of the skin surface, nor is it allowed to contain any pectoralis, chest wall, or lung (figure courtesy of RTOG 0413/NSABP B-39) [19]

care possible, it is recommended that physicians utilize external-beam APBI within the context of an established clinical trial whenever possible. If such a trial is not available, clinicians should utilize strict patient selection, thoroughly discuss the investigational nature of external-beam APBI, and employ the treatment principles discussed herein.

18.5 Conclusions

External-beam approaches to partial breast irradiation have many advantages, and most patients treated on the recent large US randomized trial (RTOG 0413/NSABP B-39) were treated with such techniques. Considerable research has been conducted to evaluate the impact of external-beam APBI on disease control, toxicity, and cosmetic outcomes. As such studies mature, caution is warranted, and patients are best treated in the setting of clinical protocols that allow us to further optimize dose, fractionation, and technique. Undoubtedly, external-beam approaches to APBI hold much promise; it is our responsibility to ensure that we continue to develop our understanding by offering this option to appropriately selected patients in ways that allow us to refine its application and maximize its safety and tolerability.

References

1. Ribeiro GG, Dunn G, Swindell R, Harris M, Banerjee SS. Conservation of the breast using two different radiotherapy techniques: interim report of a clinical trial. Clin Oncol (R Coll Radiol). 1990;2(1):27–34. Available at: http://www.ncbi.nlm.nih.gov/pubmed/2261385. Accessed 18 Nov 2014.
2. Ribeiro GG, Magee B, Swindell R, Harris M, Banerjee SS. The Christie Hospital breast conservation trial: an update at 8 years from inception. Clin Oncol (R Coll Radiol). 1993;5(5):278–83. Available at: http://www.ncbi.nlm.nih.gov/pubmed/8305334. Accessed 3 Nov 2014.
3. Dodwell DJ, Dyker K, Brown J, et al. A randomised study of whole-breast vs tumour-bed irradiation after local excision and axillary dissection for early breast cancer. Clin Oncol (R Coll Radiol). 2005;17(8):618–22. Available at: http://www.ncbi.nlm.nih.gov/pubmed/16372487. Accessed 3 Nov 2014.
4. Formenti SC, Hsu H, Fenton-Kerimian M, et al. Prone accelerated partial breast irradiation after breast-conserving surgery: five-year results of 100 patients. Int J Radiat Oncol Biol Phys. 2012;84(3):606–11. doi:10.1016/j.ijrobp.2012.01.039.
5. Wernicke AG, Gidea-Addeo D, Magnolfi C, Fenton-Kerimian M, Goldberg J, Formenti SC. External beam partial breast irradiation following breast-conserving surgery: preliminary results of cosmetic outcome of NYU 00–23. Int J Radiat Oncol. 2006;66(3):S32. doi:10.1016/j.ijrobp.2006.07.083.
6. Harris JR, Levene MB, Svensson G, Hellman S. Analysis of cosmetic results following primary radiation therapy for stages I and II carcinoma of the breast. Int J Radiat Oncol Biol Phys. 1979;5(2):257–61. Available at: http://www.ncbi.nlm.nih.gov/pubmed/110740. Accessed 19 Feb 2015.
7. Baglan KL, Sharpe MB, Jaffray D, et al. Accelerated partial breast irradiation using 3D conformal radiation therapy (3D-CRT). Int J Radiat Oncol Biol Phys. 2003;55(2):302–11. Available at: http://www.ncbi.nlm.nih.gov/pubmed/12527042. Accessed 17 Feb 2015.
8. Vicini FA, Remouchamps V, Wallace M, et al. Ongoing clinical experience utilizing 3D conformal external beam radiotherapy to deliver partial-breast irradiation in patients with early-stage breast cancer treated with breast-conserving therapy. Int J Radiat Oncol Biol Phys. 2003;57(5):1247–53. Available at: http://www.ncbi.nlm.nih.gov/pubmed/14630258. Accessed 17 Nov 2014.
9. Vicini F, Arthur D, Polgar C, Kuske R. Defining the efficacy of accelerated partial breast irradiation: the importance of proper patient selection, optimal quality assurance, and common sense. Int J Radiat Oncol Biol Phys. 2003;57(5):1210–3. Available at: http://www.ncbi.nlm.nih.gov/pubmed/14630252. Accessed 17 Feb 2015.
10. Shah C, Wilkinson JB, Lanni T, et al. Five-year outcomes and toxicities using 3-dimensional conformal external beam radiation therapy to deliver accelerated partial breast irradiation. Clin Breast Cancer. 2013;13(3):206–11. doi:10.1016/j.clbc.2012.09.020.
11. Vicini F, Winter K, Wong J, et al. Initial efficacy results of RTOG 0319: three-dimensional conformal radiation therapy (3D-CRT) confined to the region of the lumpectomy cavity for

stage I/II breast carcinoma. Int J Radiat Oncol Biol Phys. 2010;77(4):1120–7. doi:10.1016/j.ijrobp.2009.06.067.
12. Chafe S, Moughan J, McCormick B, et al. Late toxicity and patient self-assessment of breast appearance/satisfaction on RTOG 0319: a phase 2 trial of 3-dimensional conformal radiation therapy-accelerated partial breast irradiation following lumpectomy for stages I and II breast cancer. Int J Radiat Oncol Biol Phys. 2013;86(5):854–9. doi:10.1016/j.ijrobp.2013.04.005.
13. Taghian AG, Kozak KR, Doppke KP, et al. Initial dosimetric experience using simple three-dimensional conformal external-beam accelerated partial-breast irradiation. Int J Radiat Oncol Biol Phys. 2006;64(4):1092–9. doi:10.1016/j.ijrobp.2005.09.042.
14. Galland-Girodet S, Pashtan I, MacDonald SM, et al. Long-term cosmetic outcomes and toxicities of proton beam therapy compared with photon-based 3-dimensional conformal accelerated partial-breast irradiation: a phase 1 trial. Int J Radiat Oncol Biol Phys. 2014;90(3):493–500. doi:10.1016/j.ijrobp.2014.04.008.
15. Recht A, Ancukiewicz M, Alm El-Din MA, et al. Lung dose-volume parameters and the risk of pneumonitis for patients treated with accelerated partial-breast irradiation using three-dimensional conformal radiotherapy. J Clin Oncol. 2009;27(24):3887–93. doi:10.1200/JCO.2008.20.0121.
16. Berrang TS, Olivotto I, Kim D-H, et al. Three-year outcomes of a Canadian multicenter study of accelerated partial breast irradiation using conformal radiation therapy. Int J Radiat Oncol Biol Phys. 2011;81(5):1220–7. doi:10.1016/j.ijrobp.2010.07.2003.
17. Aaronson NK, Bartelink H, van Dongen JA, van Dam FS. Evaluation of breast conserving therapy: clinical, methodological and psychosocial perspectives. Eur J Surg Oncol. 1988;14(2):133–40. Available at: http://www.ncbi.nlm.nih.gov/pubmed/3360154. Accessed 17 Nov 2014.
18. Rodríguez N, Sanz X, Dengra J, et al. Five-year outcomes, cosmesis, and toxicity with 3-dimensional conformal external beam radiation therapy to deliver accelerated partial breast irradiation. Int J Radiat Oncol Biol Phys. 2013;87(5):1051–7. doi:10.1016/j.ijrobp.2013.08.046.
19. Radiation Therapy Oncology Group. NSABP Protocol B-39/RTOG Protocol 0413: A randomized phase III study of conventional whole breast irradiation (WBI) versus partial breast irradiation (PBI) for women with stage 0, I, or II breast cancer. Available at: http://www.rtog.org/ClinicalTrials/ProtocolTable/StudyDetails.aspx?study=0413.
20. Lei RY, Leonard CE, Howell KT, et al. Four-year clinical update from a prospective trial of accelerated partial breast intensity-modulated radiotherapy (APBIMRT). Breast Cancer Res Treat. 2013;140(1):119–33. doi:10.1007/s10549-013-2623-x.
21. Leonard C, Carter D, Kercher J, et al. Prospective trial of accelerated partial breast intensity-modulated radiotherapy. Int J Radiat Oncol Biol Phys. 2007;67(5):1291–8. doi:10.1016/j.ijrobp.2006.11.016.
22. Rusthoven KE, Carter DL, Howell K, et al. Accelerated partial-breast intensity-modulated radiotherapy results in improved dose distribution when compared with three-dimensional treatment-planning techniques. Int J Radiat Oncol Biol Phys. 2008;70(1):296–302. doi:10.1016/j.ijrobp.2007.08.047.
23. Liss AL, Ben-David MA, Jagsi R, et al. Decline of cosmetic outcomes following accelerated partial breast irradiation using intensity modulated radiation therapy: results of a single-institution prospective clinical trial. Int J Radiat Oncol Biol Phys. 2014;89(1):96–102. doi:10.1016/j.ijrobp.2014.01.005.
24. Jagsi R, Ben-David MA, Moran JM, et al. Unacceptable cosmesis in a protocol investigating intensity-modulated radiotherapy with active breathing control for accelerated partial-breast irradiation. Int J Radiat Oncol Biol Phys. 2010;76(1):71–8. doi:10.1016/j.ijrobp.2009.01.041.
25. Hepel JT, Tokita M, MacAusland SG, et al. Toxicity of three-dimensional conformal radiotherapy for accelerated partial breast irradiation. Int J Radiat Oncol Biol Phys. 2009;75(5):1290–6. doi:10.1016/j.ijrobp.2009.01.009.
26. Leonard KL, Hepel JT, Hiatt JR, Dipetrillo TA, Price LL, Wazer DE. The effect of dose-volume parameters and interfraction interval on cosmetic outcome and toxicity after

3-dimensional conformal accelerated partial breast irradiation. Int J Radiat Oncol Biol Phys. 2013;85(3):623–9. doi:10.1016/j.ijrobp.2012.06.052.
27. Bourgier C, Acevedo-Henao C, Dunant A, et al. Higher toxicity with 42 Gy in 10 fractions as a total dose for 3D-conformal accelerated partial breast irradiation: results from a dose escalation phase II trial. Radiat Oncol. 2012;7:141. doi:10.1186/1748-717X-7-141.
28. Olivotto IA, Whelan TJ, Parpia S, et al. Interim cosmetic and toxicity results from RAPID: a randomized trial of accelerated partial breast irradiation using three-dimensional conformal external beam radiation therapy. J Clin Oncol. 2013;31(32):4038–45. doi:10.1200/JCO.2013.50.5511.
29. Whelan TJ, Levine M, Julian J, Kirkbride P, Skingley P. The effects of radiation therapy on quality of life of women with breast carcinoma: results of a randomized trial. Ontario Clinical Oncology Group. Cancer. 2000;88(10):2260–6. Available at: http://www.ncbi.nlm.nih.gov/pubmed/10820347. Accessed 17 Nov 2014.
30. Levine MN, Guyatt GH, Gent M, et al. Quality of life in stage II breast cancer: an instrument for clinical trials. J Clin Oncol. 1988;6(12):1798–810. Available at: http://www.ncbi.nlm.nih.gov/pubmed/3058874. Accessed 17 Nov 2014.
31. Shumway D, Kapadia N, Do T, et al. Development of a photonumeric scale for acute radiation dermatitis in breast cancer patients. Int J Radiat Oncol Biol Phys. 2014;90(1):238. doi:10.1016/j.ijrobp.2014.06.008.
32. Jagsi R, Haffty BG. External-beam accelerated partial-breast irradiation: exploring the limits of tolerability. J Clin Oncol. 2013;31(32):4029–31. doi:10.1200/JCO.2013.51.1717.
33. Weed DW, Edmundson GK, Vicini FA, Chen PY, Martinez AA. Accelerated partial breast irradiation: a dosimetric comparison of three different techniques. Brachytherapy. 2005;4(2):121–9. doi:10.1016/j.brachy.2004.12.005.
34. Yarnold J, Ashton A, Bliss J, et al. Fractionation sensitivity and dose response of late adverse effects in the breast after radiotherapy for early breast cancer: long-term results of a randomised trial. Radiother Oncol. 2005;75(1):9–17. doi:10.1016/j.radonc.2005.01.005.
35. Yarnold J, Bentzen SM, Coles C, Haviland J. Hypofractionated whole-breast radiotherapy for women with early breast cancer: myths and realities. Int J Radiat Oncol Biol Phys. 2011;79(1):1–9. doi:10.1016/j.ijrobp.2010.08.035.
36. Bentzen SM, Yarnold JR. Reports of unexpected late side effects of accelerated partial breast irradiation--radiobiological considerations. Int J Radiat Oncol Biol Phys. 2010;77(4):969–73. doi:10.1016/j.ijrobp.2010.01.059.
37. Livi L, Buonamici FB, Simontacchi G, et al. Accelerated partial breast irradiation with IMRT: new technical approach and interim analysis of acute toxicity in a phase III randomized clinical trial. Int J Radiat Oncol Biol Phys. 2010;77(2):509–15. doi:10.1016/j.ijrobp.2009.04.070.
38. Livi L, Meattini I, Marrazzo L, et al. Accelerated partial breast irradiation using intensity-modulated radiotherapy versus whole breast irradiation: 5-year survival analysis of a phase 3 randomised controlled trial. Eur J Cancer. 2015. doi:10.1016/j.ejca.2014.12.013.
39. Trombetta M, Julian TB, Kim Y, Werts ED, Parda D. The allegheny general modification of the Harvard Breast Cosmesis Scale for the retreated breast. Oncology (Williston Park). 2009;23(11):954–6. Available at: http://www.ncbi.nlm.nih.gov/pubmed/19947346. Accessed 17 Feb 2015.
40. Wolmark N, Curran WJ, Vicini F, et al. Response to "Unacceptable cosmesis in a protocol investigating intensity-modulated radiotherapy with active breathing control for accelerated partial-breast irradiation" (Int J Radiat Oncol Biol Phys 2010;76:71–78) and "Toxicity of three-dimensional conformal radiotherapy for accelerated partial breast irradiation" Int J Radiat Oncol Biol Phys 2009;75:1290-1296). Int J Radiat Oncol Biol Phys. 2010;77(1):317. doi:10.1016/j.ijrobp.2009.12.033; author reply 318.
41. Kozak KR, Katz A, Adams J, et al. Dosimetric comparison of proton and photon three-dimensional, conformal, external beam accelerated partial breast irradiation techniques. Int J Radiat Oncol Biol Phys. 2006;65(5):1572–8. doi:10.1016/j.ijrobp.2006.04.025.

42. Bush DA, Slater JD, Garberoglio C, Yuh G, Hocko JM, Slater JM. A technique of partial breast irradiation utilizing proton beam radiotherapy: comparison with conformal x-ray therapy. Cancer J. 2007;13(2):114–8. doi:10.1097/PPO.0b013e318046354b.
43. Moon SH, Shin KH, Kim TH, et al. Dosimetric comparison of four different external beam partial breast irradiation techniques: three-dimensional conformal radiotherapy, intensity-modulated radiotherapy, helical tomotherapy, and proton beam therapy. Radiother Oncol. 2009;90(1):66–73. doi:10.1016/j.radonc.2008.09.027.
44. Wang X, Amos RA, Zhang X, et al. External-beam accelerated partial breast irradiation using multiple proton beam configurations. Int J Radiat Oncol Biol Phys. 2011;80(5):1464–72. doi:10.1016/j.ijrobp.2010.04.052.
45. Bush DA, Do S, Lum S, et al. Partial breast radiation therapy with proton beam: 5-year results with cosmetic outcomes. Int J Radiat Oncol Biol Phys. 2014;90(3):501–5. doi:10.1016/j.ijrobp.2014.05.1308.
46. Chang JH, Lee NK, Kim JY, et al. Phase II trial of proton beam accelerated partial breast irradiation in breast cancer. Radiother Oncol. 2013;108(2):209–14. doi:10.1016/j.radonc.2013.06.008.
47. Pezner RD, Patterson MP, Hill LR, et al. Breast retraction assessment: an objective evaluation of cosmetic results of patients treated conservatively for breast cancer. Int J Radiat Oncol Biol Phys. 1985;11(3):575–8. Available at: http://www.ncbi.nlm.nih.gov/pubmed/3972667. Accessed 24 Feb 2015.
48. Taghian AG, Kozak KR, Katz A, et al. Accelerated partial breast irradiation using proton beams: Initial dosimetric experience. Int J Radiat Oncol Biol Phys. 2006;65(5):1404–10. doi:10.1016/j.ijrobp.2006.03.017.

Part IV
Intra-operative Radiotherapy

Chapter 19
Patient Selection for IORT

Eleanor Harris, William Small Jr., and Stephen R. Grobmyer

Contents

Intraoperative radiotherapy (IORT) for breast cancer has been shown in a number of studies to be safe and efficacious in selected women with early stage breast cancer undergoing breast-conserving surgery (lumpectomy) (see Tables 19.1 and 19.2). Breast IORT includes a variety of technical methods which primarily involve delivery of a single high dose of radiation to the periphery of the lumpectomy bed, usually given at the time of surgery, or in some studies as a second planned procedure shortly after the lumpectomy. It is a specific form of partial breast irradiation with associated selection criteria. Breast IORT, like breast brachytherapy, requires special equipment and training in order to deliver the radiation therapy. There are several devices in use for the delivery of breast IORT, each of which is associated with clinical trials using that technology. As with all other modalities for partial breast irradiation, thorough appreciation of the scientific rationale, supporting studies, and clinical considerations helps to guide appropriate selection criteria. In current use for breast IORT, there are two technologies using 50 kV (soft) X-rays, the INTRABEAM Intraoperative Radiotherapy (Carl Zeiss Meditec, Dublin, CA) and Axxent Electronic Brachytherapy System (Xoft, San Jose, CA). Alternately, there

E. Harris, MD (✉)
Department of Radiation Oncology, Brody School of Medicine, East Carolina University, 600 Moye Blvd, Greenville, NC 27855, USA
e-mail: harrisel@ecu.edu

W. Small Jr., MD
Department of Radiation OncologyStritch School of Medicine, Loyola University Chicago, 2160 S 1st Avenue, Maguire Center, RM 2932, Maywood, IL 60153, USA
e-mail: WMSMALL@lumc.edu

S.R. Grobmyer, MD, FACS
Department of Surgery, Cleveland Clinic, 9500 Euclid Ave./A81, Cleveland, OH 44195, USA
e-mail: grobmys@ccf.org

D.W. Arthur et al. (eds.), *Short Course Breast Radiotherapy: A Comprehensive Review of Hypofractionation, Partial Breast, and Intra-Operative Irradiation*,
DOI 10.1007/978-3-319-24388-7_19

Table 19.1 Selection criteria for IOERT in prospective studies using any electron beam technologies

Author/ year	Number patients	Technique	Dose	Median follow-up	Ages/ median (years)	ER+/PR+	Tumor size	Nodal status	Other criteria	In breast recurrence	Breast cancer survival	Overall survival
Veronesi [1] ELIOT, 2013	1305	Mobile linac	21 Gy	5.8 yr	48–75/NS	91 %/80 %	<2.5 cm	Any	None	5 yr: 4.4 % (EBRT = 0.4 %)	97.9 %	96.8 %
Hanna [2] 2014	152	Linear accelerator	21 Gy	50.7 mos	>40/58	92 %/92 %	≤3.0 cm	N0	IDC; unicentric by MRI	5 yr: 3.7 %	92.5 %	97.8 %
Cedolini [3] 2014	73	Mobile linac	21 Gy	72 mos	48–80/60	NS (Luminal A = 68.5 %)	<3.0 cm	N0-N1mic	IDC; margin > 5 mm	5 yr 2 %	NS	98.7 %
Lemanski [4] 2013	42	Linear accelerator	21 Gy	72 mos	≥65/72	ER+ required	T0-T1	N0	IDC; margins > 2 mm; No EIC or LVI	5 yr: 9.5 %	92.7 %	100 %
Osti [5] 2013	110	Linear accelerator	21 Gy	27 mos	>48/66	95.5 %/95.5 %	<2.5 cm	N0-N1	Postmenopausal; no EIC	3 yr: 2.7 %	92.9 %	97.3 %
Sawaki [6] 2012	32	Mobile linac	21 Gy	26 mos	>50/	NS	<2.5 cm	N0	Negative margins; no EIC	2 yr: 0	100 %	100 %
Dessena [7] 2011	30	Mobile linac	21 Gy	11.7 mos	≥35/51.7	NS	≤2.5 cm	cN0	Grade 1–2; ILC allowed	1 yr: 0	100 %	100 %
Veronesi [8] 2001	84	Mobile linac	17–21 Gy	8 mos	>32/58	85 %/72 %	≤2.5 cm	NS	No EIC	1 yr 0	99 %	NS

IDC invasive ductal carcinoma, *ER* estrogen receptor, *PR* progesterone receptor, *NS* not stated, *Yr* year, *mos* months, *Gy* gray, *EIC* extensive intraductal component, *LVI* lymphovascular space invasion, *ILC* invasive lobular cancer

Table 19.2 Selection criteria for IORT with 50 kV in prospective studies using electron technologies

Author/year	Number patients	Technique	Dose	Median follow-up	Ages/ median (years)	ER+/PR+	Tumor size	Nodal status	Other	In breast recurrence	Breast cancer survival	Overall survival
Vaidya, TARGIT-A [9] 2014	3451	INTRABEAM	20 Gy	29 mos	≥45/63	90 %/71 %	Not specified (84 %<2 cm)	N0-N1	No ILC	5 yr 3.3 %	98.9 %	96.1 %
Bitterman [10] 2014	468	INTRABEAM	20 Gy	3 year minimum	>60/70	NS	T1	cN0	IDC	3 yr: 0.8 % (crude)	NS	NS
Elliott [11] 2011	67	INTRABEAM	5 Gy (at 10 mm)	28 mos	>50/60	NS	≤ 3.5 cm	cN0	IDC	0	98.5 % (crude)	98.5 % (crude)
Deneve [12] 2012	42	INTRABEAM	20 Gy	3 mos	>60/71	98 %/93 %	≤ 3.1 cm	cN0	No ILC; postmenopausal	0	NS	NS

IDC invasive ductal carcinoma, *ER* estrogen receptor, *PR* progesterone receptor, *NS* not stated, *Yr* year, *mos* months, *Gy* gray, *EIC* extensive intraductal component, *LVI* lymphovascular space invasion, *ILC* invasive lobular cancer are mobile electron accelerators, including Mobetron (IntraOp Medical Corporation, Sunnyvale, CA), NOVAC, and LIAC (Sordina IORT Technologies SpA, Vincenza, Italy).

Relative biological effectiveness (RBE = $D_{x/}D$) is a comparison of the severity of radiation-induced damage for a given dose (D) relative to a reference radiation (D_x) for a given biological endpoint, such as cell survival, chromosome aberration, or DNA damage. Cobalt-60 or 6 megavoltage (MV) are often used as the reference radiation in experimental systems. It has been well established for several decades that the relative RBE of photons increases with decreasing energy [13]. Evidence shows that this occurs because the energy of the secondary electrons emitted decreases with a commensurate increase in linear energy transfer (LET) [14]. Several experimental systems using cell survival techniques have demonstrated increased biological effects from low-energy X-rays. Brenner et al. calculated the RBE of low-energy photons at clinically relevant doses. They showed an RBE for 40 kilovoltage (kV) photons to range from 1.53 at the source to 1.4 at a depth of 20 mm (compared to cobalt-60). These authors noted that RBE increases with decreasing dose, so actual RBE increases with depth. This results in a slower falloff with dose of the biologically weighted dose at any given depth. A recent literature review reported RBE for 10 % cell survival from different experimental systems and cell types for low-energy X-rays (range 10–240 kV) ranging between 1.1 and 1.7 [15]. The RBE of low-energy electronic brachytherapy sources was estimated by Reniers et al. to be enhanced by 40–50 % over Co^{60} or Ir^{192} and similar to the low-energy gamma rays emitted by I^{125} [16].

Specific experiments have been conducted using 50 kV X-ray devices. Spadinger et al. compared the RBE of selected low LET radiation modalities relative to cobalt-60, including 50 kVp X-rays, assaying survival in two normal cell lines at dose ranges up to 10 Gy [17]. For 55 kVp, RBE varied from 1.2 to 1.3 at low and higher doses. Astor et al., compared cell survival data from the Photon Radiosurgery System (PRS) calibrated at 50 kV to 6 MV photons [18]. For 50 kV and 0.05 % cell survival, the authors measured an RBE of 1.9 for Chinese hamster (normal) cells and RBE of 1.4 for human glioblastoma cells. The RBE for the 50 kV X-rays also increased with depth: at 1 mm RBE = 1.2 and at 4 mm = 1.9. Liu et al. radiated cells in a water-equivalent phantom device with the INTRABEAM 4 cm spherical applicator, a 50 kV surface therapy machine and 6 MV photons as reference radiation, using a clonogenic inactivation assay for normal human and tumor cell lines [19]. This study showed an RBE for 50 kV X-rays at 8 mm depth ranged from 1.26 to 1.42 for the various cell lines. Each of the studies described used a different X-ray source, and use of filters, shielding, or applicators varied.

Herskind et al. used the linear-quadratic formula to model the RBE of 50 kV X-rays converted to an equivalent fractionated dose of 2 Gy (EQD2) as a function of depth [20]. The probability of local control was also estimated from the dose-response relationship fitted to clinical data. The authors postulated that a "sphere of equivalence" resulted from an increased local control probability in the high-dose region closer to the applicator surface that partly compensated for lower local control probability at greater distances from the applicator. The local control rates that were estimated were thus approximately equivalent to that of conventionally fractionated external beam irradiation, but with a different spatial distribution.

The higher RBE for low-energy X-rays may result in higher tumor control rates in the relevant range of tissue, which corresponds to the clinically relevant tissue in selected patients. Clinical data, including the randomized trials discussed in this section, are consistent with this concept. Any form of partial breast irradiation by definition leaves some proportion of the breast tissue unirradiated; therefore, thorough understanding of the strengths and limitations of different techniques is important for clinicians to consider when selecting patient for whom partial breast irradiation with IORT or any modality is recommended.

The INTRABEAM® system (Zeiss) delivers a low-energy photon beam from a compact mobile X-ray unit with electronic control that has been in clinical use since 1999 [21]. The miniaturized accelerator produces an electron beam in the main housing unit that is accelerated to the tip of a drift tube. An isotropic point source of low-energy 50 kVp maximum voltage X-rays is generated. This system was originally designed for single fraction IORT and is calibrated to be used at a single isotropic dose rate and output factor. IORT is delivered using either reusable solid-state spherical applicators of sizes ranging from 1.5 to 5 cm diameter, and treatment time runs 20–35 min depending upon the applicator used. The applicator is placed into the lumpectomy cavity and the tissue is approximated to the surface of the applicator circumferentially for treatment using a purse-string suture and is then removed after treatment delivery, when the incision is closed as usual.

The Axxent® System (Xoft Inc., Sunnyvale, CA) is an electronic brachytherapy platform that became clinically available in 2009 [22]. The radiation source is a miniature, electronic, high-dose-rate low-energy X-ray tube integrated into a flexible multi-lumen catheter. It produces X-rays of a 40–50 kVp energy range at the catheter tip and a mean energy of 26.7 kV. The system includes a mobile controller for power and is equipped with a user interface. The Axxent system was originally designed as alternative to Ir-192 balloon brachytherapy, intended for fractionated balloon-based APBI, and to have variable currents and voltages in order to change the dose rate and depth properties. Treatment planning consists of a dwell time calculation for a specified dose and depth with system calibration for each treatment. The source itself is disposable, used for only 10 fractions and for breast IORT; disposable balloons in varying spherical and ellipsoidal sizes (3–6 cm spherical and 5–6 × 7 cm elliptical) are available, with a treatment time of under 10 min. Both of these systems may be used in an unshielded operating room, with topical shielding available. Since these devices contain no radioactive source, a radioactive material license is not required, and the devices are not subjected to regulation by the Nuclear Regulatory Commission but must be registered by a state regulatory agency.

The mobile electron accelerators produce electrons of energies from 3 to 12 MeV and are used to treat the lumpectomy cavity in the breast using an applicator or cone inserted into the cavity at the time of the surgery. The units can be used in an unshielded operating room and can be transported among different locations (see AAPM Report 92 [23]). Since electrons are more penetrating than low-energy X-rays, the breast tissue is mobilized and shields are inserted into the deep aspect of the cavity to shield the intrathoracic structures. Typically, a dose of 20 Gy using the appropriate electron energy for the depth required is delivered. Personnel must leave the operating room due to the exposure from the radiation delivery. This modality for irradiation is referred to as intraoperative electron radiation therapy (IOERT).

As is discussed in detail in this section, there are two large prospective randomized trials for IORT, the TARGiT-A trial [9] and the ELIOT trial [1]. TARGiT-A compared standard whole-breast radiation (EBRT) to single-dose IORT (TARGIT) using the Zeiss INTRABEAM technology. The trial enrolled 3451 patients from 33 centers in 10 countries from 2000 to 2012 using a non-inferiority statistical design. The study employed a risk-adapted design that anticipated the possibility of finding adverse pathologic features on final pathology and mandated whole-breast radiation after IORT when such features were present. The study prespecified two strata for IORT during the lumpectomy (prepathology) or as a second procedure after the initial surgery (postpathology) and so was able to compare the impact of timing of IORT on outcomes.

To be eligible for TARGiT-A [24], women had to be age 45 years or older and suitable for wide local excision of unifocal invasive ductal carcinoma based on preoperative exam and imaging studies. Three adverse features mandating whole-breast radiation after IORT on the experimental arm were specified in the core protocol: final excision margins <1 mm, extensive in situ component, or invasive lobular carcinoma. Patients with positive margins underwent re-excision then external beam radiation. In addition, individual participating centers could prospectively in their treatment policies (decided upon before enrolling any patients) specify additional adverse features to prompt their use of whole-breast radiation. The statistical plan anticipated use of whole-breast radiation after IORT in 15 % of patients enrolled on the IORT arm. In the most recent analysis, it was reported that 15 % of patients in the IORT arm also received whole-breast radiation, including 22 % in the prepathology and 3.6 % of the postpathology strata. Most women enrolled had favorable cancers, including ≤2 cm (87 %), grade 1–2 (85 %), node negative (84 %), estrogen receptor positive (93 %), and mammographically detected (63 %). At a median follow-up of 2.5 years for the whole cohort, for the primary endpoint in breast recurrence (IBR), there was a 2 % difference between EBRT (1.3 %) and TARGiT (3.3 %), which was within the prespecified non-inferiority margin of 2.5 %. In the prepathology stratum, the IBR difference was 1.1 % for EBRT and 2.1 % for TARGIT. In the postpathology stratum, the IBR difference was 1.7 % EBRT and 5.4 % TARGIT. The investigators suggest that the prepathology timing is thus the preferred option. Overall deaths were lower in the TARGIT arm (3.9 %) compared to the EBRT arm (5.3 %). Toxicity was similar between the two arms for hematoma requiring treatment, postoperative infection, delayed wound healing, and any major toxicity. There was more seroma requiring more than three aspirations after IORT than after whole-breast radiation (2.1 % vs. 0.8 %) and more RTOG grade 3–4 toxicities after whole-breast radiation than after IORT (2.1 % vs. 0.5 %). Given the different beam energy and dose rate, the TARGIT trial data may not be directly applicable to treatments delivered with the Xoft system.

The ELIOT study, using a mobile electron device, was conducted at the Institute Milan and randomized 1305 women from 2000 to 2007 between external whole-breast irradiation (EBRT) of 50 Gy whole breast plus a 10-Gy tumor bed boost or single-dose electron IOERT of 21 Gy. The study used equivalence statistical design, with an equivalence margin for local recurrence of 7.5 % in the IOERT group. To be eligible for the ELIOT trial, women with stage I-II invasive breast cancer age 48–75 years old, with a maximum tumor diameter of 2.5 cm suitable for breast-conserving surgery, could be randomized. There was no additional whole-breast radiation used and no other exclusion criteria or adaption of treatment for any adverse pathologic features on final pathology. Most women recruited had favorable cancers, including estrogen receptor positive (90 %), Her2 negative (97 %), and node negative (74 %). At a median follow-up of 5.8 years, in breast recurrence occurred in 0.4 % in the EBRT arm and 4.4 % in the IOERT arm, which was within the prespecified equivalence margin, and with no difference in 5-year overall survival (96.8 % and 96.9 %, respectively). All skin side effects significantly favored the IOERT group, while a higher incidence of fat necrosis was seen after IOERT than after whole-breast radiation. There were no differences in breast fibrosis, retraction, pain, or burning. The investigators suggest that the in breast recurrence rate could be improved with stricter selection criteria and potentially by the use of additional external beam radiation in selected patients. According to their analyses, risk factors for local recurrence with IOETRT included tumor size >2 cm, high grade, four or more positive nodes, and triple negative histology.

There are several smaller phase I and II institutional studies of breast IORT using either the INTRABEAM device or intraoperative electrons (see Tables 19.1 and 19.2). Several institutional studies have confirmed lower rates of pain and skin toxicity and no increased seroma rate with IORT compared to whole-breast external beam irradiation, similar to the two randomized trials.

Factors other than local control may influence patient and provider selection of breast cancer therapy. Corica et al. performed a survey of Western Australia health professionals treating breast cancer patients and found that between 3 and 7.5 % found IORT an unacceptable option at any risk of local recurrence, 18–21 % found it acceptable at equivalent risk to whole-breast radiation, and 56–59 % deemed it acceptable with a 1–3 % increased risk [25]. Alvarado et al. conducted a patient preference survey between breast IORT and fractionated whole-breast external beam irradiation, also by varying increases in 10-year local recurrence risk [26]. This study found that patients accepted a median additional local recurrence risk for IORT of 2.3 %, with 91 % accepting IORT if equivalent or with some additional risk compared to whole-breast radiation. A quality of life study was performed by Welzel et al. on a subgroup of German patients enrolled in the TARGIT-A trial, using the EORTC QLQ-C30 and BR23 instruments [27]. Patients receiving IORT alone reported significantly less general pain, less breast and arm symptoms, and better role functioning than patients receiving whole-breast radiation.

The studies described guide selection criteria for breast IORT, as do published guidelines and consensus statements for appropriate selection of patients for partial breast irradiation. The widely followed American Society for Radiation

Oncology (ASTRO) consensus guideline [28] published in 2009 did not include criteria specifically for breast IORT, and the randomized trials studying IORT have been published since that statement was written. When considering selection criteria for IORT, it seems reasonable to reference the selection criteria for APBI, as well as consider the eligibility criteria used in the TARGIT-A and ELIOT studies as informed by their respective results. The TARGIT investigators recommend using their criteria and including whole-breast radiation as per protocol for adverse pathologic features. The ELIOT investigators suggest that stricter criteria for IOERT should likely be applied, with omission of those with higher-risk features or with the additional of whole-breast radiation when those features are present on final pathology. Because radiation is delivered at the time of lumpectomy in most cases of IORT or IOERT, selection criteria must be based on the information available prior to surgery or intraoperatively.

A recent retrospective large study involving data from 19 US centers characterized patients being selected for IORT using INTRABEAM. Most US centers are treating patients with invasive ductal carcinoma, tumor size <2 cm, hormone receptor positive, and clinically node negative [29]. Patients with tumors >2 cm have been treated, but issues related to cosmesis (due to larger required volume of tissue removal) and risk for margin-positive lumpectomy (due to larger tumor size) should be taken into account in the decision to pursue IORT in these patients. Much less data available on the treatment of patients with invasive lobular carcinoma or DCIS though treating patients with these histologies have been reported. The decision to treat patients with these histologies should occur in the context of a fully informed discussion regarding the limited available data on outcomes in these settings. Tumor multicentricity is an exclusion criteria for breast IORT. Preoperative breast MRI can be useful in detecting sites of occult multicentric breast cancer and is used by some centers in the North America[19], although the preoperative use of MRI in this context is controversial.

There are technical considerations that should also be considered in selection of patients for IORT with INTRABEAM or Xoft devices which are placed within the lumpectomy cavity. Very small breast size can restrict the technical ability to place the applicators safely within the cavity. Intraoperatively, patients in whom conformity between the applicator and surrounding breast tissue cannot be achieved should not receive IORT with these devices. Similarly, if adequate skin spacing between the skin and applicator as determined by intraoperative breast ultrasound cannot be achieved, then breast IORT with these devices should not be performed due to increased risk of skin toxicity.

There are other factors which should be considered in selection of patients with IORT including prior history of breast irradiation, the setting of local recurrence of breast cancer, collagen vascular disease, and breast implants. There is some limited data available to suggest that IORT may be safely offered in these settings [30], but the risks and benefits should be fully discussed with patients as part of the informed consent process.

The recommendation for additional whole-breast radiation after IORT or IOERT may be considered an inconvenience to some patients and will be associated with the higher toxicity of radiating this larger volume. Therefore, careful preoperative and intraoperative assessment may be warranted to limit the use of subsequent EBRT after IORT. Such assessment could include preoperative axillary imaging with ultrasound or other modalities to assess for suspicious nodes. MRI was not commonly used in the IORT trials or any other trials of APBI and is not routinely recommended, but thorough imaging with high-quality mammogram and ultrasound is certainly necessary. Intraoperative assessment of the sentinel node and of excision margins may further reduce unexpected findings on postoperative pathology (Moffitt study here). Certainly, women being offered IORT or IOERT at the time of lumpectomy should be specifically counseled for the indications for whole-breast radiation after IORT during the informed consent process and be willing to undergo further treatment as warranted by final pathologic findings, or be aware of the potential risks of forgoing additional treatment. While this process is similarly required for any patient being offered partial breast radiation, the particular processes and recommendations associated with breast IORT or IOERT should be specifically addressed and patient preference taken into account in the decision-making process.

References

1. Veronesi U, Orecchia R, Maisonneuve P, et al. Intraoperative radiotherapy versus external radiotherapy for early breast cancer (ELIOT): a randomised controlled equivalence trial. Lancet Oncol. 2013;14(13):1269–77.
2. Hanna SA, de Barros AC, de Andrade FE, Bevilacqua JL, Piato JR, Pelosi EL, Martella E, da Silva JL, Carvalho Hde A. Intraoperative radiation therapy in early breast cancer using a linear accelerator outside of the operative suite: an "image-guided" approach. Int J Radiat Oncol Biol Phys. 2014;89:1015–23.
3. Cedolini C, Bertozzi S, Seriau L, Londero AP, Concina S, Moretti E, Padovani R, Pasqualucci A, Ceschia T, Risaliti A. Feasibility of conservative breast surgery and intraoperative radiation therapy for early breast cancer: a single-center, open, non-randomized, prospective pilot study. Oncol Rep. 2014;31:1539–46.
4. Lemanski C, Azria D, Gourgon-Bourgade S, Gutowski M, Rouanet P, Saint-Aubert B, Ailleres N, Fenoglietto P, Dubois JB. Intraoperative radiotherapy in early-stage breast cancer: results of the montpellier phase II trial. Int J Radiat Oncol Biol Phys. 2010;76:698–703.
5. Osti MF, Carnevale A, Bracci S, Amanti C, Lombardi A, Maggi S, DE Sanctis V, Valeriani M, Enrici RM. Exclusive electron intraoperative radiotherapy in early-stage breast cancer: a monoinstitutional experience. Anticancer Res. 2013;33:1229–35.
6. Sawaki M, Sato S, Noda S, Idota A, Uchida H, Tsunoda N, Kikumori T, Aoyama Y, Ishihara S, Itoh Y, Imai T. Phase I/II study of intraoperative radiotherapy for early breast cancer in Japan. Breast Cancer. 2012;19:353–9.
7. Dessena M, Dessi M, Demontis B, Grosso LP, Porru S, Meleddu GF, Lay G, Murenu G, Amichetti M, Di Martino L. Exclusive intra-operative radiation therapy (IORT) for early stage breast cancer: pilot study of feasibility. G Chir. 2011;32:104–9.
8. Veronesi U, Orecchia R, Luini A, Gatti G, Intra M, Zurrida S, Ivaldi G, Tosi G, Ciocca M, Tosoni A, De Lucia F. A preliminary report of intraoperative radiotherapy (IORT) in limited-stage breast cancers that are conservatively treated. Eur J Cancer. 2001;37:2178–83.
9. Vaidya JS, Wenz F, Bulsara M, Tobias JS, Joseph DJ, Keshtgar M, Flyger HL, Massarut S, Alvarado M, Saunders C, Eiermann W, Metaxas M, Sperk E, Sütterlin M, Brown D, Esserman

L, Roncadin M, Thompson A, Dewar JA, Holtveg HM, Pigorsch S, Falzon M, Harris E, Matthews A, Brew-Graves C, Potyka I, Corica T, Williams NR, Baum M, TARGIT Trialists' Group. Risk-adapted targeted intraoperative radiotherapy versus whole-breast radiotherapy for breast cancer: 5-year results for local control and overall survival from the TARGIT-A randomised trial. Lancet. 2014;383(9917):603–13.
10. Bitterman A, Shiloni E, Goldman I, Hanna-Zaknun R, Davidovich S, Kramer A, Ben-Shahar Y, Steiner M. Intraoperative radiotherapy (IORT) in early breast cancer. Harefuah. 2014;153:460–2.
11. Elliot RL, Deland M, Head JF, Elliott MC. Accelerated partial breast irradiation: initial experience with the Intrabeam System. Surg Oncol. 2011;20:73–9.
12. Deneve JL, Hoefer Jr RA, Harris EE, Laronga C. Accelerated partial breast irradiation: a review and description of an early North American surgical experience with the intrabeam delivery system. Cancer Control. 2012;19:295–308.
13. ICRU. The quality factor in radiation protection ICRU Report 40. Bethesda: International Commission on Radiation Units and Measurements; 1986.
14. Brenner DJ, Leu C-S, Beatty JF, Shefer RE. Clinical relative biological effectiveness of low energy X-rays emitted by miniature X-ray devices. Phys Med Biol. 1999;44:323–33.
15. Nikjoo H, Lindborg L. RBE of low energy electrons and photons. Phys Med Biol. 2010;55:R65–109.
16. Reniers B, Liu D, Rusch T, Verhaegen F. Calculation of relative biological effectiveness of a low-energy electronic brachytherapy source. Phys Med Biol. 2008;53(24):7125–35.
17. Spadinger I, Palcic B. The relative biological effectiveness of 60Co gamma-rays, 55 kVp X-rays, 250 kVp X-rays, and 11 MeV electrons at low doses. Int J Radiat Biol. 1992;61(3):345–53.
18. Astor MB, Hilaris BS, Gruerio A, Varricchione T, Smith D. Preclinical studies with the photon radiosurgery system (PRS). Int J Radiat Oncol Biol Phys. 2000;47(3):809–13.
19. Liu Q, Schneider F, Ma L, Wenz F, Herskind C. Relative biological effectiveness (RBE) of 50 kV X-rays measured in a phantom for intraoperative tumor-bed irradiation. Int J Radiat Oncol Biol Phys. 2013;85(4):1127–33.
20. Herskind C, Griebel J, Kraus-Tiefenbacher U, Wenz F. Sphere of equivalence–a novel target volume concept for intraoperative radiotherapy using low-energy X rays. Int J Radiat Oncol Biol Phys. 2008;72(5):1575–81.
21. http://www.zeiss.com/meditec/en_de/products/oncology/intrabeam-for-breast-cancer/intrabeam.html. Accessed 15 May 2015.
22. http://www.xoftinc.com/. Accessed 15 May 2015.
23. http://aapm.org/pubs/reports/RPT_92.pdf. Accessed 15 May 2015.
24. Vaidya JS, Joseph DJ, Tobias JS, Bulsara M, Wenz F, Saunders C, Alvarado M, Flyger HL, Massarut S, Eiermann W, Keshtgar M, Dewar J, Kraus-Tiefenbacher U, Sütterlin M, Esserman L, Holtveg HM, Roncadin M, Pigorsch S, Metaxas M, Falzon M, Matthews A, Corica T, Williams NR, Baum M. Targeted intraoperative radiotherapy versus whole breast radiotherapy for breast cancer (TARGIT-A trial): an international, prospective, randomised, non-inferiority phase 3 trial. Lancet. 2010;376(9735):91–102.
25. Corica T, Joseph D, Saunders C, Bulsara M, Nowak AK. Intraoperative radiotherapy for early breast cancer: do health professionals choose convenience or risk? Radiat Oncol. 2014;9:33.
26. Alvarado MD, Conolly J, Park C, Sakata T, Mohan AJ, Harrison BL, Hayes M, Esserman LJ, Ozanne EM. Patient preferences regarding intraoperative versus external beam radiotherapy following breast-conserving surgery. Breast Cancer Res Treat. 2014;143:135–40.
27. Welzel G, Hofmann F, Blank E, Kraus-Tiefenbacher U, Hermann B, Sutterlin M, Wenz F. Health-related quality of life after breast-conserving surgery and intraoperative radiotherapy for breast cancer using low-kilovoltage X-rays. Ann Surg Oncol. 2010;17 Suppl 3:359–67.
28. Smith BD, Arthur DW, Buchholz TA, Haffty BG, Hahn CA, Hardenbergh PH, Julian TB, Marks LB, Todor DA, Vicini FA, Whelan TJ, White J, Wo JY, Harris JR. Accelerated partial

breast irradiation consensus statement from the American Society for Radiation Oncology (ASTRO). Int J Radiat Oncol Biol Phys. 2009;74(4):987–1001.
29. Valente S, et al. North American Experience with intraoperative radiation using low-kilovoltage X-rays for breast cancer: initial report of TARGIT-R (Retrospective). Ann Surg Onc. 2015;22(1 Suppl):S16.
30. Keshtgar MR, Vaidya JS, Tobias JS, Wenz F, Joseph D, Stacey C, Metaxas MG, Keller A, Corica T, Williams NR, Baum M. Targeted intraoperative radiotherapy for breast cancer in patients in whom external beam radiation is not possible. Int J Radiat Oncol Biol Phys. 2011;80(1):31–8.

Chapter 20
Physics of Intraoperative Radiotherapy for the Breast

Firas Mourtada

Contents

20.1 Introduction

Traditional intraoperative radiotherapy (IORT) utilizes either linear-accelerator electrons or high-dose-rate (HDR) radionuclide-based devices. IORT delivers a single large dose or as a boost in situ in the operating room. These modalities require special shielding of the operating room and extensive radiation safety logistics, hence only a few large centers adopted such approaches. Recently, the development of miniature soft X-ray-producing electronic brachytherapy sources (50 kVp or less) eliminated such burden with less regulatory requirements, making it more attractive for clinics to add IORT as an option. Other advantage of IORT is that less overall time is needed for a course of therapy since the single high-dose fraction in the operating room (delivered within 20–50 min) is much shorter than external beam fractionated radiotherapy. In this chapter, we describe the two "electronic brachytherapy" (eBx) systems currently available: the Zeiss INTRABEAM and the

F. Mourtada, PhD, FAAPM
Department of Radiation Oncology, Helen Graham Cancer Center, 4701 Olgetown-Stanton Rd Ste 1110, Newark 19713, DE, USA

Helen F. Graham Cancer Center, Christiana Care Health System, Newark, Delaware, USA

Division of Medical Physics, Department of Radiation Oncology, Kimmel Cancer Center, Thomas Jefferson University, Philadelphia, USA

Department of Radiation Physics, UT MD Anderson Cancer Center, Houston, Texas, USA
e-mail: FMourtada@christianacare.org

D.W. Arthur et al. (eds.), *Short Course Breast Radiotherapy: A Comprehensive Review of Hypofractionation, Partial Breast, and Intra-Operative Irradiation*,
DOI 10.1007/978-3-319-24388-7_20

Xoft Axxent systems that are FDA approved for breast IORT. Quality assurance (QA) tasks and dosimetric uncertainty issues are also discussed. As of this writing, there are no societal guidelines for electronic brachytherapy QA. However, the AAPM TG-72 "intraoperative radiation therapy using mobile electron linear accelerators" have useful information about radiation protection, machine commissioning, and logistics [1]. Other current AAPM guidelines that should also be consulted prior to initiating an eBt IORT program are TG-43: dosimetry of interstitial brachytherapy sources [2, 3], TG-56: code of practice of brachytherapy physics [4], TG-59: HDR Brachytherapy Treatment Delivery [5], TG-61: AAPM protocol for 40–300 kV X-ray beam dosimetry in radiotherapy and radiobiology [6], and TG-186: model-based dose calculation methods in brachytherapy beyond the TG-43 formalism [7].

20.2 Basic Physics Description of Currently Available IORT Systems

20.2.1 INTRABEAM® System

The INTRABEAM eBx system (Carl Zeiss Meditec AG, Jena, Germany) received US FDA approval for IORT in 1999. The INTRABEAM eBx source (XRS 4) is a miniaturized accelerator that has a maximum potential of 50 kVp potential and up to 40 microA cathode filament current. The XRS 4 consists of an electron gun, electron acceleration cavity, and two bending magnets, which guide the electrons through the 10-cm long × 3.2-mm diameter probe toward the gold target. Bremsstrahlung X-rays are generated isotopically. Details of the XRS 4 construction details can be found in the literature (Dinsmore et al.) [8]. The XRS unit has an internal radiation monitor (IRM) to insure beam output constancy during treatment.

The INTRABEAM spherical applicators with several sizes are available for breast IORT. The sphere solid body is made from a biocompatible polyetherimide (PEI: $C_{37}H_{24}O_6N_2$), with physical density of 1.27–1.51 g/cm^3. The sphere has 5.6 mm dia. Cavity in the center allows the probe of the XRS X-ray source to fit firmly for breast IORT procedures. PEI melting point is 350 °C, thus suitable for standard steam sterilization cycles ($n = 100$). Eight sphere diameters are provided ranging from 1.5 to 5.0 cm in 0.5 cm increment to allow for the best fit to size of tumor cavity at time of excision. Spheres with diameter less than 3.5 cm have an additional aluminum layer inside the cavity to harden the beam spectrum.

Other equipment are the floor stand and cart, both designed to work in the sterile OR environment and for easy mobility and mounting of the entire control unit and QA dosimeter.

20.2.1.1 INTRABEAM System Quality Assurance

QA should be performed within 24 h prior to patient treatment. Required tests include verification of beam symmetry and dose output.

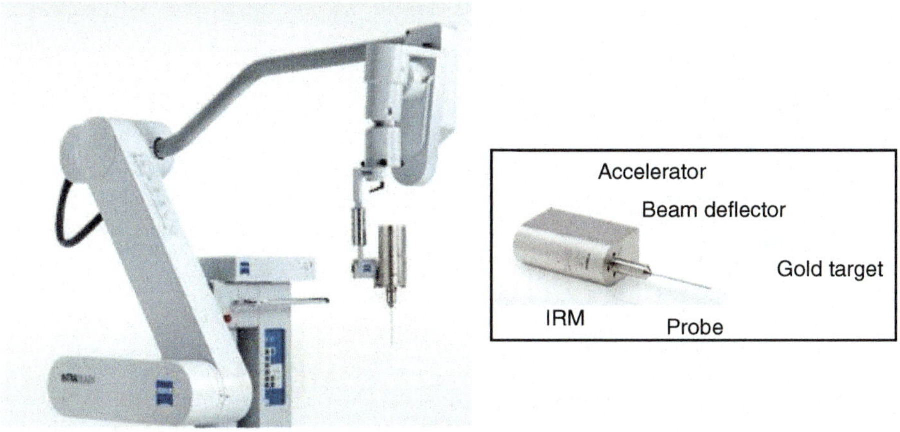

Fig. 20.1 XRS X-ray source of the INTRABEAM System. *IRM* internal radiation monitor. Overall dimensions: 70×175×110 mm (width×height×length) and weight 1.6 kg (Permission from Carl Zeiss Meditec AG, Jena, Germany)

Symmetry is verified using a vendor-supplied device with five photodiode array, four diodes located at 90° intervals, and one long probe axis (Fig. 20.1). The system software adjusts the current of the bending magnets to minimize the variance among the diodes.

For dose output consistency, prior to a clinical case, the IRM count rate is cross-checked with an independent ion chamber. During treatment, the IRM rate is continuously monitored by the software, and if deviations over 10 % are detected, automatic adjustment of the treatment time is applied. The output is displayed on the treatment monitor of the control unit and thus enables continuous monitoring throughout the treatment. Necessary fine-tuning is performed automatically.

Optional QA tests for the INTRABEAM system are the probe straightness integrity test and the bending current verification test. A special device called PIACH (probe adjuster/ionization chamber holder) which attaches to the probe (Fig. 20.2) can be rotated around its axis. Details of the tests are provided in the manufacturer's instructions for use.

At initial system commissioning and at annual calibration, the dose rate as a function of depth should be verified using a soft X-ray ionization chamber in a 3D water phantom. Verification for each clinically used voltage and current (i.e., beam quality) should be verified. Both ion chamber and electrometer should be calibrated every 2 years as recommended by AAPM TG 51 [4]. The vendor provides as an option a water phantom, INTRABEAM Water Phantom (shielded with leaded glass), to enable the physicist to accurately position the tip of the XRS 4 miniaturized accelerator relative to an ionization chamber in water. The accurate positioning and precise propagation of the source (±0.1-mm) ensure verification of the depth dose curve with or without an applicator, making it possible to measure the depth dose curve for initial system commissioning and annual QA verification.

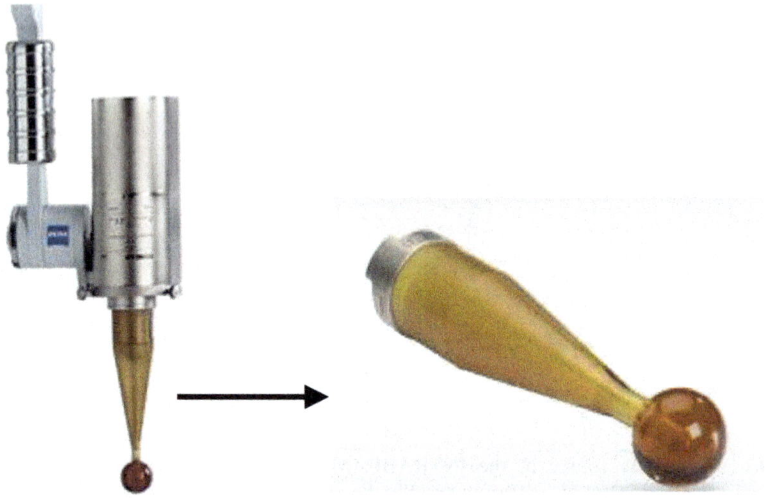

Fig. 20.2 INTRABEAM spherical applicator. The sphere solid body is made from a biocompatible polyetherimide (PEI: C37H24O6N2), with physical density of 1.27–1.51 g/cm^3 and 350 °C melting point. The sphere has 5.6-mm dia. cavity in the center to allow the probe of the XRS X-ray source to fit firmly for breast IORT procedures (Permission from Carl Zeiss Meditec AG, Jena, Germany)

20.2.1.2 INTRABEAM Shielding Considerations

It has been reported that at 2 m from the INTRABEAM source (unshielded), the exposure rate is about 15 mR/h [9]. A mobile-shielded panel and or a leaded apron is sufficient to reduce radiation exposure to background levels. This should allow the OR staff to remain with the patient during irradiation. Basic ALARA (as low as reasonably achievable) rules should always be used to reduce personnel exposure.

20.2.2 Xoft® Axxent® Electronic Brachytherapy (eBx) System

The Xoft Axxent Electronic Brachytherapy (Xoft Inc., Fremont, CA) utilizes a miniaturized X-ray source to deliver high-dose-rate (HDR) radiation for IORT treatments. This approach has a clear advantage over radionuclide-based IORT sources such as Ir-192 and Co-60, whereas the eBx source can be turned on or off and thus requires minimal shielding in the OR. The Xoft System received FDA clearance in 2005 for breast cancer treatment and in 2009 for IORT. The Xoft Axxent System main components are the Axxent controller, the Axxent X-ray source, Axxent cooling tube set, well chamber/electrometer, and optional FlexiShield and Rigid Shield (Fig. 20.3). Special applicators are also provided for the breast, cervix, endometrium, and skin.

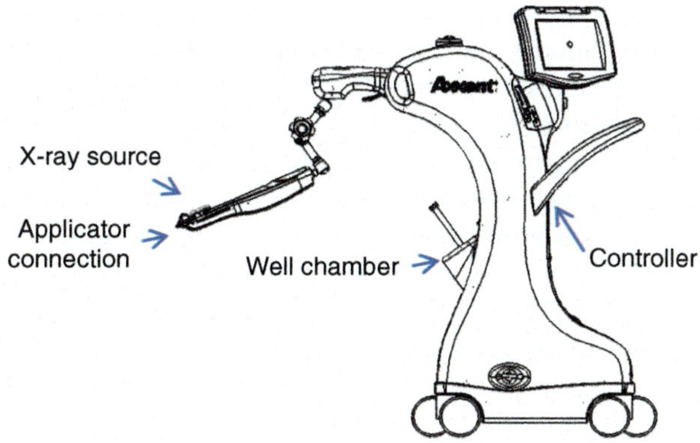

Fig. 20.3 Xoft Electronic Brachytherapy System (Permission from Xoft)

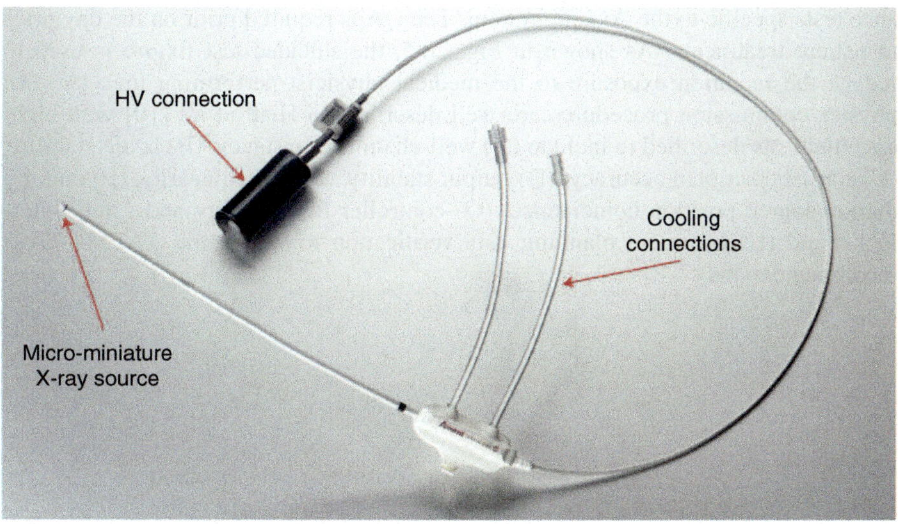

Fig. 20.4 Xoft Axxent X-ray source (Permission from Xoft)

The controller includes high voltage supply, filament current, and circulates cooling water to the X-ray source. It moves the X-ray source in a stepped, linear manner through the applicator, based on pullback dwell times and dwell positions provided by the operator. The source is a miniaturized X-ray tube, operating at 50 kV, located at the tip of a cooling catheter assembly that delivers radiation in a stepped linear manner to provide conformal doses through the applicator directly to the tissue (Fig. 20.4). Only the Axxent X-ray source is compatible with and may be used with the Axxent controller.

The X-ray source is a non-sterile, disposable device intended to deliver intracavitary radiation. Sources are provided to customers on an annual contract basis, similar to how Ir-192 sources are provided with brachytherapy source contracts. Source life varies based on usage patterns at each facility, but on average, sources are changed out monthly. Sources can be quickly and easily replaced by customer personnel within a few minutes – it is not necessary to have the manufacturer's service personnel onsite to perform the source replacement procedure. The Xoft source is water-cooled. The cooling tubing set and cooling pump circulate water through the source catheter. Any interruption in flow is detected by the flow sensor, which signals the Controller to stop producing X-rays until the flow restriction is remedied.

For breast IORT, the Axxent source is positioned inside the Axxent balloon applicator. Three sizes of Axxent balloon applicators are available (3–4 cm dia., 4–5 cm dia., and 5–6 cm dia.) as shown in Fig. 20.5.

20.2.2.1 Xoft System Quality Assurance

The Axxent Physics Accessories Kit provides QA tools to perform quality assurance tests specific to the Axxent system. The QA is required prior on the day prior to patient treatments. As shown in Fig. 20.5, the shielded test fixture is used to reduce the radiation exposure to the medical physicist performing the QA. The physics commission procedures are well described in Hiatt et al. [10] with eight essential tests described to include (A) well-chamber constancy, (B) beam stability, (C) source positional accuracy, (D) output stability, (E) timer linearity, (F) dummy marker/source position coincidence, (G) controller functionality and safety interlocks, and (H) treatment planning data verification following the AAPM TG-43 recommendations [2, 3].

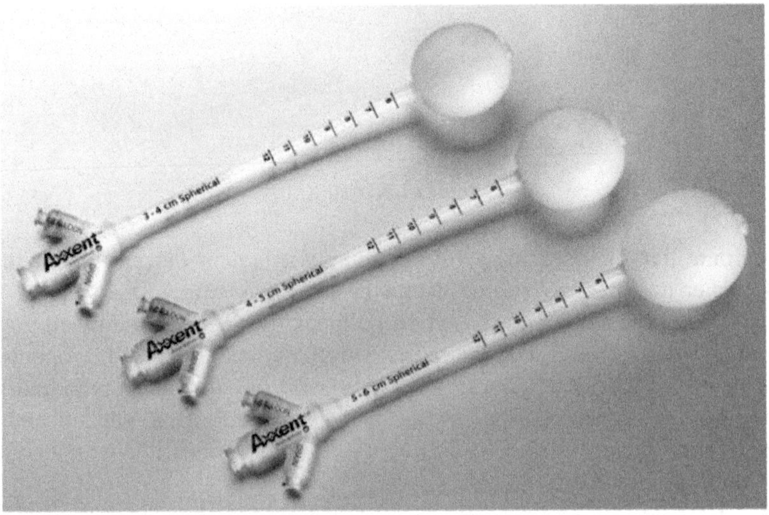

Fig. 20.5 Axxent balloon applicators. Three sizes are available (3–4 cm dia., 4–5 cm dia., and 5–6 cm dia.) (Permission from Xoft)

20.2.2.2 XOFT Shielding Considerations

Similar to the INTRABEAM shielding requirement discussed above, the Xoft system requires minimal shielding in the OR room for IORT procedures. Xoft provides the FlexiShield® drape (a 15-inch flexible drape of 0.4-mm lead equivalent) placed over the breast. Rusch et al. have shown exposure rate reduction from 15 to 1 mR/h to the OR personnel when using this drape [11]. Using in-house-designed phantoms, Safigholi et al. evaluated radiation exposure rates in the vicinity of the Axxent device for the breast and reported an exposure of 200 mR/h at 30 cm from the Axxent balloon inside the breast cavity [12]. To reduce the exposure levels, they used mobile lead shields which reduced exposure by about 95 %.

20.2.2.3 Breast IORT Dosimetric Considerations

Typical intraoperative electronic brachytherapy prescription dose is 20 Gy (for both INTRABEAM and Axxent sources) in a single fraction prescribed to the external surface of the spherical applicator. The dose gradient within the first 1 cm of tissue is severe, resulting in delivering ~5 and ~10 Gy at 1-cm tissue depth for the INTRABEAM and Axxent systems, respectively. Treatment time is on the order of 20–50 min (Table 20.1). The radiobiological factors for single fraction IORT are discussed in Chaps. 19, 21, 22.

The INTRABEAM dose calculation method is fairly simplified 1D calculation from a single source position, where for a given prescription dose, the dwell time is calculated based on a reference dose rate in water provided by the vendor and a correction factor obtained during the calibration process. The radial dose-rate function in tissue is calculated from the in-water dose-rate function without the applicator by multiplication with correction factors (ATFs), defined as the ratio between the dose rates in the presence and in the absence of the applicator as a function of the radius, r (distance from the target).

The Xoft Axxent dose calculation method is based on the AAPM TG-43 method. Rivard et al. determined the Xoft Axxent source model S700 TG-43 dosimetry parameters from measurements and calculations in water at 40, 45, and 50 kV settings using the MCNP5 Monte Carlo code, a parallel plate ionization chamber, and a high-purity germanium (HPGe) detector for photon spectra measurements [13]. Currently commercial treatment planning systems using TG-43 method can be used to commission the Xoft source in a similar fashion to other HDR or LDR sources.

Table 20.1 Basic summary of IORT commercial units and source available on the US market

	Source	Rx dose @ surface (Gy)	Dose @ 1-cm depth (Gy)	Treatment time (min)	APBI applicator
INTRABEAM (Zeiss)	50 kVp X-rays	20	5	20–50 min	Solid spherical
Axxent (Xoft)	50 kVp X-rays	20	10	15–25	Balloon catheter

It should be noted that TG-43 dosimetry for low-energy sources is calculated for water. The recently updated guidelines for dosimetry in brachytherapy per AAPM TG-186 have recommended the use of model-based dosimetry calculations as a replacement for TG-43 [7]. TG-186 highlights shortcomings in the water-based approach in TG-43, particularly for low-energy brachytherapy sources. Landry et al. [14] investigated the sensitivity of Monte Carlo (MC) dose calculations to uncertainties in human tissue composition for a range of low photon energy brachytherapy sources: ^{125}I, ^{103}Pd, ^{131}Cs, and the Axxent eBt source. The simulations suggest that dose distributions in breast tissue differ from water and are influenced by density, mean tissue composition, and patient-to-patient composition variations. Dose variations of up to 30 % from water for 70 % adipose/30 % gland breast were found, and the variability of the breast composition adds a ±10 % dose uncertainty. Such dosimetric uncertainty is due to the dominance of the photoelectric effect in this energy range and its large variation due to variations of tissue effective atomic number. The authors concluded that imaging tools providing more accurate estimates of elemental compositions such as dual-energy CT would be beneficial.

Recently, White et al. performed a Monte Carlo study of the Xoft Axxent in several breast tissue density and composition and different dose reporting methods and compared to TG-43-based plans [15]. Results were calculated using two dose reporting methods, dose to water ($D_{w,m}$) and dose to medium ($D_{m,m}$), for the heterogeneous simulations. All results were compared against TG-43-based dose distributions and evaluated using dose ratio maps and DVH metrics. Changes in skin and PTV dose were highlighted. Based on a prescription dose of 34 Gy, the average D90 to PTV was reduced by between ~4 and ~40 %, depending on the scoring method, compared to the TG-43 result. Maximum skin dose is also reduced by 10–15 % due to the absence of backscatter not accounted for in TG-43. The balloon applicator also contributed to the reduced dose. The authors concluded that TG-186-based calculations produce results that are different from TG-43 for the Axxent source. The differences depend strongly on the method of dose reporting. This study emphasized the importance of backscatter to peak skin dose. More robust dose calculation engines such as Monte Carlo are in development to account for patient geometries, tissue heterogeneities, and applicator for low-energy brachytherapy sources [15]. Early adopters of eBt for breast IORT should realize such dosimetric uncertainties when comparing clinical trial results.

References

1. Beddar AS, Biggs PJ, Chang S, et al. Intraoperative radiation therapy using mobile electron linear accelerators: report of AAPM Radiation Therapy Committee Task Group No. 72. Med Phys. 2006;33:1476–89.
2. Nath R, Anderson LL, Luxton G, et al. Dosimetry of interstitial brachytherapy sources: recommendations of the AAPM Radiation Therapy Committee Task Group No. 43. American Association of Physicists in Medicine. Med Phys. 1995;22:209–34.
3. Rivard MJ, Coursey BM, DeWerd LA, et al. Update of AAPM Task Group No. 43 Report: a revised AAPM protocol for brachytherapy dose calculations. Med Phys. 2004;31:633–74.

4. Nath R, Anderson LL, Meli JA, et al. Code of practice for brachytherapy physics: report of the AAPM Radiation Therapy Committee Task Group No. 56. American Association of Physicists in Medicine. Med Phys. 1997;24:1557–98.
5. Kubo HD, Glasgow GP, Pethel TD, et al. High dose-rate brachytherapy treatment delivery: report of the AAPM Radiation Therapy Committee Task Group No. 59. Med Phys. 1998;25:375–403.
6. Ma CM, Coffey CW, DeWerd LA, et al. AAPM protocol for 40-300 kV x-ray beam dosimetry in radiotherapy and radiobiology. Med Phys. 2001;28:868–93.
7. Beaulieu L, Carlsson Tedgren A, Carrier JF, et al. Report of the Task Group 186 on model-based dose calculation methods in brachytherapy beyond the TG-43 formalism: current status and recommendations for clinical implementation. Med Phys. 2012;39:6208–36.
8. Dinsmore M, Harte KJ, Sliski AP, et al. A new miniature x-ray source for interstitial radiosurgery: device description. Med Phys. 1996;23:45–52.
9. Park CC, Yom SS, Podgorsak MB, et al. American Society for Therapeutic Radiology and Oncology (ASTRO) Emerging Technology Committee report on electronic brachytherapy. Int J Radiat Oncol Biol Phys. 2010;76:963–72.
10. Hiatt J, Cardarelli G, Hepel J, et al. A commissioning procedure for breast intracavitary electronic brachytherapy systems. J Appl Clin Med Phys. 2008;9:2775.
11. Rusch T, Axelrod S, Smith P. Performance of Xoft FlexiShield flexible X-ray shielding in laboratory tests and in a goat mammary model. In: 47th annual meeting of the American Association of Physicists in Medicine, Seattle, WA; 2005.
12. Safigholi H, Faghihi R, Jashni SK, et al. Characteristics of miniature electronic brachytherapy x-ray sources based on TG-43U1 formalism using Monte Carlo simulation techniques. Med Phys. 2012;39:1971–9.
13. Rivard MJ, Davis SD, DeWerd LA, et al. Calculated and measured brachytherapy dosimetry parameters in water for the Xoft Axxent X-Ray Source: an electronic brachytherapy source. Med Phys. 2006;33:4020–32.
14. Landry G, Reniers B, Murrer L, et al. Sensitivity of low energy brachytherapy Monte Carlo dose calculations to uncertainties in human tissue composition. Med Phys. 2010;37:5188–98.
15. White SA, Landry G, Fonseca GP, et al. Comparison of TG-43 and TG-186 in breast irradiation using a low energy electronic brachytherapy source. Med Phys. 2014;41:061701.

Chapter 21
A Risk-Adapted Approach to Breast Radiation Using Targeted Intraoperative Radiotherapy (TARGIT)

Jayant S. Vaidya, Jeffrey S. Tobias, Frederik Wenz, Samuele Massarut, Max Bulsara, Christobel Saunders, Henrik Flyger, Michael Alvarado, Wolfgang Eiermann, Tammy Corica, David Joseph, and Michael Baum

---

Professor J.S. Vaidya, MBBS MS DNB FRCS PhD (✉)
Professor of Surgery and Oncology, Clinical Trials Group, Division of Surgery and Interventional Science, University College London, 132 Hampstead Road, London, UK
e-mail: jayantvaidya@gmail.com http://www.jayantvaidya.org; http://www.targit.org.uk

Professor J.S.Tobias
Department of Clinical Oncology, University College London Hospitals, London, UK

Professor F. Wenz
Department of Radiation Oncology, University Medical Centre Mannheim, University of Heidelberg, Heidelberg, Germany

S. Massarut
Department of Surgery, Centro di Riferimento Oncologico, Aviano, Italy

Professor M. Bulsara
Department of Biostatistics, University of Notre Dame, Fremantle, WA, Australia

Professor C. Saunders
School of Surgery, University of Western Australia, Perth, WA, Australia

H. Flyger
Department of Breast Surgery, University of Copenhagen, Copenhagen, Denmark

M. Alvarado
Department of Surgery, University of California, San Francisco, CA, USA

Professor W. Eiermann
Department of Gynecology and Obstetrics, Red Cross Hospital, Munich, Germany

T. Corica • Professor D. Joseph
Department of Radiation Oncology, Sir Charles Gairdner Hospital, Perth, WA, Australia

Professor M. Baum
Clinical Trials Group, Division of Surgery and Interventional Science, University College London, London, UK

D.W. Arthur et al. (eds.), *Short Course Breast Radiotherapy: A Comprehensive Review of Hypofractionation, Partial Breast, and Intra-Operative Irradiation*,
DOI 10.1007/978-3-319-24388-7_21

Contents

Whole-organ detailed three-dimensional pathological analysis of mastectomy specimens vis-à-vis the results of breast-conserving surgery trials demonstrates a remarkable phenomenon: in addition to the main tumor, the mastectomy specimen often reveals multiple foci of cancer distributed widely in the breast volume. This is in contrast with the location of a local recurrence, which mostly occurs in the area around the original tumor – thus, it makes sense to focus radiation only around the original tumor. Based on this insight, the targeted intraoperative radiotherapy technique and the device to deliver it were developed in the late 1990s, the first case treated at the Middlesex Hospital, University College London, UK, on 2 July 1998. Pilot studies confirmed feasibility and safety, and in March 2000, the TARGIT-A randomized trial was launched.

One of the reasons for the localization of in-breast recurrence in the immediate areas around the original tumor might be the loss of heterozygosity in the morphologically normal cells around the tumor [1]. Another speculative reason might be the wound fluid that bathes the tumor bed. Surgical wound fluid has been shown to have a stimulatory effect on tumor cells – stimulating their growth, motility, and invasiveness. "Temporal miss" – the really important delay in delivering radiotherapy – probably occurs in the few hours/days immediately after surgery when the tumor bed bathes in wound fluid. Translational research has shown that TARGIT IORT abrogates such potentially harmful effect of wound fluid [2].

TARGIT delivers a physical dose of 20 Gy to the surface of the tumor bed, in the cavity produced by excision of tumor tissue, using a spherical applicator (the Intrabeam® system; Carl Zeiss Meditec, Germany), while the patient is anesthetized for primary surgery. The technique itself has FDA approval and CE mark for clinical use in any part of the body. Unlike the Novac-7 system being used in the Italian ELIOT trial, TARGIT does not require extensive dissection of skin flaps and chest wall away from the breast disc and is delivered to undisturbed fresh well-vascularized tumor bed. The low-energy X-rays (50 kV) used in TARGIT means that unlike other methods of PBI, the volume of tissue that receives very high doses of radiation is small; therefore, external beam whole breast radiotherapy (EBRT) can be safely added. The heart and the lungs do not receive any significant irradiation during TARGIT IORT; it does not require complicated CT planning, nor does a particular tumor location make a patient ineligible. Adoption of TARGIT IORT has been estimated to reduce healthcare costs by a significant degree.

The TARGIT-A trial (http://www.targit.org.uk) was slow to recruit initially, but soon gathered pace and completed its initial goal of 2232 patients in 2010, when the first results were published. The trial closed in June 2012 after recruitment of 3451 patients from 33 centers in 11 countries in Europe, the USA, and Australia. The 5-year results of local recurrence and the first analysis of survival was presented as a late-breaking paper in the San Antonio Breast Cancer Conference in December 2012 followed by the publication of the full paper in the Lancet. The primary outcome was absolute difference in local recurrence, with a non-inferiority margin of 2.5 %. The secondary outcomes included toxicity, breast cancer-specific mortality, and non-breast-cancer mortality. For the primary outcome of local recurrence in the conserved breast, TARGIT was found to be non-inferior to EBRT overall and in women given TARGIT with initial surgery (the prepathology stratum) ($n=2298$). With delayed TARGIT (postpathology stratum, $n=1153$) the between-group difference was larger than 2.5 %, and non-inferiority was not established. In a planned subgroup analysis for allowing better case selection, progesterone (PgR) receptor status was found to be the only predictor of outcome: hormone-responsive patients (PgR positive) had very similar local recurrence with TARGIT during lumpectomy or EBRT 5-year rates (1.4% vs 1.2%). Grade 3 or 4 radiotherapy toxicity was significantly reduced with TARGIT. Overall, breast cancer mortality was much the same between groups, but to date, there were significantly fewer non-breast-cancer deaths with TARGIT, attributable to fewer deaths from cardiovascular causes and other cancers, leading to a trend in reduced overall mortality in the TARGIT arm. The trial concluded that for selected patients with breast cancer (women who are 45 years of age and older with unifocal hormone-sensitive invasive ductal carcinoma that is up to 3.5 cm in size), TARGIT concurrent with lumpectomy within a risk-adapted approach is as effective and safe alternative to postoperative EBRT.

TARGIT IORT is being used in over 250 centers worldwide and is included as the part of the many national guidelines. Pilot studies that suggest that a tumor bed boost with TARGIT might be superior to EBRT boost [3]. This is being tested in the TARGIT-B randomized trial in women with higher risk of local recurrence; it is recruiting in 20 centers already. The results of the TARGIT-A and TARGIT-B trials could bring true individualization of radiotherapy treatment for breast cancer.

21.1 Individualizing Local Treatment for Breast Cancer

It took the mammoth effort of 26,000 women in 36 randomized trials to be meta-analyzed in the Oxford Overview [4–7] to make the move from radical mastectomy described by William Halsted more than 100 years ago [8] to breast-conserving therapy that is considered the norm today. As we stand on these giants' shoulders, the next step – the real paradigm shift – to a local therapy truly localized to the tumor and its environs at least in selected patients, might be easier. However, as generations change, change is not always easy and the lessons from the past are often forgotten.

In this chapter, we shall give a synopsis of its rationale followed by details about the intraoperative approach of delivering partial breast radiotherapy.

The dogma of 3–6 weeks of postoperative radiotherapy after breast-conserving surgery for all patients is one of the main obstacles in widespread utilization of breast-conserving surgery. The radiotherapy schedule is inconvenient for patients and contributes substantially to the unacceptable waiting lists experienced in many oncology departments worldwide. While making decisions about which operation to choose, recurrence, radiation therapy, and rapid recovery are the main factors women are concerned about [9]. Consequently, if radiation can be completed at the time of the surgery, then two significant concerns will be addressed, and perhaps fewer women will feel obliged to choose mastectomy just because they live far away from a radiotherapy facility [10] or wish to avoid prolonging their treatment.

Furthermore, it has been estimated that the externally delivered boost dose misses target volume in 24–80 % of cases [11, 12]. Thus, a large proportion of local recurrences could be attributed to this "geographical miss." This could be even more important today in the age of oncoplastic surgery when there is extensive remodeling of breast to achieve a better cosmetic result. In this situation, it is very difficult to delineate the tumor bed even with markers such as gold seeds. This can result either in complete missing of the target or a "precautionary" overtreatment by enlargement of the boost field. Delivering radiotherapy immediately after tumor excision with the TARGIT approach, before remodeling occurs, could ensure that the radiotherapy (boost or alone) is delivered to the correct target.

A delay in delivery of radiotherapy either because of a long waiting list or because chemotherapy is given first may jeopardize its effectiveness [13, 14], although this has been difficult to substantiate. The really important delay may however be the one that occurs immediately after surgery. We have found that the tumor bed is a rich microenvironment that promotes proliferation, migration, and invasion [2, 15, 16]. Targeting this microenvironment at the right time could be crucially important. We would like to call missing this window of opportunity a "temporal miss" analogous to its spatial counterpart. Finally, whole breast irradiation carries the risks of acute and long-term complications such as erythema, fatigue, prolonged discomfort, radiation pneumonitis, rib fracture, cardiovascular effects, and carcinogenesis that could compromise the long-term benefit from postoperative radiotherapy [6, 17]. Finally, it is also difficult to measure the effect of the stress of taking a prolonged course of radiation – which might inadvertently have a small albeit important effect on the woman's general health.

It is possible that local recurrence may be facilitated by a local field defect. The morphologically normal cells surrounding breast cancer demonstrate a loss of heterozygosity, which is often identical to that of the primary tumor [1]. In addition, aromatase activity in the index quadrant is higher than other quadrants [18], and estrogen has the potential to stimulate mutagenesis, growth, and angiogenesis [19, 20]. Patients with ipsilateral breast tumor recurrence (IBTR) has an increased risk of carrying the mutant p53 gene (23 % vs. 1 %) [21] and, young patients (<40 years) with IBTR have a disproportionately increased risk (40 %) of carrying a deleterious BRCA1/2 gene mutation [22]. This suggests that local recurrence is probably related to background genetic instability. It appears that a dynamic interaction between the local factors (such as aromatase) present in the breast parenchyma, the systemic hormonal milieu, and genetic instability will determine the risk and location of local recurrence, in addition to the biology of the excised primary tumor.

The location of recurrence in the breast with respect to site of the primary tumor shows an interesting distribution. Between 80 and 100 % of early breast recurrences occur in the quadrant that harbored the primary tumor which is in contrast to the findings of three-dimensional analysis of mastectomy specimens [23, 24] which reveal that 63 % of breasts harbor occult cancer foci and 80 % of these are situated remote from the index quadrant. It therefore appears that these widespread and occult multifocal/multicentric cancers in other quadrants of the breast remain dormant for a long time and have a low risk of causing clinical tumors. This is corroborated by the fact that although there is a high frequency (20 % in young (median age 39) women and 33 % in women between 50 and 55) of tumors found in breasts when analyzed in autopsy studies [25], the frequency of clinical breast cancer in the population is considerably lower.

Arguably, in the EORTC study [26], only 56 % of local recurrences are reported to have occurred in the original tumor bed. In fact, a further 27 % recurred diffusely throughout the breast including the tumor bed, leaving 29 % recurrences outside the index quadrant. However, patients in this study received intensive mammographic follow-up that might have unearthed subclinical occult tumors in other quadrants of unproven clinical significance.

21.2 Radiotherapy Has a Dual Benefit: Both the Seed and the Soil

It appears that local recurrence occurs in the index quadrant, whether or not radiotherapy is given [27–29] and irrespective of clear margins. Of the breast-conserving trials that have tested the effect of radiotherapy, patients in the NSABP-B06 [30], Ontario [31], Swedish [32], and Scottish [33] trials had less extensive surgery compared with the Milan III trial [34]. The recurrence rate in the control arm of the Milan III trial, in which the tumors were smaller and excision was considerably wider, was low (8.8 % vs. 24–27 % in other trials) albeit at the cost of cosmesis. Nevertheless, radiotherapy reduced it even further and at the same proportional rate as in other trials. If local recurrence had been caused by residual disease only, then radiotherapy would have affected a much larger proportional reduction in those patients with positive margins or less extensive surgery, but radiotherapy is just as effective in patients with negative margins suggesting that radiotherapy may have an effect on the soil rather than the seed [35].

Thus, radiotherapy may have a dual effect of inhibiting the growth of genetically unstable cells around the primary tumor and of making the whole breast tissue less conducive to growth [35]. This idea has been supported by translational research during intraoperative radiotherapy performed at the Centro di Riferimento di Oncologia, Aviano, Italy [2], demonstrating for the first time that radiotherapy could be exerting its beneficial effect via an effect on the tumor microenvironment. We found that the wound fluid collected in the 24 h following surgical wide local excision of cancer stimulates breast cancer cell lines to proliferate, migrate, and invade into Matrigel. On the other hand, the fluid collected from wounds that had received targeted intraoperative radiotherapy did not have such an effect. Thus, if a tumor bed boost is delivered immediately after the operation using the TARGIT IORT approach, it could be superior to the conventional external beam boost that suffers from a temporal and possibly a geographical miss.

Systemic therapies such as aromatase inhibitors or ovarian suppression may achieve a similar effect on the microenvironment through reduction of estrogen concentration in the breast and may have a synergistic effect with radiotherapy [36]. Thus, with increasing use of systemic therapy, intraoperative radiotherapy to the tissues surrounding the primary tumor might be all the radiotherapy that is necessary, and such an approach may solve many of the problems of postoperative radiotherapy discussed earlier and may allow many more women with breast cancer to conserve their breast.

21.3 The Surgical technique of TARGeted Intraoperative radioTherapy (TARGIT) using the Intrabeam system

21.3.1 The Device Used in the TARGIT IORT technique: Intrabeam

Modern intraoperative radiotherapy devices derive benefit from miniaturization technology. No longer do we need to transport the patient to the purposed-built radiotherapy suite – the (mini) radiotherapy suite comes to the patient right in the operating room! The first device to be used for TARGIT IORT was the Intrabeam™ (Photoelectron Corporation, Lexington MA, USA) [37, 38], which is now manufactured by Carl Zeiss AG (Oberkochen, Germany) (Fig. 21.1). The two other systems of mobile linear accelerators are Mobetron system (Oncology Care Systems Group of Siemens Medical Systems, Intraop Medical Inc, Santa Clara, CA, USA) and the Novac-7 system (Hitesys SPA, Italy). Some of the characteristics of these machines are given below (Table 21.1) (taken from [35]).

The Intrabeam machine contains a miniature electron gun and electron accelerator contained in an X-ray tube which are powered by a 12-V power supply. "Soft" X-rays (50 kVp) are emitted from the point source. Tissue is kept at a distance from the source by spherical applicators to give a uniform dose. Various

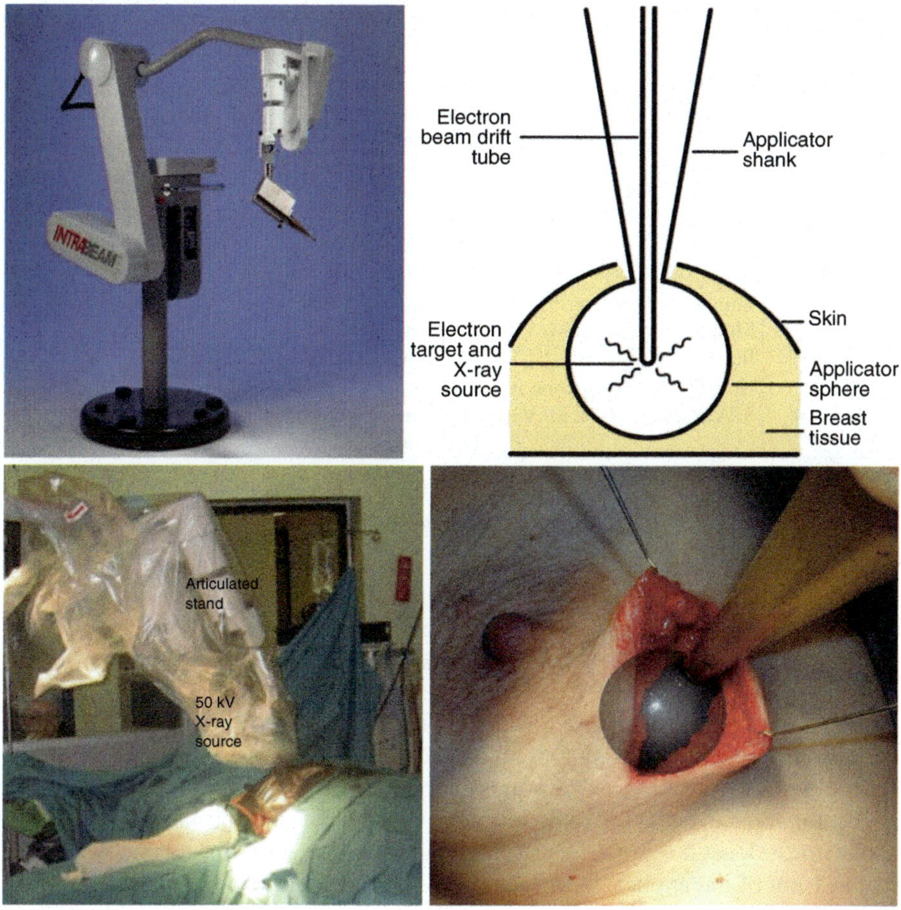

Fig. 21.1 The TARGIT technique. The Intrabeam device (*top left*) and a schematic diagram showing how the spherical applicator fits into the tumor bed (*top right*). Intraoperative radiotherapy being delivered in the operation theater (*bottom left*) and a close-up of the spherical applicator in the tumor bed (*bottom right*) (Taken from Vaidya et al. [40])

sizes of applicator spheres are available to suit the size of the surgical cavity. The precise dose rate depends on the diameter of the applicator and the energy of the beam, both of which may be varied to optimize the radiation treatment. For example, a dose of 18–20 Gy at applicator surface, i.e., the tumor bed, can be delivered in about 25–35 min with a 3.5-cm applicator. The quick attenuation of the radiation minimizes the need for radiation protection to the operating personnel. Usually, the operating team leaves the room, but the anesthetist (and anyone else interested in observing the procedure) sits behind a mobile lead shield that prevents exposure. The technique has been previously described in detail [39], and an operative video is available on the Internet (https://www.youtube.com/watch?v=GVlHGpvRf8A).

Table 21.1 Some characteristics of intraoperative radiotherapy systems

Device	Company	Radiation type	Dose	Weight (kg)	Modification of operating room
Intrabeam	Carl Zeiss AG, Germany	Soft X-rays at 50 Kv	Physical dose of 20Gy next to the applicator (with a quick attenuation) over 25–30 min. Setting up time is about 10–12 min	1.8	Not usually required
Mobetron	Intraop Medical Inc, USA	Electrons at 4–12 MeV	20 Gy physical dose in 3–5 min. Setting up time is about 20 min	1275	Necessary
Novac-7	Hitesys SPA, Italy	Electrons at 4–12 MeV	20 Gy physical dose in 3–5 min Setting up time is about 20 min	650	Necessary

21.3.2 TARGIT IORT Surgical Technique (Fig. 21.1)

In the operating room, wide local excision of the primary tumor is carried out in the usual manner, with a margin of normal breast tissue. After the lumpectomy, it is important to achieve complete hemostasis, because even a small amount of bleeding in the 20–25 min during which radiotherapy is being delivered can distort the cavity enough to considerably change the dosimetry. Different size applicators are tried until one is found that fits snugly within the cavity. A purse string suture needs to be skillfully placed: it must pass through the breast parenchyma and appose it to the applicator surface, but at the same time, it must not bring the dermis too close to the applicator surface. It is important to protect the dermis, which should not be brought within 1 cm of the applicator surface. Fine prolene sutures can be used to slightly retract the skin edge away the applicator. However, complete eversion of the skin or using self-retaining retractors will increase the separation from the applicator so much that it would jeopardize the radiation dose and risk under treatment. The shaft does not emit any radiation, and there is no need to use a wet gauze to separate the wound from the shaft – this could separate the target subcutaneous breast tissues from the applicator surface and reduce the therapeutic radiation. In patients undergoing sentinel node sampling with immediate cytological or histological evaluation (so that complete axillary clearance can be carried out at the same sitting), TARGIT IORT can often be delivered while the surgical team waits for this result without wasting operating room time. With this elegant approach, the pliable breast tissue around the cavity of surgical excision wraps around the radiotherapy source, i.e., the target is "conformed" to the source. This simple, effective technique avoids the unnecessarily complex and sophisticated techniques of using interstitial implantation of radioactive wires or the even more complex techniques necessary for conformal radiotherapy by external beams with multi-leaf collimators from a linear accelerator. It eliminates "geographical miss" and delivers radiotherapy at the earliest possible time after surgery. The quick attenuation of the radiation dose protects normal tissues and allows the treatment to be carried out in unmodified operating theaters. Thus, in theory, the biological effect and cosmetic outcome could be improved.

The surgical part of the TARGIT IORT technique is simple and does *not* require extensive dissection around the breast, separating it from the skin anteriorly and the chest wall posteriorly, that is necessary to give intraoperative radiotherapy with other devices such as the Novac-7 used in the ELIOT trial. This means that it can be administered even under local anesthetic [41].

21.4 Randomised Clinical Trials of TARGIT Technique Using Intrabeam System

Based on the hypothesis that index quadrant irradiation is sufficient, in July 1998 we introduced the technique of targeted intraoperative radiotherapy (TARGIT) [37–39] delivered as a single dose using low-energy X-rays, targeted to the peritumoral tissues from within the breast using the Intrabeam device. In patients with small, hormone-positive breast cancers, which are now becoming the majority, this could be the sole radiotherapy treatment. The TARGIT-A trial tested whether single dose TARGIT IORT within a risk-adapted approach was non-inferior to conventional whole breast radiotherapy over several weeks. The TARGIT-B trial is testing whether a TARGIT IORT tumour bed boost is superior to externally delivered post-operative tumour bed boost in women who are either younger than 45 years or have a higher risk of local recurrence.

21.5 TARGIT IORT as the Sole Radiation Treatment within a Risk-Adapted Approach: The TARGIT-A Randomised Trial (Fig. 21.2)

TARGIT-A trial recruited 3451 patients between 24 March 2000 and June 2012. In this prospective, randomized, non-inferiority trial, women aged 45 years or older with invasive ductal breast carcinoma undergoing breast-conserving surgery were enrolled from 33 centers in 11 countries. Patients were randomly assigned in a 1:1 ratio to receive TARGIT or whole breast EBRT, with blocks stratified by center and by timing of delivery of targeted intraoperative radiotherapy: randomization occurred either before lumpectomy (the immediate (prepathology) stratum, TARGIT simultaneous with lumpectomy) or after lumpectomy (the delayed (postpathology) stratum, TARGIT given subsequently by reopening the wound). Such stratification allowed easier operation theater logistics and a more stringent case selection, but needed a reoperation to reopen the wound to give TARGIT as delayed procedure. Postoperative discovery of predefined factors (e.g., lobular carcinoma) could trigger addition of EBRT to TARGIT (in an expected 15 % of patients), making the experimental arm the risk-adapted approach, vis-a-vis the control arm which followed a

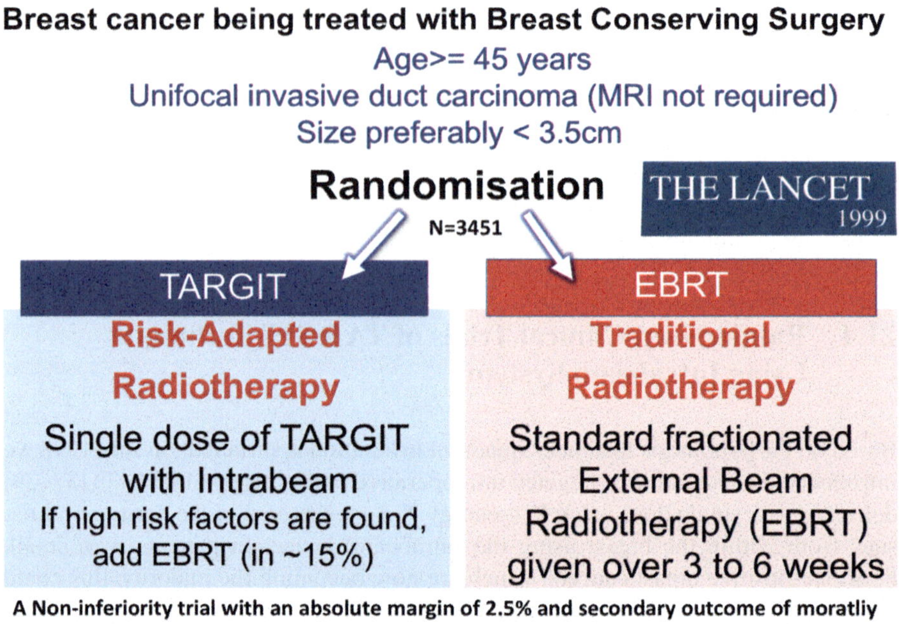

Fig. 21.2 TARGIT-A trial schema

one-size-fits-all policy. The primary outcome was absolute difference in local recurrence in the conserved breast, with a prespecified non-inferiority margin of 2.5% prespecified analyses included outcomes as per timing of randomization in relation to lumpectomy. Secondary outcomes included complications and mortality. A planned analyses were performed in 2010 after the initial accrual of 2232 patients [42] and again in 2012 after closure of the trial with an accrual of 3451 patients. For the second analysis, standard tests for non-inferiority were performed, and at this time for a log rank test for difference in survival, the significance level for p value was set at 0.01 for local recurrence as this was a second analysis for local recurrence and at 0.05 for mortality. In 2010, it was calculated that the number of participants needed to prove non-inferiority was 585.

For subgroup analysis, it was hypothesized that hormone sensitivity might be predictive of response to TARGIT and decided to analyze whether the response to radiotherapy in the TARGIT-A trial was dependent on hormone receptor responsiveness using progesterone receptor status as its marker, before the data were unblinded for the 2012 analysis. The effect of hormone sensitivity using progesterone receptor (PgR) status; timing of randomization/delivery of TARGIT; age; tumor grade; ER status; Her-2 status; presence of DCIS; margin status, whether screen detected or not; lymph-vascular invasion; and node status on the outcome were assessed in a Cox proportional hazard model.

The main analyses were also performed on patients in the prepathology stratum who were randomized in the first 8 years in the TARGIT-A trial. Details of some other analyses are also discussed here: the effect of omission of EBRT on (a) recurrence of breast cancer in quadrants of breast other than the index quadrant – the original hypothesis and on (b) axillary recurrence, (c) whether a beneficial effect of irradiation of tumor bed on the patient's microenvironment could contribute to the difference in non-breast-cancer mortality, (d) whether the higher threshold for margin positivity in the German cohort to add EBRT-improved outcomes, and (e) health economics.

21.5.1 Main Findings

These findings were published in the Lancet [40]. One thousand seven hundred twenty-one patients were randomized to TARGIT and 1730 to EBRT. Supplemental EBRT after TARGIT was necessary in 15.2 % [239 of 1571] of patients who received TARGIT (21.6 % prepathology, 3.6 % postpathology). Three thousand four hundred fifty-one patients had a median follow-up of 2 years and 5 months (IQR 12–52 months), 2020 of 4 years, and the first 1222 randomized patients (the earliest cohort, i.e., those randomized in the first 8 years of the trial) had a median follow-up of 5 years.

21.5.1.1 Five-Year Analysis of Local Recurrence and Survival

The test of non-inferiority in terms of control of local recurrence in the conserved breast found that TARGIT was non-inferior to EBRT for the whole trial (Pnon-inferiority=0.00000012) and for the prepathology stratum (Pnon-inferiority=0.0000000013), but not the postpathology stratum ($P_{non\text{-}inferiority}$=0.06640).

For the first 1222 patients randomized in the trial, the median follow-up was 5 years and the test for non-inferiority results found that TARGIT was non-inferior to EBRT in terms of local recurrence in the conserved breast when both strata were taken together $P_{non\text{-}inferiority}$=0.040), and for the prepathology stratum (Pnon-inferiority=0.00914), but not for the postpathology stratum ($P_{non\text{-}inferiority}$=0.35108).

The 5-year estimated risk for local recurrence in the conserved breast was 3.3 % (95 % CI 2.1–5.1) for TARGIT and 1.3 % (0.7–2.5) for EBRT. TARGIT simultaneously with lumpectomy (prepathology, $n=2298$) had much the same rate of local recurrence in the conserved breast as EBRT: 2.1 % (1.1–4.2) versus 1.1 % (0.5–2.5; $p=0.31$). With delayed TARGIT (postpathology, $n=1153$), the between-group difference in local recurrence was larger than 2.5 % (TARGIT 5.4 % [3.0–9.7] vs EBRT 1.7 % [0.6–4.9]; $p=0.069$).

Overall, breast cancer mortality was much the same between groups (2.6 % [1.5–4.3] for TARGIT vs 1.9 % [1.1–3.2] for EBRT; $p=0.56$), but there were significantly fewer non-breast-cancer deaths with TARGIT (1.4 % [0.8–2.5] vs 3.5 % [2.3–5.2]; $p=0.0086$), attributable to fewer deaths from cardiovascular causes and other cancers. Overall mortality was 3.9 % (2.7–5.8) for TARGIT versus 5.3 % (3.9–7.3) for EBRT ($p=0.099$).

For the preferred option of using TARGIT during initial lumpectomy, the breast cancer mortality was similar (TARGIT 17 deaths vs. EBRT 15 deaths, 5-year rates, 3.3 % [1.9–5.8] vs. 2.7 % [1.5–4.6], $p=0.72$, non-breast-cancer mortality was 12 patients for TARGIT and 27 patients for EBRT (1.3 %, [0.7–2.8] vs. 4.4 % [2.8–6.9], $p=0.016$). Overall mortality was numerically lower by 2.3 % with TARGIT 4.6 % [1.8–6.0] vs. 6.9 % [4.3–9.6], $p=0.12$. In this stratum when TARGIT is given simultaneously with lumpectomy, the 5-year survival without local recurrence was TARGIT 93.9 % (95 %CI 90.9–95.9) vs. EBRT 92.5 % (95 %CI 89.7–94.6), p value $=0.35$. These data are used to create a pictogram to help patients and doctors to make a shared well-informed decision about using TARGIT IORT during lumpectomy (Fig. 21.3) [43].

There were 817 patients randomized in the first 8 years of the trial in the prepathology stratum. The median follow-up was 5.01 years. For local recurrence in the conserved breast, TARGIT was non-inferior to EBRT ($P_{non\text{-}inferiorty}=0.00914$). The 5-year Kaplan-Meier estimated risks were statistically not different for local recurrence TARGIT 1.8 % (95 % CI 0.84–4.2) vs. EBRT 0.84 %(0.3–2.6), $p=0.32$, and for deaths from breast cancer TARGIT 3.9 % (2.3–6.7) vs. EBRT 3.0 % (1.7–5.4), $p=0.34$. There were significantly fewer deaths from causes other than breast cancer with TARGIT 1.9 % (0.9–3.9) vs. EBRT 5.1 %(3.2–8.0), $p=0.04$. It should be noted that the number needed to

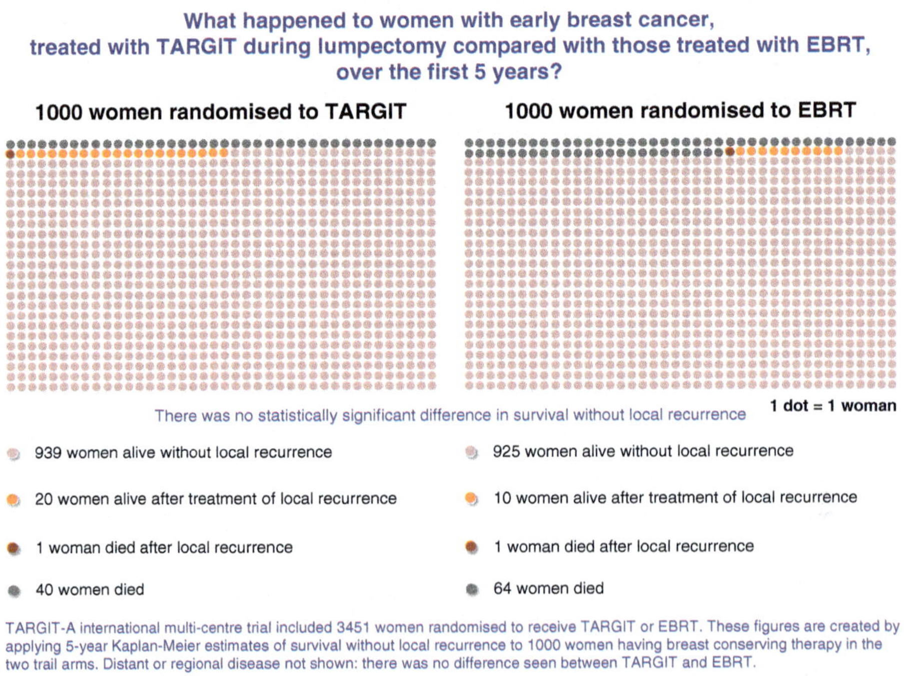

Fig. 21.3 A pictogram to help patients and doctors to make a shared well-informed decision about using TARGIT IORT during lumpectomy

prove non-inferiority was calculated to be 585, and therefore, this earliest cohort of 817 patients has enough power to draw reliable conclusions.

21.5.1.2 Local Toxicity

The frequency of any complications and major toxicity was similar in the two groups (for major toxicity, TARGIT, 37 [3.3 %] of 1113 vs. EBRT, 44 [3.9 %] of 1119; $p=0.44$). Radiotherapy toxicity (Radiation Therapy Oncology Group grade 3) was lower in the TARGIT group (six patients [0.5 %]) than in the EBRT group (23 patients [2.1 %]; $p=0.002$). In the second analysis in 2012, among complications 6 months after surgery, wound-related complications were much the same between groups, but grade 3 or 4 skin complications were significantly reduced with TARGIT (four of 1720 vs 13 of 1731, $p=0.029$).

21.5.2 Subgroup Analysis

In PgR-positive cases ($n=2462$), there was no significant difference between the two arms (TARGIT vs. EBRT) in terms of the 5-year risk of local recurrence 2.3 %(1.3–4.3) vs. 1.49 %(0.75–3.0) $p=0.51$, while in PgR-negative cases, local recurrence was higher in the TARGIT arm 7.0 %(3.5–13.6) vs. 0.5 %(0.1–3.7) $p=0.017$. In the large group of 1625 PgR-positive cases in the prepathology stratum, breast cancer control with TARGIT was similar to EBRT (5-year risk of local recurrence 1.4 %(0.5–3.9) vs. 1.2 %(0.5–2.9) $p=0.77$ and breast cancer mortality: 1.78 %(0.7–4.4) vs. 1.98 %(0.94–4.2) $p=0.9$) while mortality from other causes was reduced with TARGIT 1.59 %(0.7–3.4) vs. 4.51 %(2.8–7.3), $p=0.04$, leading to a 3.1 % reduction in overall mortality 3.3 %(1.83–6.04) vs. 6.4 %(4.3–9.6), $p=0.08$. Margin status was a predictive factor only in the EBRT arm. Other factors did not influence the outcomes.

21.5.3 Other Analyses

a. *Other quadrant recurrences*: 94.4 % of cases in the TARGIT-A trial did not have a preoperative MRI. Seven hundred ninety-three patients in the prepathology stratum randomized to TARGIT had only TARGIT as their radiotherapy. With 2098 women years of follow-up, there were nine recurrences in the conserved breast. The 5-year local recurrence rate in those who received TARGIT alone was 2.7 % (95 % CI 1.3–5.5), which was not different from the whole prepathology cohort randomized to TARGIT 2.1 % (1.1–4.2). In these 793 patients, one would expect 63 % (i.e., 500) of patients to have additional foci of cancer in their breasts, and 80 % of these (i.e., 400) should be in quadrants other than the index quadrant. In reality, seven patients had recurrence in the scar, six had new contralateral cancers, and 2 had cancers growing in other quadrants – implying that the remaining potential 398 foci had remained dormant. Among 935 patients who received whole breast radiotherapy, the same number of cancers ($n=2$) occurred in other quadrants, and there were five new contralateral cancers. Therefore, cancer foci in breast that are away from the site of the primary tumor remained dormant and behaved no differently from those in the contralateral breast. They also appeared to be unaffected by whole breast radiotherapy. This analysis from the randomized TARGIT-A trial further vindicates the initial hypothesis upon which the trial was predicated and provides evidence supporting partial breast irradiation.

b. *Axillary recurrence*: We found that omission of EBRT did not increase axillary recurrence when analyzed as per treatment received: the number of axillary recurrences were 5/1613 when EBRT was not given vs. 6/1762 when EBRT was given; 5-year risks 0.68 %[95 %CI 0.28–1.6] vs. 0.82 %[0.34=2.02], hazard ratio 0.84[0.26–2.74, $p=0.8$].

c. *Reduction in non-breast-cancer mortality as a potential beneficial effect of TARGIT*: We found that among the 1730 patients randomized to receive EBRT, the 8 cardiac deaths were not significantly different from the 12 estimated based on age, sex, and follow-up period. Most interestingly, there were no deaths from non-breast-cancer causes in the TARGIT+EBRT group compared with 24 in the EBRT group 0/218 vs. 24/892, log-rank $p=0.012$. Although the numbers are small and follow-up relatively short, these data may suggest that EBRT toxicity can lead to excess non-breast-cancer deaths, or that there is a local effect of TARGIT on the tumor bed caused by inhibiting the cancer-stimulating cytokines, which may spill over to reduce systemic inflammatory response to trauma and have significant long-term systemic beneficial effects, that might be protective against cardiac and cancer mortality [44]. This hypothesis seems farfetched. However, it is testable, and the TARGIT-B trial (see below) provides the ideal experimental model (TARGIT-Boost+EBRT vs EBRT Boost+EBRT) to test it.

d. *Adequacy of 1 mm as threshold for negative margin*: Additional EBRT was given in nearly twice the number of patients in the TARGIT arm in the German centers (prompted by the higher limit of 10-mm tumor-free margin) compared with the rest of the trial population (31.3 % (96/306) vs. 17.4 %(123/706). However, the 5-year local recurrence rate in the German cohort was not lower than the rest of the world: German 2.6 % (95 % CI 0.87–7.8) vs. rest of the world 1.9 % (95 % CI 0.81–4.5). Therefore, a policy of adding EBRT after TARGIT only when the margin is less than 1 mm appears appropriate.

e. *Health economic analyses*: Suggest that if TARGIT were given instead of EBRT in suitable patients, it would significantly reduce costs to the healthcare providers. The estimates vary between £65 million GBP in the UK to $1.4 billion USD in the USA over 5 years. Furthermore, each patient who avoids EBRT would save between £402 and £957 depending on whether they would have used public transport or their own car (2011 prices).

f. *Cosmetic and breast-related quality of life outcomes*: TARGIT-A trial participants from the post-pathology stratification in Western Australia participated in a cosmesis and quality of life sub-study. There was a trend for greater proportions of TARGIT patients self-reporting an Excellent/Good result compared to EBRT patients, but the difference was not statistically significant. TARGIT patients fared better than EBRT patients in breast-related quality of life and clinically significant differences were seen at the 6-month and 1-year time points (data presented in 9th Intrabeam User Meeting, Germany 2015).

g. *Patient Preference*: Hypothetical patient preference studies have consistently shown that patients are willing to trade risk of local recurrence for the convenience and different side effect profile of IORT. Posttreatment, 65 % of surveyed TARGIT-A patients considered IORT an acceptable treatment option even with a higher risk [45], and 83 % of recently diagnosed patients yet to have any radiotherapy felt the same way (data presented in 9th Intrabeam User Meeting, Germany 2015). Hypothetically, if all treatment modalities offered equivalent outcomes, 13 % of pretreatment patients chose EBRT, 26 % chose IORT as separate procedure, and 61 % chose IORT during lumpectomy as their preferred option.

21.5.4 Summary of TARGIT-A Trial Results

In cases selected as per the TARGIT-A trial protocol, TARGIT during lumpectomy compared with EBRT results in non-inferior local control, similar mortality from breast cancer, and statistically significantly reduced mortality from non-breast-cancer causes.

Subgroup analysis found that PgR status influenced the outcome of patients overall and those randomized to TARGIT; margin status influenced the outcome of those randomized to EBRT. Other patient or tumor factors had no significant influence on the outcome of patients randomized in the two arms. It appears that hormone receptor positivity identifies a group in which local control with TARGIT during lumpectomy is very similar to EBRT.

Other analyses provide further evidence supporting limited irradiation and suggest new hypothesis as well as demonstrating the cost-effectiveness of TARGIT. For appropriate use of TARGIT IORT, we have developed an app for use on both iOS and Android smartphone systems. It can be found on the respective app stores by searching for “TARGIT decision.”

The Adequacy of Follow-Up Several large randomized trials of radiotherapy have found that the effect of radiotherapy is on local recurrence in mostly in the first 2–3 years and almost all of it is seen in the first 5 years. A difference seen at 5 years does not increase with longer follow-up of up to 25 years. Therefore, these results are based on sufficient number of patients (1222 patients with a median follow-up of 5 years) whose follow-up that is long enough to allow a change of practice. However, as breast cancer is a chronic illness, we are committed to longer follow-up (the protocol aims for a 10-year follow-up of all patients) for ethical, moral, scientific, and academic reasons, as with higher number of events, which will accrue with time, could allow for a more in-depth analyses and refinement of our understanding.

21.5.5 Conclusion from the TARGIT-A Trial

For patients with breast cancer selected as per the TARGIT-A trial protocol (women who are 45 years of age and older with unifocal hormone sensitive invasive ductal carcinoma that is up to 3.5 cm in size), TARGIT concurrent with lumpectomy within a risk-adapted approach is as effective and safer alternative to postoperative EBRT.

21.6 TARGIT IORT as a Tumor Bed Boost: The TARGIT-B Trial (Fig. 21.4)

In the pilot studies in the UK the USA, Australia, Germany, and Italy testing the feasibility and safety of the technique, TARGIT IORT was used as "boost" dose [46, 47] and also received whole breast EBRT. This was not a low-risk group. A third of the patients were younger than 51 years, 57 % of cancers were between 1 to 2 cm, (21 % >2 cm), 29 % had a grade 3 tumor, and 29 % were node positive. Among these 300 cases, the 5-year actuarial recurrence rate was 1.73 % (SE 0.77). This compares very favorably with the recurrence rates achieved in recent trials of radiotherapy (see Table 21.2) despite having a cohort of patients with a worse prognosis. It appears that given as a boost, TARGIT IORT yields very low recurrence rates. TARGIT is already used a standard option for the routine tumor bed boost in many centers and is in the German radiation oncology guidelines of the year 2008. While we recognize that TARGIT boost is at least equivalent to conventional EBRT boost, we believe that there is pathological, biological (geographical and temporal accuracy), mathematical modeling, and clinical evidence to suggest that it is likely to be superior. Therefore, the TARGIT-Boost trial, funded by the UK Department of Health (Health Technology Assessment programme) is currently recruiting patients

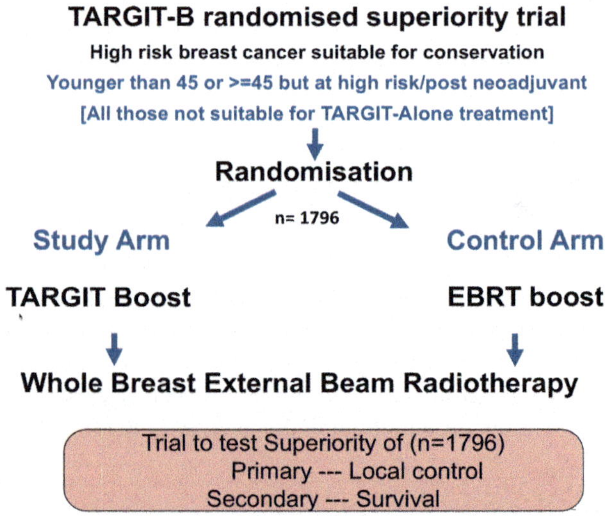

Fig. 21.4 TARGIT-B trial schema

Table 21.2 Comparison of TARGIT IORT Boost with recent clinical trial data

High-risk factors	EORTC boost [8]	START-B trial [9]	TARGIT boost
Young age	37 % (<=50)	21 % (<50)	32 % (<50)
% >1 cm	75 %	86 %	78 %
% Grade 3	N/A	23 %	29 %
% Node + ve %	21 %	23.6 %	29 %
Recurrence rate at 5 years	**4.3 %**	**2.8 %**	**1.73 %**

from over 20 centers. This trial is aimed to ascertain whether a TARGIT-Boost yields a lower recurrence rate than EBRT Boost in higher-risk or young patients.

21.7 Conclusion

Over 250 centers in 31 countries around the world already use TARGIT IORT, and over 15,000 patients have been treated with the TARGIT technique. It is already in many national guidelines and approval for NHS funding for its use is underway. Unlike most other "new" treatments, this one may be actually be less expensive than the current standard!

Mere novelty and the convenience of new technology should not come in the way of its proper scientific assessment before it is used for standard care. Randomized clinical trials are essential to test this revolutionary approach. And, when randomized trials are performed, one should take heed of the results and allow them to change our prior, albeit long-held notions.

We believe that the future for local treatment of breast cancer could be tailored to the needs of the patient and the tumor. The patient, the surgeon, and the radiation oncologist will be able to choose from several well-tested approaches. This may mean not just wider availability of breast-conserving therapy, but also that small incremental benefits from targeted and tailored treatment may reduce morbidity and even mortality.

References

1. Deng G, Lu Y, Zlotnikov G, Thor AD, Smith HS. Loss of heterozygosity in normal tissue adjacent to breast carcinomas. Science. 1996;274(5295):2057–9.
2. Belletti B, Vaidya JS, D'Andrea S, Entschladen F, Roncadin M, Lovat F, Berton S, Perin T, Candiani E, Reccanello S, Veronesi A, Canzonieri V, Trovo MG, Zaenker KS, Colombatti A, Baldassarre G, Massarut S. Targeted intraoperative radiotherapy impairs the stimulation of breast cancer cell proliferation and invasion caused by surgical wounding. Clin Cancer Res (An Official Journal of the American Association for Cancer Research). 2008;14(5):1325–32.
3. Vaidya JS, Baum M, Tobias JS, Wenz F, Massarut S, Keshtgar M, Hilaris B, Saunders C, Williams NR, Brew-Graves C, Corica T, Roncadin M, Kraus-Tiefenbacher U, Sutterlin M, Bulsara M, Joseph D. Long-term results of targeted intraoperative radiotherapy (TARGIT) boost during breast-conserving surgery. Int J Radiat Oncol Biol Phys. 2011;81(4):1091–7.

4.Early Breast Cancer Trialists' Collaborative Group (EBCTCG). Effect of radiotherapy after breast-conserving surgery on 10-year recurrence and 15-year breast cancer death: meta-analysis of individual patient data for 10,801 women in 17 randomised trials. Lancet. 2011;378(9804):1707–16.
5.Early Breast Cancer Trialists' Collaborative Group. Effects of radiotherapy and of differences in the extent of surgery for early breast cancer on local recurrence and 15-year survival: an overview of the randomised trials. Lancet. 2005;366(9503):2087–106.
6.Early Breast Cancer Trialists' Collaborative Group. Favourable and unfavourable effects on long-term survival of radiotherapy for early breast cancer: an overview of the randomised trials. Lancet. 2000;355(9217):1757–70.
7.Early Breast Cancer Trialists' Collaborative Group. Effects of radiotherapy and surgery in early breast cancer. An overview of the randomized trials. N Engl J Med. 1995;333(22):1444–55.
8.Halsted WS. The results of operations for the cure of cancer of the breast performed at The Johns Hopkins Hospital from June 1889 to January 1894. Johns Hopkins Hospital Reports. 1894;4:297–350.
9.Katz SJ, Lantz PM, Janz NK, Fagerlin A, Schwartz K, Liu L, Deapen D, Salem B, Lakhani I, Morrow M. Patient involvement in surgery treatment decisions for breast cancer. J Clin Oncol. 2005;23(24):5526–33.
10. Athas WF, Adams-Cameron M, Hunt WC, Amir-Fazli A, Key CR. Travel distance to radiation therapy and receipt of radiotherapy following breast-conserving surgery. J Natl Cancer Inst. 2000;92(3):269–71.
11. Sedlmayer F, Rahim HB, Kogelnik HD, Menzel C, Merz F, Deutschmann H, Kranzinger M. Quality assurance in breast cancer brachytherapy: geographic miss in the interstitial boost treatment of the tumor bed. Int J Radiat Oncol Biol Phys. 1996;34(5):1133–9.
12. Machtay M, Lanciano R, Hoffman J, Hanks GE. Inaccuracies in using the lumpectomy scar for planning electron boosts in primary breast carcinoma. Int J Radiat Oncol Biol Phys. 1994;30(1):43–8.
13. Wyatt RM, Beddoe AH, Dale RG. The effects of delays in radiotherapy treatment on tumour control. Phys Med Biol. 2003;48(2):139–55.
14. Mikeljevic JS, Haward R, Johnston C, Crellin A, Dodwell D, Jones A, Pisani P, Forman D. Trends in postoperative radiotherapy delay and the effect on survival in breast cancer patients treated with conservation surgery. Br J Cancer. 2004;90(7):1343–8.
15. Massarut S, Baldassare G, Belleti B, Reccanello S, D'Andrea S, Ezio C, Perin T, Roncadin M, Vaidya JS. Intraoperative radiotherapy impairs breast cancer cell motility induced by surgical wound fluid. J Clin Oncol. 2006;24(18S):10611.
16. Baldassarre G, Belleti B, Vaidya JS, D'Andrea S, Roncadin M, Perin T, Trova MG, Candiani E, Veronesi A, Colombatti A, Massarut S. Intraoperative radiotherapy (IORT) impairs surgical wound-stimulated breast cancer cell invasion. J Clin Oncol. 2007;25(18S):21139.
17. Rutqvist LE, Johansson H. Mortality by laterality of the primary tumour among 55,000 breast cancer patients from the Swedish Cancer Registry. Br J Cancer. 1990;61(6):866–8.
18. O'Neill JS, Elton RA, Miller WR. Aromatase activity in adipose tissue from breast quadrants: a link with tumour site. Br Med J (Clin Res Ed). 1988;296(6624):741–43.
19. Nakamura J, Savinov A, Lu Q, Brodie A. Estrogen regulates vascular endothelial growth/permeability factor expression in 7,12-dimethylbenz(a)anthracene-induced rat mammary tumors. Endocrinology. 1996;137(12):5589–96.
20. Lu Q, Nakmura J, Savinov A, Yue W, Weisz J, Dabbs DJ, Wolz G, Brodie A. Expression of aromatase protein and messenger ribonucleic acid in tumor epithelial cells and evidence of functional significance of locally produced estrogen in human breast cancers. Endocrinology. 1996;137(7):3061–8.
21. Turner BC, Gumbs AA, Carbone CJ, Carter D, Glazer PM, Haffty BG. Mutant p53 protein overexpression in women with ipsilateral breast tumor recurrence following lumpectomy and radiation therapy. Cancer. 2000;88(5):1091–8.
22. Turner BC, Harrold E, Matloff E, Smith T, Gumbs AA, Beinfield M, Ward B, Skolnick M, Glazer PM, Thomas A, Haffty BG. BRCA1/BRCA2 germline mutations in locally recurrent

breast cancer patients after lumpectomy and radiation therapy: implications for breast-conserving management in patients with BRCA1/BRCA2 mutations [see comments]. J Clin Oncol. 1999;17(10):3017–24.
23. Vaidya JS, Vyas JJ, Chinoy RF, Merchant N, Sharma OP, Mittra I. Multicentricity of breast cancer: whole-organ analysis and clinical implications. Br J Cancer. 1996;74(5):820–4.
24. Baum M, Vaidya JS. Molecular staging of cancer [letter; comment]. Lancet. 1997;350(9082):962.
25. Nielsen M, Thomsen JL, Primdahl S, Dyreborg U, Andersen JA. Breast cancer and atypia among young and middle-aged women: a study of 110 medicolegal autopsies. Br J Cancer. 1987;56(6):814–9.
26. Bartelink H, Horiot JC, Poortmans P, Struikmans H, Van den Bogaert W, Barillot I, Fourquet A, Borger J, Jager J, Hoogenraad W, Collette L, Pierart M, European Organization for Research and Treatment of Cancer Radiotherapy and Breast Cancer Groups. Recurrence rates after treatment of breast cancer with standard radiotherapy with or without additional radiation. N Engl J Med. 2001;345(19):1378–87.
27. Clark RM, Wilkinson RH, Mahoney LJ, Reid JG, MacDonald WD. Breast cancer: a 21 year experience with conservative surgery and radiation. Int J Radiat Oncol Biol Phys. 1982;8(6):967–79.
28. McCulloch PG, MacIntyre A. Effects of surgery on the generation of lymphokine-activated killer cells in patients with breast cancer. Br J Surg. 1993;80(8):1005–07.
29. Clarke DH, Martinez AA. Identification of patients who are at high risk for locoregional breast cancer recurrence after conservative surgery and radiotherapy: a review article for surgeons, pathologists, and radiation and medical oncologists [see comments]. J Clin Oncol. 1992;10(3):474–83.
30. Fisher B, Anderson S, Redmond CK, Wolmark N, Wickerham DL, Cronin WM. Reanalysis and results after 12 years of follow-up in a randomized clinical trial comparing total mastectomy with lumpectomy with or without irradiation in the treatment of breast cancer. N Engl J Med. 1995;333(22):1456–61.
31. Clark RM, Whelan T, Levine M, Roberts R, Willan A, McCulloch P, Lipa M, Wilkinson RH, Mahoney LJ. Randomized clinical trial of breast irradiation following lumpectomy and axillary dissection for node-negative breast cancer: an update. Ontario Clinical Oncology Group. J Natl Cancer Inst. 1996;88(22):1659–64.
32. Liljegren G, Holmberg L, Bergh J, Lindgren A, Tabar L, Nordgren H, Adami HO. 10-Year results after sector resection with or without postoperative radiotherapy for stage I breast cancer: a randomized trial [see comments]. J Clin Oncol. 1999;17(8):2326–33.
33. Forrest AP, Stewart HJ, Everington D, Prescott RJ, McArdle CS, Harnett AN, Smith DC, George WD. Randomised controlled trial of conservation therapy for breast cancer: 6-year analysis of the Scottish trial. Scottish Cancer Trials Breast Group [see comments]. Lancet. 1996;348(9029):708–13.
34. Veronesi U, Luini A, Del Vecchio M, Greco M, Galimberti V, Merson M, Rilke F, Sacchini V, Saccozzi R, Savio T. Radiotherapy after breast-preserving surgery in women with localized cancer of the breast [see comments]. N Engl J Med. 1993;328(22):1587–91.
35. Vaidya JS, Tobias JS, Baum M, Keshtgar M, Joseph D, Wenz F, Houghton J, Saunders C, Corica T, D'Souza D, Sainsbury R, Massarut S, Taylor I, Hilaris B. Intraoperative radiotherapy for breast cancer. Lancet Oncol. 2004;5(3):165–73.
36. Azria D, Larbouret C, Cunat S, Ozsahin M, Gourgou S, Martineau P, Evans DB, Romieu G, Pujol P, Pelegrin A. Letrozole sensitizes breast cancer cells to ionizing radiation. Breast Cancer Res. 2005;7(1):R156–63.
37. Vaidya JS, Baum M, Tobias JS, D'Souza DP, Naidu SV, Morgan S, Metaxas M, Harte KJ, Sliski AP, Thomson E. Targeted intra-operative radiotherapy (Targit): an innovative method of treatment for early breast cancer. Ann Oncol (Official Journal of the European Society for Medical Oncology/ESMO). 2001;12(8):1075–80.
38. Vaidya JS, Baum M, Tobias JS, Houghton J. Targeted intraoperative radiothearpy (TARGIT)-trial protocol. Lancet. 1999. http://www.thelancet.com/protocol-reviews/99PRT-47.

39. Vaidya JS, Baum M, Tobias JS, Morgan S, D'Souza D. The novel technique of delivering targeted intraoperative radiotherapy (Targit) for early breast cancer. Eur J Surg Oncol (The Journal of the European Society of Surgical Oncology and the British Association of Surgical Oncology). 2002;28(4):447–54.
40. Vaidya JS, Wenz F, Bulsara M, Tobias JS, Joseph DJ, Keshtgar M, Flyger HL, Massarut S, Alvarado M, Saunders C, Eiermann W, Metaxas M, Sperk E, Sutterlin M, Brown D, Esserman L, Roncadin M, Thompson A, Dewar JA, Holtveg HM, Pigorsch S, Falzon M, Harris E, Matthews A, Brew-Graves C, Potyka I, Corica T, Williams NR, Baum M, TARGIT Trialists' Group. Risk-adapted targeted intraoperative radiotherapy versus whole-breast radiotherapy for breast cancer: 5-year results for local control and overall survival from the TARGIT-A randomised trial. Lancet. 2014;383(9917):603–13.
41. Vaidya JS, Walton L, Dewar J. Single dose targeted intraoperative radiotherapy (TARGIT) for breast cancer can be delivered as a second procedure under local anaesthetic. World J Surg Oncol. 2006;4:2.
42. Vaidya JS, Joseph DJ, Tobias JS, Bulsara M, Wenz F, Saunders C, Alvarado M, Flyger HL, Massarut S, Eiermann W, Keshtgar M, Dewar J, Kraus-Tiefenbacher U, Sutterlin M, Esserman L, Holtveg HM, Roncadin M, Pigorsch S, Metaxas M, Falzon M, Matthews A, Corica T, Williams NR, Baum M. Targeted intraoperative radiotherapy versus whole breast radiotherapy for breast cancer (TARGIT-A trial): an international, prospective, randomised, non-inferiority phase 3 trial. Lancet. 2010;376(9735):91–102.
43. Vaidya JS, Bulsara M, Wenz F, Joseph D, Saunders C, Massarut S, Flyger H, Eiermann W, Alvarado M, Esserman L, Falzon M, Brew-Graves C, Potyka I, Tobias J, Baum M. Pride, Prejudice, or Science – attitudes towards the results of the TARGIT-A trial of targeted intraoperative radiotherapy for breast cancer. Int J Radiat Oncol Biol Phys. 2015;92(3):491–7.
44. Vaidya JS, Bulsara M, Wenz F. Ischemic heart disease after breast cancer radiotherapy. N Engl J Med. 2013;368(26):2526–7.
45. Corica T, Nowak A, Saunders C, Bulsara M, Joseph D. Patient preferences for adjuvant radiotherapy in early breast cancer – an Australian Sub-study of the International TARGIT Trial. Eur J Cancer. 2012;48(Suppl 1):S187: Abstract 482.
46. Vaidya JS, Baum M, Tobias JS, Wenz F, Massarut S, Keshtgar M, Hilaris B, Saunders C, Williams N, Brew-Graves C, Corica T, Roncadin M, Kraus-Tiefenbacher U, Sutterlin M, Bulsara M, Joseph D. Long term results of targeted intraoperative radiotherapy (Targit) boost during breast conserving surgery. Int J Radiat Oncol Biol Phys. 2011;81(4):7.
47. Vaidya JS, Baum M, Tobias JS, Massarut S, Wenz F, Murphy O, Hilaris B, Houghton J, Saunders C, Corica T, Roncadin M, Kraus-Tiefenbacher U, Melchaert F, Keshtgar M, Sainsbury R, Douek M, Harrison E, Thompson A, Joseph D. Targeted intraoperative radiotherapy (TARGIT) yields very low recurrence rates when given as a boost. Int J Radiat Oncol Biol Phys. 2006;66(5):1335–8.

Chapter 22
Intraoperative Technique with Electrons

Claire Lemanski and David Azria

Contents

Intraoperative radiation therapy (IORT) is based on a single dose of ionizing radiation delivered during surgery, affording a very precise application of a high dose to a precise target volume, with a minimal exposure to healthy tissues which are usually moved or protected during the procedure. IORT delivered with electrons was developed in the late 1970s and was initially dedicated to deep-seated or radioresistant tumors (such as with pancreatic cancer, retroperitoneal sarcomas) or locoregional pelvic relapses in previously irradiated volumes.

This technique requires trained teams and specific equipment and has been available only in isolated institutions until the last decade. However, today IORT is slowly experiencing a new "birth" with its developing role in early-stage breast cancer. In this indication, IORT offers utmost precision in the delineation of the treatment volume and the sparing of normal breast tissue leading to an optimal cosmetic result.

Two independent observations provide support for the concept of intraoperative delivery of post lumpectomy radiation. First, breast cancer has demonstrated a high sensitivity to high doses per fraction [1], and IORT offers the unique opportunity to deliver extremely high doses in one procedure and a time of optimal oxygenation of the tumor bed and better radiosensitivity. Second, it has also been hypothesized that

C. Lemanski (✉) • D. Azria
Department of Radiation Oncology and Medical Physics, I.C.M. Institute Regional du Cancer Montpellier, Montpellier Cedex 5 34298, France
e-mail: Claire.Lemanski@icm.unicancer.fr; azria@valdorel.fnclcc.fr

D.W. Arthur et al. (eds.), *Short Course Breast Radiotherapy: A Comprehensive Review of Hypofractionation, Partial Breast, and Intra-Operative Irradiation*,
DOI 10.1007/978-3-319-24388-7_22

immediate irradiation during surgery abrogates the proliferative cascade induced by the surgical wound healing on the tumor microenvironment [2]. While an interesting concept observed in vitro, these data need to be confirmed in clinical ongoing research [3]. Today, the growing use of IORT for the treatment of breast cancer is greatly facilitated by the safety and efficacy demonstrated by the accelerated partial-breast irradiation (APBI) treatment concept [4–6] and the technical development of lightweight mobile accelerators with simplified use, delivering 50 kV photons or electrons. Within the general concept of APBI, IORT explores dose delivery acceleration to its extreme with its very seductive one fraction scheme.

22.1 Equipment

The differences in equipment depend on the history of each center. In Montpellier, we had the ability to initiate and develop IORT for breast cancer very early with initiation in the late 1980s. We had the advantage of having a treatment machine already in place that was originally dedicated for IORT for gastrointestinal tumors and complex pelvic relapses. This treatment machine was a linear accelerator, Saturne 20 of Varian™, able to deliver electron beams with energy ranging from 6 to 13 MeV. Additionally, it was ideally located in a sealed bunker within an operating theater.

With this setup, the anesthetized patient was moved over to the accelerator at the appropriate time during the surgical procedure and treatment dose delivered to the defined target. This privileged and unique situation in Europe and North America, at that time, was reserved for only a few treatment teams that were usually invested in IORT for deep tumors with a multidisciplinary aggressive and specific treatment approach.

At the end of the 1990s, new lightweight and mobile accelerators were available and able to deliver electron beams with energies ranging from 3 to 10 MeV. The machine mobility allowed both the surgery and IORT to be performed with the patient in one position on the operating table, avoiding the need to move the patient to the accelerator. Radiation protection for the physicians and operating room personnel requires the addition of mobile barriers around the operating table to provide needed shielding, and all personnel are required to leave the room at the time of treatment.

22.1.1 Radiosurgical Modalities and IORT Procedure

The technique is straightforward and quite simple, but, is based on optimal cooperation between the surgeons and radiation oncologists.

The tumor removal is realized in the same way as any standard breast surgery: Lumpectomy is performed with a direct incision, centered on the tumor in lesions located in the outer aspects of the breast or a periareolar incision with lesions located in inner/medial locations. The excision extends deeply to the fascia of the pectoralis major muscle.

IORT requires dedicated personnel for the intraoperative pathology specimen handling and evaluation. At the time of tumor removal, the specimen must be analyzed during the surgical procedure for size and histology and to ensure margins are not involved. This allows for immediate re-excision if necessary. Axillary lymph node dissection or sentinel node sampling is classically performed [7–9].

Following confirmation of appropriate surgical excision, treatment with electrons is delivered through long cylindrical collimators that are very different from the spherical applicators used with photons. Glandular tissue surrounding the excision cavity is surgically mobilized, from the fascia and from the skin, to expose the limits of the resection cavity to the radiation field. The target is temporarily approximated by sutures to maintain its location within the radiation planning target volume [7].

A shielding device may be added at this time in order to protect underlying organs. If necessary, a dedicated 5-mm-thick lead disk (available in various diameters) is then inserted between the pectoral muscle and the mobilized gland. In our experience, these protective devices are only used for inferior left-breast tumors. In this unique situation the customized shielding is used in order to protect the heart and the anterior coronary arteries. The need is most appropriate in thin patients with a small breast when we estimate that the thickness of the gland and thoracic wall is small enough that additional shielding is needed to avoid unnecessary and potentially toxic radiation dose delivery to the heart. The applicator tubes are then placed under visual control by the radiation oncologist in conjunction with the surgeon to encompass the entire tumor bed so as to avoid a geographical miss. The collimator diameter (ranging in our experience from 40 to 60 mm) is selected to offer the perfect coverage of the entire tumor bed plus a safe margin and is placed directly in contact with the mobilized gland. The skin is then assured and maintained to be out of the radiation field with the use of Beckman spacers and, if necessary, with additional sterile gauze creating an additional tissue-equivalent barrier. This further protects the skin from the low-energy electrons scattered around the collimator's edges.

The gland thickness is measured with a needle, perpendicularly inserted through the gland mobilized down to the fascia of the pectoralis major muscle, and based on this thickness the appropriate electron energy is chosen to assure the target is covered with the intended dose.

The patient is then moved into the appropriate location and the applicator connected to the accelerator. As discussed, the need for patient movement can be avoided today in centers equipped with mobile electron accelerators available directly in the operative room.

The dose is then prescribed, according to the indication (boost or APBI). The duration of the actual radiation dose delivery depends on the equipment and on the level of energy, but remains much shorter as compared to the delivery of IORT with 50 kV photons. Typical intraoperative electron treatment times vary between 3 and 10 min.

Once the full dose has been delivered, the patient is then brought back to the surgical room (as in our arrangement) or the accelerator removed from the surgical area (in the case of mobile accelerator use). The case is then moved toward completion with the temporary sutures cut and the applicator removed. The tumor cavity is then remodeled and the incision closed in a conventional fashion. Typically, there is no drain placed and no perioperative antibiotic prophylaxis specifically prescribed for the IORT procedure.

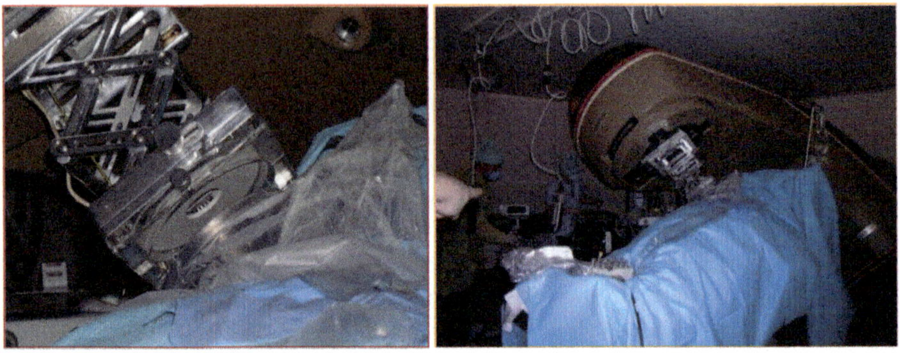

22.2 Physics and Dose

The linear accelerator used for IORT provides multiple variations to allow an optimal personalization of the treatment.

There is a range of applicators with diameters up to 100 mm; however, where at our institution the maximal tumor size is restricted to ≤30 mm, we are selecting an applicator between 40 and 60 mm diameter. The angle of approach can be flat or 15–45° with the use of a movable arm allowing for a patient unique setup for ideal coverage of the tumor bed.

Additionally, there is a range of energy levels available for the electron beam. The collection is machine dependent with a range from 6 to 13 MeV for the linear accelerator-based IORT or from 3 to 12 MeV for the three Italian mobile accelerators Novac™, 7 Liac™, and Mobetron™.

The electrons offer a very homogenous dose. A dose of 10Gy is prescribed to the depth of the 90% isodose line when used as a boost and then followed with a dose of 50Gy with the addition of external-beam whole-breast radiotherapy (WBRT). When IORT is used as the only form of adjuvant radiotherapy, a 21 Gy dose is delivered to the target.

22.2.1 Treatment Results

22.2.1.1 Electrons for Boost

When the IORT is used as a boost, it is always followed with the addition of standard 50 Gy to the whole-breast target. This treatment approach can be used for all the tumors suitable for breast-conserving therapy according to the classic selection criteria. IORT delivers, in this case, a high dose in the region with the highest probability of recurrence.

Started in 1989 in Montpellier and then in Italy and Austria, the results after using IORT as a boost have been reported with mature results [10]. However, it should be noted that no phase III trial has been ever conducted.

In 2006, we published the first retrospective cohort with a median follow up of 9 years (range 5–15 years). The IORT boost was delivered at the time of surgical resection with a median dose of 10 Gy and then followed with 50 Gy WBRT. Among 50 patients, two experienced late local relapses (10 %) occurring 8 and 14 years after the surgery. Cosmetic results were good to excellent [7].

With similar patient selection and treatment approach, an Austrian retrospective match-pair analysis between 188 patients treated with external-beam boost was compared to 188 similar patients treated with an IORT boost This publication observed a reduction of the 4-year local recurrence rate with the use of IORT, 4–0 %, and appeared to be confirmed in the reporting of the 10-year local recurrence rate, from 7.2 to 1.6 % [11].

A retrospective pooled analysis was recently published by the International Society of Intraoperative Radiotherapy (ISIORT) to evaluate the long-term results of the IORT boost strategy [12]. 1109 patients from Austria, Germany, Italy, and France received an IORT boost, median 10 Gy dose, at the time of surgery followed by 50–54 Gy WBRT. 60 % of this patient cohort was considered to have at least one high risk factor for local failure: age <45, high-grade tumor >20 mm, or node involvement. Despite this high-risk group of patients, only 16 in-breast recurrences were observed with a median follow-up of 6 years (range 12–150 months) translating to a 6-year local relapse rate of 0.8 %. In multivariate analysis, only high-grade tumor appeared to be predictive of local recurrence.

Two phase II trials are exploring the possibility of further accelerating the dose delivery scheme by combining IORT boost and hypofractionated whole-breast irradiation in cases where IORT alone is not suitable. A multicenter phase II trial, HIOB – hypofractionated whole-breast irradiation following intraoperative electron boost – has been initiated and conducted by the ISORT (http://www.clinicaltrials.gov/ct2/Show/NCT01343459?term=hiob&rank=1). It will explore the addition of the acceleration of the whole-breast irradiation scheme (15 fractions of 2.7 Gy WBRT after a 10 IORT boost) in a non-randomized prospective fashion. An Italian phase II trial has also been completed that tested the same question, but follow-up is limited at this time [13].

22.2.1.2 Electrons for Partial-Breast Irradiation

Despite the limited published data documenting a benefit of overall survival, adjuvant radiotherapy is systematically recommended after breast-conserving surgery in many European countries. This occurs independent of stage or age and based predominantly on the increased rate of in-breast tumor recurrence (IBTR) over time in the absence of radiotherapy in conjunction with the likelihood of patients diagnosed after 65 years who have an extended life expectancy and lived long enough to experience recurrence.

Intraoperative radiotherapy has few side effects and thus might be an attractive option for some low-risk patients. One way to improve the acceptability of external radiotherapy is then to reduce the number of fractions and the volume of the irradiated breast, therefore shortening overall treatment time. Studies with at least 10 years of median follow-up have confirmed that hypofractionation in radiotherapy for breast cancer is safe and effective [14, 15]. However, the maximal possibility of reduced overall treatment time is offered by IORT and its one-shot procedure.

Delivering radiotherapy in one day reduces the overall cost and time dedicated to the radiotherapy treatment for active women with the reduction of toxicity. Additionally, IORT has reduced waiting lists in many centers [16].

Both European and American Societies for brachytherapy have published guidelines defining selection criteria for patients suitable for APBI [17, 18]. For these patients, APBI could be considered routine practice and possible criteria that could help guide the use of IORT.

In a very selected population, a French phase II trial was completed between 2004 and 2007 evaluating IORT with electrons for APBI. ASTRO guidelines were followed allowing women >65 years of age who had T1N0 estrogen receptor-positive tumors to be enrolled. With 6-year median follow-up, the local relapse rate has been reported as 9 %, 5-year disease-free survival as 92.7 %. Three true local relapses, located in the same quadrant with similar histology or higher grade, occurred late in follow-up at 25, 54, and 60 months after the IORT procedure. This confirms the absolute necessity of needing extended follow-up and mature results when evaluating APBI. All of the patients are alive without disease, with good to excellent cosmetic results in 93 %, as judged similarly by both patient and physician evaluation [19, 20].

The first and unique phase III trial comparing IORT APBI to standard WBRT has been conducted in Italy and published in 2013. This large trial (ELIOT – Electrons for Intra-Operative Treatment) enrolled a select population of 1305 patients who were randomized after quadrantectomy to receive either WBRT (50 Gy in 25 fractions followed by a boost to the surgical bed of 10 Gy in five fractions using external electron beam) or intraoperative radiotherapy with electrons (21 Gy in one fraction to the tumor bed using 6–9 MeV energies prescribed to the 90 % isodose depth). Using a non-inferiority hypothesis, local recurrence of less than 7.5 % in the intraoperative radiotherapy group was deemed to show equivalent efficacy compared with whole-breast irradiation. The primary endpoint was ipsilateral breast tumor recurrence (IBTR). After median follow-up of 5.8 years, the 5-year event rate for IBTR was 4.4 % (95 % CI 2.7–6.1) with intraoperative radiotherapy and 0.4 % (0.0–1.0) with whole-breast irradiation. Thus, the rate of local recurrence with intraoperative radiotherapy was within the specified equivalence margin, but was significantly worse than that for whole-breast irradiation.

Thought-provoking information gained from these results relates to the site of IBTR. The authors distinguished true local relapses from new ipsilateral breast tumors outside the index quadrant. Occurrence of true local relapses ($p=0.0003$), local relapses outside the index quadrant ($p=0.0001$), and axillary or regional lymph node metastases ($p=0.03$) was all significantly increased in the IORT arm. Of 35 local recurrences in the intraoperative radiotherapy group, 14 (40 %) occurred outside the index quadrant, and 21 (60 %) were true local recurrences. In a multivariable analysis, tumor size, the presence of four or more positive nodes, a poorly differentiated tumor, and triple-negative subtype were associated with increased likelihood of IBRT.

22.3 Toxicity and Cosmetic Results

The various electron-based series of IORT do not report consistent side effects. We initiated the incorporation of IORT boost for breast cancer treatment in 1989 and published in 2006 with a long, 9-year median follow-up (range 5 to 15 years) [7], and our phase II trial of exclusive IORT delivered for APBI was reported with 6-year follow-up [20].

Both series reported a very low rate of late side effects, and good to excellent cosmetic results were reported in 93 % of the patients at 5 years when treated with IORT only. In this experience there was minimal change in breast size and breast shape (86 % and 89 %, respectively) Telangiectasia or skin color change was not appreciated. It is interesting to note that as a result of optimal sparing of normal tissue, the excellent results were independent of the breast size, when large breasts may present with worse cosmetic results after external irradiation [20].

The skin was spared of late effects, and necrosis was avoided based on a careful sparing of the subcutaneous vessels during the mobilization of the gland around the tumor bed [5, 7, 8, 20]. This large surgical mobilization results in the expected appearance of frequent and totally asymptomatic radiological changes, due to cytosteatonecrosis in a large number of patients (approximately 70 % in our experience). But these mammograms are easily managed by trained radiologists and rarely require a biopsy for pathologic evaluation.

22.3.1 Limits and Advantages of Electrons for IORT

22.3.1.1 Evaluation of the Disease

IORT techniques are often criticized as a technique that does not allow image verification of the target and target volume coverage [21]. However, more appropriate challenge is to define the treatment volume during the operation based on clinical appreciation and on the accuracy of the direct histological analysis. In the case of a discrepancy where the definitive histological result reveals a more extensive tumor or involved margins as compared to the intraoperative assessment, the only solution is a reoperation. A radical approach or, more frequently, a second tumorectomy coupled with an adjuvant external whole-breast irradiation follows. In our experience this occurs in approximately 8–10 % of patients. This risk adaptive strategy allows treatment of all patients in an optimized way, with an ability to follow with appropriately tailored treatment if needed. Therefore, there is no risk of under treating even in this subgroup of women with more extensive disease. For the other 90 %, the APBI is realized in a very attractive one-shot procedure.

22.3.1.2 Dose

Treatment dose has been empirically chosen in all the series using electrons; however, unlike studies using 50 kV photons, these chosen doses differ between levels used for APBI and for [12]. The choice of 21 Gy for APBI was arrived through an Italian dose escalation study demonstrating its safety [22]. It should be noted that it is not possible to use linear quadratic formalism to estimate the biological equivalent dose of either the 10 Gy (for boost) or 21 Gy (as sole adjuvant treatment) fraction and that they were initiated empirically and continue based on long follow-up carcinologic results and tolerability.

The use of intraoperative normal tissue shielding devices has been based on clinical estimation and approximation: The thickness of the thoracic wall and gland cannot be precisely measured, and the dose falloff characteristics are only estimated on characteristics including the energy of electrons and the diameter of the applicator. Based on modern radiotherapy dose delivery methods, this estimation seems outdated [21].

In response to these estimations and level of uncertainty, we incorporated a method of dose measurement into our phase II trial evaluating IORT as sole treatment. In this trial, a systematic in vivo dosimetry was introduced for all treatments. The PTW type 911 semiconductor detector was placed in the middle of the target volume serving to measure the dose delivered. Recognizing the need for a quality assurance program for all IORT procedures, we chose this quality index as our primary endpoint and demonstrated that there was an acceptable difference of <20 % between the prescribed and measured doses with good reproducibility of the technique [15].

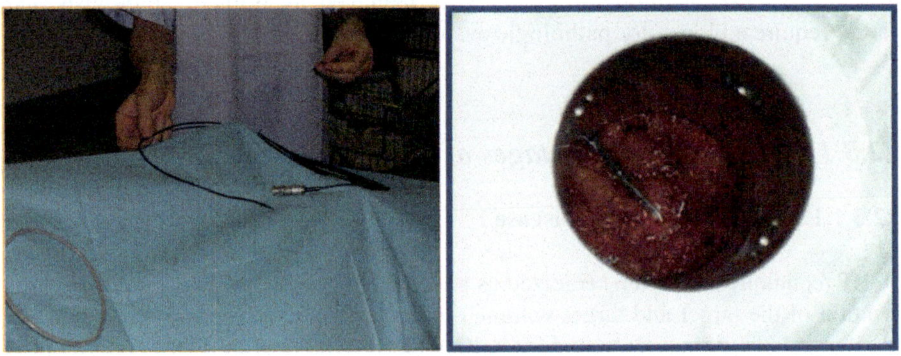

22.3.1.3 Treatment Outcome

Despite the lack of published phase III studies, the results for IORT as a boost are mature and with long follow-up with very encouraging low local relapse rates. In fact, the lowest published with any technique. Similar in application, the phase III TARGIT B trial, conducted in the UK employs a 20 Gy boost delivered by 50 kV photons.

APBI continues to face skepticism regardless of the technique evaluated. The ELIOT trial has heightened this doubt, reporting higher local relapse rate in the IORT arm as compared to standard WBRT. There are many potential explanations for these results. The first is the lack of information addressing the rate of involved margins and the rate of second surgery. This is a frequent criticism of intraoperative radiotherapy, but can be easily managed. In the event of discovering more advanced disease after intraoperative radiotherapy (discovery of involved margins or any adverse histological features on the definitive pathology report – high grade, multifocality, lymph vessel invasion, extensive intraductal disease, triple-negative phenotype, or involvement of axillary lymph nodes), a second surgery is required with the addition of postoperative whole-breast external-beam irradiation. We consider this as a designed strategy of adaptive risk.

In ELIOT the addition of whole-breast irradiation has been realized in only 5 % (31 of 647) of patients; this appears to be relatively low considering the high rate of high-grade tumors (20 %), involved nodes (26 %), lobular tumors (8 %), nonluminal tumors (10 %), and T2 stage (10 %). Interpretation of the effect of additional whole-breast irradiation is also difficult, because the ELIOT protocol specified additional irradiation only for patients with four or more positive axillary nodes. Surprisingly, additional irradiation was only delivered to the affected breast in both studies, whereas in clinical practice, the breast and both the supraclavicular and internal mammary chain nodes are irradiated.

The median follow-up of ELIOT is 5.8 years and too short to draw definitive conclusions about the risk of breast cancer death, particularly in patients selected outside the ASTRO recommendations. True local recurrences appear with a median follow-up of 5 years after primary treatment; therefore, it remains important to evaluate these trials with long-term follow-up, and adequate long-term results are needed to confirm the safety of APBI. It should be noted, however, that long-term follow-up with brachytherapy as APBI has been updated with 10-year follow-up with equivalent local control as compared to WBRT [6].

22.3.1.4 Cosmetic Results and Quality of Life

IORT offers significant advantages over external-beam 3D-conformal radiotherapy by avoiding the low doses delivered with the multiple field setups. The ability to spare the skin and subcutaneous tissue in the vicinity of the operative bed avoids possible late localized fibrosis and leads to a preservation of breast contour.

Moreover, it should to be noted that combining surgery and radiation at the same time offers the opportunity to proceed with immediate oncoplastic surgery, which partly explains the excellent cosmetic results of various series. When evaluated, the scores for body image are very high [19].

For APBI, scores for quality of life (QOL) are also rated as very good, with very few mood disorders or anxiety reported. Evaluation of autonomy by ADL (activities of daily living) and IADL (Lawton instrumental activities of daily living) questionnaires indicates excellent performance and behavior levels of sociobiological functions in older patients after single-dose delivery of IORT [19].

1 Cosmetic Results for Boost

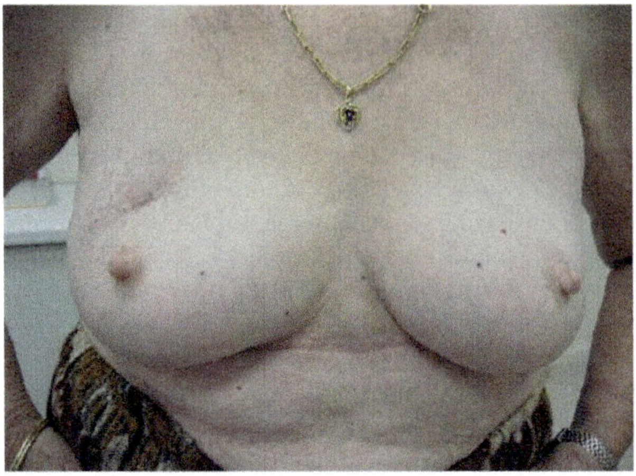

Patient treated with intraoperative radiotherapy boost (left breast) and external electron boost (right breast) for two early breast cancers in 1995 and 2000, respectively.

We observe Grade 2 telangiectasia within the external boost field and no late side effect in the IORT boost

2 Cosmetic Results for IPAS

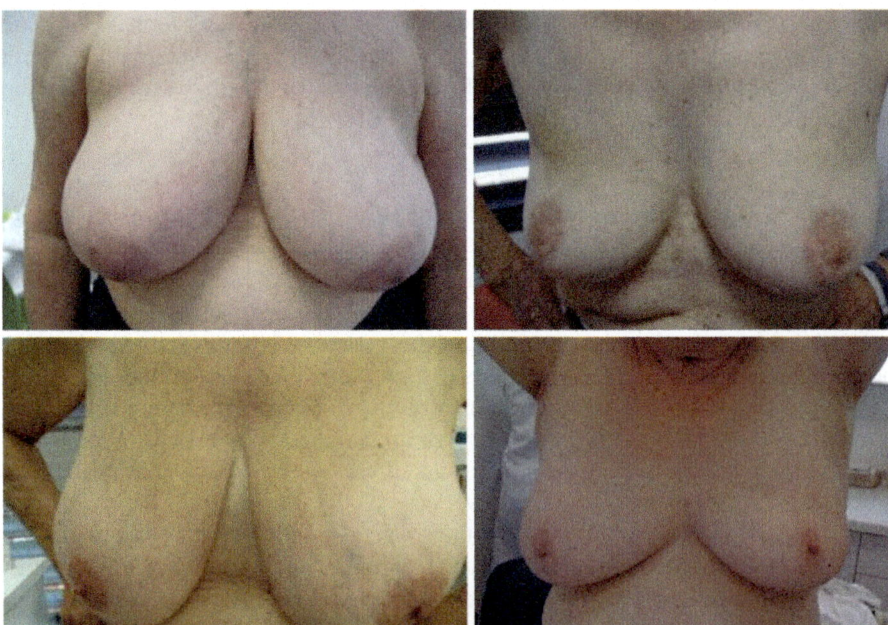

4 patients treated with Electrons for APBI. 6 years follow-up

22.3.1.5 Cost

Reducing the 6 weeks of daily radiotherapy to one fraction delivered during surgery will dramatically reduce the cost of adjuvant breast radiotherapy. A medico-economic prospective study is ongoing in France to evaluate its impact on health-care resources and public health.

The cost of the adjuvant irradiation and the distance to radiation therapy equipment will no longer be a major consideration when choosing between breast-conserving therapy, mastectomy, or even totally omitting adjuvant irradiation due to treatment delivery barriers [23, 24].

22.3.1.6 Equipment

Electron beam offers an optimal, homogeneous dose treatment option for IORT. Initiated with large, stationary, and cumbersome classical linear accelerators, the technique has today moved to more convenient, mobile accelerator. This change explains the noted growth of IORT and adoption of IORT with several hundred centers already equipped in Europe with mobile intraoperative treatment machines.

Although the radiation protection of the operating theater dedicated to IORT is simple, it remains an important aspect of this technique due to the risk of scattered radiation and forces the use of leaded barriers and the exit of staff during the treatment delivery. Depending on the country, laws and constraints dictated by nuclear safety authorities vary widely. There are many centers now equipped in Italy, with centers now found in Germany and the United States. Interesting, the French health authorities have not yet authorized the use of mobile electron accelerators outside of a bunker. This partially explains why many French centers today are equipped with small 50 kV accelerators.

22.4 Conclusion

IORT, after decades of confined use among highly specialized teams, has recently gained a lot of interest. Numerous teams have now adopted this treatment technique and have demonstrated its feasibility and safety. Patient satisfaction among treated patients remains high [20], and there appears to be a short learning curve with new treatment teams.

In general, this treatment approach offers significant advantages exemplified by precise target volume delineation through a reinforced collaboration between surgeon and radiation oncologist. Additionally, proper patient selection and technique provides optimal local control and with the ability to avoid skin and adjacent mammary gland irradiation, the best cosmetic results are realized.

APBI delivered by IORT offers the unique opportunity to complete radiotherapy with a “one-shot procedure,” the maximal example of treatment acceleration.

However, for success, IORT requires a very strict oncologic approach and adherence to international selection criteria. However, as final pathology is not available, an important aspect of the overall treatment approach success is to follow through with WBRT when definitive results show unfavorable factors and therefore transform the intended APBI to a standard treatment and the dose delivered during the surgery into a boost. This adaptive risk strategy must be strictly observed to achieve overall success in every woman treated.

The choice of using IORT electrons offers a dose homogeneity and a larger choice in the modulation of treatment depth to account for varying target thickness. However, these advantages are accompanied by the requirement of the use of a larger degree of mammary gland surgical mobilization and the need for radioprotection in the surgery theater.

Today, more and more teams are becoming equipped with mobile electrons, as the technique is appealing to both physicians and patients. New indications of APBI are under exploration through ongoing clinical trials.

Iconography

Equipment

Linac Accelerator Saturne

PTW semi-conductor detector used for *in vivo* dosimetry for electrons IORT, placed at the center of the circular target volume

References

1. Fowler JF. The linear-quadratic formula and progress in fractionated radiotherapy. Br J Radiol. 1989;62:679–94.
2. Belletti B, Vaidya JS, D'Andrea S, et al. Targeted intraoperative radiotherapy impairs the stimulation of breast cancer cell proliferation and invasion caused by surgical wounding. Clin Cancer Res. 2008;14:1325–32.
3. Vaidya JS, Baldassarre G, Massarut S. Beneficial effects of intraoperative radiotherapy on tumor microenvironment could improve outcomes (Int J Radiat Oncol Biol Phys 2008;72:1575–1581). Int J Radiat Oncol Biol Phys. 2009;74:976; author reply 976–977.
4. Vaidya JS, Wenz F, Bulsara M, et al. Risk-adapted targeted intraoperative radiotherapy versus whole-breast radiotherapy for breast cancer: 5-year results for local control and overall survival from the TARGIT-A randomised trial. Lancet. 2014;383:603–13.
5. Veronesi U, Orecchia R, Maisonneuve P, et al. Intraoperative radiotherapy versus external radiotherapy for early breast cancer (ELIOT): a randomised controlled equivalence trial. Lancet Oncol. 2013;14:1269–77.
6. Polgár C, Fodor J, Major T, et al. Breast-conserving therapy with partial or whole breast irradiation: ten-year results of the Budapest randomized trial. Radiother Oncol. 2013;108:197–202.
7. Lemanski C, Azria D, Thezenas S, et al. Intraoperative radiotherapy given as a boost for early breast cancer: long-term clinical and cosmetic results. Int J Radiat Oncol Biol Phys. 2006;64:1410–5.
8. Intra M, Luini A, Gatti G, et al. Surgical technique of intraoperative radiation therapy with electrons (ELIOT) in breast cancer: a lesson learned by over 1000 procedures. Surgery. 2006;140:467–71.
9. Orecchia R, Veronesi U. Intraoperative electrons. Semin Radiat Oncol. 2005;15:76–83.

10. Sedlmayer F, Reitsamer R, Fussl C, et al. Boost IORT in breast cancer: body of evidence. Int J Breast Cancer. 2014;2014:1–6.
11. Reitsamer R, Peintinger F, Kopp M, et al. Local recurrence rates in breast cancer patients treated with intraoperative electron-boost radiotherapy versus postoperative external-beam electron-boost irradiation. A sequential intervention study. Strahlenther Onkol. 2004;180:38–44.
12. Fastner G, Sedlmayer F, Merz F, et al. IORT with electrons as boost strategy during breast conserving therapy in limited stage breast cancer: long term results of an ISIORT pooled analysis. Radiother Oncol. 2013;108:279–86.
13. Ivaldi GB, Leonardi MC, Orecchia R, et al. Preliminary results of electron intraoperative therapy boost and hypofractionated external beam radiotherapy after breast-conserving surgery in premenopausal women. Int J Radiat Oncol Biol Phys. 2008;72:485–93.
14. Haviland JS, Owen JR, Dewar JA, et al. The UK Standardisation of Breast Radiotherapy (START) trials of radiotherapy hypofractionation for treatment of early breast cancer: 10-year follow-up results of two randomised controlled trials. Lancet Oncol. 2013;14:1086–94.
15. Whelan TJ, Pignol J-P, Levine MN, et al. Long-term results of hypofractionated radiation therapy for breast cancer. N Engl J Med. 2010;362:513–20.
16. Bartelink H, Arriagada R. Hypofractionation in radiotherapy for breast cancer. Lancet. 2008;371:1050–2.
17. Smith BD, Arthur DW, Buchholz TA, et al. Accelerated partial breast irradiation consensus statement from the American Society for Radiation Oncology (ASTRO). Int J Radiat Oncol Biol Phys. 2009;74:987–1001.
18. Polgár C, Limbergen EV, Pötter R, et al. Patient selection for accelerated partial-breast irradiation (APBI) after breast-conserving surgery: recommendations of the Groupe Européen de Curiethérapie-European Society for Therapeutic Radiology and Oncology (GEC-ESTRO) breast cancer working group based on clinical evidence (2009). Radiother Oncol. 2010;94:264–73.
19. Lemanski C, Azria D, Gourgon-Bourgade S, et al. Intraoperative radiotherapy in early-stage breast cancer: results of the Montpellier phase II trial. Int J Radiat Oncol Biol Phys. 2010;76:698–703.
20. Lemanski C, Azria D, Gourgou-Bourgade S, et al. Electrons for intraoperative radiotherapy in selected breast-cancer patients: late results of the Montpellier phase II trial. Radiat Oncol. 2013;8:191.
21. Khan AJ, Dale RG, Arthur DW, et al. Ultrashort courses of adjuvant breast radiotherapy: wave of the future or a fool's errand? Cancer. 2012;118:1962–70.
22. Luini A, Orecchia R, Gatti G, et al. The pilot trial on intraoperative radiotherapy with electrons (ELIOT): update on the results. Breast Cancer Res Treat. 2005;93:55–9.
23. Lazovich DA, White E, Thomas DB, et al. Underutilization of breast-conserving surgery and radiation therapy among women with stage I or II breast cancer. JAMA. 1991;266:3433–8.
24. Schroen AT. Impact of patient distance to radiation therapy on mastectomy use in early-stage breast cancer patients. J Clin Oncol. 2005;23:7074–80.

Part V
Emerging Treatment Approaches

Chapter 23
Ultrashort Courses of Breast Radiotherapy

Atif J. Khan, Stuti Ahlawat, Laurie Kirstein, and Sharad Goyal

Contents

23.1 Clinical Background

In this brief chapter, we will consider reported and in-progress attempts at compressing the duration of adjuvant accelerated partial-breast irradiation (APBI) beyond the usual 4–5 treatment days with 8–10 fractions. As has been reviewed elsewhere, APBI involves treating the surgical cavity with a 1–2 cm margin, thus reducing the volume of breast tissue by up to 50 % using various radiotherapeutic

A.J. Khan, MD (✉) • S. Ahlawat, MD • S. Goyal, MD
Department of Radiation Oncology, Rutgers Cancer Institute of New Jersey, Rutgers Robert Wood Johnson Medical School, 195 Little Albany Street, New Brunswick, NJ 08903, USA
e-mail: atif.j.khan@rutgers.edu

L. Kirstein, MD
Department of Surgery, Rutgers Cancer Institute of New Jersey, New Brunswick, NJ USA

Department of Surgery, Rutgers Robert Wood Johnson Medical School, New Brunswick, NJ USA

D.W. Arthur et al. (eds.), *Short Course Breast Radiotherapy: A Comprehensive Review of Hypofractionation, Partial Breast, and Intra-Operative Irradiation*, DOI 10.1007/978-3-319-24388-7_23

methods. Technical approaches of APBI include multi-catheter interstitial brachytherapy, balloon catheter brachytherapy, external 3D conformal external-beam radiotherapy (3D-CRT), and intraoperative radiotherapy (IORT). To date, the body of available literature supports the hypothesis that APBI is a safe, well-tolerated therapy in selected women and appears to be equivalent to WBI in terms of efficacy and ultimate breast cosmesis [1–5]. A further progression of the APBI literature has been the recent interest in extremely short courses of adjuvant radiotherapy; these efforts will be discussed presently. Although there are dedicated chapters for IORT and preoperative single-fraction radiotherapy, we will review these briefly for the purpose of drawing comparisons.

23.2 Intraoperative Radiotherapy

23.2.1 TARGIT (Targeted Intraoperative Radiotherapy)

Intraoperative radiation therapy is the ultimate in short-course radiotherapy—the entire course of treatment is delivered in a single fraction using some type of intraoperative applicator. Of current reported intraoperative experiences, the TARGIT-A trial is the largest. This approach employs the Intrabeam device (Carl Zeiss, Oberkochen, Germany) which uses an intraoperative spherical applicator to deliver a single dose of 20 Gy at the applicator surface with 50 kV x-rays. This high surface dose attenuates to a dose of 5 Gy at 1 cm [6]. The TARGIT trialists have cited the following as their rationale for an intraoperative approach: (1) the breast harbors multicentric foci which however remains clinically dormant and without consequence [7], (2) 85–90 % of "true" local recurrences occur around the lumpectomy cavity [8, 9], (3) local recurrences after fractionated radiotherapy occur at least partially because of microenvironmental factors that encourage proliferation [10], and (4) the low therapeutic dose of TARGIT is offset by the high relative biologic effect (RBE) of a 50 kV x-ray beam (RBE of 1.5 at 1 cm) [7]. The RBE is a term that accounts for different biological effects (for a given biological endpoint) resulting from various types of radiation. The authors first conducted a trial in which the identical intraoperative treatment (20 Gy at surface) was delivered as a boost followed by whole-breast external-beam radiation therapy (EBRT) in a prospective cohort of 300 treated breasts [11]. With a median follow-up of 60.5 months, 8 ipsilateral breast tumor recurrences were reported (crude failure rate of 2.7 % and 5-year Kaplan-Meier estimate of 1.73 %). Based on these results, the trialists launched the TARGIT-A trial for lower risk patients to test the efficacy of single-fraction treatment compared to fractionated whole-breast EBRT and the TARGIT-B trial to test the equivalence of TARGIT delivered as a boost in higher risk patients.

Updated findings of the TARGIT-A trial were recently published [12]. A total of 3451 women were randomized to either fractionated whole-breast radiotherapy (with or without a boost) or to intraoperative radiotherapy at a dose of 20 Gy at the applicator surface. Patients were stratified into two strata: 2/3 of patients were treated in the prepathology stratum where women had lumpectomy and intraoperative RT at the same sitting, while the remaining women (post-pathology stratum) were taken back to the OR for the TARGIT treatment after final pathology had been reviewed. The investigators predefined a 2.5 % absolute non-inferiority margin with a background 5-year local recurrence rate of 6 %. The trialists also estimated that 15 % of patients assigned to TARGIT would ultimately have pathological features that would warrant additional whole-breast EBRT, although these adverse features were not strictly outlined for the treating sites. The median age of patients was 63 (interquartile range 57–69), 87 % of tumors were under 2 cm, and 84 % were grade 1 or 2; over 93 % of tumors were ER positive. Although the trial allowed node-positive patients, 84 % of patients were node negative. Approximately 80 % of patients received systemic therapy. The median follow-up of the entire group was 2 years and 5 months; 2020 patients had a median of 4-year follow-up. The 5-year LR rates were 3.3 % vs. 1.3 % favoring the EBRT arm ($p=0.042$). In the prepathology stratum, the corresponding numbers were 2.1 % vs. 1.1 %. In the post-pathology stratum, the results were much worse: 5.4 % vs. 1.7 %. The true significance and correct interpretation of these local failure numbers has been heavily contested and was the subject of a remarkable exchange of the correspondence in the Lancet's letters to the editor. To the TARGIT trialists, the differences are insignificant and did not meet the predetermined threshold of inferiority, thus ushering in a new era of "pragmatic radiotherapy." However, a more critical review of the data leads one to the opposite conclusion. Professor Jack Cuzik's letter to the editor is particularly notable for both the substance of the criticism and the fact that he chaired the Data Monitoring Committee for the TARGIT trial and resigned due to the reporting methods of the trialists. Professor Cuzik notes that the authors misuse the non-inferiority criterion, which requires that the upper limit of the confidence intervals for the respective 5-year local failure survival estimates be below the chosen threshold (2.5 % in this study). Using this criterion, the upper limit of the respective CIs for TARGIT vs. EBRT is 5.1 % vs. 2.5 %, thus exceeding the pre-specified threshold. The fact that non-inferiority is rejected with just 2.4 years worth of follow-up is particularly telling. To circumvent this, the authors instead use crude rates and a binomial proportions analysis of 5-year local recurrence. However, this analysis can only be done if all subjects have had 5 years worth of follow-up—in the TARGIT trial only 611/3451 had completed 5 years of follow-up. In addition, 21 % of TARGIT patients in the prepathology stratum received whole-breast radiotherapy. Thus it seems conceivable that this contamination of signal in the prepathology stratum would render make the results less interpretable. In contrast, the post-pathology stratum represents a clearer test of the two techniques. The post-pathology group is confirmed to be a favorable cohort of patients, and yet the TARGIT-treated group has a LF curve that mimics trial arms with no adjuvant radiotherapy at all. This in fact is consistent with the sub-therapeutic doses one expects with this technology.

A separate issue raised by the TARGIT trialists is the seemingly higher rates of non-breast cancer mortality in the EBRT group, driven reportedly by higher rates of cardiovascular morbidity. In the context of a large randomized trial, a finding such as this should be taken seriously. Notably, the difference exists only in the pre-pathology stratum. Given the incredulously short time latency for a lethal effect attributed to whole-breast irradiation, and the unwillingness of the trialists to report details of dosimetry, laterality, and cardiac morbidities, one can only assume that the finding is due to imbalances not accounted for in the pre-randomization screening.

In summary, while the TARGIT strategy is truly novel and is already the subject of a clinical trial involving thousands of women, it has been prematurely presented as "practice changing" and the fundamentals of the TARGIT trial have repeatedly been called into question. The deviation from established trial fundamentals appears to be decidedly unsound and calls into question how randomized trials are selected and how peer review for even prominent medical journals is handled. The kV-source technology used in the TARGIT trial produces a sub-therapeutic dose in the treatment volume at risk for residual, and, based on the trial results, we are seeing this inadequacy of treatment. The difference is clear in the post-pathology stratum where the two arms are compared most directly, but even in the entire cohort the criterion for non-inferiority is rejected. The authors appear to be carefully curating the data to fit their eager agenda of practice change and willfully ignoring the many legitimate issues raised by prominent thought leaders.

23.2.2 ELIOT (Intraoperative Radiotherapy with Electrons)

The Milan group has been studying the utility of intraoperative radiotherapy with electrons (ELIOT). The ELIOT technique, while similar in intent to TARGIT, is a strikingly different treatment. After a lumpectomy, the breast tissue in the flap is undermined and mobilized and approximated within the operative field. Thus both the superficial and deep layers of the lumpectomy cavity are placed in the beam's eye view of a Perspex cylindrical "cone" applicator. An intraoperative dose of 21 Gy is prescribed to the 90 % isodose line and delivered with 3–12 MeV electrons to encompass the tumor bed [13]. The appropriate electron energy is selected based on a measurement of breast thickness in the clinical target volume. The Italian group arrived at this dose using linear quadratic formalism, but used an alpha/beta ratio of 10 for breast cancer control. They tested the concept in a dose-escalation study, demonstrating its safety [14]. This led to the launch of the randomized ELIOT trial of whole-breast RT versus IORT which was recently reported. 1305 cases were randomized, 654 to the whole-breast arm, and 651 to the ELIOT arm [15]. With a median follow-up of approximately 6 years, the 5-year ipsilateral breast tumor recurrence rate was 4.4 % in the ELIOT arm and 0.4 % in the whole-breast arm ($p<0.0001$). The corresponding 5-year "true" local recurrence rates were 2.5 vs. 0.4 % ($p=0.0003$). Significantly higher rates of fat necrosis were seen with ELIOT (14 % vs. 7 %, $p=0.04$).

With the ELIOT approach, a homogenous dose is delivered to a target volume that is more consistent with the target volumes treated in the accumulated APBI literature. Notably, the authors concede in the latest paper that a 21 Gy dose in a single fraction is equivalent to 131 Gy in 2 Gy equivalents when an alpha/beta ratio of 4 is used. Thus the higher rates of fat necrosis are not surprising at all. The clinical fat necrosis rate in the ELIOT randomized trial was 14 % compared to about 2.3 % reported with balloon device-based APBI. This is almost certainly because the ELIOT dose is almost double the 2 Gy equivalent dose of fractionated courses of APBI.

Why then is the treatment less efficacious in the face of such high doses? The ELIOT approach is agnostic to final pathology findings; no "remedial" treatment was offered to women found to have positive margins or positive lymph nodes. In this way it was a much more appropriate and pure comparison of whole-breast RT and intraoperative radiotherapy. The impact of positive margins on local failure is well documented. Margin status from the primary lumpectomy specimens is not reported in the ELIOT data (nor is it reported in the TARGIT paper); however approximately 25 % of patients in both groups were node positive, with approximately 5 % with pN1b disease (>3 positive nodes). The ELIOT experience thus amply highlights the perils of poor patient selection, a feature that is inherent and inescapable in the concept of intraoperative radiotherapy. To summarize, the ELIOT experience as reported in their randomized trial is fraught with not one but two major reasons for pessimism—suboptimal tumor control and higher toxicity.

Before moving on, it is important to make one additional observation regarding intraoperative therapy. Neither the TARGIT nor the ELIOT techniques allow image verification of target volume coverage or dose to organs at risk. Although unlikely, it is certainly not impossible that a deep-seated lumpectomy bed could bring an applicator in close proximity to a critical organ or structure without the treating physicians ever realizing it. Although the intraoperative approaches do often include an attempt to undermine the breast to introduce shielding devices, this exercise is still not image verified and may cause more breast trauma. In any case, the very idea of treating a volume of tissue based on dose falloff characteristics of a particular photon/electron energy and a particular-sized applicator ("lookup table"-style treatment) seems to be outdated in the current era of 3D planning.

23.3 Preoperative Radiotherapy

Accelerated preoperative partial-breast irradiation is a novel treatment paradigm in which the treatment sequence is altered and patients receive stereotactic, image-guided radiotherapy before their scheduled lumpectomy—treatment can be delivered in a single or a few fractions. The potential advantages of such an approach are obvious. The treatment convenience of a single fraction is similar to intraoperative therapy. By irradiating an intact, in vivo lesion with an image-guided approach, the issue of volume reconstruction during postoperative APBI planning is obviated. The total lack of image guidance for organs at risk seen with intraoperative therapy is circumvented. Preoperative treatment volumes may be smaller and there may be biological advantages to treating a well-vascularized tumor. Finally, the treatment offers a unique opportunity to study the radiation response of high single-fraction doses.

Bondiau and colleagues in Nice reported results from their institutional pilot trial of preoperative hypofractionated APBI [16]. The intent of this trial was to add a short course of preoperative RT to patient receiving neoadjuvant chemotherapy. Patients were treated during the 2nd of 6 planned cycles of chemotherapy. Briefly, four fiducials were placed under ultrasound guidance to localize the tumor, followed by a treatment planning CT scan. MRI was performed separately to aid in contouring. However, MRIs were taken in the prone position, while treatment planning CTs were in the supine position. A robotic stereotactic radiosurgery system was used to deliver two dose levels to a total of 6 patients. Four patients received 19.5 Gy in 3 fractions of 6.5 Gy and two patients received 22.5 Gy in 3 fractions of 7.5 Gy. Surgery was performed 4–8 weeks after chemotherapy per standard of care and postoperative RT was delivered to 50 Gy in 2 Gy fractions. There were two clinical complete responses (CRs) and one pathological CR. Skin toxicity as measured at multiple time points by clinical exam, calorimetry, dermoscopy, and thickening on ultrasound revealed minimal toxicity. This study demonstrated that high-fraction external-beam radiotherapy to the breast was feasible and associated with acceptable early toxicity.

Horton and Hwang recently reported first results from an institutional, prospective, dose-escalation phase I trial of women with low-risk cT1N0 invasive ductal carcinoma or DCIS < 2 cm treated with single-fraction preoperative APBI [17]. A treatment planning MRI scan was performed in the Department of Radiation Oncology for most patients ($n = 21$) but also in outside diagnostic facilities ($n = 11$). Thirty patients were scanned in the prone position with arms up. Prior to treatment, patients had on-board kv and cone-beam CT imaging. RT was prescribed at either 15, 18, or 21 Gy to cohorts of 8 patients to probe the maximum tolerated dose. Lumpectomy occurred within 10 days of RT. Radiation response on MRI and paraffin-embedded samples were analyzed for correlative analyses.

A total of 32 women were enrolled. 3 women received additional whole-breast RT. No DLTs were observed at a median follow-up of 23 months. Imaging correlates demonstrated post-radiation vascular permeability on MRI and induction of inflammatory gene signature in a 27 gene set that was dose-dependent. All patients treated with single-fraction therapy had good or excellent cosmesis. Three patients who had additional WBRT did not do as well, with one patient developing two grade 3 toxicities, one with a wound infection, and all three with fair or poor cosmesis.

Additional preoperative APBI has been reported from a Danish group [18] and a similar study is ongoing at the University of Maryland (NCT01014715). These are not discussed here as they are not "shortened" from the conventional APBI schedules. The preoperative radiotherapy experience is a novel departure from the standard APBI methods that attempts to address certain problems inherent in postoperative APBI. However, the preoperative approach creates a new set of issues that have yet to be addressed. Foremost among these is the issue of target delineation. CT-based planning, even with fiducial guidance, is unlikely to clearly delineate GTVs. MRIs are typically acquired in the prone position. Thus, fusion of MRI and CT will require complex deformable registration techniques. A simple, rigid registration to clips will be hard to justify unless at least three clips are placed in each case for localization. Alternatively, dedicated MRI-based treatment planning will be needed. Thus, although the pioneers of preoperative APBI have cited its simplicity, brevity, and cost-savings as a primary rationale, the reality is that preoperative APBI will likely require either routine MRI simulation or complex soft tissue fusion of MRI and CT images, advanced immobilization techniques for supinely planned breasts, heavy involvement of a breast radiologist, pre-image verification with cone-beam or other 3D imaging, and complex multibeam, stereotactic treatment planning and advanced robotic tumor tracking. These considerations are not particularly practical and will be a barrier to adoption, especially in resource-constrained economies.

23.4 Postoperative Experiences of Highly Abbreviated Radiotherapy

23.4.1 Extremely Hypofractionated Partial-Breast Radiotherapy

Vermeulen and colleagues have reported a small series of stereotactic radiosurgery delivered by CyberKnife to 9 patients [19]. Two of these patients received 30 Gy in 5 fractions while the rest received the usual 34 Gy in 10 fractions. With a median follow-up of 7 months, observed toxicities were modest. This paper illustrates the general challenges associated with external-beam stereotactic approaches. Patients were simulated and treated in the supine position using implanted gold fiducials used for planning and tracking. Earlier data in a technical communication had demonstrated that titanium markers could be unreliable due to contrast loss when superimposed by bony structures of the thorax. Patient positioning in CT and MRIs had to be extensively optimized using custom-designed immobilization devices. In summary, like all stereotactic implementations, post-op SBRT to the breast requires close attention to detail and significant investment of resource.

With a similar intent, the Beaumont group reported on a cohort of 45 patients treated with 4 fractions of 7 Gy over 2 days using a single-lumen MammoSite (TM, Hologic) device [20]. With a median follow-up of 3.7 years and a minimum follow-up of 2 years, only grade 1 and 2 toxicities were reported. The most common toxicities were fat necrosis (18 %) and asymptomatic seroma (42 %). Three patients had rib fractures.

Given the landscape of reported literature for ultrashort-course radiotherapy, our group wanted to develop a strategy that accounted for the shortcomings of IORT and preoperative RT. An ideal treatment strategy would still be delivered over 1 or 2 days, but (1) allow for full pathology review before treatment assignment, (2) be image guided, (3) cover an at-risk volume that is supported by evidence, (4) rely on accepted radiobiological modeling, and (5) have some preexisting data on dose constraints for toxicity. We addressed most of these issues in our multi-site, prospective, nonrandomized dose-escalation study to determine the safety and feasibility of delivering APBI with the Contura MLB balloon catheter (Bard, Irvine, CA) in a short-course, 2-day fashion. This was a "schedule-seeking" study of 3 patient cohorts, each with 30 patients. Treatment began with 4 fractions of 7 Gy delivered twice daily over 2 days. If predefined toxicities were below threshold within a 6-month follow-up period (i.e., in a cohort of 30 patients $\leq$ 10 in-breast complications > grade 2 and $\leq$ 1 non-breast complication > grade 2 occur), the dose prescription was elevated to the next level; 3 fractions of 8.25 Gy were to be delivered over 2 days. Again, in the absence of unacceptable toxicities, the dose prescription was planned to escalate to the final fractionation schedule of 2 fractions of 10.25 Gy, delivered over 2 days. We defined very conservative dosimetric criteria for acceptability: maximum skin and rib dose to not exceed 100 % of prescription dose and V150 and V200 to not exceed 40 and 10 cc, respectively. We reported first results from patients treated with 7 Gy × 4, demonstrating the dosimetric feasibility of this approach and no greater than grade 2 toxicity. One breast infection and 2 cases each of fat necrosis and symptomatic seromas were seen. This trial was suspended due to lack of funding after enrollment of the second dose cohort (8.25 Gy × 3, EQD2 of 60 Gy). We are launching a new successor trial of 200 women who will be treated to 7.5 Gy × 3 fractions (EQD2 of 50 Gy) delivered over 2 or 3 days. The primary endpoint is toxicity rate exceeding grade 2.

23.4.2 Extremely Hypofractionated Whole-Breast Radiotherapy

Although one may be tempted to restrict these high-fraction doses to partial-breast volumes, several investigators have also delivered large fractions to whole-breast volumes. Single weekly fractions appear to be safe and can shorten treatment time. Dragun et al. reported a phase II of once-weekly hypofractionated WBI [21]. Patients with stage 0–II breast cancer after undergoing lumpectomy with negative margins were treated with 30 Gy to the breast with 6 Gy weekly fractions over 5 weeks. Patients were not allowed to undergo elective nodal radiation. In their series of 42 patients, the authors report any grade ≥2 toxicity rate of 42.8 %. They report only 1 grade 3 toxicity related to narcotic use. Furthermore, patient reported outcomes of breast pain, edema, and swelling all decreased to baseline within 1 month [21].

Similarly, Rovea et al. also delivered once-weekly HF WBI, 30–32.5 Gy given in 5 weekly fractions to older patients (mean age 80 years) after lumpectomy [22]. Their retrospective review of consecutively treated patients with a median follow-up of 46.5 months revealed 3- and 5-year local control rates 99.5 % and 98 %, respectively. Acute grade 2 skin toxicity was observed in 4.8 %, grade 3 in 1 %, and grade 4 in 0.3 %. Late skin toxicity included grade 2 in 6.5 % and grade 3 in 4.3 % of the patients. Cosmetic results were good to excellent in 86.4 % of patients [22].

The once-weekly concept is being tested in a randomized trial by the UK trialists led by Yarnold. The UK FAST trial has completed enrolled to a three-arm trial of 50 Gy in 2 Gy fractions vs. 28.5 Gy in 5.7 Gy once-weekly fractions vs. 30 Gy in 6 Gy once weekly all delivered over 5 weeks. Patients were eligible for enrollment if they had node-negative breast cancer measuring 3 cm or less and age ≥50 years old after BCS. The primary endpoint is 2-year change in breast appearance. Although the trial is currently in follow-up, the early results indicate that 30 Gy over 5 weeks had worse breast appearance outcomes when compared to 28.5 and 50 Gy. With a median follow-up 37.3 months, the early results show 2 local relapses and 23 deaths [23]. It will be crucial to see mature data of this very important trial.

The UK FAST-Forward trial is the successor trial to the UK FAST and aims to assess shortening the weekly fractionation schedule even further. The control arm of the trial is 40 Gy in 15 fractions. The experimental arms include 27 Gy in 5 fractions of 5.4 Gy vs. 26 Gy in 5 fractions of 5.2 Gy given over 5 consecutive days. A 10 or 16 Gy boost may be added to the surgical scar or lumpectomy site. The experimental schedule attempts to shorten treatment time for whole-breast RT even further, down to a single work week. The primary endpoint is ipsilateral tumor control.

23.5 Conclusions

Extremely short courses of partial and whole-breast radiotherapy, delivered preoperatively, intraoperatively, and postoperatively, are natural directions of investigation in the realm of breast radiotherapy. It is also natural for innovation to be met with skepticism and debate. The UK and Italian investigators are to be commended for initiating the discourse on a treatment strategy that has significant implications for both patients and payers. Their efforts, perhaps somewhat flawed, are at least partly responsible for the shortened radiotherapy studies of APBI and whole-breast irradiation currently being investigated. It is imperative that we frame the correct questions and attempt to resolve them with well-designed clinical trials.

References

1. Chen PY, et al. Long-term cosmetic results and toxicity after accelerated partial-breast irradiation: a method of radiation delivery by interstitial brachytherapy for the treatment of early-stage breast carcinoma. Cancer. 2006;106:991–9. doi:10.1002/cncr.21681.
2. Chen PY, et al. Four-year efficacy, cosmesis, and toxicity using three-dimensional conformal external beam radiation therapy to deliver accelerated partial breast irradiation. Int J Radiat Oncol Biol Phys. 2010;76:991–7, doi: S0360-3016(09)00424-6 [pii]. 10.1016/j.ijrobp.2009.03.012.
3. Vicini FA, et al. Interim cosmetic results and toxicity using 3D conformal external beam radiotherapy to deliver accelerated partial breast irradiation in patients with early-stage breast cancer treated with breast-conserving therapy. Int J Radiat Oncol Biol Phys. 2007;69:1124–30, doi:S0360-3016(07)00759-6 [pii]. 10.1016/j.ijrobp.2007.04.033.

4. Goyal S, et al. Factors associated with optimal cosmetic results at 36 months in patients treated with accelerated partial breast irradiation (APBI) on the American Society of Breast Surgeons (ASBrS) MammoSite Breast Brachytherapy Registry Trial. Ann Surg Oncol. 2009;16:2450–8. doi:10.1245/s10434-009-0561-y.
5. Khan AJ, et al. Local control, toxicity, and cosmesis in women younger than 50 enrolled onto the American Society of Breast Surgeons MammoSite Radiation Therapy System registry trial. Ann Surg Oncol. 2009;16:1612–8. doi:10.1245/s10434-009-0406-8.
6. Vaidya JS, et al. TARGeted Intraoperative radiotherapy (TARGIT): an innovative approach to partial-breast irradiation. Semin Radiat Oncol. 2005;15:84–91, doi:S1053429604001419 [pii].
7. Vaidya JS, et al. Intraoperative radiotherapy for breast cancer. Lancet Oncol. 2004;5:165–73.
8. Clark RM, et al. Randomized clinical trial to assess the effectiveness of breast irradiation following lumpectomy and axillary dissection for node-negative breast cancer. J Natl Cancer Inst. 1992;84:683–9.
9. Veronesi U, et al. Radiotherapy after breast-preserving surgery in women with localized cancer of the breast. N Engl J Med. 1993;328:1587–91. doi:10.1056/NEJM199306033282202.
10. Belletti B, et al. Targeted intraoperative radiotherapy impairs the stimulation of breast cancer cell proliferation and invasion caused by surgical wounding. Clin Cancer Res. 2008;14:1325–32, doi:14/5/1325 [pii]. 10.1158/1078-0432.CCR-07-4453.
11. Vaidya JS, et al. Long-term results of targeted intraoperative radiotherapy (targit) boost during breast-conserving surgery. Int J Radiat Oncol Biol Phys. 2011;81:1091–7, doi:S0360-3016(10)03043-9 [pii]. 10.1016/j.ijrobp.2010.07.1996.
12. Vaidya JS, et al. Targeted intraoperative radiotherapy versus whole breast radiotherapy for breast cancer (TARGIT-A trial): an international, prospective, randomised, non-inferiority phase 3 trial. Lancet. 2010;376:91–102, doi:S0140-6736(10)60837-9 [pii]. 10.1016/S0140-6736(10)60837-9.
13. Orecchia R, Veronesi U. Intraoperative electrons. Semin Radiat Oncol. 2005;15:76–83.
14. Luini A, et al. The pilot trial on intraoperative radiotherapy with electrons (ELIOT): update on the results. Breast Cancer Res Treat. 2005;93:55–9.
15. Veronesi U, et al. Intraoperative radiotherapy versus external radiotherapy for early breast cancer (ELIOT): a randomised controlled equivalence trial. Lancet Oncol. 2013;14:1269–77. doi:10.1016/S1470-2045(13)70497-2.
16. Bondiau PY, et al. Robotic stereotactic radioablation concomitant with neo-adjuvant chemotherapy for breast tumors. Int J Radiat Oncol Biol Phys. 2009;75:1041–7. doi:10.1016/j.ijrobp.2008.12.037.
17. Horton JK, Blitzblau RC, Yoo S, et al. Preoperative Single-Fraction Partial Breast Radiation Therapy: A Novel Phase 1, Dose-Escalation Protocol With Radiation Response Biomarkers. International journal of radiation oncology, biology, physics 2015;92:846–55.
18. van der Leij F, et al. First results of the preoperative accelerated partial breast irradiation (PAPBI) trial. Radiother Oncol. 2015;114:322–7. doi:10.1016/j.radonc.2015.02.002.
19. Vermeulen S, et al. Accelerated partial breast irradiation: using the CyberKnife as the radiation delivery platform in the treatment of early breast cancer. Front oncol. 2011;1:43. doi:10.3389/fonc.2011.00043.
20. Wilkinson JB, et al. Four-year results using balloon-based brachytherapy to deliver accelerated partial breast irradiation with a 2-day dose fractionation schedule. Brachytherapy. 2012;11:97–104. doi:10.1016/j.brachy.2011.05.012.
21. Dragun AE, et al. A phase 2 trial of once-weekly hypofractionated breast irradiation: first report of acute toxicity, feasibility, and patient satisfaction. Int J Radiat Oncol Biol Phys. 2013;85:e123–8. doi:10.1016/j.ijrobp.2012.10.021.
22. Rovea P, et al. Once-weekly hypofractionated whole-breast radiotherapy after breast-conserving surgery in older patients: a potential alternative treatment schedule to daily 3-week hypofractionation. Clin Breast Cancer. 2015;15(4):270–6. doi:10.1016/j.clbc.2014.12.011.
23. Agrawal RK, et al. First results of the randomised UK FAST trial of radiotherapy hypofractionation for treatment of early breast cancer (CRUKE/04/015). Radiother Oncol. 2011;100:93–100. doi:10.1016/j.radonc.2011.06.026.

Chapter 24
Breast Conservation Therapy Without Capsular Contracture in Augmented Women Using Interstitial Brachytherapy

Robert R. Kuske

Contents

24.1 Scope of the Problem

The number of women who are diagnosed with breast cancer in the presence of breast augmentation is increasing each year. As it is known that silicone or saline implants do not cause breast cancer [9], the increase is the direct result of the rising number of breast augmentation surgeries that are being performed per year (Fig. 24.1). For the past 20 years, breast augmentation has been one of the most common surgical procedures in the United States, Brazil, and other countries [1]. There are regional differences in the USA, with more implants inserted in California, Arizona, New York, and Florida than in Wisconsin, Nebraska, or Alabama, for example. Women who had their implants a decade or more ago at young ages are now at the age when their risk of breast cancer is significant. Oncologists are seeing more patients who have had breast augmentation each year, and there is little in the literature providing guidance on treatment management. Indeed, the surgical literature suggests mastectomy and reconstruction as the preferred treatment because of the high risk of complications after whole breast external beam radiotherapy. This recommendation is disappointing to most of these women, as they have already

R.R. Kuske, MD, FAACE
Radiation Oncology, Virginia G. Piper Cancer Center, Arizona Center for Cancer Care, 10460 N. 92nd St., Suite 101, Scottsdale, AZ 85258, USA
e-mail: rkuske@breastmd.com

D.W. Arthur et al. (eds.), *Short Course Breast Radiotherapy: A Comprehensive Review of Hypofractionation, Partial Breast, and Intra-Operative Irradiation*,
DOI 10.1007/978-3-319-24388-7_24

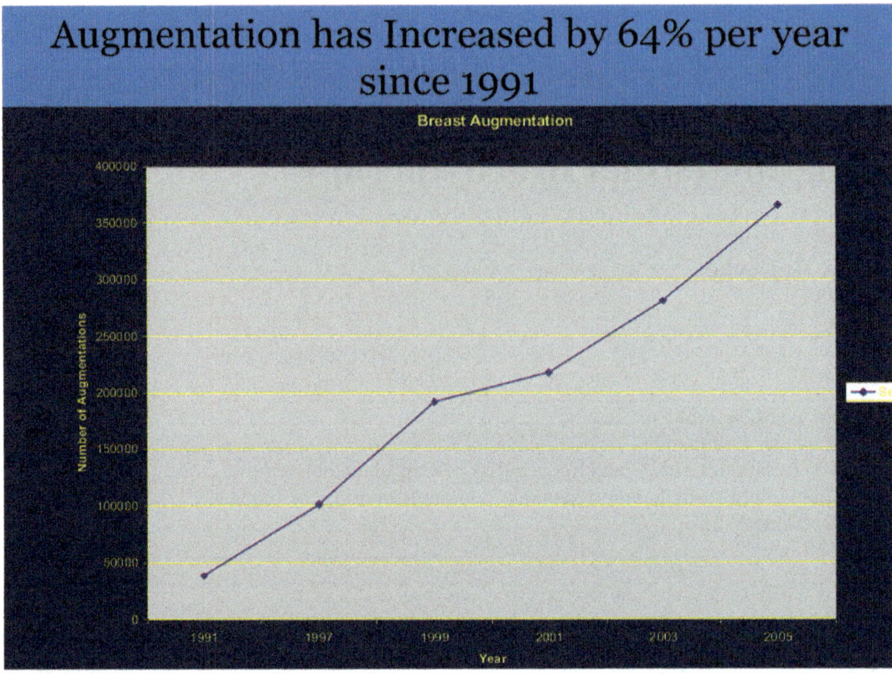

Fig. 24.1 Rate of breast augmentation over time

declared their priority on cosmesis by the fact that they have had breast augmentation in the first place. Retaining the option of breast conservation after the diagnosis of breast cancer despite having implants would provide these women with the opportunity for remaining whole, preserving a sensate breast with smaller scars, and maintaining quality of life.

Neil Handel and Melvin Silverstein reported a capsular contracture rate of 55 % after whole breast irradiation in the presence of breast augmentation [2, 3]. This high rate of capsular contracture and subsequent reparative surgery has led many surgeons and their plastic and reconstructive surgery colleagues to recommend mastectomy followed by reconstruction as the best treatment for early-stage breast cancer in women with implants.

Without implants, breast conservation therapy is considered the preferred method of early-stage breast cancer treatment because survival rates are equivalent to mastectomy and allows women to remain whole [4]. Stage for stage, breast conservation should be offered to women with breast augmentation as well. Preventing capsular contracture is key to expanding breast conservation in this growing population of women. This goal has been the focus of our 20-year investigation into a technique that minimizes the risk of symptomatic capsular contracture, presented later in this chapter.

What is the magnitude of this problem? With approximately 400,000 women undergoing breast augmentation per year in the USA alone and one in eight of these women eventually expected to be diagnosed with breast cancer, in the future we have the potential to encounter as many as 50,000 cases per year of newly diagnosed breast cancer in women with breast implants.

24.2 Capsular Contracture

Foreign objects in the human body usually provoke an inflammatory and fibrotic response from the immune system. Fibroblasts and white blood cells are programmed to "wall off" the bullet, splinter, breast implants, or other nonnative intruders. Breast implants are either silicone gel or saline inside a silicone shell. The interface between human tissue and the implant is silicone, because the element that is chemically closest to carbon is silicone. Consequently, the immune response is dampened because the silicone surface is not regarded as exceptionally foreign by the body.

Radiotherapy also provokes an inflammatory and fibrotic response from the immune system. As cells and tissues are injured by ionizing radiation, there is an initial inflammatory response, later followed by healing in the form of varying degrees of fibrosis.

The combination of breast implants and radiotherapy frequently causes "spherical fibrosis" or collagen wrapping around the implants [5] (Fig. 24.2). This process has been termed "capsular contracture" and can be mild, moderate, or severe. Just as a healing wound contracts over time, pulling the edges of the skin closer together, the fibrosis tightens around the implant over time.

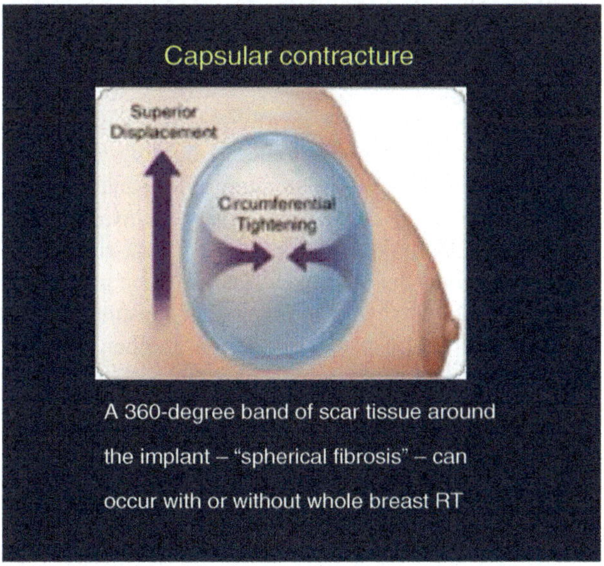

Fig. 24.2 Spherical fibrosis, capsular contracture (Ref. [5])

Table 24.1 Baker classification system for capsular contracture [5]

1. The implant is soft, with symmetrical size and shape
2. There is some firmness of the implant, and it is firmer, but no visible deformity
3. The implant is noticeably harder, and there is distortion of the breast size and shape
4. The implant can be seen and is fixed and hard and retracted superiorly toward the clavicle

Capsular contracture around breast implants occurs without radiotherapy as well and is estimated to be clinically detectable after breast augmentation approximately 15 % of the time. It can be asymptomatic or cause problems for the woman such as hardening, pain from pressure on the ribs or nerves, or gradual movement of the implant superiorly toward the clavicle. The degree of capsular contracture can be rated on a Baker Score [6] (Table 24.1).

It remains unclear why the combination of breast augmentation and whole breast radiotherapy is a super-additive effect for capsular contracture. The fibrosis that is seen is more pronounced than what has been reported with either the breast implant or the radiotherapy alone. It has been suggested that the 360° exposure of the entire implant to therapeutic doses of radiation is a contributory factor to high rate of symptomatic capsular contracture following traditional whole breast irradiation.

24.3 RT Techniques That Could Reduce Risk of Capsular Contracture

If one accepts the hypothesis that circumferential exposure of the breast implant results in the increased incidence of capsular contracture, then the breast-conserving solutions would be: (1) lumpectomy alone without breast irradiation or (2) partial breast irradiation.

Lumpectomy alone for invasive breast cancer carries with it a 25–35 % risk of ipsilateral breast tumor recurrence, according to many randomized and nonrandomized reports in the medical literature. Meta-analysis has proven a survival advantage for breast irradiation after a lumpectomy for invasive breast cancers [10]. Lumpectomy alone for DCIS likewise carries a significant risk of local recurrence without radiotherapy, and half the recurrences are invasive cancer. For most women, withholding breast irradiation to avoid an increase in capsular contracture is not a viable option.

Mastectomy and reconstruction is another option, but it is difficult to reliably predict prior to surgery which patients will still require radiotherapy postmastectomy because of yet unknown pathologic findings, positive axillary nodes, close/positive surgical margins, or other adverse pathology. In addition, despite the advent of skin and nipple-sparing mastectomies, this represents more extensive surgery with longer scars and loss of sensitivity, and the long-term cosmetic outcomes are variable and in general not as favorable as with breast conservation therapy.

The partial breast irradiation options are listed in Table 24.2. IORT is given in a single large fraction at the time of the lumpectomy or reexcision. Typically,

Table 24.2 Partial breast irradiation options

In the presence of breast augmentation
1. Intraoperative radiotherapy (IORT)
A. Electron beam
B. Soft x-rays
2. 3-d-conformal external beam radiotherapy (3-d-CRT)
3. Single-entry brachytherapy devices
A. Balloon catheters with or without multi-lumens
B. Strut-based catheters
4. Interstitial multicatheter brachytherapy

20–21 Gy is delivered to a variable depth and volume of tissue depending on the technique utilized. Radiation exposure to the implant is of little consequence since it is an inanimate object.

Balloon and strut-based brachytherapy is rarely possible because of the limited space usually present between the skin and the surface of the implant. It is common to have only 1.5–2.5 cm of tissue beneath the skin in front of the implant. A paucity of breast tissue is why these patients originally elect to have breast augmentation, and the tissue that is present tends to thin out over time from tightness and the upward pressure of the augmentation implant.

Approximately 10 % of augmented women with breast cancer can undergo single-entry devices (Fig. 24.3). Eligible women include those who have gained considerable weight since the implants were placed, or women who have peripheral tumor locations such as the axillary tail of Spence or beyond the boundaries of the implant (Fig. 24.4).

The most predictable and reliable technique is CT-guided "pinch view" interstitial brachytherapy, details to follow. The thin catheters that are used are able to fit into small spaces with limited tissue, follow the curvature of the implant, treat whatever margin around the surgical edge that is deemed necessary, and allow the ability to shape the dose cloud and limit the skin or rib dose.

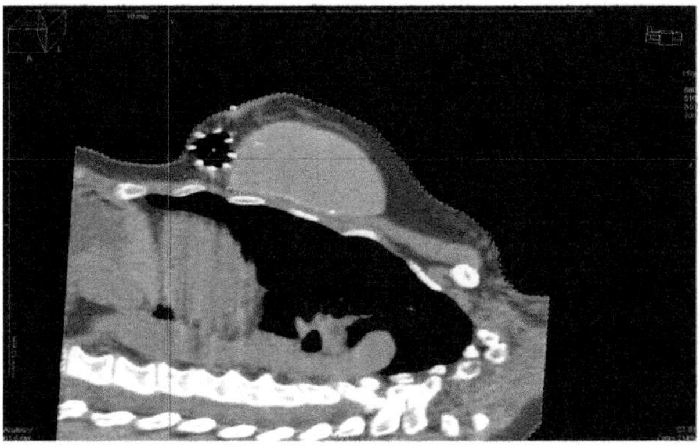

Fig. 24.3 Strut-based brachytherapy in an augmented woman just above the inframammary fold of the left breast

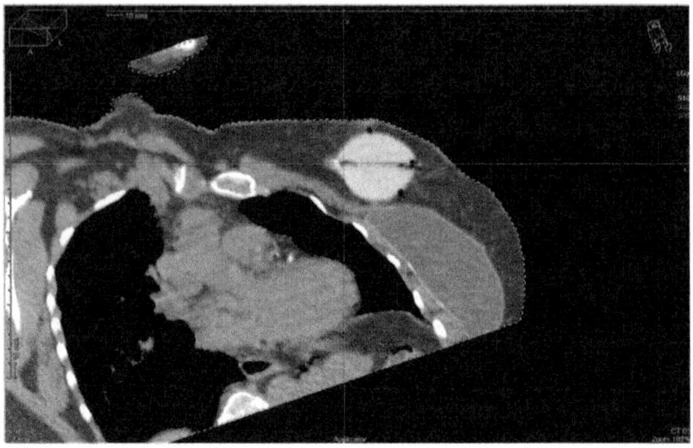

Fig. 24.4 Balloon brachytherapy in the axillary tail of Spence, well above the augmentation implant

24.4 Interstitial Brachytherapy Technique without Rupturing the Implant

The technique of image-guided interstitial brachytherapy catheter insertion requires a CT simulator (present in most Radiation Oncology Departments since the year 2000) or access to a CT scanner in diagnostic radiology, brachytherapy treatment planning software, contouring skills, a brachytherapy template, and strong medical physics support. With these elements, and the technique described below, a neophyte can perform the same brachytherapy as the author with reproducible target-volume coverage.

On the day of consultation in the radiation oncology office, breast ultrasound is performed in order to detect a seroma or postoperative changes, confirm that a target is present, measure the size and shape of the surgical cavity, and note the relation of the cavity to the augmentation implant. The implant surface is seen as a double white line on ultrasound. When a seroma is clearly seen, the radiation oncologist can visualize the lumpectomy cavity in 3 dimensions, allowing preplanning.

With oncoplastic lumpectomy techniques, a fusion of breast cancer surgery with plastic surgical principles, the cavity is usually closed. The oncoplastic surgeon reshapes the remaining breast tissue and approximates the cavity walls. With oncoplasty, pre-procedure ultrasound is rarely helpful, and a pre-procedure CT is then needed in radiation oncology or radiology to ensure that a target is present. Surgical colleagues will mark the cavity wall with clips or a 3-d marking device to facilitate target definition for brachytherapy, especially if oncoplasty is employed.

No general anesthesia or conscious sedation is necessary. The addition of this does add expense and complexity and is unnecessary with good local anesthesia . Alternatively, 1 h before the procedure, the patient is asked to take a narcotic pain reliever (e.g., Nucynta, Percocet, or Vicodin) and an anxiolytic/muscle relaxer (e.g., Valium or lorazepam) (Table 24.3).

The patient is positioned supine or partly decubitus on the CT table in radiation oncology, usually with the ipsilateral arm comfortably at her side. Wide antiseptic skin prep covers the entire breast. Sterile towels and drapes surround the breast and shield the head of the patient.

Table 24.3 Local anesthetic formulae and preoperative medications

Skin wheal:
35 cc 1 % lidocaine with epinephrine
2 cc 8.4 % sodium bicarb
35 cc Lactated Ringer's solution
Tumescent:
25 cc 2 % lidocaine with epinephrine
3 cc 8.4 % sodium bicarb
215 cc Lactated Ringer's solution
mEq sodium bicarbonate
Average amount injected per case:
30 cc skin wheal mixture through a 27 G needle, 1.25 inches long, and 10 cc syringe, on each side of the template.
150 cc tumescent mixture through a 25 G needle, 1.5 inches long and 10 cc syringe, on each side of the template
Pre-op meds:
Nucynta 50 mg taken p.o. 1 h before
Valium 5 mg taken p.o. 1 h before
Topical EMLA cream: 30 g applied under plastic wrap 1 h before the procedure

The breast is massaged for several minutes to loosen it off the augmentation implant and facilitate bunching the breast tissue up and away from the implant. The lumpectomy site is palpated, with the ultrasound or CT images as a reference, to help plan template orientation. The breast tissue at the lumpectomy site must be bunched up while the implant is pushed in the reverse direction, similar to Eklund or "pinch view" or "push back" mammography that is standard breast imaging for women with implants. Note that the thickness of the breast tissue may be only 1.5 cm in the relaxed state before pinching, but the thickness increases to 3–4 cm after bunching.

Mastisol or Tincture of benzoin is applied to the skin surface where the template will be touching to prevent template slippage. With one hand, the breast is strongly lifted up and away from the augmentation implant, and the implant pushed backward, while the breast brachytherapy template (Fig. 24.5) is positioned. The front and back plates are closed with moderate compression so that the deep plane is as close to the augmentation implant as feasible. Side clamps are attached to the template to make the plates parallel.

The surgical assistant holds the template against the augmentation to prevent slippage, while the radiation oncologist chooses 3 holes for anchoring needles that are shallow and safely away from the implant to avoid puncture. These holes are chosen to be in the target volume. A skin wheal is raised on both the proximal and distal sides with half-strength buffered local anesthetic, and dilute and buffered tumescent local anesthetic is injected along the chosen pathway (Table 24.3). Thin 27 G needles are used for the skin wheal and a 25 G for the tumescent. The three anchoring needles are inserted without CT guidance, with care to ensure that they remain perpendicular to the plane of the template as they traverse the breast, exiting the large hole on the back template.

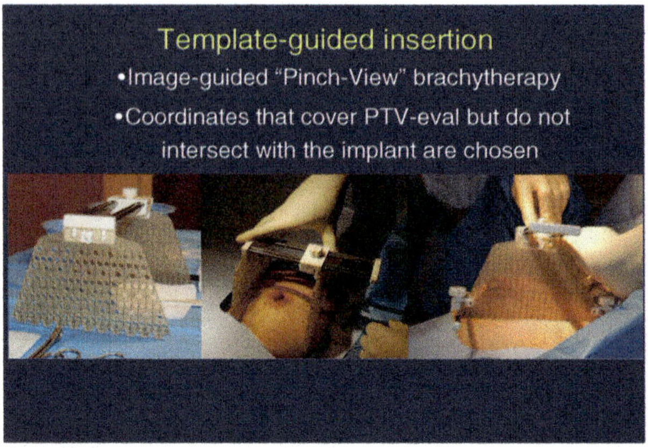

Fig. 24.5 The breast brachytherapy template

After the 3 anchoring needles, the template will not slip and will maintain its position relative to the augmentation implant. A breast CT without contrast is obtained while the template is attached. These images are exported to a computer with 3-d brachytherapy treatment planning software.

Image guidance is a key to the success of this procedure. On each slice, the medical physicist or dosimetrist, under the supervision of the radiation oncologist, contours the implant, skin, and lumpectomy edges. The software then expands the cavity volume by 1.5–2 cm in all directions, except for 5 mm from the implant and 5 mm from the skin surface, creating a modified planning treatment volume (PTV-eval).

The software renders a 3-dimensional picture of the breast on the computer monitor, and these images are rotated until the front and back template holes are aligned. The physicist then outlines the maximum cross-sectional area of the PTV-eval using a catheter marking tool in the software, so the target volume is displayed on each CT slice in the Z-plane. The physicist also outlines the surface of the implant and the skin, so that they are displayed on the "needles eye view" when the templates are aligned. The CT slices are then scrolled in the Z-plane on the computer monitor until the large holes on the back template are in view.

With the PTV-eval, skin, and implant displayed (Fig. 24.6), it is simple to choose coordinates of template holes that are within or just beyond the PTV-eval but do not intersect with the implant + 5 mm or the go outside the skin surface (Fig. 24.7). Skin wheal and tumescent local anesthetic as described above are then injected. After all local anesthetic is injected, a thick guiding template is attached to the front plate (over the 3 anchoring needles) to force each 19 G brachytherapy needle insertion to be perfectly parallel and straight. You can also manually guide each needle insertion instead, foregoing the thick guiding template.

Initially, it is helpful, to obtain a CT at this point to assure that the needles are placed correctly. The template is then disassembled, and only the needles remain in place with the breast relaxed from compression. You will notice that the rows come closer together after the template is removed and compression relaxed. The deep row

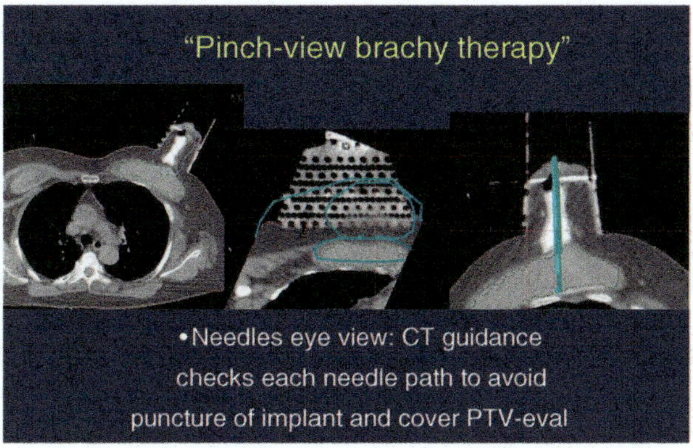

Fig. 24.6 Image-guided needle insertion with the implant, skin, PTV-eval, and holes of the template displayed

Fig. 24.7 Diagram of the template with the chosen holes marked

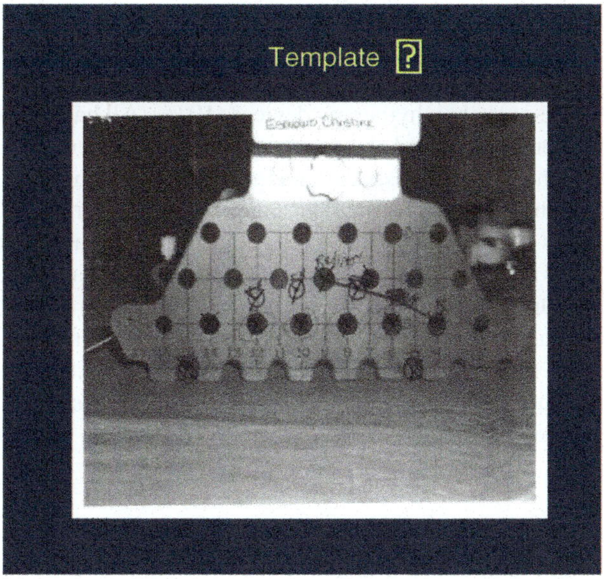

will also "fall back" to the surface of the implant. Additional freehand needles can be inserted to cover any gaps in coverage, if necessary, being careful to manually push the implant away from the needle's pathway and keep the needles parallel.

The needles are then exchanged for polyethylene catheters secured with buttons and trimmed to proper length. Patient is provided a break and returns 2 h later, after any swelling has dissipated, for the treatment planning CT. The first treatment is delivered on the following day allowing time for CT-based 3-d treatment planning.

Certain dosimetric guidelines are routine. Commonly used fractionation schemes are presently 34 Gy in 10 b.i.d. fractions over 5 treatment days or 34 Gy in 8 b.i.d. fractions over 4 treatment days. It is recommended to limit the skin dose, as defined here as skin surface, to ≤100 % of prescribed dose with a goal of 95 % of the prescribed dose delivered to 95 % of the PTV-eval. The dose homogeneity index achieved is typically 10 % less than what we see with non-augmented breasts, 75–80 %, but rarely below 70 %. The 150 % isodose lines may touch, but not coalesce. If the brachytherapy does not meet these guidelines, additional needles are inserted under local anesthetic to improve coverage and homogeneity.

The catheters are removed minutes after the 8th or 10th and final high-dose brachytherapy treatment. No local anesthetic or narcotic is required, since the catheters are removed easily without significant resistance or discomfort.

The patient is seen 7–10 days after catheter extraction to ensure there are no wound complications or healing delays.

24.5 Outcomes

The author has treated more than 250 women with breast augmentations with select breast cancers over the past 20 years with interstitial brachytherapy (90 %) or single-entry brachytherapy devices (10 %). All had lumpectomy and axillary dissection or sentinel node biopsy to complete breast conservation surgery. Selection criteria have been consistent and uniform, with tumors less than or equal to 3 cm that have been excised with clear margins (no ink on tumor), and zero to three axillary nodes positive without extracapsular extension, accepted.

As reported at the annual meeting of the American Society of Therapeutic Radiology and Oncology (ASTRO) [7], 10 % of patients were noted to have Baker 2–4 capsular contracture at the time of consultation before treatment of her breast cancer. Less than 5 % experience new or additional capsular contracture is seen after interstitial brachytherapy. Cosmetic outcome has been superior to that seen with brachytherapy for non-augmented women. Tumor control has been 95 % at 7 years median follow-up.

24.6 Summary

The advantages to APBI in this population extend beyond convenience. It allows each patient to retain her breast and breast augmentation implant. It reduces radiation exposure to only the affected part of the breast in the vicinity of the original tumor site. It minimizes dose to the lung, heart, chest wall, ribs, and normal breast or nodal tissue. Note that the implant acts as a spacer, further separating internal organs from radiation exposure. In women with augmentation, the radiation dose cloud does not encompass the entire implant, eliminating circumferential irradiation of the entire implant. When we embarked on the initial clinical trial, we hypothesized that brachytherapy would prevent the spherical fibrosis that causes capsular contracture.

Capsular contracture is spherical fibrosis caused by circumferential exposure of the foreign body implant by whole breast irradiation (Fig. 24.8). Patients know this as "painful hardening of the implant" (Fig. 24.9). It can be seen without radiotherapy as well and is a known risk of breast augmentation.

In many cancer types treated in radiation oncology, image guidance and tighter conformal radiation fields have improved tumor control rates and decreased toxicity [8]. Breast brachytherapy is an example of an advance in dose delivery that conforms precisely to the target volume, minimizing exposure of normal tissues. The rapid dose fall-off, inherent in the physics of brachytherapy, is especially attractive in the treatment of women with augmented breasts. The prescription dose is at the periphery, so the dosimetry follows the biology of breast cancer cell density gradient. The

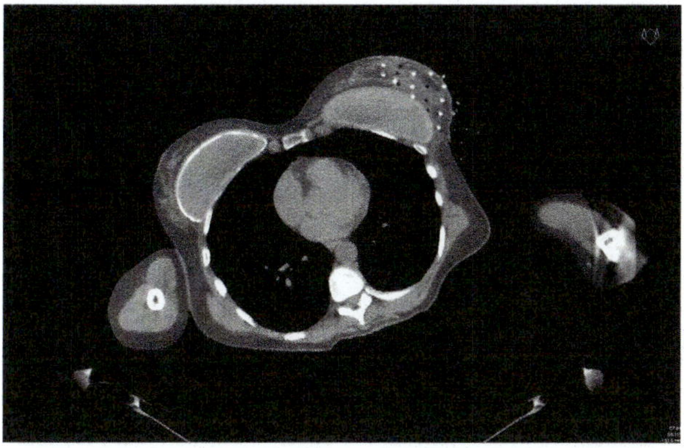

Fig. 24.8 CT evidence for severe capsular contracture 15 years after whole breast RT on the right, with brachytherapy for a metachronous left breast cancer. Note the calcified plaque surrounding the right implant, with no evidence for capsular contracture on the left

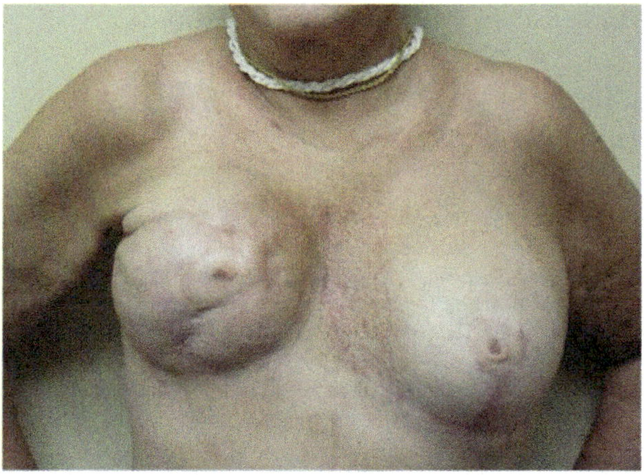

Fig. 24.9 Right-sided Baker 4 capsular contracture 7 years following external beam radiotherapy after prior augmentation and mastopexy with keyhole and inverted-T incisions bilaterally

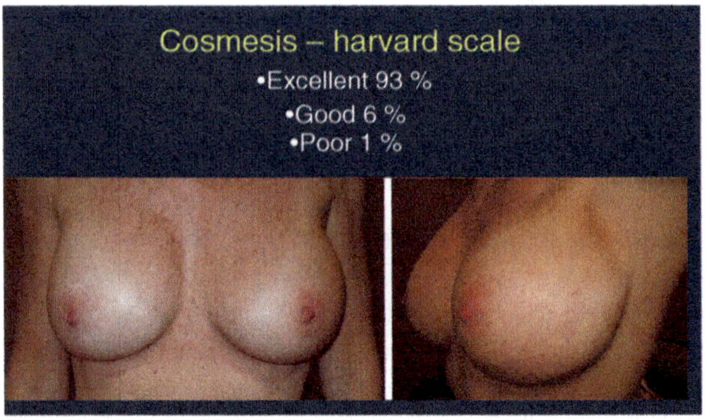

Fig. 24.10 Excellent cosmetic outcome 5 years after multicatheter brachytherapy APBI in the presence of augmentation

tissue inside that dose envelope is ~15 % higher dose, providing an inherent boost closer to the epicenter of where the cancer started. Since only a small surface area of the implant is exposed to significant ionizing radiation, scar tissue does not envelope the silicone or saline implant. The risk of capsular contracture is significantly reduced, and the cosmetic outcomes are excellent/good in over 90 % of cases (Fig. 24.10).

The "pinch view" image-guided technique described in this chapter utilizes a commercially available template and 3-d treatment planning software. The method is simple, safe, and reproducible from one institution to the next. Long-term data [7] supports the conclusion that interstitial breast brachytherapy may be the treatment of choice for select women with early-stage breast cancer in the presence of breast augmentation.

Acknowledgements The author would like to acknowledge the efforts of Rezwan Chowdhury, MD, a former brachytherapy fellow who now practices in British Columbia, Canada, and who presented the first augmentation paper at our national meeting. I am also grateful for breast surgeons and my practice colleagues who have supported the brachytherapy studies and program since its inception. Kristina Allen is noted for her administrative assistance for these patients. Margaret Snyder, RN, collected and analyzed the data.

References

1. International Society of Aesthetic Plastic Surgery. ISAPS international survey on aesthetic/cosmetic procedures performed in 2011. http://www.isaps.org/files/html-contents/Downloads/ISAPS%20Results%20-%20Procedures%20in%202011.pdf.
2. Handel N. The Effect of Silicone implants on the diagnosis, prognosis, and treatment of breast cancer. Plast Reconstr Surg. 2007;120(7 Suppl 1):81S–93.
3. Handel N, Silverstein MJ. Breast cancer diagnosis and prognosis in augmented women. Plast Reconstr Surg. 2006;118(3):587–93; discussion 594–6.
4. NIH consensus conference: treatment of early-stage breast cancer. JAMA. 1991;265:391.

5. Macadam S. Capsular contracture [ONLINE]. 2015. Available at: http://drsheinamacadam.com/surgical-definitions/. Accessed 03 Apr 15.
6. Spear SL, Baker JL. Classification of capsular contracture after prosthetic breast reconstruction. Plast Reconstr Surg. 1995;96(5):1119–23.
7. Kuske R, Chowdhury R, Snyder M, et al. Accelerated partial breast irradiation for select breast cancers in the presence of augmentation. Int J Radiat Oncol Biol Phys. 2012;84(3 Suppl):S87.
8. Dawson LA, Sharpe MB. Image-guided radiotherapy: rationale, benefits, and limitations. Lancet Oncol. 2006;7(10):848–58.
9. FDA Update on the Safety of Silicone Gel-filled Breast Implants, June 2011, Center for Devices and Radiological Health, U.S. Food and Drug Administration. www.fda.gov/downloads/MedicalDevices/Products and Medical Procedures/Implants and Prosthetics/Breast Implants/ucm260090.pdf.
10. Early Breast Cancer Trialists' Group (2005). Effects of radiotherapy and of differences in the extent of surgery for early breast cancer on local recurrence and 15-year survival: an overview of the randomized trials. Lancet 366:2097–2106.

Chapter 25
Noninvasive Image-Guided Breast Brachytherapy (NIBB)

Jaroslaw T. Hepel

Contents

25.1 Introduction and Background

Over the last several decades, the field of radiation oncology has strived to achieve more conformal and targeted treatments with the goal to decrease morbidity and improve patient quality of life. For early-stage breast cancer, accelerated partial-breast irradiation (APBI) has been a significant advance in this regard. However, the conventional APBI techniques are not optimal for all patients [1]. Interstitial multi-catheter brachytherapy is sophisticated and adaptable to even the most difficult tumor bed and breast geometry [2, 3]. However, the complexity of this implant procedure has limited its use to select high-volume centers. Furthermore, the invasive nature of this approach is not acceptable to some women. Intracavitary brachytherapy is a technically simplified implant which has resulted in a broader user base [4]. However, the simplified dosimetry of these implants limits this technique in

J.T. Hepel, MD, F.A.C.R.O
Department of Radiation Oncology, Rhode Island Hospital
Warren Alpert Medical School of Brown University, Providence, RI
e-mail: jhepel@lifespan.org

D.W. Arthur et al. (eds.), *Short Course Breast Radiotherapy: A Comprehensive Review of Hypofractionation, Partial Breast, and Intra-Operative Irradiation*,
DOI 10.1007/978-3-319-24388-7_25

situations of complicated tumor bed geometry especially when oncoplastic tissue rearrangement is performed. Additionally, this technique remains invasive and requires the percutaneous catheter to remain in place for the duration of the therapy. This again is not acceptable to some women. Three-dimensional conformal external-beam radiation therapy (3D-CRT) is a noninvasive approach to APBI. However, unlike the interstitial and intracavitary approaches, uncertainties related to daily set-up errors and intrafraction patient, breast, and respiratory motions require additional margin expansion to ensure appropriate treatment of the at-risk tissues surrounding the lumpectomy cavity. This results in significantly larger treatment volumes. Several studies have shown increased rates of late toxicity and fair-to-poor cosmetic outcomes with this technique [5–8]. And these suboptimal outcomes have been correlated with treatment volumes [5].

Noninvasive image-guided breast brachytherapy (NIBB) is a novel APBI technique and holds potential advantages over other APBI techniques. Similar to interstitial and intracavitary brachytherapy, NIBB has the advantage of delivering radiation to the tumor bed with a high degree of precision. This is accomplished by employing breast immobilization and mammographic-like image guidance for each radiation treatment. However, unlike interstitial and intracavitary brachytherapy, NIBB is completely noninvasive making this approach more acceptable to patients not willing to undergo percutaneous catheter placement. The inconvenience and discomfort of managing an indwelling catheter or catheters is eliminated, as is the risk of instrumentation-related infection. Also, oncoplastic reconstruction to enhance the cosmetic outcomes of surgery can be performed with NIBB as long as the tissues at risk are appropriated marked with surgical clips or other fiducials. Furthermore, unlike the 3D-CRT technique, NIBB does not require an additional large margin expansion. With breast immobilization and image guidance, the inaccuracies related to set-up errors and patient or breast motion are essentially eliminated. Additionally, the breast compression used for immobilization displaces nontarget breast tissue out of the irradiation field. This results in further reduction in target and irradiated volumes, thereby reducing the risk of toxicities associated with larger treatment volumes. Altogether, this makes NIBB an attractive and promising approach for the delivery of APBI [9].

25.2 NIBB Technique

25.2.1 AccuBoost System

NIBB is delivered using the AccuBoost™ brachytherapy system (Fig. 25.1) (Advanced Radiation Therapy, Inc., Tyngsboro, MA). This commercially available system was designed and has been FDA cleared to deliver partial-breast irradiation. The system utilizes a pair of breast compression and immobilization plates, onboard kV imaging, targeting grids, and a series of specialized applicators. Radiation is delivered using a high-dose rate (HDR) Ir-192 source via remote afterloader.

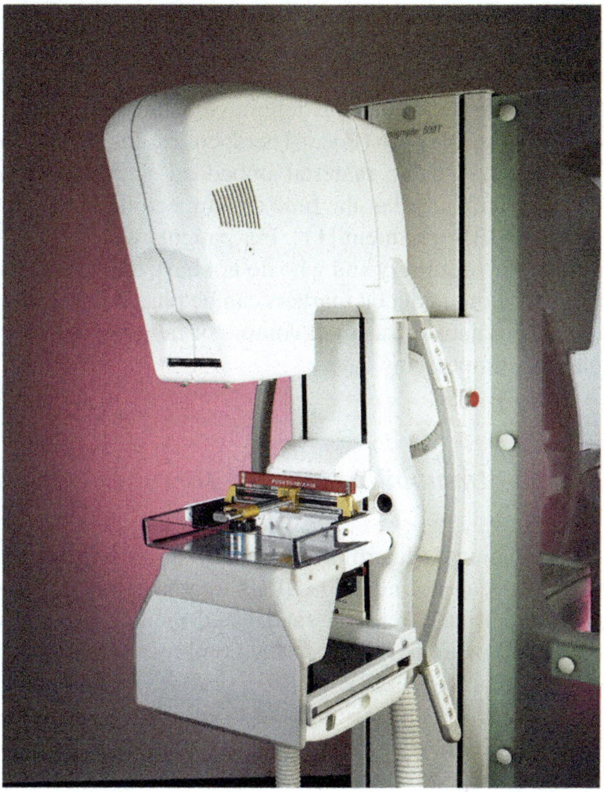

Fig. 25.1 The AccuBoost system

25.2.2 Simulation

In order to be deemed a good candidate for the NIBB technique, the patient's tumor bed needs to be able to be positioned between the compression plates, the entire tumor bed should be identifiable on AccuBoost imaging, and the intended target volume should be able to be encompassed by one of the available applicators. In addition, breast compression achieving a separation of $\leq$8 cm has been recommended to limit skin dose when NIBB is used for APBI.

To evaluate a patient's candidacy for the NIBB technique, pretreatment simulation is performed. Often, a CT simulation is performed first. CT simulation is not required for the NIBB technique, but it is very useful to evaluate the position and configuration of the tumor bed, delineate the number of surgical clips, and assess the relationship of surgical clips or markers to the tumor bed, skin, and chest wall. This information helps to guide optimal patient/breast position and to ensure that the entire tumor bed is visualized on AccuBoost imaging.

Simulation on the AccuBoost system is then performed. Patients are positioned upright, either seated or standing, with breast compression and mammography-like imaging performed sequentially in two orthogonal axes. Using AccuBoost imaging, the tumor bed is identified. This can be accomplished using postsurgical changes; however, the entire tumor bed is only well defined in about half of patients using this method alone. The use of surgical clips, placed at the time of lumpectomy, has been shown to be very helpful in defining the tumor bed [10]. Alternatively, other markers can be used. BioZorb (Focal Therapeutics, Inc., Aliso Viejo, CA) is a helical marker made of resorbable material imbedded with six metallic fiducial markers. This device is implanted at the time of lumpectomy and can be used to define the tumor bed for NIBB treatment [11]. For patients who did not have clips or markers place at the time of surgery and who do not have a well-defined tumor bed by postsurgical changes alone, fiducial markers can be placed percutaneously using CT or US guidance. Alternatively, a small volume of radiopaque contrast material can be injected into the lumpectomy cavity.

25.2.3 Immobilization and Target Localization

Once a patient is determined to be an appropriate candidate for the NIBB technique, treatment can be initiated. NIBB treatment is delivered via two orthogonal axes, typically oriented cranial-caudal and medial-lateral. For each treatment axis, the breast is positioned between the compression plates and immobilized with gentle compression (Fig. 25.2a). This procedure is similar to mammography except that the extent of compression is less. The goal of compression is to achieve a stable breast position and should be tailored to patient comfort. Once immobilized, a mammography-like image using 30 kV x-rays is obtained. This high-contrast, high-resolution image is used to localize the tumor bed and to select applicators for treatment. The selected pair of applicators needs to encompass the intended target volume (Fig. 25.2b). The clinical target volume (CTV) should include the tumor bed with an appropriate margin to account for microscopic disease spread. A CTV margin of 1.0 cm around the lumpectomy cavity limited by the chest wall and skin has been used consistent with other APBI techniques. With appropriate breast immobilization, a stable position of the breast and tumor bed can be achieved. Therefore, in the initial NIBB APBI phase II trial, no additional margin for the planning target volume (PTV) was used. However, a small margin expansion of 1–5 mm can be considered.

25.2.4 Applicators and Applicator Selection

Once the patient is immobilized and the target is defined on imaging, an appropriately sized and shaped pair of applicators is selected to encompass the PTV. Three generations of applicators have been developed (Fig. 25.3). First-generation applicators consist of natural-round and D-shaped applicators. Each of these applicators is designed with a circular channel at the base through which a HDR Ir-192 source

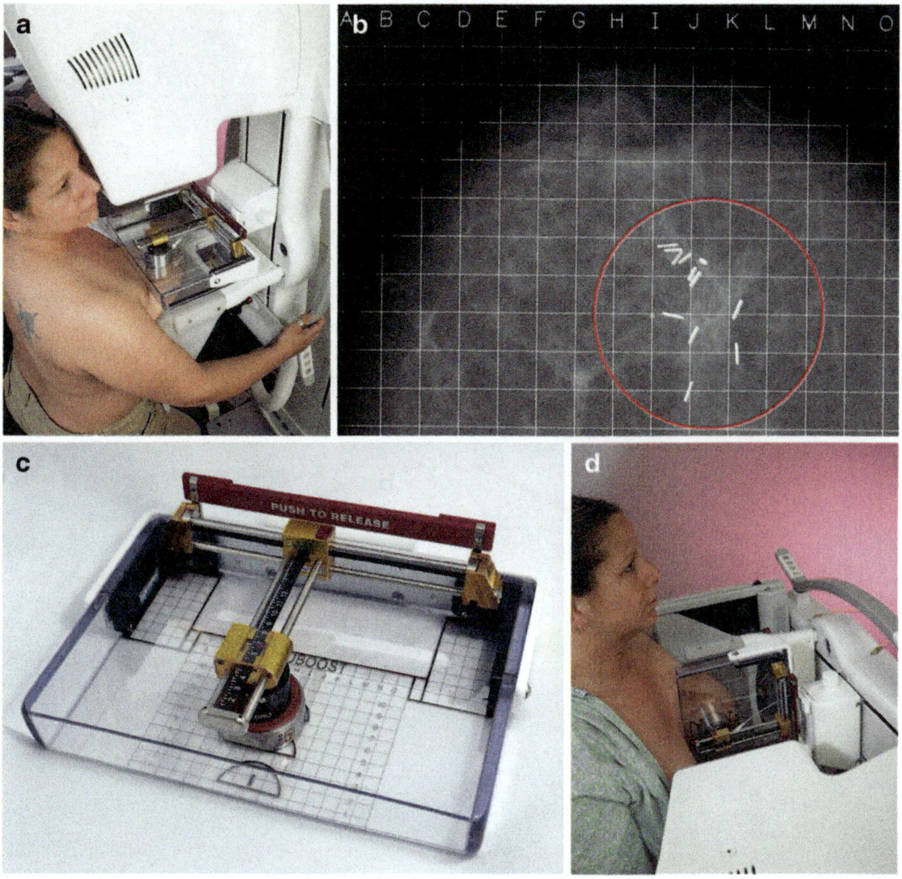

Fig. 25.2 NIBB technique. (**a**) Breast immobilization with compression in the cranial-caudal axis. (**b**) AccuBoost imaging demonstrating tumor bed identification, applicator size selection to encompass the PTV, and tumor bed localization using the targeting grid. (**c**) Applicator positioning on either side of the compression plates according to targeting grid location. (**d**) Breast immobilization in the orthogonal axis with medial-lateral compression

travels (Fig. 25.4). The tungsten shielding of the applicator collimates and directs the Ir-192 photon emission at the tumor bed in a beam-like projection [12]. Second-generation, conical-round applicators were developed to decrease both the skin dose and treatment time. These applicators have a central cone shield which reduced skin scatter yet maintains dose at depth (Fig. 25.5) [13]. Second-generation applicators are optimized to maximally reduce skin dose (skin-dose optimized – SDO) or to maximally decrease treatment time (dose-rate optimized – DRO). Third-generation, conical-round applicators were developed with beveled-wedge shielding at the posterior wall. This allows for closer positioning of the applicator to the chest wall in order to better encompass deep-seated tumors. These are also available in both DRO

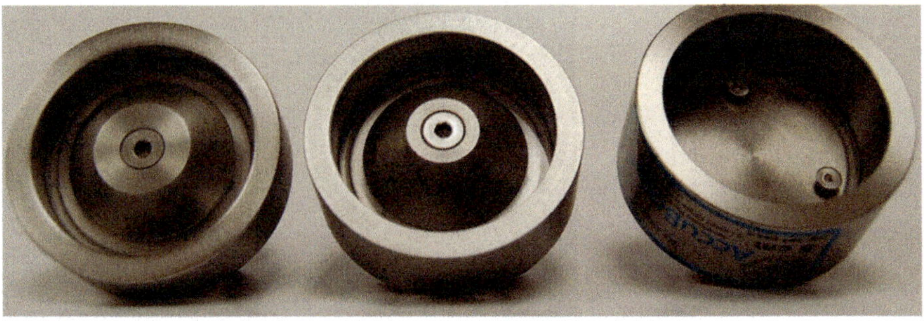

Fig. 25.3 AccuBoost applicators. From left to right: 5 cm second-generation conical-round applicator (DRO), 5 cm second-generation conical-round applicator (SDO), and 5 cm first-generation natural-round applicator

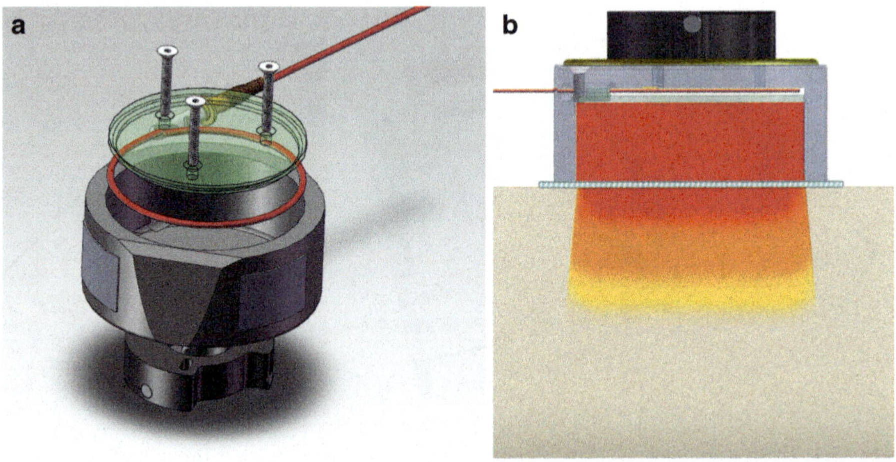

Fig. 25.4 AccuBoost applicator schematic. (a) Circular channel at the base of each applicator allows for passage of HDR Ir-192 source. (b) Photon emissions from the Ir-192 source are collimated by the applicator in a beam-like projection

and SDO configuration. For APBI, SDO applicators are recommended as these minimize skin dose. All three generations of round applicators are available in 5, 6, 7, and 8 cm sizes, and first-generation D-shaped applicator is available in 4.5, 5.3, and 6.0 cm sizes. Second-generation D-shaped applicators with DRO and SDO configuration are in development.

25.2.5 Treatment Delivery

Once a pair of applicators is selected, the applicator positions are determined using the image localization grid. The applicators are attached to the corresponding position on either side of the compression plates (Fig. 25.2c). The use of two applicators

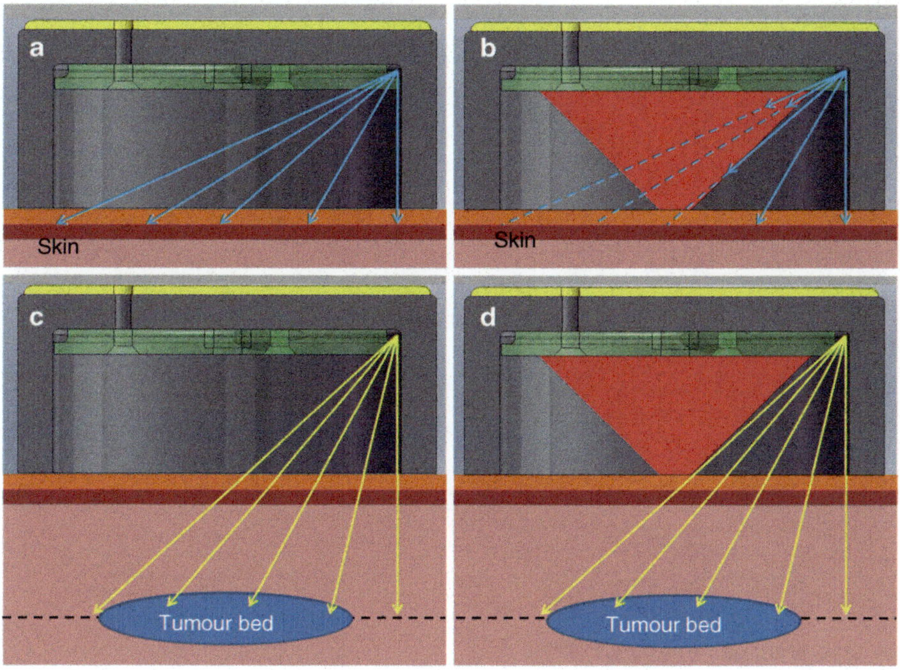

Fig. 25.5 Schematic of a second-generation applicator demonstrating reduction in surface dose while maintaining dose at depth by using a central conical shield (**b, d**) as compared with a first-generation applicator (**a, c**)

allows for treatment to be delivered in a parallel-opposed fashion. Once each applicator is positioned, it is then attached to a HDR Ir-192 remote afterloader for treatment delivery. Currently, source dwell positions are symmetrically distributed at 1.0 cm intervals along the circular channel at the base of each applicator. Dwell times at each position are likewise equivalent to generate a symmetric beam-like projection. Using a planning nomogram, the dwell times are determined to deliver the intended prescription dose.

After completion of treatment in one axis, breast compression is released, and the process is repeated along the orthogonal axis (Fig. 25.2d). The use of two orthogonal axes for each fraction results in conformal dose distribution to the target volume, decreased dose to skin, and decreased dose to nontarget breast tissue as compared to treatment utilizing a single axis (Fig. 25.6).

25.2.6 Dose Prescription

A prescription dose of 34.0 Gy in ten fractions was used in the initial phase II trial evaluating NIBB APBI [14]. Treatment can be delivered either twice daily over 1 week or once daily over 2 weeks. Twice-daily treatments should be at least 6 h apart

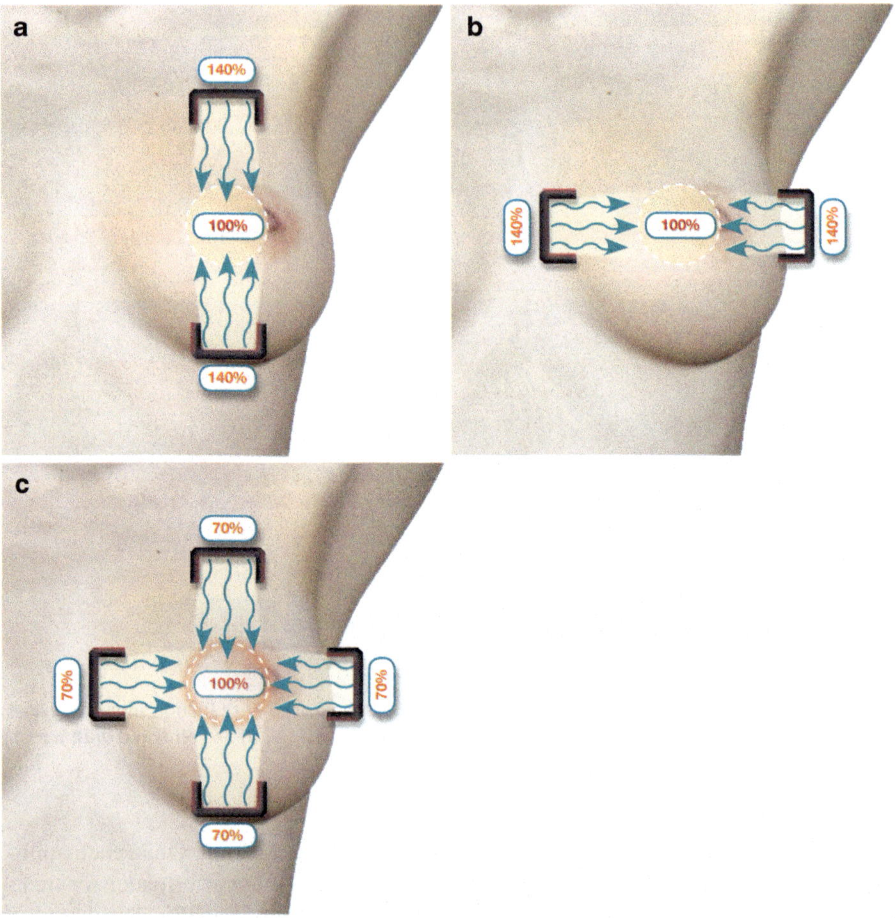

Fig. 25.6 Schematic of NIBB treatment. Sequential compression and treatment in the cranial-caudal axis (**a**) followed by medial-lateral axis (**b**). (**c**) The use of two orthogonal axes for treatment results in conformal dose distribution to the tumor bed with relative sparing of superficial skin dose and nontarget breast tissue

to allow adequate time for normal tissue repair between fractions. The treatment dose is prescribed to the midplane between the paired applicators (100 % isodose line). This dose and fractionation was based on dose schedules used with other brachytherapy techniques for APBI.

More recently, dosimetric evaluation has shown that the NIBB technique results in dose heterogeneity across the target volume that is intermediate to that which is typical of interstitial or intracavitary brachytherapy and that which is typical of external-beam 3D-CRT [15]. As such, equivalent uniform dose (EUD) calculations have been performed comparing NIBB, interstitial brachytherapy, intracavitary brachytherapy, and 3D-CRT [16]. This work has suggested that a mild increase (5.8 %) in prescription dose for NIBB to 36.0 Gy in ten fractions would result in an

EUD that more closely approximates that which is achieved with other APBI techniques. At Tufts and Brown Universities, we have implemented this dose modification for future protocols.

As with other APBI techniques, shorter and more convenient treatment schedules are being explored. It is quite clear that the twice-daily schedule commonly employed is not convenient for patients. In the initial NIBB APBI trial, the choice of daily versus BID treatment was based on patient preference, and only one quarter of patients elected for BID treatment [14]. Therefore, a shorter schedule that is delivered daily would be ideal. Currently, a prospective phase II trial evaluating a schedule of 28.5 Gy in five daily fractions is accruing patients [17].

25.3 Dosimetry and Treatment Planning

Treatment planning for NIBB has been performed using 2D planning of each individual treatment axis. Patient specific 3D planning is not currently available. Mammography-like imaging is used to generate high-contrast, high-quality images for localization of the tumor bed, and positioning of applicators is used at the time of treatment delivery. Composite dosimetry between the two orthogonal treatment axes has been challenging with this technique as a result of the extent of tissue deformity from one compressed state to a unique compressed state in the orthogonal plane. Commercially available software for deformable image registration at this time cannot accurately co-register image sets obtained in these two divergent states.

In order to evaluate the dose distribution using NIBB, composite 3D dosimetry has been generated using several methods. The simplest of these methods uses a fixed tissue model which assumes no tissue compression or deformity. This model has shown that the summated dose between the two orthogonal treatment axes results in coverage of the target volume by the prescription dose with relative sparing of nontarget tissues (Fig. 25.7). This simple model, however, ignores the complexity of tissue deformity which will influence dose distribution. Thus to evaluate the effect of tissue deformity, a more robust deformable model was created [18]. This model uses finite element analysis (FEA) incorporating known planar stress loading tissue biomechanics and an elasticity coefficient specific to breast tissue. This deformable FEA model was then used to simulate NIBB treatment via two sequential orthogonal compression axes. Monte Carlo benchmarking for validation has shown agreement with dose deviation within 2 %. A comprehensive evaluation of the effect of target size, target location, extent of breast compression, applicator size, and applicator type within a clinically relevant range was performed (Fig. 25.8). In most situations examined, greater than 95 % of the PTV was covered by greater than 95 % of the prescription dose. In the remaining "worst-case" scenarios, minimum coverage was maintained at greater than 90 % of the PTV, which was covered by greater than 90 % of the prescription dose.

To further evaluate the 3D dosimetry of NIBB, Sioshansi et al. performed a modeling study of composite dosimetry using patient-specific CT data sets. For this

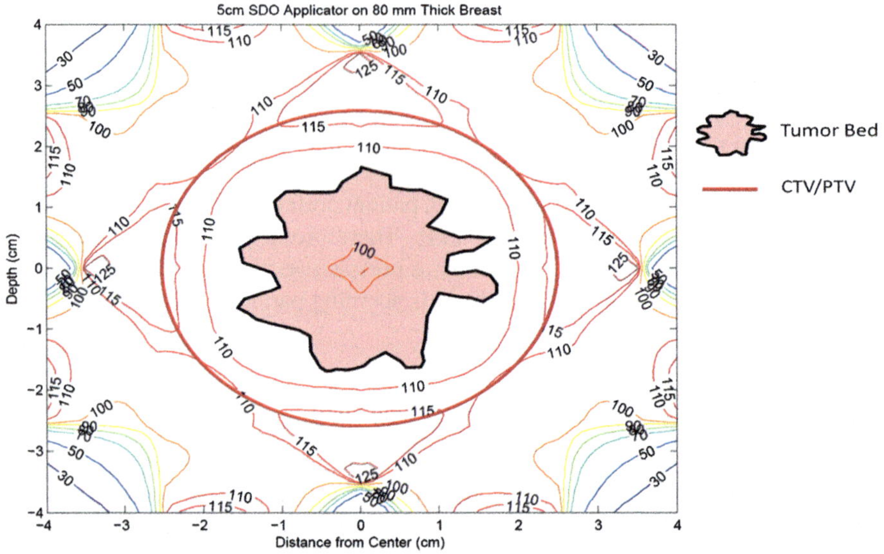

Fig. 25.7 Fixed dosimetry model assuming no tissue compression or deformity. Example of central plane composite dose distribution of sequential irradiation in two orthogonal treatment axes using 5 cm round applicators at 8 cm separation. The isodose distribution demonstrates coverage of the PTV with the prescription dose

study, patients underwent CT imaging with breast compression simulating NIBB treatment. Dosimetric comparison between NIBB and 3D-CRT techniques for the delivery of APBI was performed (Fig. 25.9) [15]. This comparison showed good target coverage by the prescription dose for both NIBB and 3D-CRT techniques. The PTV V90 was 96 % and 100 %, respectively. However, PTV volumes were 50 % smaller with the NIBB technique, which resulted in significantly lower doses delivered to normal tissues. The maximum skin dose was 10 % lower with NIBB. Similarly, the chest wall and lung maximum doses were lower by factors of 3.0 and 4.8, respectively. The dose distribution was more heterogeneous for NIBB compared with 3D-CRT, but less heterogeneous than other brachytherapy techniques.

Aside from target coverage, another important consideration when using a relatively low-energy brachytherapy source externally to treat a target at depth is the dose delivered to the skin. Skin dose using NIBB is minimized in several ways including using two orthogonal axes for each treatment, ensuring that there was no significant skin overlap between treatment axes, and limiting breast separation with compression to ≤8 cm. Although the optimal skin dose constraint for this technique is not yet known, using these restrictions, the maximum skin dose is expected to be <100 % of the prescription dose. Doses to the chest wall or structures deep to the chest wall, e.g., heart and lung, are not expected to be a concern using the NIBB technique as the treatment axes are tangential to the chest wall. The resulting dose to the chest wall is expected to be significantly less than prescription dose in all scenarios. This has been confirmed by direct measurements [19].

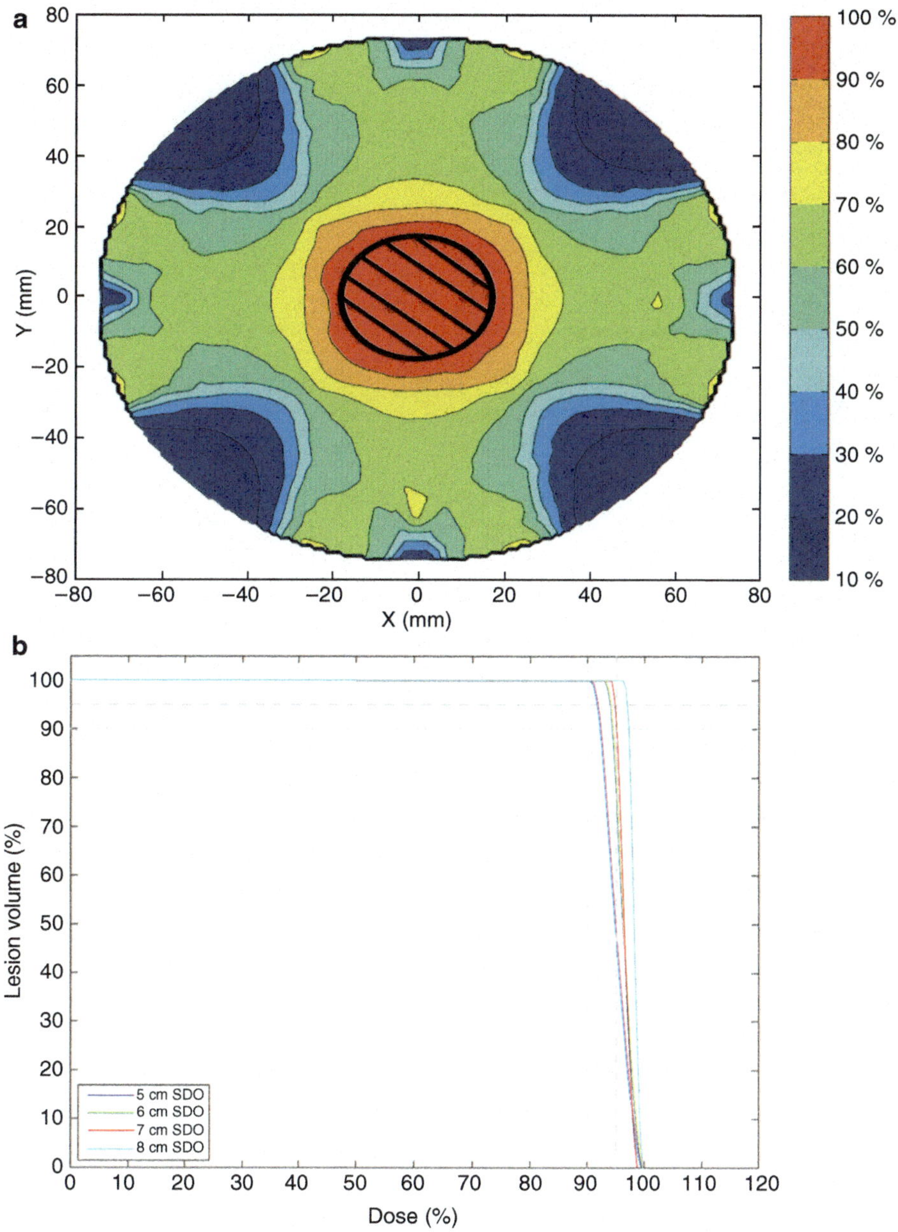

Fig. 25.8 Fine element biomechanical model. Example treatment of a 3.5 cm target treated sequential in two orthogonal axes using second-generation round SDO applicators. (**a**) Composite central plane dose distribution of treatment with a 5 cm applicator with compression from 12 to 6 cm along each axis. Graphs demonstrating composite dose volume histograms evaluating the effect of (**b**) applicators size, (**c**) extent of breast compression, and (**d**) target central axis offset on resulting PTV coverage

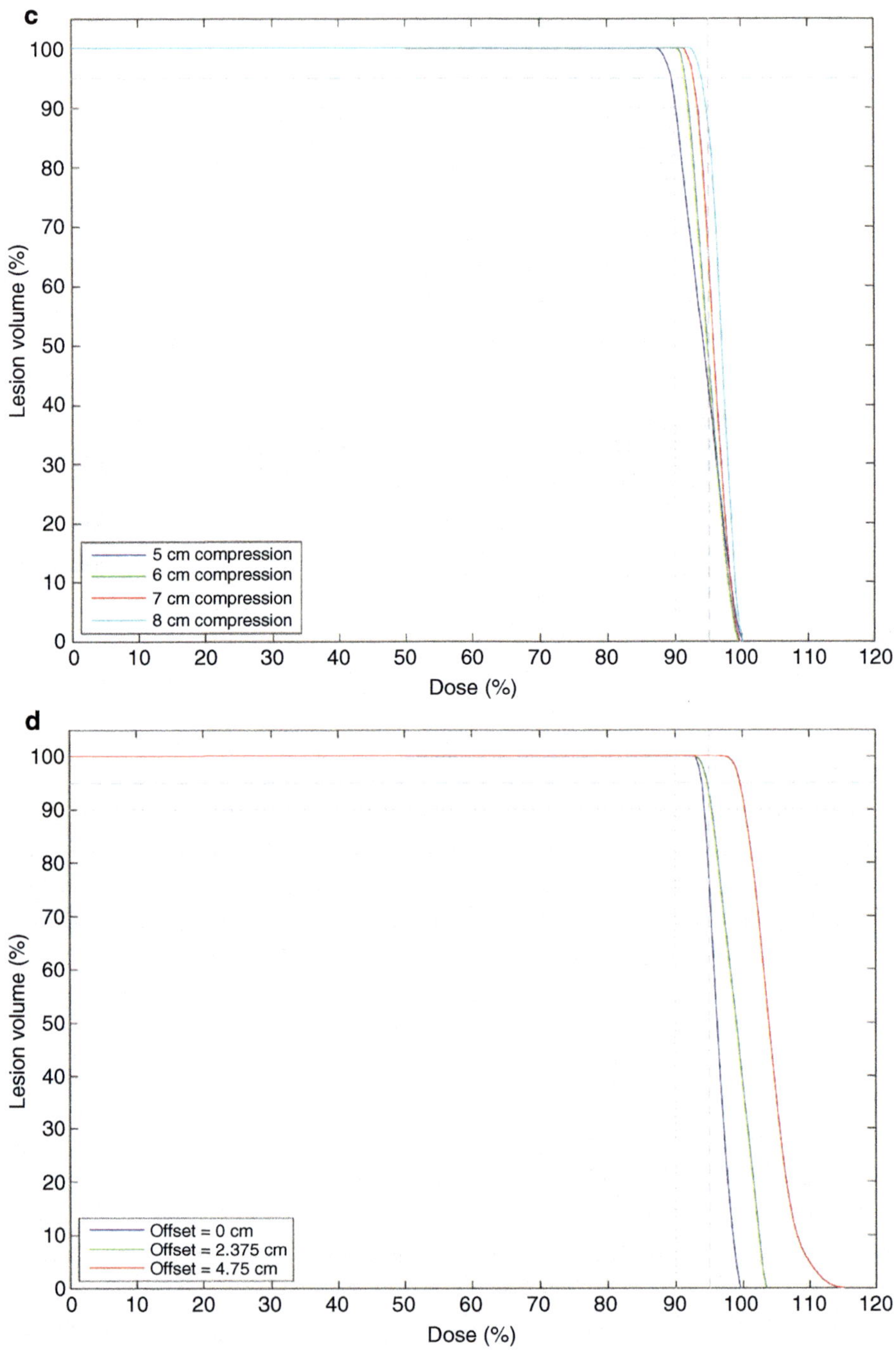

Fig. 25.8 (continued)

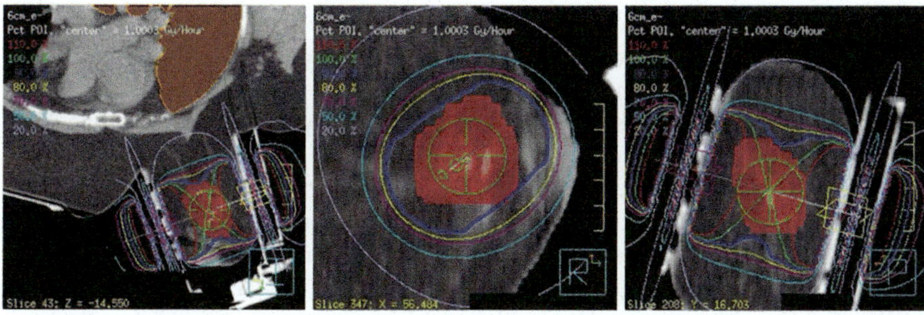

Fig. 25.9 Dosimetry model using CT data of patients simulated with breast compression and modeled dose distribution of NIBB applicators [15]

25.4 Clinical Results

Early clinical experience with the NIBB technique was in the setting of the delivery of tumor bed boost in conjunction with whole-breast radiation therapy. A multi-institutional registry study demonstrated initial feasibility of this technique [20]. One hundred and forty six patients received a boost to the tumor bed in 5–7 fractions using NIBB. Treatment was well tolerated. A minority of patients reported discomfort with compression when NIBB was delivered before or during whole-breast irradiation. Discomfort was, however, common (59 %) when NIBB boost was performed after completion of whole-breast irradiation as might be expected. Acute skin toxicity was reported to be mild with only 1 patient developing a grade 3 acute reaction. Early analysis of late toxicity revealed no grade 3 or greater events. Cosmetic outcome at 6 months was excellent, good, and fair/poor in 62 %, 38 %, and 0 %, respectively. This registry trial has recently been updated. In 341 patients, good-to-excellent cosmetic outcome has been maintained in 96.7 % of patients, and there continues to be no late grade 3 or greater skin or subcutaneous toxicity reported [21]. The freedom from recurrence has been 98.5 %.

Single institutional experience from Brown University using NIBB for boost has also has been analyzed [22]. In 144 women treated, acute skin reaction was grade 2 in 58 % and grade 3 in 4 %. There was no significant grade 3 or greater late skin or subcutaneous toxicity noted. Good-to-excellent cosmetic outcome was seen in 98.4 % of patients. To compare the outcomes of NIBB boost to boost using either external-beam electrons or photons, a match-pair analysis was performed. Treated patients were matched in a 1–2 fashion with respect to age, stage, chemotherapy use, dose, and fractionation. A total of 141 patients were analyzed of which 47 received NIBB boost and 94 received electron or photon boost. NIBB was associated with a trend for a decreased rate of acute moist desquamation and a statistically significant decreased rate of late skin and subcutaneous toxicity [22].

This successful experience using NIBB to deliver boost irradiation led to the investigation of NIBB as a sole treatment modality for delivery of APBI. A prospective multi-institutional phase II trial was initiated which has now completed accrual.

Patients were enrolled between 2011 and 2013. Patient eligibility was in accordance to the American Brachytherapy Society consensus guidelines for APBI [23]. Patients received APBI using the NIBB technique to a dose of 34 Gy delivered in ten fractions. Treatment was delivered either twice daily over 1 week or once daily over 2 weeks. The choice of daily versus twice-daily treatment in this trial was based on patient preference. A total of 40 evaluable patients were enrolled. The median age was 68 years (range 50–92 years). Mean tumor size was 1.1 cm (range 0.3–3.0 cm) with two thirds invasive carcinoma and one third DCIS. All patients were node negative. Most (93 %) were postmenopausal. By ASTRO guidelines for APBI, 47.5 % were considered "suitable" and 52.5 % were considered "cautionary" [24]. Treatment was delivered daily in 72 % and twice daily in 28 %. All patients completed protocol treatment [9]. The average treatment time per axis was 14 min (5–20 min), and the average time from start of first treatment axis to completion of orthogonal axis was 43 min (30–63 min). Discomfort with treatment was mild with a median score of 1 on a standard ten-point pain scale. Acute skin reaction was mild in most patients with the majority of patients having no skin reaction or mild erythema. Grade 2 skin reaction developed in 28 % of patients. No patient developed significant moist desquamation or grade 3 or greater acute skin toxicity. Analysis of acute skin toxicity revealed that the rate of grade 2 skin reaction was associated with both breast separation upon compression ($p<0.01$) and applicator type ($p=0.001$) [14]. Grade 2 skin reaction was seen in 62.5 % using first-generation applicator, 33.3 % using a combination of first- and second-generation applicators, and 0 % using only second-generation applicators. At a median follow-up of 15 months (range 6–24 months), no patient has developed late grade 2 or greater toxicity. The most commonly observed late toxicity was mild hyperpigmentation (grade 1) which typically resolved with extended follow-up. No significant skin or subcutaneous fibrosis toxicity or fatness necrosis was observed. Four patients developed grade 1 telangiectasia. The resulting cosmetic outcome at last follow-up was good-to-excellent in 97.5 % of patients. The freedom from ipsilateral breast tumor recurrence was 97.5 %, with one patient developing recurrence outside the treatment volume. This trial's initial results are encouraging and results will be updated as the data matures. Additionally, a NIBB APBI registry trial is ongoing with the aim to evaluating results of this technique across a broad base of users. Results of this registry trial are not yet available.

25.5 Future Directions

Although NIBB to deliver APBI in ten fractions is a convenient method to deliver adjuvant radiation as part of a breast-conserving therapy approach, it is not yet ideal in terms of convenience. From the experience of the initial NIBB APBI trial, it became clearly evident that patients do not find twice-daily treatment convenient, with only a quarter of patients elected this schedule. However, APBI delivered over 2 week only provides a marginal convenient benefit over a hypofractionated whole-breast regimen delivered in 3 weeks. Therefore, to evaluate a shorter and more convenient treatment schedule for the NIBB technique, a trial evaluating a short-course schedule consisting of 28.5 Gy in five daily fractions has been initiated and is currently accruing patients. This and other studies to identify the most appropriate yet convenient dosing schedule will be beneficial.

Another area in need of further investigation is to address the current lack of patient-specific 3D planning. The challenge for 3D planning is twofold. First, current methods do not allow acquisition of 3D imaging data in the treatment position. Second, the significant degree of tissue deformity between compression axes has been a challenge to create composite dosimetry. Future work in advancing both deformable image registration software and deformable modeling is needed.

25.6 Conclusion

NIBB holds promise as an alternative method to deliver APBI. This technique has advantages of being noninvasive, yet maintaining precision in targeting the tumor bed by employing breast immobilization and image guidance. Like all other APBI techniques, NIBB is not superior in all clinical situations. However, NIBB may prove a very useful technique at the disposal of the treating physician to help tailor treatment to the individual patient's clinical situation and personal preferences.

References

1. Hepel JT, Wazer DE. A comparison of brachytherapy techniques for partial breast irradiation. Brachytherapy. 2012;11(3):163–75.
2. Arthur DW, Winter K, Kuske RR, et al. A phase II trial of brachytherapy alone after lumpectomy for select breast cancer: tumor control and survival outcomes of RTOG 95–17. Int J Radiat Oncol Biol Phys. 2008;72(2):467–73.
3. Hepel JT. Late toxicity and cosmetic outcomes related to interstitial multi-catheter brachytherapy for partial breast irradiation. Brachytherapy. 2014;13(1):23–6.
4. Shah C, Badiyan S, Ben Wilkinson J, et al. Treatment efficacy with accelerated partial breast irradiation (APBI): final analysis of the American Society of Breast Surgeons MammoSite(®) breast brachytherapy registry trial. Ann Surg Oncol. 2013;20(10):3279–85.
5. Hepel JT, Tokita M, MacAusland SG, et al. Toxicity of three-dimensional conformal radiotherapy for accelerated partial breast irradiation. Int J Radiat Oncol Biol Phys. 2009;75(5):1290–6.
6. Leonard KL, Hepel JT, Hiatt JR, et al. The effect of dose-volume parameters and interfraction interval on cosmetic outcome and toxicity after 3-dimensional conformal accelerated partial breast irradiation. Int J Radiat Oncol Biol Phys. 2013;85(3):623–9.
7. Jagsi R, Ben-David MA, Moran JM, et al. Unacceptable cosmesis in a protocol investigating intensity-modulated radiotherapy with active breathing control for accelerated partial-breast irradiation. Int J Radiat Oncol Biol Phys. 2010;76:71–8.
8. Olivotto IA, Whelan TJ, Parpia S, et al. interim cosmetic and toxicity results from RAPID: a randomized trial of accelerated partial breast irradiation using three-dimensional conformal external beam radiation therapy. J Clin Oncol. 2013;31(32):4038–45.

9. Hepel JT, Hiatt JR, Sha S, et al. The rationale, technique, and feasibility of partial breast irradiation using non-invasive image-guided breast brachytherapy (NIBB). Brachytherapy. 2014;13(5):493–501.
10. Hepel JT, Leonard KL, Hiatt JR, et al. Factors influencing eligibility for breast boost using noninvasive image-guided breast brachytherapy. Brachytherapy. 2014;13(6):579–83.
11. Smith LA, Kuske RR, Cross MJ. Improved targeting of the lumpectomy cavity using a spiral 3-D marker. Int J Rad Oncol Bio Phys. 2014;90(1S):S276.
12. Rivard MJ, Melhus CS, Wazer DE, et al. Dosimetric characterization of round HDR 192Ir AccuBoost applicators for breast brachytherapy. Med Phys. 2009;36:5027–32.
13. Yang Y, Melhus CS, Sioshansi S, et al. Treatment planning of a skin-sparing conical breast brachytherapy applicator using conventional brachytherapy software. Med Phys. 2011;38(3):1519–25.
14. Hepel JT, Leonard KL, Sha S, et al. Non-invasive image-guided breast brachytherapy (NIBB) to deliver accelerated partial breast irradiation (APBI): analysis of acute toxicity and early outcomes. Int J Rad Oncol Bio Phys. 2014;90(1S):S136.
15. Sioshansi S, Rivard MJ, Hiatt JR, et al. Dose modeling of noninvasive image-guided breast brachytherapy in comparison to electron beam boost and three-dimensional conformal accelerated partial breast irradiation. Int J Radiat Oncol Biol Phys. 2011;80(2):410–6.
16. Leonard KL, Rivard MJ, Wazer DE, et al. Prescription dose evaluation for APBI with noninvasive image-guided breast brachytherapy using equivalent uniform dose. Brachytherapy. 2015;14(4):496–501.
17. www.clinicaltrials.gov. NCT01961531.
18. Rivard MJ, Ghadyani HR, Bastien AD, et al. Multi-axis dose accumulation of noninvasive image-guided breast brachytherapy through biomechanical modeling of tissue deformation using the finite element method. J Contemp Brachytherapy. 2015;7(1):55–71.
19. Hiatt JR, Rava PS, Leonard KL, et al. Chest wall dose assessment in patients treated using non-invasive image-guided breast brachytherapy APBI. Brachytherapy. 2013;12(2):S47.
20. Hamid S, Rocchio K, Arthur D, et al. A multi-institutional study of feasibility, implementation, and early clinical results with noninvasive breast brachytherapy for tumor bed boost. Int J Radiat Oncol Biol Phys. 2012;83:1374–80.
21. Schuster JM, Chipko C, Saraiya S, et al. Update on a multi-institutional study of noninvasive breast brachytherapy for tumor bed boost: cosmesis and tumor control. Brachytherapy. 2014;13:S19.
22. Leonard KL, Hepel JT, Styczynski JR, et al. Breast boost using noninvasive image-guided breast brachytherapy vs. external beam: a 2:1 matched-pair analysis. Clin Breast Cancer. 2013;13:455–9.
23. Shah C, Vicini F, Wazer DE, et al. The American Brachytherapy Society consensus statement for accelerated partial breast irradiation. Brachytherapy. 2013;12(4):267–77.
24. Smith BD, Arthur DW, Buchholz TA, et al. Accelerated partial breast irradiation consensus statement from the American Society for Radiation Oncology (ASTRO). Int J Radiat Oncol Biol Phys. 2009;74(4):987–1001.

Chapter 26
APBI (Accelerated Partial Breast Irradiation) for in Breast Recurrence Following WBI

Jean-Michel Hanoun-Levi

Contents

26.1 Introduction

Breast cancer represents the most frequent cancer among women with an estimated incidence of 1.38 million new cancer cases diagnosed in 2008 (23 % of all cancers) and ranks second overall (10.9 % of all cancers) [1]. The risk of breast cancer recurrence for a given patient depends on a variety of factors, including patient age, inherited susceptibility, tumor characteristics, type of treatment for the original tumor (e.g., surgery and/or radiation therapy), and other lifestyle factors such as obesity and alcohol consumption. In the 1980s and the 1990s, the ipsilateral breast tumor recurrence (IBTR) rates were reported to be 8–19 % in the 10 years following initial diagnosis and treatment [2]. In the early twenty-first century, the local recurrence rates after completion of adjuvant therapy are still about 10 and 20 % at 10 and 15 years, respectively [3]. The concept of breast-conservative treatment (BCT) as the management of primary breast cancer was proposed by Veronesi et al. [4] at the Cancer Institute of Milan at the end of the 1970s. From the beginning, the Italian team considered BCT to be based on the association of conservative surgery with

J.-M. Hanoun-Levi, MD, PhD
Department of Radiation Oncology, Antoine Lacassagne Cancer Center – University of Nice-Sophia, Nice, France
e-mail: jean-michel.hannoun-levi@nice.unicancer.fr

D.W. Arthur et al. (eds.), *Short Course Breast Radiotherapy: A Comprehensive Review of Hypofractionation, Partial Breast, and Intra-Operative Irradiation*,
DOI 10.1007/978-3-319-24388-7_26

postoperative radiation therapy (RT) of the whole breast. Veronesi et al. [5] reported with a 20-year follow-up the results of a randomized trial confirming that the long-term survival rate among women who undergo BCT was equivalent to that among women who undergo mastectomy. At the same time, Fisher et al. [6] highlighted the critical role of adjuvant RT in the case of conservative surgery. Regarding the local treatment strategy for IBTR after BCT, salvage mastectomy is currently considered as the gold standard approach. However, in regard to the conservative treatment philosophy for primary breast cancer, should mastectomy still remain the unique salvage treatment in the case of an IBTR?

By definition, an IBTR is considered as a local recurrence occurring within the breast which was initially conservatively treated with surgery followed with postoperative whole breast irradiation. However, because it is often difficult to determine whether an IBTR is a true recurrence of the primary tumor or a new primary developing within the treated breast, it is probably better to refer to the IBTR as a 2nd ipsilateral breast cancer event (IBCE). This also allows us to label possibly a 3rd IBCE, should it occur. Furthermore, the local treatment of a 2nd IBCE typically excludes addressing the previously managed ipsilateral axilla. Three different salvage options are primarily described in the literature: (1) salvage mastectomy, (2) second breast-conserving surgery alone (i.e., without re-irradiation), and (3) second breast-conserving surgery with re-irradiation. This chapter focuses on salvage conservative treatment combining lumpectomy and accelerated partial breast re-irradiation (APBrI).

26.2 Patient Selection Criteria for Second BCT

Patient selection criteria for a second attempt at BCT (2nd BCT) have been critically analyzed. Kurtz et al. [7] have shown that size of the recurrent tumor (>20 mm), time interval between primary tumor and 2nd IBCE (<36 months), and less than four involved lymph nodes (when axillary dissection was performed) were considered as prognostic factors for DFS (multivariate analysis). Furthermore, these authors showed that the rate of 2nd local recurrence (3rd IBCE) was significantly correlated with margin and hormone receptor status (univariate analysis). Alpert et al. [8] considered patients amenable to 2nd BCT if the recurrence was localized on mammogram and physical examination and had a pathologic size <3 cm, without skin or lymphovascular invasion and with <3 positive nodes. Ishitobi et al. [9] reported the clinical outcome of 78 patients who presented with a 2nd IBCE treated conservatively with second lumpectomy alone. With a median follow-up of 40 months, the authors noted a 5-year second local recurrence-free survival rate of 78.8 %, and they consider hormonal status (positive estrogen receptors) as a significantly independent predictive factor for second local recurrence-free survival. The time interval between 2nd IBCE and primary tumor was an independent prognostic factor for OS with a cut-off ranging from 24 to 36 months [10, 11]. More recently, the Breast Cancer Working Group of the GEC-ESTRO retrospectively analyzed a cohort of 217 pts who underwent salvage lumpectomy plus APBrI for a 2nd IBCE [12]. On univariate analysis, age at the time of 2nd IBCE (≤55 vs >55 years; $p=0.035$), histological grade (I–II vs III; $p=0.0003$), and hormonal receptor status (HR+ vs HR-, i.e., OR-/PR-; $p=0.001$) were prognostic factors for a 3rdIBCE, while pathological size (≤20 vs >20 mm; $p=0.03$), number of brachytherapy planes (=1 vs ≥2; $p=0.0003$), and number of brachytherapy needles (≤5 vs >5; $p=0.01$) were prognostic factors for distant metastases. For overall survival, pathological size ($p=0.007$), histological grade ($p=0.009$), hormonal receptor status ($p=0.01$), and number of planes ($p=0.004$) were considered as prognostic factors in univariate analysis. On multivariate analysis, prognostic factors included the histological grade ($p=0.008$) for 3rd IBCE, pathological size ($p=0.03$) and number of planes ($p=0.002$) for distant metastases, and histological grade ($p=0.02$) and number of planes ($p=0.009$) for OS.

26.3 Technical Considerations

Currently, there are many different APBI techniques available for partial breast re-irradiation for treatment of a 2nd IBCE following whole breast irradiation. These include intraoperative radiotherapy (IORT) techniques (electrons – or 50 Kv x-ray photons) or postoperative partial breast irradiation techniques (brachytherapy or external beam RT). Brachytherapy techniques include both intracavitary devices and multicatheter interstitial approaches (Fig. 26.1). In the case of APBrI, all these different technical options are described in the literature (except IORT with electrons) with interstitial brachytherapy still remaining the most popular method. Interstitial brachytherapy has the advantage of being able to be conformed to any target, performed intra- or postoperatively and can be delivered with either low [13–16], pulsed [17], or high-dose rate (HDR) brachytherapy [12, 18, 19]. Due to radioprotection and dose optimization considerations, HDR interstitial brachytherapy is currently considered standard of care. Furthermore, this technique allows for an outpatient procedure leading to a comfortable and acceptable treatment for the patient. The brachytherapy balloon technique has been recently described [20] *as well as* intraoperative RT using 50 Kv X-photons [21]. External beam RT was initially reported using electron beams [22], but the use of photon beams has been recently investigated by the RTOG in a prospective phase II clinical trial [23].

For APBI as well as for APBrI, the delineation of the target volume remains a critical point. Whatever the APBrI technique used, clips within or outlining the tumor bed represent an important point for this delineation. Recently, the Breast Cancer Working Group of GEC-ESTRO proposed some recommendations to define and delineate the target in case of APBI using multicatheter interstitial brachytherapy [24]. Briefly, five different steps are described:

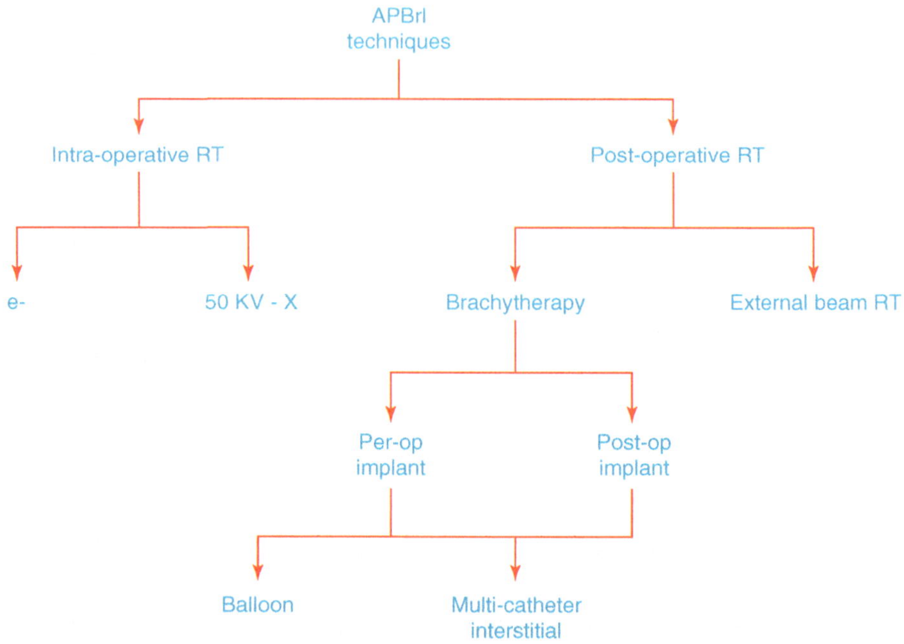

Fig. 26.1 Accelerated and partial breast re-irradiation techniques

1. Detailed knowledge about the primary surgical procedure (particularly about type of surgery, use/number and location of surgical clips, tumor bed-related position of the skin scar), pathologic details (size of resection, margins in six directions), and preoperative imaging (mammography and/or MRI and/or ultrasound) is obligatory.
2. Identification of the tumor location and translation of this information into a current CT imaging data set.
3. Calculation of the size of safety margins needed to cover the CTV (clinical target volume) in all six directions.
4. Definition of the target – CTV / PTV (planning target volume).
5. Delineation of the target – CTV / PTV according to defined rules.

For interstitial brachytherapy, the rules of implantation must follow the Paris system recommendations [25]. It is important to implant (if possible) at least two planes with a minimum number of 10–12 catheters. For PDR or HDR brachytherapy, dosimetric planning should be done based on CT-based 3D imaging. Dose-volume adaptation can be performed automatically with dedicated software or using graphical optimization. Dose-volume histogram (DVH) analysis should confirm that the prescribed dose covers 90 % of the PTV, with an acceptable dose nonuniformity ratio (DNR): V150/V100 ≤0.35 (preferably ≤0.30). The maximum surface skin dose should be ≤70 % of the prescribed dose. To assure optimal dose homogeneity and reduction of focal areas of excessive dose, it is recommended that the confluence of two adjacent V200% isodose volumes or a V200% isodose volume with diameter >10 mm be avoided.

Regarding the prescribed dose for HDR brachytherapy, the protocols used for APBI were empirically reported for APBrI: 34 Gy (3.4 Gy/fraction delivered BID over 5 consecutive days) or 32 Gy (4 Gy/fraction over 4 consecutive days) while for PDR brachytherapy, a total dose of 46–50 Gy delivered at a rate of 0.50–0.80 Gy/h, 1 pulse/h, 24 h/day. In the case of balloon-based brachytherapy, the same HDR dose protocol has been described [20]. For IORT, a total dose of 14.7–20 Gy has been proposed [21]. However, in contrast to the brachytherapy and IORT experience where dose fractionation schemes used for APBI were then used for APBrI, the RTOG 1014 protocol introduced a new dose fractionation scheme with the goal of gaining a radiobiologic advantage to avoid soft tissue late effects. In this protocol, the use of external beam partial breast irradiation for APBrI has been explored; 45 Gy was delivered in a hyperfractionated approach using 1.5 Gy BID, separated by at least 6 h and given in 15 consecutive working days [23].

26.3.1 Clinical Data for Second Breast-Conserving Surgery with APBrI

For re-irradiation for a 2nd BCT, interstitial brachytherapy has been the most commonly applied technique using either low (LDR) [13–16], pulsed (PDR) [17], or high-dose rate (HDR) brachytherapy [18–20]. External beam re-irradiation based on electron therapy of the tumor bed [22] or intraoperative radiation therapy (IORT) using 50 kV photons [21] was also reported. Re-irradiation technical features and related clinical outcomes are presented in Table 26.1. In the case of interstitial brachytherapy, the 3rd IBCE rate was approximately 10 % (range, 0–26 %). The 5-year DFS rate was 60 % (range, from 31 to 85 %), while the 5-year OS rate was approximately 75 % (range, from 50 to 89 %). Grade 3–4 complication rates were about 8 % (range, 3–11 %), and cosmetic results acceptable as excellent/good in 70 % of cases (range, 53–100 %). Maulard et al. [13] have retrospectively compared their results in cases of 2nd IBCE, sole salvage brachytherapy (LDR 60–70 Gy) with 2nd BCT with postoperative brachytherapy (LDR 30 Gy). Tumors treated with salvage brachytherapy alone were statistically larger. The authors reported a rate of 3rd IBCE of 26 and 17 % after surgery plus brachytherapy and brachytherapy alone, respectively. Hannoun-Levi et al. [14] have retrospectively analyzed a series of 69 patients who underwent a 2nd BCT for 2nd IBCE using LDR brachytherapy. Two groups of patients were compared regarding the delivered dose (30 vs. 46 Gy) and the number of planes used (1 vs. 2). The authors showed that the 3rd IBCE rate was lower in cases of a higher delivered dose and larger irradiated volume. Using PDR brachytherapy combined with a 2nd lumpectomy for 2nd IBCE, Kauer-Dorner et al. [17] reported an actuarial 5-year 2nd local control rate of 93 % with a mean follow-up of 57 months (2 patients experienced a 3rd IBCE). Five-year DFS and OS were 77 and 87 %, respectively. Grade 3–4 late side effects were 7 %, while cosmetic outcome was excellent to fair in 76 %. Regarding quality of life, the authors reported that mean scores of scales and items of QLQ-BR23 (breast cancer-specific quality of life questionnaire) were comparable to primary breast-conserving therapy. Guix

Table 26.1 Clinical outcome results after second breast-conservative surgery combining with re-irradiation for 2nd ipsilateral breast cancer event

Authors	pts[a]	MFU (months)	IT	Dose (Gy)	3rd IBCE (%)	5-year DFS (%)	5-year OS (%)	G3-4 Tox (%)	Exc/good CR (%)
Maulard et al. [13]	15	48	ILB	30	26	31	61	8	53
	23	36	ILB[b]	60–70	17	41	50	–	–
Deutsch et al. [22]	39	63	e-TB	50	21	68	78	NA	69
Hannoun-Levi et al. [14]	24	50	ILB	30	25	69	92	10	NA
	45	50	ILB	46	11	–	–	–	–
Kraus-Tiefenbacher et al. [21]	15	26	IORT	14.7–20	0	NA	NA	0	82
Chadha et al. [15]	15	36	ILB	30–45	7	NA	100[c]	0	100
Trombetta et al. [16]	21	40	ILB	45–50	5	NA	NA	10	92
Guix et al. [18]	36	89	IHB	30	3	64[d]	97[d]	0	NA
Hannoun-Levi et al. [19]	42	21	IHB	34	2	NA	NA	3	97
Kauer-Dorner et al. [17]	39	57	IPB	56	7	77	87	7	76
GEC-ESTRO [12]	217	47	ILB/IPB/IHB	46/50/32	4	85	89	11	85
Trombetta et al. [20]	18	40	BHB	34	11	–	–	6	

[a]*pts* number of patients, *MFU* median follow-up, *IT* irradiation technique, *ILB* interstitial low-dose rate brachytherapy, *IORT* intraoperative radiation therapy, *IHB* interstitial high-dose rate brachytherapy, *IPB* interstitial pulse-dose rate brachytherapy, *BHB* balloon high-dose rate brachytherapy, *e-TB* electron therapy to the tumor bed, *3rd IBCE* third ipsilateral breast cancer event rate, *DMFS* distant metastasis-free survival, *DFS* disease-free survival, *CSS* cause-specific survival, *OS* overall survival, *NA* not available

[b]Without second lumpectomy

[c]3-year DFS

[d]10-year DFS/10-year OS

et al. [18] have retrospectively analyzed a series of patients who were treated with 2nd BCT and interstitial HDR brachytherapy. With a median follow-up of 89 months, corresponding to the longest follow-up, the authors reported 10-year DFS and OS rates of 64 and 97 %, respectively. In this series, no grade 3–4 complications were observed. More recently, the GEC-ESTRO (Groupe Européen de Curiethérapie (GEC) and the European Society for Radiotherapy & Oncology (ESTRO)) Breast Cancer Working Group presented the results of an international multicentric retrospective study of 217 patients with 2nd IBCE who underwent a 2nd BCT combining salvage lumpectomy plus interstitial brachytherapy [12]. The authors reported an actuarial 5- and 10-year 2nd local recurrence rate of 5.6 and 7.2 %, respectively, while the actuarial 5- and 10-year distant metastasis rates were 9.6 and 19.1 %, respectively. Actuarial 5- and 10-year OS rates were 88.7 and 76.4 %, respectively.

26.4 APBrI vs. Salvage Mastectomy or Lumpectomy

26.4.1 Salvage Mastectomy Alone

Currently, the only available studies comparing APBrI, salvage mastectomy, and lumpectomy alone are retrospective and/or comparative reports; there are no prospective, randomized phase III trials. The local recurrence rate after radical mastectomy performed as sole salvage therapy for 2nd IBCE after initial BCT was about 10–15 % (range, 3–32 %) [10, 26–34]. After salvage radical mastectomy, the 10-year disease-free survival (DFS) rate was about 40–45 % (range, 32–47), while overall survival (OS) was about 70 % (range, 61–84) and 65 % (range, 58–69) at 5 and 10 years, respectively (Table 26.2). Voogd et al. [30] reported the results of a retrospective study focusing on 266 patients with local recurrence in the breast. Of all patients, 85 % underwent salvage mastectomy, 8 % underwent local excision, and 7 % received systemic treatment only or remained untreated. Local recurrences detected by mammography alone were smaller than those detected by physical examination ($p=0.04$). With a 5-year median follow-up from the salvage treatment, the metastatic recurrence-free survival rate was 47 % (95 % CI, 40–53 %). Skin involvement, the extent of recurrence (< or = 10 mm vs. >10 mm), and both lymph node status and histological grade of the primary disease were strong predictors for distant metastases in patients with invasive recurrence.

26.4.2 Second Breast-Conserving Surgery Alone

Because a patient who underwent BCT for the primary breast tumor wishes often to be conservatively treated for the 2nd IBCE, several teams have published the results of retrospective studies analyzing the feasibility and the clinical outcome of second

Table 26.2 Clinical outcome results after salvage mastectomy for 2nd ipsilateral breast cancer event

Authors	[a]pts	MFU (months)	3rd IBCE (%)	10-year DMFS (%)	5-year DFS (%)	5-year OS (%)
Kurtz et al. [7]	66	84	12	NA	NA	NA
Fowble et al. [26]	52	25	NA	NA	59	84
Osborne et al. [27]	46	28	15	NA	55	76
Cajucoum et al. [28]	25	52	32	NA	51	65
Abner et al. [29]	123	39	6	NA	41	NA
Voogd et al. [30]	266	60	25	47	NA	61
Salvadori et al. [31]	134	NA	4	55[b]	NA	70
Doyle et al. [11]	112	44	3	47	NA	69[c]
Huang et al. [32]	126	NA -	12	45	NA	58[c]
Alpert et al. [8]	116	244	7	32	NA	66[c]

[a]*pts* number of patients, *MFU* median follow-up, *3rd IBCE* third ipsilateral breast cancer event rate, *DMFS* distant metastasis-free survival, *DFS* disease-free survival, *CSS* cause-specific survival, *OS* overall survival, *NA* not available
[b]4-year DMFS
[c]10-year OS

Table 26.3 Clinical outcome results after second breast-conservative surgery *without* postoperative re-irradiation for 2nd ipsilateral breast cancer event

Authors	[a]pts	MFU (months)	3rd IBCE (%)	10-year DMFS (%)	10-year CSS (%)	10-year OS (%)
Kurtz et al. [10]	50	51	32	NA	64	42
Abner et al. [29]	16	39	31	NA	NA	NA
Dalberg et al. [33]	17	NA	12.5	NA	NA	NA
Salvadori et al. [31]	57	NA	19	80[b]	NA	85[c]
Alpert et al. [8]	30	244	7	24	61	58
Ishitobi et al. [9]	78	40	21	NA	NA	NA

[a]*pts* number of patients, *MFU* median follow-up, *3rd IBCE* third ipsilateral breast cancer event rate, *DMFS* distant metastasis-free survival, *DFS* disease-free survival, *CSS* cause-specific survival, *OS* overall survival, *NA* not available
[b]4-year DMFS
[c]5-year OS

breast-conserving surgery used as sole therapy (i.e., without postoperative re-irradiation) [7, 9, 31, 34, 35]. In these studies, the second tumor recurrence rate was about 20 % (range, 7–32 %), while the 10-year cause-specific survival and overall survival rates were 60 % (range, 61–64 %) and 50 % (range, 42–58 %) respectively (Table 26.3).

26.5 Further Steps and Controversies

One of the most important controversies associated with a 2nd IBCE is the risk of systemic disease. This risk is correlated with the pathologic features of the 2nd IBCE but also with the notion that the risk relates to whether the 2nd IBCE is actually a true recurrence (TR) or a new primary (NP) tumor. Both the pathologic and location information of the 2nd IBCE as it compares to the original primary tumor is considered as well as the time interval between primary and recurrent tumor [34]. Indeed, this time interval was reported as an independent prognostic factor for DFS and OS with a cut-off ranging from 24 to 36 months [7, 32]. New molecular approaches are proposed to refine more precisely the 2nd IBCE features between NP and TR [35, 36]. Although there is a significant level of proof supporting breast conservation treatment as an appropriate treatment option for primary breast cancer [5, 6], there is comparatively less supporting evidence for a breast-conserving approach for a 2nd IBCE, and therefore salvage mastectomy should still be considered the standard treatment for these patients. Could breast-conservative treatment be considered for women presenting with 2nd IBCE considering that they have already undergone surgery, whole breast irradiation, and possibly systemic therapies for the original primary tumor? The literature is beginning to suggest that this may be a reasonable alternative when patients wish to avoid mastectomy when proper selection and attention to anticipated cosmetic outcome are considered. Additionally, published experiences support the need for the addition of APBrI following breast-conserving surgery if 2nd BCT is pursued.

References

1. Breast cancer incidence and mortality worldwide in 2008 summary. http://globocan.iarc.fr/Pages/fact_sheets_cancer.aspx. Accessed 03.03.15.
2. DeVita, Vincent T; Lawrence, Theodore S; Rosenberg, Steven A, DeVita, Hellman, and Rosenberg's cancer : principles & practice of oncology 8th ed. Philadelphia : Wolters Kluwer/Lippincott Williams & Wilkins, c2008.
3. Brewster AM, Hortobagyi GN, Broglio KR, et al. Residual risk of breast cancer recurrence 5 years after adjuvant therapy. J Natl Cancer Inst. 2008;100:1179–83.
4. Veronesi U. New trends in the treatment of breast cancer at the Cancer Institute of Milan. AJR Am J Roentgenol. 1977;128:287–9.
5. Veronesi U, Cascinelli N, Mariani L, et al. Twenty-year follow-up of a randomized study comparing breast-conserving surgery with radical mastectomy for early breast cancer. N Engl J Med. 2002;347:1227–32.
6. Fisher B, Anderson S, Bryant J, et al. Twenty-year follow-up of a randomized trial comparing total mastectomy, lumpectomy, and lumpectomy plus irradiation for the treatment of invasive breast cancer. N Engl J Med. 2002;347:1233–41.

7. Kurtz JM, Jacquemier J, Amalric R, et al. Is breast conservation after local recurrence feasible? Eur J Cancer. 1991;27:240–4.
8. Alpert TE, Kuerer HM, Arthur DW, et al. Ipsilateral breast tumor recurrence after breast conservation therapy: outcomes of salvage mastectomy vs. salvage breast-conserving surgery and prognostic factors for salvage breast preservation. Int J Radiat Oncol Biol Phys. 2005;63:845–51.
9. Ishitobi M, Komoike Y, Nakahara S, et al. Repeat lumpectomy for ipsilateral breast tumor recurrence after breast conserving treatment. Oncology. 2011;81(5–6):381–6.
10. Kurtz JM, Amalric R, Brandone H, et al. Results of wide excision for mammary recurrence after breast-conserving therapy. Cancer. 1988;61:1969–72.
11. Doyle T, Schultz DJ, Peters C, et al. Long-term results of local recurrences after breast conservation treatment for invasive breast cancer. Int J Radiat Oncol Biol Phys. 2001;51:74–80.
12. Hannoun-Levi JM, Resch A, Gal J, et al., GEC-ESTRO Breast Cancer Working Group. Accelerated partial breast irradiation with interstitial brachytherapy as second conservative treatment for ipsilateral breast tumour recurrence: multicentric study of the GEC-ESTRO Breast Cancer Working Group. Radiother Oncol. 2013;108:226–31.
13. Maulard C, Housset M, Brunel P, et al. Use of perioperative or split-course interstitial brachytherapy techniques for salvage irradiation of isolated local recurrences after conservative management of breast cancer. Am J Clin Oncol. 1995;18:348–52.
14. Hannoun-Levi JM, Houvenaeghel G, Ellis S, et al. Partial breast irradiation as second conservative treatment for local breast cancer recurrence. Int J Radiat Oncol Biol Phys. 2004;60:1385–92.
15. Chadha M, Feldman S, Boolbol S, et al. The feasibility of a second lumpectomy and breast brachytherapy for localized cancer in a breast previously treated with lumpectomy and radiation therapy for breast cancer. Brachytherapy. 2008;7:22–8.
16. Trombetta M, Julian TB, Bhandari T, et al. Breast conservation surgery and interstitial brachytherapy in the management of locally recurrent carcinoma of the breast: the Allegheny General Hospital experience. Brachytherapy. 2008;7:29–36.
17. Kauer-Dorner D, Pötter R, Resch A, et al. Partial breast irradiation for locally recurrent breast cancer within a second breast conserving treatment: alternative to mastectomy? Results from a prospective trial. Radiother Oncol. 2012;102:96–101.
18. Guix B, Lejárcegui JA, Tello JI, et al. Exeresis and brachytherapy as salvage treatment for local recurrence after conservative treatment for breast cancer: results of a ten-year pilot study. Int J Radiat Oncol Biol Phys. 2010;78:804–10.
19. Hannoun-Levi JM, Castelli J, Plesu A, et al. Second conservative treatment for ipsilateral breast cancer recurrence using high-dose rate interstitial brachytherapy: preliminary clinical results and evaluation of patient satisfaction. Brachytherapy. 2011;10:171–7.
20. Trombetta M, Hall M, Julian TB. Long-term followup of breast preservation by re-excision and balloon brachytherapy after ipsilateral breast tumor recurrence. Brachytherapy. 2014;13:488–92.
21. Kraus-Tiefenbacher U, Bauer L, Scheda A, et al. Intraoperative radiotherapy (IORT) is an option for patients with localized breast recurrences after previous external-beam radiotherapy. BMC Cancer. 2007;7:178.
22. Deutsch M. Repeat high-dose external beam irradiation for in-breast tumor recurrence after previous lumpectomy and whole breast irradiation. Int J Radiat Oncol Biol Phys. 2002;53:687–91.
23. Arthur DW, et al. RTOG 1014 radiation Therapy in Treating women with Locally Recurrent Breast Cancer Previously Treated with Repeat Breast-Preserving Surgery. https://www.rtog.org/ClinicalTrials/ProtocolTable/StudyDetails.aspx?action=openFile&FileID=6358.
24. Strnad V, Van Limbergen E, Hannoun-Levi JM, et al., on behalf of Working Group Breast Cancer of GEC-ESTRO. Recommendations from GEC ESTRO Breast Cancer Working Group (I): target definition and target delineation for accelerated or boost Partial Breast Irradiation

using multicatheter interstitial brachytherapy after breast conserving closed cavity surgery. Radiother Oncol. 2015;115(3):342–8.
25. Pierquin B, Dutreix A, Paine CH, et al. The Paris system in interstitial radiation therapy. Acta Radiol Oncol Radiat Phys Biol. 1978;17:33–48.
26. Fowble B, Solin LJ, Schultz DJ, et al. Breast recurrence following conservative surgery and radiation: patterns of failure, prognosis, and pathologic findings from mastectomy specimens with implications for treatment. Int J Radiat Oncol Biol Phys. 1990;19:833–42.
27. Osborne MP, Borgen PI, Wong GY, et al. Salvage mastectomy for local and regional recurrence after breast-conserving operation and radiation therapy. Surg Gynecol Obstet. 1992;174:189–94.
28. Cajucoum CC, Tsangaris TH, Nemoto T, et al. Results of salvage mastectomy for local recurrence after breast-conserving surgery without radiation therapy. Cancer. 1993;71:1774–9.
29. Abner AL, Recht A, Eberlein T, et al. Prognosis following salvage mastectomy for recurrence in the breast after conservative surgery and radiation therapy for early-stage breast cancer. J Clin Oncol. 1993;11:44–8.
30. Voogd AC, van Tienhoven G, Peterse HL, et al., for the Dutch Study Group on Local Recurrence after Breast Conservation. Local recurrence after breast conservation therapy for early stage breast carcinoma: detection, treatment, and outcome in 266 patients. Cancer. 1999;85:437–46.
31. Salvadori B, Marubini E, Miceli R, et al. Reoperation for locally recurrent breast cancer in patients previously treated with conservative surgery. Br J Surg. 1999;86:84–7.
32. Huang E, Buchholz TA, Meric F, et al. Classifying local disease recurrences after breast conservation therapy based on location and histology: new primary tumors have more favorable outcomes than true local disease recurrences. Cancer. 2002;95:2059–67.
33. Dalberg K, Mattsson A, Sandelin K, et al. Outcome of treatment for ipsilateral breast tumor recurrence in early-stage breast cancer. Breast Cancer Res Treat. 1998;49:69–78.
34. Panet-Raymond V, Truong PT, McDonald RE, et al. Rue recurrence versus new primary: an analysis of ipsilateral breast tumor recurrences after breast-conserving therapy. Int J Radiat Oncol Biol Phys. 2011;81:409–17.
35. Vicini FA, Antonucci JV, Goldstein N, et al. The use of molecular assays to establish definitively the clonality of ipsilateral breast tumor recurrences and patterns of in-breast failure in patients with early-stage breast cancer treated with breast-conserving therapy. Cancer. 2007;109:1264–72.
36. Bollet MA, Servant N, Neuvial P, et al. High-resolution mapping of DNA breakpoints to define true recurrences among ipsilateral breast cancers. J Natl Cancer Inst. 2008;100:48–58.

Chapter 27
Preoperative Partial Breast

Yvonne M. Mowery, Cedric X. Yu, and Janet K. Horton

Contents

27.1 Introduction

Accelerated partial breast irradiation (APBI) is an evolving alternative to whole breast irradiation (WBI) for treatment of low-risk, early-stage breast cancer. This approach offers improved patient convenience and potentially decreased cost through shorter treatment time. Additionally, irradiation of a smaller target volume may lead to reduced dose to surrounding normal tissues. Published data with at least 5-year follow-up indicate similar efficacy with APBI compared to WBI for a carefully selected patient subset [1–10].

Toxicity outcomes have also typically been favorable for brachytherapy, intraoperative, and external-beam (EBRT) partial breast irradiation techniques [1–5, 7–12].

Y.M. Mowery • J.K. Horton, MD (✉)
Department of Radiation Oncology, Duke University Medical Center, Durham, NC, USA
e-mail: janet.horton@duke.edu

C.X. Yu
Department of Radiation Oncology, University of Maryland, Baltimore, MD, USA

D.W. Arthur et al. (eds.), *Short Course Breast Radiotherapy: A Comprehensive Review of Hypofractionation, Partial Breast, and Intra-Operative Irradiation*,
DOI 10.1007/978-3-319-24388-7_27

Early reports from one phase III trial in which 73 % of patients received external-beam PBI revealed low rates of toxicity [13]. However, other prospective studies utilizing intensity-modulated radiation therapy (IMRT) or three-dimensional conformal radiation therapy (3D-CRT) to deliver APBI have demonstrated suboptimal cosmetic outcomes [14, 15]. In addition, the only currently published phase III trial evaluating EBRT APBI noted fair/poor cosmesis in a significantly larger proportion of patients receiving APBI as compared to whole breast treatment (29 versus 17 %, $p < 0.001$) [16]. These suboptimal outcomes have been suggested to be linked to the large target volumes which are required postoperatively. This large target size is due, at least in part, to the difficulty in identifying residual tissue at high risk following surgical tumor resection [14, 15, 17–19]. As a result, a large and uniform margin must be placed around the postoperative seroma cavity, leading to nontrivial volumes of breast receiving prescription (9–26 %) and half prescription (34–49 %) doses [20].

Delivery of radiation prior to surgical resection is an alternative technique that utilizes in situ targeting to minimize the volume of unaffected breast tissue receiving the prescription dose. Although the optimal margin for this technique is not well defined, the small size of the intact tumor relative to the typical postoperative seroma (Fig. 27.1) makes it unlikely that postoperative target volumes can be reduced to a level comparable to that seen in the preoperative setting. In addition to potential clinical advantages, the preoperative approach provides a unique opportunity in breast cancer to study the imaging and molecular effects of radiation on breast tumors and the surrounding normal tissue.

Preoperative efforts thus far have focused on the ubiquitous linear-accelerator-based techniques available to nearly all radiation oncology providers. Intraoperative or brachytherapy APBI typically provide a more conformal dose distribution compared to EBRT, but both require specialized equipment and training. Consequently, these methods of APBI delivery are not as widely available. By

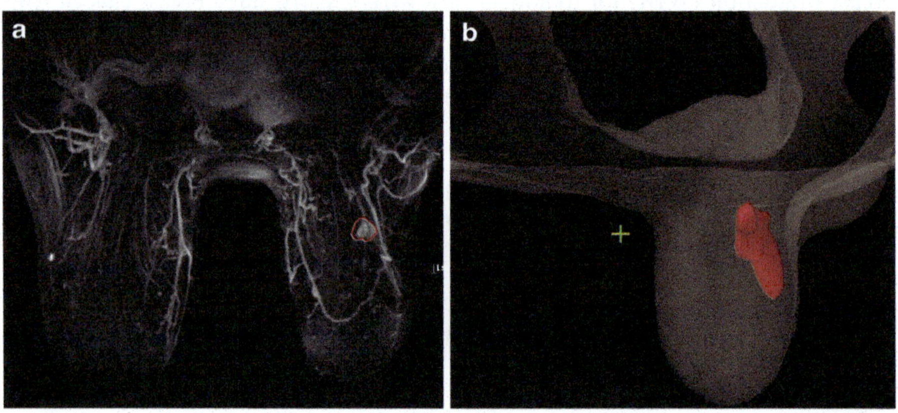

Fig 27.1 Early-stage breast cancer patient with an intact tumor (*red*) on preoperative MRI (**a**). Tumor bed on radiation treatment planning CT in the same patient following surgical resection (**b**)

contrast, most radiation oncology clinics are equipped to deliver the highly conformal EBRT necessary for preoperative APBI.

Research investigating the optimal use of preoperative APBI is ongoing; however, we anticipate that this promising technique will ultimately offer an accessible alternative to external-beam postoperative APBI in selected patients with early-stage breast cancer.

27.2 Patient Selection

Early preoperative studies have focused on the definitive use of this technique for APBI. Therefore, patient selection has mirrored postoperative APBI studies by including primarily older patients with biologically favorable tumors. These patients are likely the most appropriate group for initial testing of preoperative techniques given their generally low risk of recurrence overall.

In many instances, preoperative treatment also incorporates a contrast-enhanced breast magnetic resonance imaging (MRI). Though not always utilized in breast radiation oncology decision-making, MRI has been previously suggested as a tool to improve selection of patients for APBI. MRI is known to detect additional occult ipsilateral cancers in 23–59 % of patients [21]. Presumably these patients are at higher risk of recurrence outside the target volume with APBI and should be offered more comprehensive treatment. Though the likelihood of extensive disease in the patient population selected for APBI is low [22], MRI also serves another valuable purpose in the preoperative setting. Breast tumors can be demarcated in an imaging context that can be readily incorporated into radiation treatment planning.

Mammography and ultrasound could also be considered but require compression and lack the anatomic detail needed for treatment planning. Data is limited regarding the appropriateness of computed tomography (CT) as this modality has not routinely been utilized as a diagnostic tool in breast cancer. By contrast, breast MRI is now readily available, has been favorably correlated with pathologic tumor size (Table 27.1), and can be utilized in conjunction with typical CT-based radiation planning tools. For these reasons, MRI is a valuable addition to optimal target delineation. As such, patients unable to undergo MRI due to metallic implants or body habitus may not be ideal candidates for preoperative treatment.

Another important consideration for preoperative treatment is tumor-to-skin distance. Patients with superficial tumors who receive preoperative APBI will frequently receive close to full prescription dose in the skin. The long-term toxicity of this is not yet well understood, and in the future, carefully defined skin constraints (and omission of patients in which these cannot be met) may be required.

Even with careful selection, a few patients with unanticipated high-risk features will receive preoperative treatment. Strategies to address this postoperatively include omission of further therapy versus delivery of conventional postoperative radiation. Alternatively, a preoperative sentinel node procedure has been utilized to identify and exclude higher-risk patients [23]. Determination of preoperative nodal

Table 27.1 Correlation between tumor size delineated on MRI and pathologic assessment

Reference	*n*	Pathologic size underestimated by MRI by > 2 cm	% underestimated	% concordant	% overestimated	Factors associated with size underestimation by MRI
Grimsby et al. (2009) [44]	190	8 %[a]	15 %	53 %[b]	33 %	Nodal involvement, tumor size > 2 cm
Berg et al. (2004) [40]	96	–	5 %[c]	76 %	19 %[d]	–
Onesti et al. (2008) [47]	91	2 %[a]	2 %	79 %[e]	19 %	–
Kim et al. (2007) [53]	72	–	17 %	72 %[e]	11 %	Non-high-grade DCIS; noncomedo necrosis; DCIS without microinvasion
Lobbes et al. (2015) [45]	57	2 %	5 %	85 %[e]	9 %	–
Behjatnia et al. (2010) [48]	37	3 %	8 %	70 %[e]	22 %	Invasive lobular carcinoma
Boetes et al. (2004) [50]	36	–	14 %	75 %[e]	11 %	–
Schouten van der Velden et al. (2006) [43]	21	19 %	24 %	38 %[b]	38 %	Non-high-grade DCIS
Schmitz et al. (2010) [54]	64	25 %	52 %[f]	–	–	Extensive intraductal component
Gruber et al. (2013) [46]	121	2.5 %	–	–	–	–
Mumtaz et al. (1997) [49]	85	0 %	–	–	–	–
Cheung et al. (2004) [51]	36	0 %	–	–	–	–
Kepple et al. (2005) [52]	33	3.0 %	–	–	–	–

–, not reported

[a]Tumor size underestimation by > 1 cm based on MRI measurement

[b]Concordance indicates size discrepancy < 0.5 cm

[c]No lesion detected or foci missed on MRI that would have prompted wider surgical excision if detected

[d]Overestimation indicates lesion size overestimated by ≥ 2 cm or additional suspicious lesions noted indicating necessity of more extensive surgery than necessary based on final histopathologic findings

[e]Concordance indicates size discrepancy ≤ 1 cm

[f]Subclinical disease (mostly DCIS) located > 1 cm away from MRI-visible lesion

status is the most definitive method of selecting low-risk patients; however, it does subject patients to a second operative procedure.

27.3 Target Volume

Accurate identification of the region of breast at greatest risk for recurrence represents a major challenge in APBI. The majority of local recurrences after breast-conserving therapy for early-stage breast cancer occur in or near the tumor bed [24–29]. Therefore, typical postoperative clinical target volumes (CTV) for EBRT-based APBI consist of the lumpectomy cavity expanded by 1–1.5 cm [10, 14–16, 30]. An additional 0.5–1 cm is generally added to generate the planning target volume (PTV), accounting for setup variability and patient motion. For example, the NSABP B-39/RTOG 0413 protocol specified a 1.5 cm expansion from tumor bed to CTV with an additional 1 cm margin to PTV for 3D-conformal external-beam APBI. Similar target volumes have been used for postoperative APBI with interstitial implants [1, 31, 32]. Unfortunately, visualization of the breast tumor bed on CT is often difficult, as indicated by high interobserver variability in lumpectomy cavity contours among breast radiation oncologists [33–35]. Furthermore, poor correlation has been observed between preoperative tumor size and dimensions of the excision cavity [36]. These findings suggest that the CTV utilized in postoperative APBI may not encompass the region that is truly at highest risk for recurrence or adequately spare surrounding low-risk normal tissue.

The CTV margins for APBI are largely based on patterns of in-breast failure and pathologic studies investigating tumor extension beyond the primary focus. Older data from Holland et al. examining 282 mastectomy specimens from women with T1–T2 invasive breast cancer showed rates of invasive tumor foci beyond 2 cm from the primary tumor in 14–16 % of cases [37]. Rosen et al. showed residual invasive carcinoma in the breast in 12 % of mastectomy specimens with T1 tumors ($n = 100$) after simulated partial mastectomy with 2 cm margin around gross tumor [38]. In contrast, Vicini et al. demonstrated that residual disease was limited to <1 cm from the initial margin among >90 % of 134 cases treated initially with lumpectomy to negative margins for T1–T2 breast cancer [39], suggesting that tumor extent can be more precisely predicted with modern imaging techniques. Contrast-enhanced MRI offers a further increase in sensitivity for detection of invasive and in situ breast carcinoma [40–43]. Many, though not all, studies correlating pathologic tumor measurements with MRI-based size assessment indicate low rates of significant tumor size underestimation by MRI [44–47]. Two series demonstrated a mean size difference between MRI and histopathology of approximately 2 mm [45, 46]. On the other hand, tumor size overestimation rates as high as 38 % have been noted with MRI [43, 44]. This tradeoff is acceptable in the context of preoperative treatment in order to avoid missing the target, but it may contribute to a high rate of screen failures, i.e., patients initially thought to be eligible for preoperative APBI subsequently found to be ineligible based on

MRI. Table 27.1 illustrates the patterns of correlation between MRI estimated and final pathologic tumor size [40, 43–54].

Limited data are available regarding concordance between preoperative CT imaging and pathologic tumor size. One study has shown high correlation between CT and pathology, particularly for tumors smaller than 2 cm. In this series of 285 patients with unifocal invasive breast carcinoma, size was underestimated for 12.7 % of tumors (average 11 mm) and overestimated for 7.4 % (average 10 mm) [55]. Another study utilizing contrast-enhanced CT to assess tumor size in 144 patients showed a median deviation of 7.7 mm (range 0–60 mm) between tumor dimensions on imaging and pathology. Similar to MRI, greater deviation was noted in tumors with an extensive intraductal component [56]. CT has also been used for surgical planning, and in one multi-institutional study, the extent of excision was increased in 14 % (42 of 303 patients) based on contrast-enhanced CT scan prior to resection. Pathologically, this increase in surgical volume was appropriate in all but 3 patients. However, in almost 11 % (32 patients), the extent of disease was underestimated [57].

Van der Leij and colleagues compared pre- versus postoperative target volume delineation on CT and noted considerably less interobserver variability in the preoperative setting (Fig. 27.2) [34]. den Hartogh et al. took this a step further by comparing preoperative target delineation with both CT and MRI. High interobserver agreement was identified for both modalities in most cases but two tumors were missed entirely on CT [58]. Furthermore, the conformity index was significantly higher with MRI. Although the absolute differences are small at the gross tumor volume (GTV) level, CTV expansion amplifies these differences, resulting in distinct target volumes in patients whose tumors are difficult to identify on CT (Table 27.2). In our study at Duke University, we observed a similar finding. The mean tumor volume identified on CT scan was similar to that identified on MRI. However, the mean of the difference between the two volumes was 0.5 cm^3 (range 0–1.8 cm^3) suggesting that the target identified by CT may not be the same volume as that identified by MRI (Fig. 27.3).

Therefore, at Duke we prefer utilizing breast MRI including T1-weighted, T2-weighted, and dynamic contrast-enhanced (DCE) series for target delineation. GTV should include all areas of enhancing tumor noted on T1-weighted post-contrast MRI. T2-weighted images can be utilized to distinguish tumor from post-biopsy change. Figure 27.4 illustrates the MR and CT images from several patients treated with preoperative techniques, two in the prone position and one in supine. Although the MRI coil can distort the tissue near the chest wall in patients with larger breasts, images can still be utilized to clearly delineate the tumor location and target volume.

The optimal GTV to CTV margin for preoperative APBI is not known; however, expansions of 1.5–2 cm have been proposed [23, 59–62]. The above studies suggest that a 1.5–2 cm tumor-to-CTV margin for preoperative APBI should encompass subclinical disease in most cases, particularly given the carefully selected population eligible for APBI. Others have advocated for using a larger margin in preoperative APBI, which would partly negate the benefit of a smaller preoperative treatment

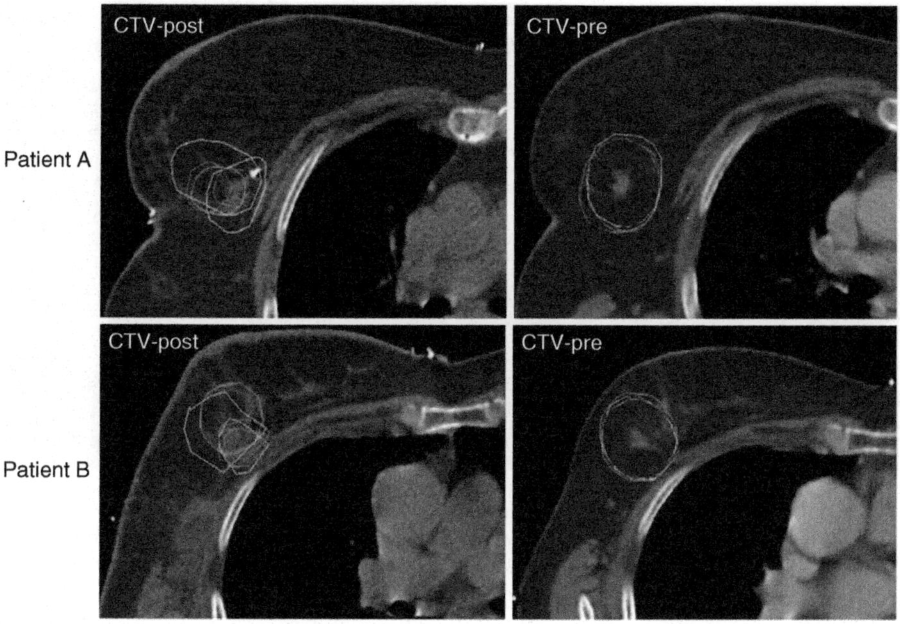

Fig 27.2 Two representative patients (**a**, **b**) with pre- and postoperative target volume delineation by 5 observers on CT. Agreement between observers is notably improved preoperatively (*right*) as compared to postoperatively (*left*) (Reproduced with permission from van der Leij et al. [23])

Table 27.2 Interobserver variability in preoperative breast tumor identification using contrast-enhanced CT or MRI

	CT		MRI		
	Median	Range	Median	Range	p-value
Mean volume (cm³)					
GTV	2.1	0.3–21.3	2.7	0.4–19.4	<0.001
CTV	48.1	27.7–137.3	59	30.4–153.1	<0.001
Conformity index					
GTV	0.56	0.11–0.83	0.61	0.37–0.78	<0.001
CTV	0.82	0.39–0.93	0.84	0.47–0.93	0.123
Mean dCOM (mm)					
GTV	1.1	0.3–12.8	1.2	0.3–3.6	0.245
CTV	1.4	0.3–13.6	1.8	0.1–4.8	0.836

Reproduced with permission from den Hartogh et al. [58]
GTV gross tumor volume, *CTV* clinical target volume, *dCOM* center of mass distance

volume relative to postoperative APBI [62]. This argument assumes that relatively uniform 1–2 cm microscopic margins are achieved postoperatively by tumor resection, leading to 2–3.5 cm margins from tumor with typical postoperative CTV expansion. In reality, microscopic margins are typically anisotropic with tumor often closely approaching one or more margins [63, 64]. Thus, the relatively small

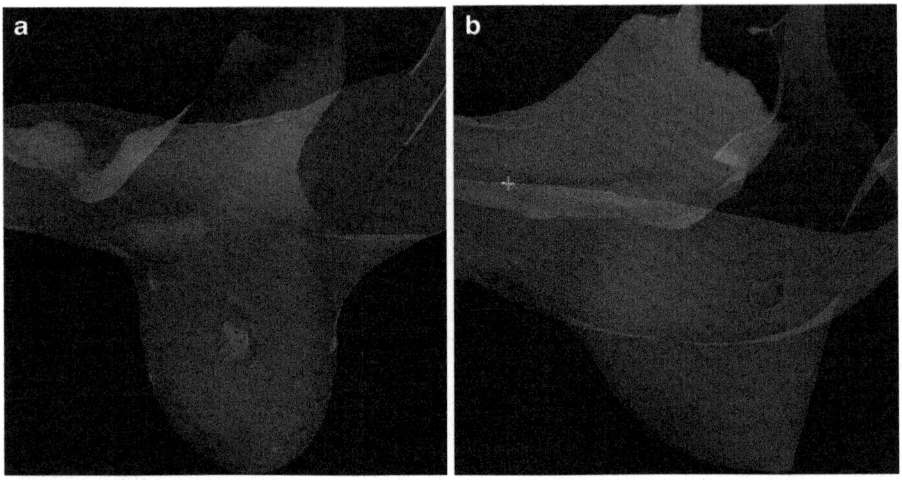

Fig 27.3 Preoperative target volume delineation based on CT (*blue*) and MRI (*red*) shown on planning CT for two patients. (**a**) Patient with suboptimal agreement between the two modalities despite similar overall target volumes. (**b**) Patient with good agreement between target volumes identified on CT and MRI

portion of the postoperative treatment volume adjacent to close margins likely provides the majority of the benefit in reducing local recurrence. Furthermore, excellent local control has been demonstrated with intracavitary brachytherapy where irradiated tissue is primarily within 1 cm of the lumpectomy margin, which equates to a similar volume to the proposed preoperative APBI CTV [65]. Finally, advances in breast imaging have improved our ability to select appropriate candidates for APBI and to accurately delineate areas at risk for disease. All of these factors likely justify a smaller target volume for preoperative APBI.

Additional margin for PTV depends on the need for interfraction reproducibility (i.e., single versus multiple fractions) and setup variability, primarily mitigated by pretreatment imaging for localization. At Duke, we use a single-fraction approach with a 0.3 cm CTV-to-PTV expansion [66]. Patient positioning is confirmed by on-board kV and cone-beam CT imaging (CBCT) using the biopsy clip as a fiducial marker (Fig. 27.5). In our series of 32 patients, we observed a mean initial shift of 1.0 cm (range 0.2–4.3). However, mean residual shift from kV to CBCT was 0.3 cm (range 0–2.1), and intrafraction motion was less than 0.3 cm in 29 of 32 patients (mean 0.2 cm, range 0–0.9). Fractionated or supine techniques are more susceptible to setup error and respiratory motion and therefore may require larger PTV expansions. However, it should be noted that even in the context of expansions equivalent to those used for postoperative external-beam APBI, investigators at the University of Maryland demonstrated a >60 % reduction in PTV in the preoperative setting. This translated into increased eligibility for APBI (93 % versus 68 %, respectively) based on NSABP B-39 dose-volume criteria [61]. Similarly, van der Leij et al. compared their preoperative PTV volumes to those in the Tufts postoperative EBRT APBI series [15]. Despite similar CTV/PTV margins and larger tumors in the van der Leij series, the mean preoperative PTV was 122 cm^3 versus 296 cm^3 postoperatively [23].

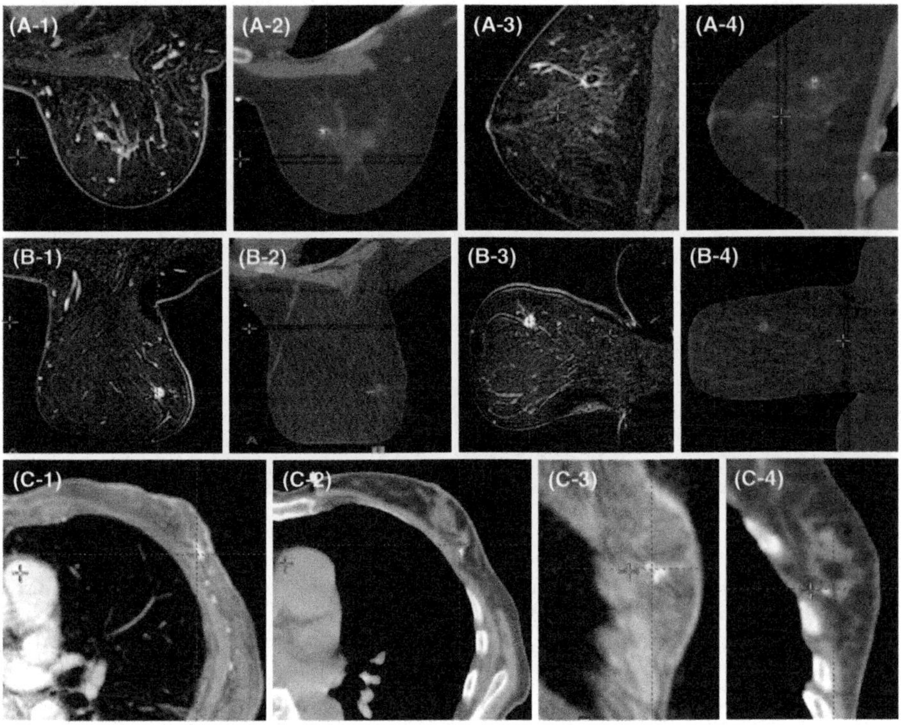

Fig 27.4 Preoperative MRI and CT images from three patients treated with preoperative APBI. Axial (*1*, *2*) and sagittal (*3*, *4*) image planes in a patient whose breast shape was similar between the two modalities (**a**), a patient who experienced significant compression from the MRI coil near the chest wall (**b**), and a patient in supine position (**c**) (Reproduced with permission from Blitzblau et al. [66])

27.4 Delivery Technique

Potential treatment techniques for preoperative APBI include 3D-CRT, IMRT, volumetric-modulated arc therapy (VMAT), and GammaPod™. The ideal technique would administer a conformal dose distribution to adequately cover the target while minimizing normal tissue dose. Reducing skin and non-target breast dose has been a focus of dosimetric optimization, given that these tissues likely play a major role in acute toxicity and long-term cosmetic outcomes. Shorter treatment delivery time would also offer the advantage of decreased intrafraction motion, potentially facilitating smaller PTV expansions. Research is ongoing to determine which techniques provide the best balance of dose conformity and homogeneity, treatment delivery time, and equipment cost/availability.

Yoo et al. recently evaluated dosimetric parameters for prone preoperative APBI plans using noncoplanar 3D-CRT, noncoplanar IMRT ($IMRT_{NC}$), coplanar IMRT ($IMRT_{CO}$), and VMAT [67]. The noncoplanar 3D-CRT and IMRT plans used four to five beams, while the coplanar IMRT plans used seven beams. The IMRT and

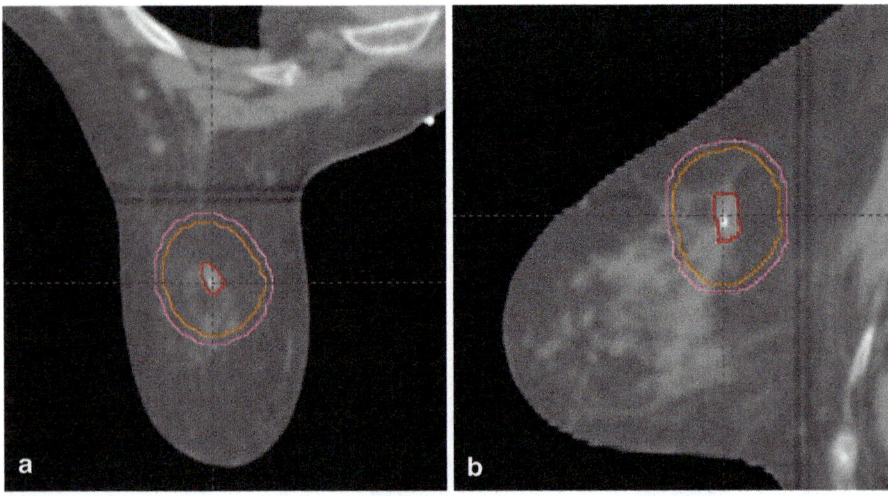

Fig 27.5 Target volume expansion for preoperative partial breast irradiation in the axial (**a**) and sagittal (**b**) planes. The GTV (*red*) is expanded by 1.5 cm to form the CTV (*orange*). An additional 3 mm (*pink*) is added for the PTV in one technique utilizing a single fraction in conjunction with pretreatment kV and CBCT imaging. Other investigators have used more generous PTV margins (Reproduced with permission from Blitzblau et al. [66])

VMAT plans were optimized to reduce skin and normal breast dose while covering >95 % of the CTV with 100 % of the prescribed dose. Dose-volume constraints and priorities are shown in Table 27.3. Skin and ipsilateral breast dose, as well as treatment delivery time, were highest with 3D-CRT plans. However, 3D-CRT also provided better target coverage and dose homogeneity than the other techniques. Overall, the $IMRT_{NC}$ and $IMRT_{CO}$ plans demonstrated similar normal tissue sparing and dose homogeneity and conformity, but estimated $IMRT_{CO}$ treatment delivery time was 1.4 min shorter. VMAT offered the shortest treatment delivery time and lowest ipsilateral V20 and V50 %; however this technique resulted in the lowest dose conformity and homogeneity. The authors concluded that IMRT plans are preferred given their excellent dose homogeneity (PTV homogeneity index 1.07–1.08), conformal target coverage (PTV conformity index 0.95–0.96), normal tissue sparing, and relatively short delivery time (Table 27.4, Fig. 27.6).

An alternative method of delivering highly conformal external-beam APBI utilizes GammaPod™, developed by Xcision Medical Systems. This device comprises the irradiation unit, breast immobilization and patient loading system, and a dedicated inverse planning system. A dual-layered vacuum-assisted cup immobilizes the breast in the prone position. This cup is embedded with fiducial markers that define a stereotactic coordinate system within which the table displacement vectors are defined. Before treatment, the patient steps onto an integrated loader that transports the patient and treatment couch from a near-vertical orientation to the prone treatment position (Fig. 27.7). While in the standing position, the patient's breast within the cup is inserted into and secured within an aperture in the couch. This

Table 27.3 Dose-volume constraints for preoperative treatment optimization using intensity-modulated or volumetric-modulated arc therapy

Structure	Dose-volume constraints	Relative priority
PTV	$D_{100} \geq 95\ \%$; $D_{max} \leq 105\ \%$	80–120
CTV	$D_{100} \geq 98\ \%$; $D_{max} \leq 102\ \%$	120–130
Skin	$D_{max} \leq 70\ \%$; $V_{50\%} \leq 2\ \%$	150–80
ILB	$V_{100\%} \leq 2–7\ \%$; $V_{50\%} \leq 10–15\ \%$; $V_{20\%} \leq 20–30\ \%$;	50
CB	$D_{max} \leq 1\ \%$;	30
Heart	$D_{max} \leq 1\ \%$;	30
ILL	$D_{max} \leq 20–30\ \%$; $V_{10\%} \leq 2–7\ \%$	30
Normal tissue	Doses between 2 mm and 2 cm from PTV boundary to fall off from 100 to 50 % of prescription	80

Reproduced with permission from Yoo et al. [67]

PTV planning target volume, *CTV* clinical target volume, *ILB* ipsilateral breast, *CB* contralateral breast, *ILL* ipsilateral lung, *Dxx* the dose to specified volume xx, *Dmax* maximum dose, *Vxx%* volume receiving xx% of prescribed dose

Table 27.4 Dosimetric comparison of preoperative external-beam treatment delivery techniques

		3D-CRT	$IMRT_{NC}$	$IMRT_{CO}$	VMAT
CTV	$V_{95\ \%}$	99.8 ± 0.4	99.5 ± 0.6[a]	99.5 ± 0.6[a]	99.5 ± 0.6[a]
	HI	1.05 ± 0.02	1.07 ± 0.04[a]	1.07 ± 0.03[a]	1.11 ± 0.04[a, b, c]
	CI	1.56 ± 0.27	1.42 ± 0.32	1.44 ± 0.30	1.60 ± 0.32
PTV	$V_{95\ \%}$	98.5 ± 1.4	96.3 ± 2.0[a]	96.5 ± 1.5[a]	96.4 ± 1.8[a]
	HI	1.05 ± 0.02	1.08 ± 0.05[a]	1.07 ± 0.04[a]	1.12 ± 0.02[a, b, c]
	CI	1.04 ± 0.17	0.95 ± 0.20	0.96 ± 0.21	1.07 ± 0.22[b, c]
Skin	$D_{10\ cm^3}$ (%)	45.9 ± 7.1	41.9 ± 5. 9[a]	43.8 ± 6.5	46.3 ± 7.42[b, c]
	$D_{1\ cm^3}$ (%)	72.9 ± 9.6	59.2 ± 10.3[a]	61.1 ± 11.9[a]	64.2 ± 11.7[a, b]
	D_{max} (%)	86.5 ± 6.7	73.7 ± 11.5[a]	74.3 ± 12.1[a]	76.3 ± 12.5[a]
ILB	$V_{20\%}$ (%)	28.5 ± 8.5	27.0 ± 7.8[a]	26.4 ± 8.3[a]	23.5 ± 7.5[a, b, c]
	$V_{50\%}$ (%)	15.3 ± 5.3	14.3 ± 3.9	14.8 ± 5.5	14.1 ± 5.6[a, c]
	$V_{100\%}$ (%)	4.3 ± 1.6	3.8 ± 1.3[a]	3.9 ± 1.4	4.4 ± 1.9[b, c]
	$D_{1\%}$ (%)	103.7 ± 1.8	103.9 ± 2.5[a]	104.0 ± 2.3[a]	105.6 ± 2.8[a]
Heart	D_{10cm^3} (%)	2.5 ± 1.7	1.8 ± 1.6[a]	1.6 ± 1.4[a]	1.3 ± 1.1[a, b, c]
CB	D_{10cm^3} (%)	1.0 ± 0.5	0.7 ± 0.3[a]	0.8 ± 0.3[a, b]	0.6 ± 0.2[a, c]
ILL	D_{10cm^3} (%)	11.4 ± 8.3	13.2 ± 10.8	11.8 ± 9.8	9.6 ± 9.9[b, c]
Dose falloff	$V_{50\%}/V_{100\%}$ of ILB	3.7 ± 0.8	3.9 ± 0.8	4.0 ± 1.1	3.3 ± 0.8[a, b, c]
Delivery time (min)		11.0 ± 1.5	9.7 ± 1.0[a]	8.3 ± 1.1[a, b]	7.0 ± 1.0[a, b, c]

Reproduced with permission from Yoo et al. [67]

[a]*p* value < 0.05 compared to 3D-CRT where *p* = the two-tailed paired *t*-test

[b]*p* value < 0.05 compared to $IMRT_{NC}$

[c]*p* value < 0.05 compared to $IMRT_{CO}$

3D-CRT 3D conformal radiation, *$IMNT_{NC}$* noncoplanar intensity-modulated radiotherapy (IMRT), *$IMRT_{CO}$* IMRT coplanar, *VMAT* volumetric-modulated arc therapy, *CTV* clinical target volume, *PTV* planning target volume, *ILB* ipsilateral breast, *CB* contralateral breast, *ILL* ipsilateral lung, *Vxx%* volume receiving xx% of prescribed dose, *HI* dose homogeneity index, *CI* conformity index, *Dxx* the dose to specified volume xx, *Dmax* maximum dose

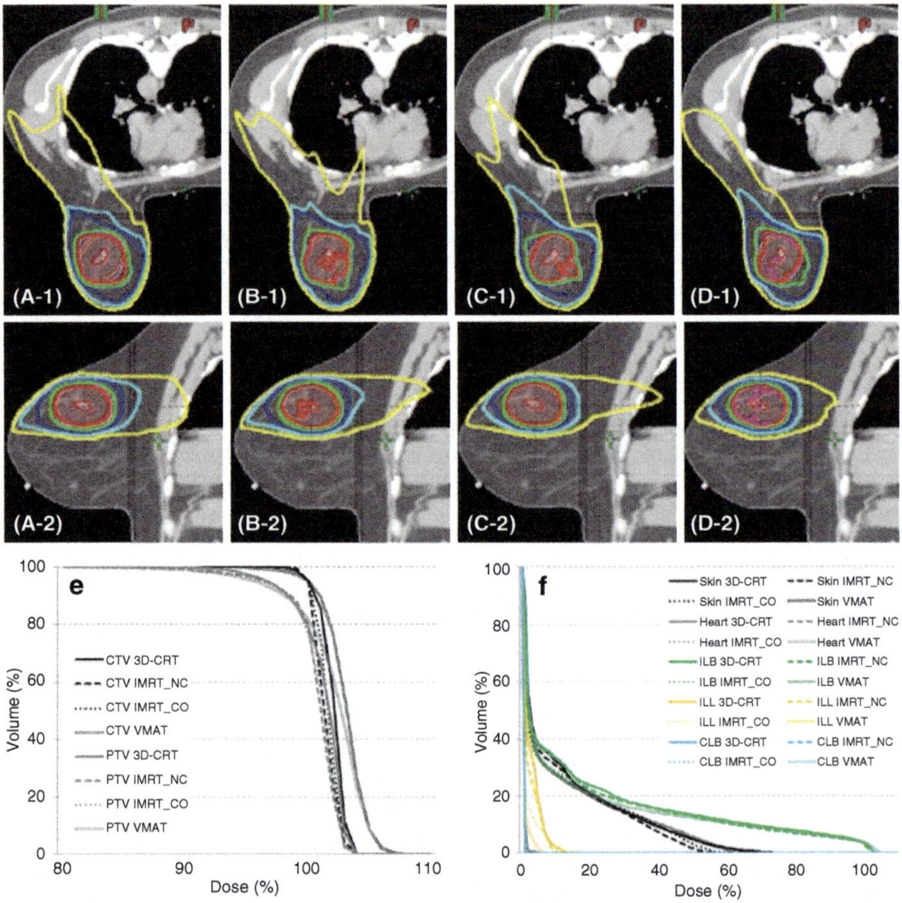

Fig 27.6 Axial (*1*) and sagittal (*2*) isodose distributions using 3D-CRT (**a**), $IMRT_{NC}$ (**b**), $IMRT_{CO}$ (**c**), and VMAT (**d**) delivery techniques. Magenta represents the 105 %, red 100 %, green 90 %, blue 50 %, cyan 30 %, and yellow 10 % isodose lines. Associated dose-volume histograms for target volumes (**e**) and normal tissue (**f**) (Reproduced with permission from Yoo et al. [67])

avoids the more awkward task of the patient climbing onto the treatment couch and inserting her breast into the aperture while prone. An adjustable foot platform is used to account for patients of different height, ensuring that the breast is at the level of the aperture. The patient loader simultaneously lifts and rotates the patient couch to the patient support table of the irradiation unit.

The irradiation unit consists of a hemispherical source carrier containing 36 Cobalt-60 sources, a tungsten collimator assembly fitting inside and concentric with the source carrier, a pair of shielding doors above the source-collimator assembly, and a dynamically controlled patient support table. The sources are blocked by 36 solid tungsten rods contained in the collimator assembly when not treating patients. Two sets of 36 collimator holes are used to create beams of either 25 mm or 15 mm

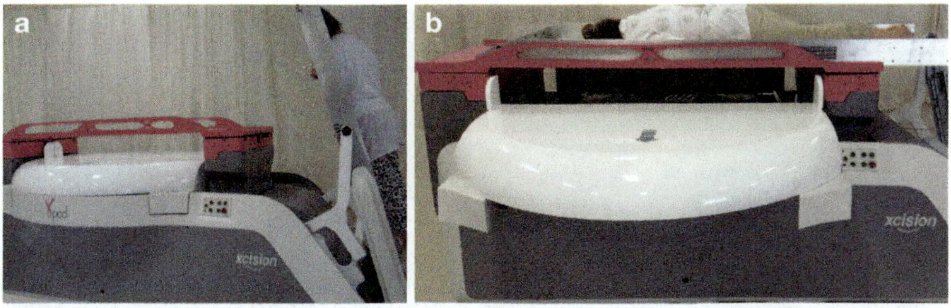

Fig 27.7 Patient in the loading position (**a**) on the GammaPod™ stereotactic radiotherapy device and in the prone position (**b**) after translation to the patient support table

diameter. The two collimator diameters can be selected by a different relative offset between the rotation angles of the collimator assembly and source carrier. Once the sources are aligned with the collimator holes of a selected size, the source carrier and collimator assembly rotate together to form 36 noncoplanar, concentric arcs focused at the isocenter. Simultaneously, the patient support table moves continuously in a large series of short vector displacements to move the focal spot and dynamically "paint" the desired dose distribution throughout the target in three dimensions [68].

Published dosimetric studies indicate that GammaPod™ has the ability to deliver highly focused uniform dose distributions to a target in the breast with fast dose falloff [69, 70]. Figure 27.8 shows typical dose distributions to a small (45 cm^3) and large (215 cm^3) target. The innermost isodose line is 100 % and the outermost is 20 %. As compared to the different intracavitary brachytherapy radiation delivery methods, GammaPod™ provides greater freedom in shaping the dose distribution using an external-beam approach. Dosimetric comparison between postoperative APBI treatment plans delivered by GammaPod™ versus intracavitary brachytherapy techniques indicates GammaPod™ delivers lower relative skin doses for targets close to the skin. For deeper targets, GammaPod™ provides a steeper dose falloff gradient beyond 1 cm from the target edge relative to brachytherapy [47]. It can either deliver a highly uniform dose to the gross tumor volume with any desired margin or deliver a differential dose to the gross tumor and its subclinical volumes. These characteristics make GammaPod™ well suited for preoperative irradiation.

Intraoperative techniques can also be utilized preoperatively. At the University of North Carolina (UNC), Kimple et al. performed a prospective trial in 71 patients with node-negative invasive ductal carcinoma (tumor <3 cm), administering a single intraoperative radiotherapy fraction immediately prior to partial mastectomy [71]. A mobile electron irradiator was used to deliver 15 gray (Gy) to the tumor with a 1.5–2 cm radial margin and the 90 % isodose line covering 1 cm deep to the tumor [72]. Preoperative ultrasound simulation was utilized to determine the optimal approach angle, electron energy, and cone size. The needle localization wire was utilized intraoperatively to identify the target and the tumor was positioned at the center of the radiation field. However, an actuarial in-breast recurrence rate of 8 %

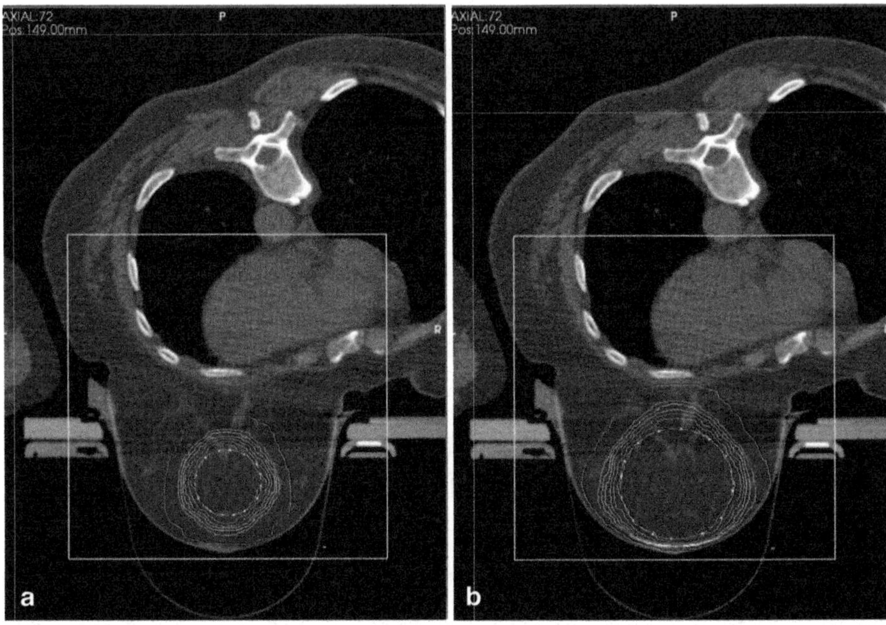

Fig 27.8 Dose distribution to a small (**a**) and large (**b**) target using the 36 rotating Cobalt-60 sources in the GammaPod™ delivery system

was noted at 3 years [71]. Therefore, additional optimization for this approach may be required and could include refined patient eligibility or intraoperative imaging for tumor localization and delineation as discussed above.

27.5 Dose/Fractionation and Efficacy

Investigators evaluating preoperative APBI have utilized a variety of approaches extrapolating from the postoperative APBI experience. In our phase I trial at Duke, women 55 or older with cT1N0 invasive carcinomas or low-/intermediate-grade ductal carcinoma in situ ≤2 cm were enrolled and received 15 Gy, 18 Gy, or 21 Gy in a single fraction [73]. The preoperative accelerated partial breast irradiation (PAPBI) trial initiated at Netherlands Cancer Institute-Antoni van Leeuwenhoek enrolled women aged 60 years and older with node-negative breast cancer and primary tumor ≤3 cm by MRI. A total dose of 40 Gy was delivered in 10 fractions over 2 weeks utilizing 3D-CRT, IMRT, or VMAT with CT guidance. Wide local excision was performed 6 weeks after completion of radiotherapy [23]. With short follow-up (median 23 months), both groups report early efficacy. In the US study, there have been no local recurrences among 32 patients, and in PAPBI, 2 out of 70 patients have had ipsilateral breast recurrences outside the radiation field.

Other dose and fractionation approaches are under investigation and are outlined in ongoing trials below. The optimal regimen for preoperative breast radiotherapy has not yet been determined. Assessment of long-term efficacy and treatment-related toxicity in ongoing clinical trials will provide additional guidance as this technique evolves.

27.6 Toxicity

Radiation prior to surgical resection is known in a variety of tumor types to increase surgical complications [74–76]. As such, treatment toxicities with preoperative APBI must be carefully assessed and reported to address this concern. Multiple factors may impact acute and long-term toxicity including the dose per fraction, total dose, dose to superficial tissues, and the interval between radiotherapy and surgical resection.

Two randomized trials, as well as the UNC intraoperative trial, have reported favorable toxicity outcomes with a large single intraoperative dose of radiation [2, 3]. However, intraoperative radiation delivery allows direct access to the tumor bed, greatly decreasing the possibility of large skin doses. Furthermore, treatment can be delivered with lower energy electrons or photons, resulting in less normal breast tissue receiving a significant portion of the prescription dose. In contrast, preoperative radiation is delivered with the skin intact to what is often a superficial breast tumor. Consequently, the skin frequently receives a high radiation dose (Fig. 27.9) which is a major potential source of acute and long-term morbidity. At Duke, we defined the skin as the first 3 mm of subcutaneous tissue and optimized the treatment plans to decrease maximum skin dose and the skin volume receiving high dose. The median maximum skin dose in our trial was 14.2 Gy (range 7.8–20.5 Gy) while at 1 cc the median was only 11.4 Gy (range 6.2–17.7) and median at 10 cm^3 was 7.1 Gy (range 3.8–11.3 Gy). Given the lack of prior experience with this approach, established normal tissue constraints were not available. However, despite these high skin doses, toxicity was limited in our experience (Table 27.5).

The optimal timing of surgical resection after radiation treatment also remains unclear. At Duke, patients underwent lumpectomy within 10 days of irradiation. In contrast, patients treated at the University of Maryland in an ongoing trial are delayed 3–4 weeks [77], and in the European PAPBI trial, 6 weeks following radiotherapy. This allows an assessment of pathologic response but may be associated

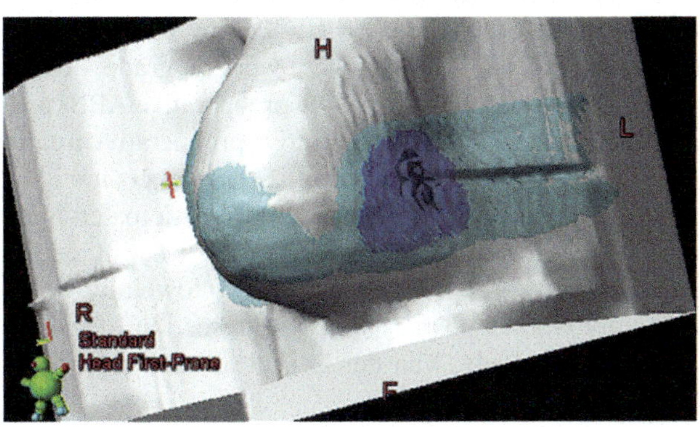

Fig 27.9 A skin surface rendering illustrating the rapid decrease in dose with increasing skin volume seen in a preoperative linear-accelerator-based treatment plan. The 10 % isodose line is represented by aqua, 30 % blue, and 50 % dark blue (Reproduced with permission from Palta et al. [59])

Table 27.5 Toxicities reported by US and European investigators evaluating two approaches to preoperative partial breast irradiation

	Total (%)	Grade 1 (%)	Grade 2 (%)	Grade 3 (%)
Horton et al.				
Fibrosis	77	65	10	3
Breast pain	48	35	13	0
Dermatitis	48	39	10	0
Persistent seroma	35	32	3	0
Skin hyperpigmentation	23	19	3	0
Breast atrophy	16	6	6	3
Skin infection	6	0	6	0
Skin ulceration	3	3	0	0
Van der Leij et al.				
Fibrosis	81	70	11	0
Breast pain	50	39	10	1
Dermatitis	44	43	1	0
Bleeding	16	0	16	0
Rib pain	16	13	3	0
Wound infection	12	3	9	0
Skin infection	11	–	–	–
Persistent seroma	10	–	–	–

–, not reported

with greater toxicity. Chaudhry et al. noted the development of symptomatic seromas in 48 % of patients (11 of 23) [77], while van der Leij et al. noted postoperative complications in 16 % (11 of 70). These included bleeding necessitating surgical intervention (2.9 % immediate; 1.4 % delayed) and wound infection (11.4 %) [23]. At Duke, we did not note any increase in postsurgical complications; however the sample size was small. All of our patients underwent a successful sentinel node procedure, and there were no incidences of serious wound infections, dehiscence, or postoperative bleeding.

Other toxicities were similar to those observed in the setting of lumpectomy and postoperative breast irradiation and were primarily grade 1 or 2. The most common findings were dermatitis, breast pain, fibrosis, and seroma (Table 27.5). Few grade 3 events were observed, and in our trial, both occurred in a patient who received postoperative whole breast radiotherapy and was subsequently diagnosed with a connective tissue disorder. There were no grade 4 or 5 toxicities.

Cosmetic outcomes following preoperative APBI are generally favorable. Patients at Duke who received only definitive preoperative treatment have all had good/excellent physician-reported cosmesis. However, cosmetic outcomes in the three patients requiring postoperative radiation for unanticipated high-risk features were fair/poor (Fig. 27.10). Although the patient number is limited, these data suggest that a large single dose of preoperative radiation followed by whole breast irradiation may significantly worsen cosmesis, despite resection of most breast tissue that was irradiated preoperatively. Van der Leij et al. also reported high rates of good/excellent

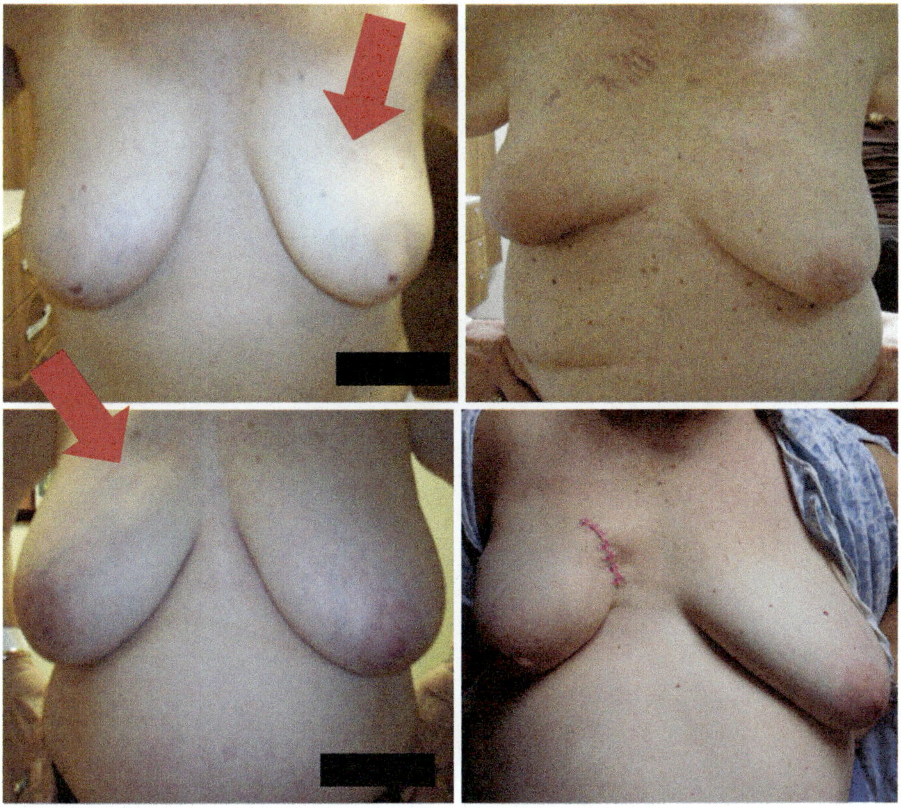

Fig 27.10 Patients treated with preoperative radiation alone ($n=29$) in a study at Duke University (*left*) had good/excellent cosmetic outcomes (*red arrows* indicate the lumpectomy cavity). Those requiring postoperative radiation (*right*, $n=3$) had fair/poor cosmetic outcomes (Reproduced with permission from Horton et al. [73])

cosmesis. Interestingly, these investigators noted that patient outcomes improved with time (Fig. 27.11). At 6 months, 77 % had good/excellent cosmetic results, but by 3 years this number had notably improved to 100 % [23]. The majority of patients in both trials rated their cosmetic outcomes as good or excellent.

27.7 Ongoing Clinical Trials

Preoperative APBI is currently under investigation in multiple clinical trials. A study at the University of Maryland is enrolling women with unifocal invasive breast carcinoma with primary tumor <3 cm and negative lymph nodes. Patients are treated to a total dose of 38.5 Gy administered twice daily in 10 fractions over 5 days. Treatment volumes are based on NSABP B39/RTOG 0413, expanding 1.5 cm

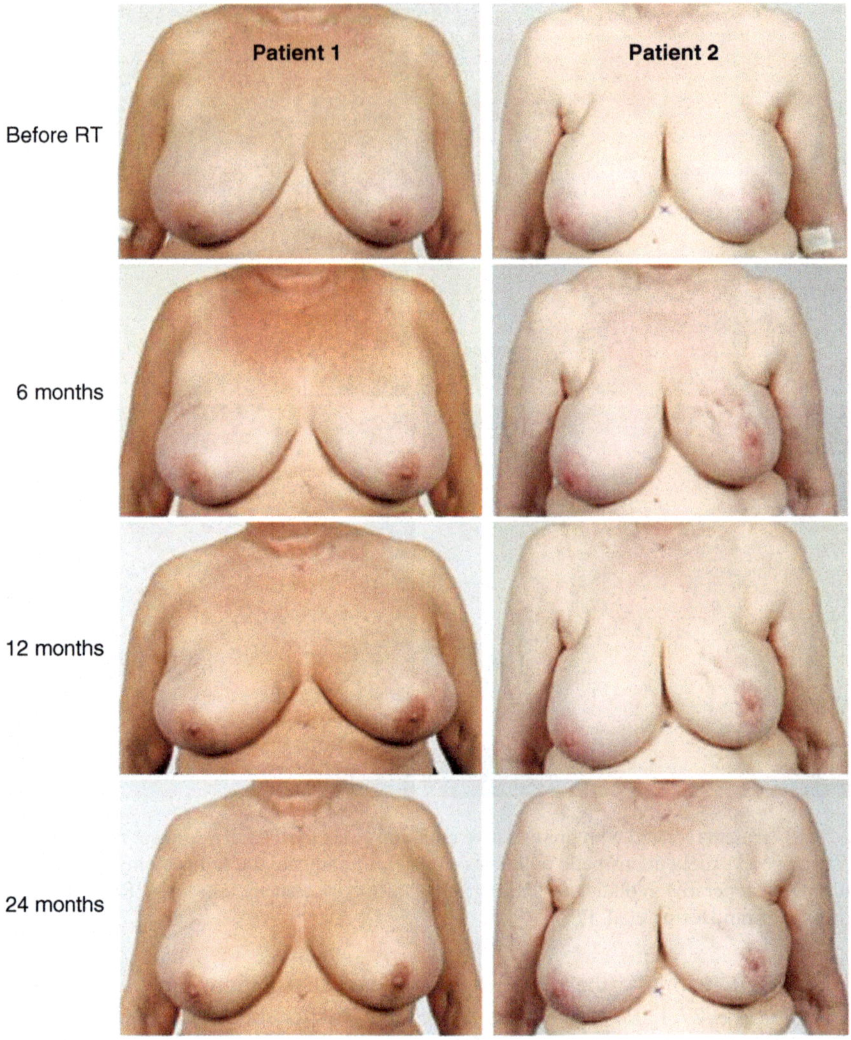

Fig 27.11 Patients on the PAPBI trial had improved cosmetic outcomes over time, increasing from 77 % with good or excellent outcomes at 6 months to 100 % at 3 years. Two patient examples are provided (Reproduced with permission from van der Leij et al. [23])

from the GTV to create the CTV with an additional 1 cm expansion to the PTV. Preliminary results indicate a complete pathologic response (morphologically or by absence of residual proliferative ability) in three of twelve patients [78].

Results have not yet been published for three preoperative APBI studies with ongoing patient recruitment. The SPORT trial ("Single Pre-Operative Radiation Therapy") is a Canadian dose-escalation study treating 10 total patients with 15, 18, or 20 Gy in a single fraction. Another prospective Canadian trial is utilizing SBRT to administer a total dose of 40 Gy in 5 fractions delivered every other day over 10–12 days to women aged 70 or older. Patients undergo breast-conserving surgery 10–12 weeks after completion of radiotherapy. The Dutch study "ABLATIVE" involves administration of a single radiotherapy dose to 25 patients and subsequent assessment of radiologic tumor response by MRI at 1 week and 2, 4, and 6 months post-radiotherapy. Breast-conserving surgery is performed 6 months after the ablative radiation treatment.

27.8 Future Directions

27.8.1 Upcoming Trials

Two additional preoperative APBI trials are not yet open for patient recruitment. The SIGNAL trial ("Stereotactic Image-Guided Neoadjuvant Ablative Radiation Then Lumpectomy") in Canada will enroll patients aged 55 and older with clinically node-negative invasive breast carcinoma. The primary tumor must measure ≤3 cm on pretreatment imaging and be located at least 1 cm from the skin surface. The GTV will be identified on CT coregistered with PET/MRI with the patient in prone position. Patients will receive a single 21 Gy dose to the GTV with margin using image-guided stereotactic body radiotherapy delivered by VMAT, followed by lumpectomy within 1 week. An upcoming trial sponsored by Ohio State University will enroll patients aged 60 and older with clinically node-negative in situ or invasive breast cancer (primary tumor ≤3 cm). MRI will be utilized to facilitate GTV contouring, and patients will be treated in the prone position. CT-guided IMRT will be utilized to treat the GTV with margin twice daily for a total of ten fractions, followed by lumpectomy within 4–6 weeks.

27.8.2 Alternative Clinical Scenarios

Preoperative whole breast irradiation is also being studied for patients with locally advanced disease. Women with node-positive breast cancer and residual disease after neoadjuvant chemotherapy are being enrolled in a clinical trial at Johns Hopkins University. In this study, veliparib and preoperative radiotherapy are administered in an effort to improve the pathologic complete response rate [79]. French investigators have also evaluated five different doses of fractionated stereotactic body radiotherapy (19.5–31.5 Gy delivered in three fractions to GTV with a 3 mm margin) as an adjunct to neoadjuvant chemotherapy for patients with locally advanced breast cancer [80]. Following surgical resection, all patients received conventional whole breast radiotherapy as well.

27.8.3 Radiation Biology

In addition, in the trial at Duke University and in the Netherlands PAPBI trial, pre- and post-radiation tissue sampling was incorporated into the preoperative trial design. Comprehensive analysis of those tissues is awaited and will provide insight into breast tumor radiation response. While initial trials focused on patients with biologically favorable tumors, incorporation of imaging and tissue correlatives in the diverse clinical scenarios above has the potential to greatly enhance our understanding of the molecular basis of radiation response in breast cancer.

27.9 Conclusions

Preoperative radiation is an area of active clinical investigation in the treatment of breast cancer. This approach has the potential to impact both short-term clinical practice and the future practice of breast radiotherapy through enhanced understanding of breast tumor radiation response.

References

1. Polgar C, Fodor J, Major T, Sulyok Z, Kasler M. Breast-conserving therapy with partial or whole breast irradiation: ten-year results of the Budapest randomized trial. Radiother Oncol. 2013;108(2):197–202. doi:10.1016/j.radonc.2013.05.008.
2. Vaidya JS, Wenz F, Bulsara M, Tobias JS, Joseph DJ, Keshtgar M, Flyger HL, Massarut S, Alvarado M, Saunders C, Eiermann W, Metaxas M, Sperk E, Sutterlin M, Brown D, Esserman L, Roncadin M, Thompson A, Dewar JA, Holtveg HM, Pigorsch S, Falzon M, Harris E, Matthews A, Brew-Graves C, Potyka I, Corica T, Williams NR, Baum M. Risk-adapted targeted intraoperative radiotherapy versus whole-breast radiotherapy for breast cancer: 5-year results for local control and overall survival from the TARGIT-A randomised trial. Lancet. 2014;383(9917):603–13. doi:10.1016/s0140-6736(13)61950-9.
3. Veronesi U, Orecchia R, Maisonneuve P, Viale G, Rotmensz N, Sangalli C, Luini A, Veronesi P, Galimberti V, Zurrida S, Leonardi MC, Lazzari R, Cattani F, Gentilini O, Intra M, Caldarella P, Ballardini B. Intraoperative radiotherapy versus external radiotherapy for early breast cancer (ELIOT): a randomised controlled equivalence trial. Lancet Oncol. 2013;14(13):1269–77. doi:10.1016/S1470-2045(13)70497-2.
4. Shah C, Badiyan S, Ben Wilkinson J, Vicini F, Beitsch P, Keisch M, Arthur D, Lyden M. Treatment efficacy with accelerated partial breast irradiation (APBI): final analysis of the American Society of Breast Surgeons MammoSite(R) breast brachytherapy registry trial. Ann Surg Oncol. 2013;20(10):3279–85. doi:10.1245/s10434-013-3158-4.
5. Shah C, Wilkinson JB, Lanni T, Jawad M, Wobb J, Fowler A, Wallace M, Chen P, Grills IS, Vicini F. Five-year outcomes and toxicities using 3-dimensional conformal external beam radiation therapy to deliver accelerated partial breast irradiation. Clin Breast Cancer. 2013;13(3):206–11. doi:10.1016/j.clbc.2012.09.020.
6. Arthur DW, Winter K, Kuske RR, Bolton J, Rabinovitch R, White J, Hanson WF, Wilenzick RM, McCormick B. A Phase II trial of brachytherapy alone after lumpectomy for select breast cancer: tumor control and survival outcomes of RTOG 95–17. Int J Radiat Oncol Biol Phys. 2008;72(2):467–73. doi:10.1016/j.ijrobp.2007.12.056.

7. Formenti SC, Hsu H, Fenton-Kerimian M, Roses D, Guth A, Jozsef G, Goldberg JD, Dewyngaert JK. Prone accelerated partial breast irradiation after breast-conserving surgery: five-year results of 100 patients. Int J Radiat Oncol Biol Phys. 2012;84(3):606–11. doi:10.1016/j.ijrobp.2012.01.039.
8. Mozsa E, Meszaros N, Major T, Frohlich G, Stelczer G, Sulyok Z, Fodor J, Polgar C. Accelerated partial breast irradiation with external beam three-dimensional conformal radiotherapy. Five-year results of a prospective phase II clinical study. Strahlenther Onkol. 2014;190(5):444–50. doi:10.1007/s00066-014-0633-1.
9. Rodriguez N, Sanz X, Dengra J, Foro P, Membrive I, Reig A, Quera J, Fernandez-Velilla E, Pera O, Lio J, Lozano J, Algara M. Five-year outcomes, cosmesis, and toxicity with 3-dimensional conformal external beam radiation therapy to deliver accelerated partial breast irradiation. Int J Radiat Oncol Biol Phys. 2013;87(5):1051–7. doi:10.1016/j.ijrobp.2013.08.046.
10. Livi L, Meattini I, Marrazzo L, Simontacchi G, Pallotta S, Saieva C, Paiar F, Scotti V, De Luca CC, Bastiani P, Orzalesi L, Casella D, Sanchez L, Nori J, Fambrini M, Bianchi S. Accelerated partial breast irradiation using intensity-modulated radiotherapy versus whole breast irradiation: 5-year survival analysis of a phase 3 randomised controlled trial. Eur J Cancer. 2015;51(4):451–63. doi:10.1016/j.ejca.2014.12.013.
11. Kuske RR, Winter K, Arthur DW, Bolton J, Rabinovitch R, White J, Hanson W, Wilenzick RM. Phase II trial of brachytherapy alone after lumpectomy for select breast cancer: toxicity analysis of RTOG 95–17. Int J Radiat Oncol Biol Phys. 2006;65(1):45–51. doi:10.1016/j.ijrobp.2005.11.027.
12. Chafe S, Moughan J, McCormick B, Wong J, Pass H, Rabinovitch R, Arthur DW, Petersen I, White J, Vicini FA. Late toxicity and patient self-assessment of breast appearance/satisfaction on RTOG 0319: a phase 2 trial of 3-dimensional conformal radiation therapy-accelerated partial breast irradiation following lumpectomy for stages I and II breast cancer. Int J Radiat Oncol Biol Phys. 2013;86(5):854–9. doi:10.1016/j.ijrobp.2013.04.005.
13. Julian TB, Costantino JP, Vicini FA, White JR, Winter KA, Arthur DW, Kuske RR, Rabinovitch R, Parda DS, Mamounas EP, Curran WJ, Wolmark N. Early toxicity results with 3D conformal external beam therapy (CEBT) from the NSABP B-39/RTOG 0413 accelerated partial breast irradiation (APBI) trial. J Clin Oncol. 2011;29:abstr 1011.
14. Liss AL, Ben-David MA, Jagsi R, Hayman JA, Griffith KA, Moran JM, Marsh RB, Pierce LJ. Decline of cosmetic outcomes following accelerated partial breast irradiation using intensity modulated radiation therapy: results of a single-institution prospective clinical trial. Int J Radiat Oncol Biol Phys. 2014;89(1):96–102. doi:10.1016/j.ijrobp.2014.01.005.
15. Leonard KL, Hepel JT, Hiatt JR, Dipetrillo TA, Price LL, Wazer DE. The effect of dose-volume parameters and interfraction interval on cosmetic outcome and toxicity after 3-dimensional conformal accelerated partial breast irradiation. Int J Radiat Oncol Biol Phys. 2013;85(3):623–9. doi:10.1016/j.ijrobp.2012.06.052.
16. Olivotto IA, Whelan TJ, Parpia S, Kim DH, Berrang T, Truong PT, Kong I, Cochrane B, Nichol A, Roy I, Germain I, Akra M, Reed M, Fyles A, Trotter T, Perera F, Beckham W, Levine MN, Julian JA. Interim cosmetic and toxicity results from RAPID: a randomized trial of accelerated partial breast irradiation using three-dimensional conformal external beam radiation therapy. J Clin Oncol. 2013;31(32):4038–45. doi:10.1200/jco.2013.50.5511.
17. Beal K, McCormick B, Zelefsky MJ, Borgen P, Fey J, Goldberg J, Cohen GN, Sacchini V. Single-fraction intraoperative radiotherapy for breast cancer: early cosmetic results. Int J Radiat Oncol Biol Phys. 2007;69(1):19–24. doi:10.1016/j.ijrobp.2007.02.010.
18. Wazer DE, Kaufman S, Cuttino L, DiPetrillo T, Arthur DW. Accelerated partial breast irradiation: an analysis of variables associated with late toxicity and long-term cosmetic outcome after high-dose-rate interstitial brachytherapy. Int J Radiat Oncol Biol Phys. 2006;64(2):489–95. doi:10.1016/j.ijrobp.2005.06.028.
19. Mellon EA, Sreeraman R, Gebhardt BJ, Mierzejewski A, Correa CR. Impact of radiation treatment parameters and adjuvant systemic therapy on cosmetic outcomes after accelerated partial breast irradiation using 3-dimensional conformal radiation therapy technique. Pract Radiat Oncol. 2014;4(3):e159–66. doi:10.1016/j.prro.2013.08.001.

20. Lei RY, Leonard CE, Howell KT, Henkenberns PL, Johnson TK, Hobart TL, Fryman SP, Kercher JM, Widner JL, Kaske T, Carter DL. Four-year clinical update from a prospective trial of accelerated partial breast intensity-modulated radiotherapy (APBIMRT). Breast Cancer Res Treat. 2013;140(1):119–33. doi:10.1007/s10549-013-2623-x.
21. Brasic N, Wisner DJ, Joe BN. Breast MR imaging for extent of disease assessment in patients with newly diagnosed breast cancer. Magn Reson Imaging Clin N Am. 2013;21(3):519–32. doi:10.1016/j.mric.2013.04.012.
22. Dorn PL, Al-Hallaq HA, Haq F, Goldberg M, Abe H, Hasan Y, Chmura SJ. A prospective study of the utility of magnetic resonance imaging in determining candidacy for partial breast irradiation. Int J Radiat Oncol Biol Phys. 2013;85(3):615–22. doi:10.1016/j.ijrobp.2012.06.014.
23. van der Leij F, Bosma SC, van de Vijver MJ, Wesseling J, Vreeswijk S, Rivera S, Bourgier C, Garbay JR, Foukakis T, Lekberg T, van den Bongard DH, van Vliet-Vroegindeweij C, Bartelink H, Rutgers EJ, Elkhuizen PH. First results of the preoperative accelerated partial breast irradiation (PAPBI) trial. Radiother Oncol. 2015. doi:10.1016/j.radonc.2015.02.002.
24. Holli K, Saaristo R, Isola J, Joensuu H, Hakama M. Lumpectomy with or without postoperative radiotherapy for breast cancer with favourable prognostic features: results of a randomized study. Br J Cancer. 2001;84(2):164–9. doi:10.1054/bjoc.2000.1571.
25. Fisher B, Anderson S, Bryant J, Margolese RG, Deutsch M, Fisher ER, Jeong JH, Wolmark N. Twenty-year follow-up of a randomized trial comparing total mastectomy, lumpectomy, and lumpectomy plus irradiation for the treatment of invasive breast cancer. N Engl J Med. 2002;347(16):1233–41. doi:10.1056/NEJMoa022152.
26. Fowble B, Solin LJ, Schultz DJ, Rubenstein J, Goodman RL. Breast recurrence following conservative surgery and radiation: patterns of failure, prognosis, and pathologic findings from mastectomy specimens with implications for treatment. Int J Radiat Oncol Biol Phys. 1990;19(4):833–42.
27. Veronesi U, Marubini E, Mariani L, Galimberti V, Luini A, Veronesi P, Salvadori B, Zucali R. Radiotherapy after breast-conserving surgery in small breast carcinoma: long-term results of a randomized trial. Ann Oncol. 2001;12(7):997–1003.
28. Liljegren G, Holmberg L, Bergh J, Lindgren A, Tabar L, Nordgren H, Adami HO. 10-Year results after sector resection with or without postoperative radiotherapy for stage I breast cancer: a randomized trial. J Clin Oncol. 1999;17(8):2326–33.
29. Clark RM, Whelan T, Levine M, Roberts R, Willan A, McCulloch P, Lipa M, Wilkinson RH, Mahoney LJ. Randomized clinical trial of breast irradiation following lumpectomy and axillary dissection for node-negative breast cancer: an update. Ontario Clinical Oncology Group. J Natl Cancer Inst. 1996;88(22):1659–64.
30. Berrang TS, Olivotto I, Kim DH, Nichol A, Cho BC, Mohamed IG, Parhar T, Wright JR, Truong P, Tyldesley S, Sussman J, Wai E, Whelan T. Three-year outcomes of a Canadian multicenter study of accelerated partial breast irradiation using conformal radiation therapy. Int J Radiat Oncol Biol Phys. 2011;81(5):1220–7. doi:10.1016/j.ijrobp.2010.07.2003.
31. Hattangadi JA, Powell SN, MacDonald SM, Mauceri T, Ancukiewicz M, Freer P, Lawenda B, Alm El-Din MA, Gadd MA, Smith BL, Taghian AG. Accelerated partial breast irradiation with low-dose-rate interstitial implant brachytherapy after wide local excision: 12-year outcomes from a prospective trial. Int J Radiat Oncol Biol Phys. 2012;83(3):791–800. doi:10.1016/j.ijrobp.2011.09.003.
32. Ott OJ, Hildebrandt G, Pötter R, Hammer J, Lotter M, Resch A, Sauer R, Strnad V. Accelerated partial breast irradiation with multi-catheter brachytherapy: Local control, side effects and cosmetic outcome for 274 patients. Results of the German–Austrian multi-centre trial. Radiother Oncol. 2007;82(3):281–6. doi:http://dx.doi.org/10.1016/j.radonc.2006.08.028.
33. Landis DM, Luo W, Song J, Bellon JR, Punglia RS, Wong JS, Killoran JH, Gelman R, Harris JR. Variability among breast radiation oncologists in delineation of the postsurgical lumpectomy cavity. Int J Radiat Oncol Biol Phys. 2007;67(1308):1299. doi:http://dx.doi.org/10.1016/j.ijrobp.2006.11.026.
34. van der Leij F, Elkhuizen PH, Janssen TM, Poortmans P, van der Sangen M, Scholten AN, van Vliet-Vroegindeweij C, Boersma LJ. Target volume delineation in external beam partial breast

irradiation: less inter-observer variation with preoperative- compared to postoperative delineation. Radiother Oncol. 2014;110(3):467–70. doi:10.1016/j.radonc.2013.10.033.
35. van Mourik AM, Elkhuizen PH, Minkema D, Duppen JC, van Vliet-Vroegindeweij C. Multiinstitutional study on target volume delineation variation in breast radiotherapy in the presence of guidelines. Radiother Oncol. 2010;94(3):286–91. doi:10.1016/j.radonc.2010.01.009.
36. den Hartogh MD, van Asselen B, Monninkhof EM, van den Bosch MA, van Vulpen M, van Diest PJ, Gilhuijs KG, Witkamp AJ, van de Bunt L, Mali WP, van den Bongard HJ. Excised and irradiated volumes in relation to the tumor size in breast-conserving therapy. Breast Cancer Res Treat. 2011;129(3):857–65. doi:10.1007/s10549-011-1696-7.
37. Holland R, Veling SHJ, Mravunac M, Hendriks JHCL. Histologic multifocality of tis, T1–2 breast carcinomas implications for clinical trials of breast-conserving surgery. Cancer. 1985;56(5):979–90. doi:10.1002/1097-0142(19850901)56:5<979::AID-CNCR2820560502>3.0.CO;2-N.
38. Rosen PP, Fracchia AA, Urban JA, Schottenfeld D, Robbins GF. "Residual" mammary carcinoma following simulated partial mastectomy. Cancer. 1975;35(3):739–47. doi:10.1002/1097-0142(197503)35:3<739::AID-CNCR2820350329>3.0.CO;2-5.
39. Vicini FA, Kestin LL, Goldstein NS. Defining the clinical target volume for patients with early-stage breast cancer treated with lumpectomy and accelerated partial breast irradiation: a pathologic analysis. Int J Radiat Oncol Biol Phys. 2004;60(3):722–30. doi:http://dx.doi.org/10.1016/j.ijrobp.2004.04.012.
40. Berg WA, Gutierrez L, NessAiver MS, Carter WB, Bhargavan M, Lewis RS, Ioffe OB. Diagnostic accuracy of mammography, clinical examination, US, and MR imaging in preoperative assessment of breast cancer. Radiology. 2004;233(3):830–49. doi:10.1148/radiol.2333031484.
41. Van Goethem M, Schelfout K, Kersschot E, Colpaert C, Verslegers I, Biltjes I, Tjalma WA, De Schepper A, Weyler J, Parizel PM. MR mammography is useful in the preoperative locoregional staging of breast carcinomas with extensive intraductal component. Eur J Radiol. 2007;62(2):273–82. doi:http://dx.doi.org/10.1016/j.ejrad.2006.12.004.
42. Hata T, Takahashi H, Watanabe K, Takahashi M, Taguchi K, Itoh T, Todo S. Magnetic resonance imaging for preoperative evaluation of breast cancer: a comparative study with mammography and ultrasonography. J Am Coll Surg. 2004;198(2):190–7. doi:http://dx.doi.org/10.1016/j.jamcollsurg.2003.10.008.
43. Schouten van der Velden AP, Boetes C, Bult P, Wobbes T. The value of magnetic resonance imaging in diagnosis and size assessment of in situ and small invasive breast carcinoma. Am J Surg. 2006;192(2):172–8. doi:10.1016/j.amjsurg.2006.02.026.
44. Grimsby GM, Gray R, Dueck A, Carpenter S, Stucky CC, Aspey H, Giurescu ME, Pockaj B. Is there concordance of invasive breast cancer pathologic tumor size with magnetic resonance imaging? Am J Surg. 2009;198(4):500–4. doi:10.1016/j.amjsurg.2009.07.012.
45. Lobbes MB, Lalji UC, Nelemans PJ, Houben I, Smidt ML, Heuts E, de Vries B, Wildberger JE, Beets-Tan RG. The quality of tumor size assessment by contrast-enhanced spectral mammography and the benefit of additional breast MRI. J Cancer. 2015;6(2):144–50. doi:10.7150/jca.10705.
46. Gruber IV, Rueckert M, Kagan KO, Staebler A, Siegmann KC, Hartkopf A, Wallwiener D, Hahn M. Measurement of tumour size with mammography, sonography and magnetic resonance imaging as compared to histological tumour size in primary breast cancer. BMC Cancer. 2013;13:328. doi:10.1186/1471-2407-13-328.
47. Onesti JK, Mangus BE, Helmer SD, Osland JS. Breast cancer tumor size: correlation between magnetic resonance imaging and pathology measurements. Am J Surg. 2008;196 (6):844–8; discussion 849–50. doi:10.1016/j.amjsurg.2008.07.028.
48. Behjatnia B, Sim J, Bassett LW, Moatamed NA, Apple SK. Does size matter? Comparison study between MRI, gross, and microscopic tumor sizes in breast cancer in lumpectomy specimens. Int J Clin Exp Pathol. 2010;3(3):303–9.

49. Mumtaz H, Hall-Craggs MA, Davidson T, Walmsley K, Thurell W, Kissin MW, Taylor I. Staging of symptomatic primary breast cancer with MR imaging. AJR Am J Roentgenol. 1997;169(2):417–24. doi:10.2214/ajr.169.2.9242745.
50. Boetes C, Veltman J, van Die L, Bult P, Wobbes T, Barentsz JO. The role of MRI in invasive lobular carcinoma. Breast Cancer Res Treat. 2004;86(1):31–7. doi:10.1023/B:BREA.0000032921.10481.dc.
51. Cheung YC, Wan YL, Lo YF, Leung WM, Chen SC, Hsueh S. Preoperative magnetic resonance imaging evaluation for breast cancers after sonographically guided core-needle biopsy: a comparison study. Ann Surg Oncol. 2004;11(8):756–61. doi:10.1245/ASO.2004.12.008.
52. Kepple J, Layeeque R, Klimberg VS, Harms S, Siegel E, Korourian S, Gusmano F, Henry-Tillman RS. Correlation of magnetic resonance imaging and pathologic size of infiltrating lobular carcinoma of the breast. Am J Surg. 2005;190(4):623–7. doi:10.1016/j.amjsurg.2005.06.028.
53. Kim do Y, Moon WK, Cho N, Ko ES, Yang SK, Park JS, Kim SM, Park IA, Cha JH, Lee EH. MRI of the breast for the detection and assessment of the size of ductal carcinoma in situ. Korean J Radiol. 2007;8(1):32–9.
54. Schmitz AC, van den Bosch MA, Loo CE, Mali WP, Bartelink H, Gertenbach M, Holland R, Peterse JL, Rutgers EJ, Gilhuijs KG. Precise correlation between MRI and histopathology – exploring treatment margins for MRI-guided localized breast cancer therapy. Radiother Oncol. 2010;97(2):225–32. doi:10.1016/j.radonc.2010.07.025.
55. Ahn SJ, Kim YS, Kim EY, Park HK, Cho EK, Kim YK, Sung YM, Choi HY. The value of chest CT for prediction of breast tumor size: comparison with pathology measurement. World J Surg Oncol. 2013;11:130. doi:10.1186/1477-7819-11-130.
56. Uematsu T, Sano M, Homma K, Shiina M, Kobayashi S. Three-dimensional helical CT of the breast: accuracy for measuring extent of breast cancer candidates for breast conserving surgery. Breast Cancer Res Treat. 2001;65(3):249–57.
57. Akashi-Tanaka S, Sato N, Ohsumi S, Kimijima I, Inaji H, Teramoto S, Akiyama F. Evaluation of the usefulness of breast CT imaging in delineating tumor extent and guiding surgical management: a prospective multi-institutional study. Ann Surg. 2012;256(1):157–62. doi:10.1097/SLA.0b013e31825b6cb1.
58. den Hartogh MD, Philippens ME, van Dam IE, Kleynen CE, Tersteeg RJ, Pijnappel RM, Kotte AN, Verkooijen HM, van den Bosch MA, van Vulpen M, van Asselen B, van den Bongard HD. MRI and CT imaging for preoperative target volume delineation in breast-conserving therapy. Radiat Oncol. 2014;9:63. doi:10.1186/1748-717X-9-63.
59. Palta M, Yoo S, Adamson JD, Prosnitz LR, Horton JK. Preoperative single fraction partial breast radiotherapy for early-stage breast cancer. Int J Radiat Oncol Biol Phys. 2012;82(1):37–42. doi:10.1016/j.ijrobp.2010.09.041.
60. Nichols EM, Dhople AA, Mohiuddin MM, Flannery TW, Yu CX, Regine WF. Comparative analysis of the post-lumpectomy target volume versus the use of pre-lumpectomy tumor volume for early-stage breast cancer: implications for the future. Int J Radiat Oncol Biol Phys. 2010;77(1):197–202. doi:http://dx.doi.org/10.1016/j.ijrobp.2009.04.063.
61. Nichols EM, Feigenberg SJ, Marter K, Cheston SB, Lasio G, Tkaczuk K, Kesmodel S, Buras R, Regine WF. Preoperative radiation therapy significantly increases patient eligibility for accelerated partial breast irradiation using 3D-conformal radiotherapy. Am J Clin Oncol. 2013;36(3):232–8. doi:10.1097/COC.0b013e3182467ffd.
62. Kim L, Shaitelman S. What is the target volume for preoperative accelerated partial breast irradiation (APBI)? In regards to Nichols et al. (Int J Radiat Oncol Biol Phys 2010;77:197–202) and Palta et al. (Int J Radiat Oncol Biol Phys 2010, in Press). Int J Radiat Oncol Biol Phys. 2011;80 (1):314–315; author reply 315–6. doi:10.1016/j.ijrobp.2010.12.038.
63. Kirby AM, Evans PM, Nerurkar AY, Desai SS, Krupa J, Devalia H, della Rovere GQ, Harris EJ, Kyriakidou J, Yarnold JR. How does knowledge of three-dimensional excision margins following breast conservation surgery impact upon clinical target volume definition for partial-breast radiotherapy? Radiother Oncol. 2010;94(3):292–9. doi:10.1016/j.radonc.2009.11.002.

64. Hanbeukers B, Borger J, van den Ende P, van der Ent F, Houben R, Jager J, Keymeulen K, Murrer L, Sastrowijoto S, van de Vijver K, Boersma L. Customized computed tomography-based boost volumes in breast-conserving therapy: use of three-dimensional histologic information for clinical target volume margins. Int J Radiat Oncol Biol Phys. 2009;75(3):757–63. doi:10.1016/j.ijrobp.2008.11.048.
65. Benitez PR, Keisch ME, Vicini F, Stolier A, Scroggins T, Walker A, White J, Hedberg P, Hebert M, Arthur D, Zannis V, Quiet C, Streeter O, Silverstein M. Five-year results: the initial clinical trial of MammoSite balloon brachytherapy for partial breast irradiation in early-stage breast cancer. Am J Surg. 2007;194(4):456–62. doi:10.1016/j.amjsurg.2007.06.010.
66. Blitzblau RC, Arya R, Yoo S, Baker JA, Chang Z, Palta M, Duffy E, Horton JK. A phase I trial of preoperative partial breast radiotherapy: patient selection, target delineation, and dose delivery. Pract Radiat Oncol. 2015;5(5):e513–20.
67. Yoo S, Blitzblau R, Yin F-F, Horton JK. Dosimetric comparison of preoperative single-fraction partial breast radiotherapy techniques: 3D CRT, noncoplanar IMRT, coplanar IMRT, and VMAT. J Appl Clin Med Phys. 2015;16(1):5126.
68. Yu CX, Shao X, Zhang J, Regine W, Zheng M, Yu YS, Deng J, Duan Z. GammaPod-a new device dedicated for stereotactic radiotherapy of breast cancer. Med Phys. 2013;40(5):051703. doi:10.1118/1.4798961.
69. Mutaf YD, Zhang J, Yu CX, Yi BY, Prado K, D'Souza WD, Regine WF, Feigenberg SJ. Dosimetric and geometric evaluation of a novel stereotactic radiotherapy device for breast cancer: the GammaPod. Med Phys. 2013;40(4):041722. doi:10.1118/1.4794477.
70. Oden J, Toma-Dasu I, Yu CX, Feigenberg SJ, Regine WF, Mutaf YD. Dosimetric comparison between intra-cavitary breast brachytherapy techniques for accelerated partial breast irradiation and a novel stereotactic radiotherapy device for breast cancer: GammaPod. Phys Med Biol. 2013;58(13):4409–21. doi:10.1088/0031-9155/58/13/4409.
71. Kimple RJ, Klauber-DeMore N, Kuzmiak CM, Pavic D, Lian J, Livasy CA, Chiu WM, Moore DT, Sartor CI, Ollila DW. Local control following single-dose intraoperative radiotherapy prior to surgical excision of early-stage breast cancer. Ann Surg Oncol. 2011;18(4):939–45. doi:10.1245/s10434-010-1392-6.
72. Kimple RJ, Klauber-DeMore N, Kuzmiak CM, Pavic D, Lian J, Livasy CA, Esler L, Moore DT, Sartor CI, Ollila DW. Cosmetic outcomes for accelerated partial breast irradiation before surgical excision of early-stage breast cancer using single-dose intraoperative radiotherapy. Int J Radiat Oncol Biol Phys. 2011;79(2):400–7. doi:10.1016/j.ijrobp.2009.10.032.
73. Horton JK, Blitzblau RC, Yoo S, Geradts J, Chang Z, Baker JA, Georgiade GS, Chen W, Siamakpour-Reihani S, Wang C, Broadwater G, Groth J, Palta M, Dewhirst MW, Barry WT, Duffy E, Chi JA, Hwang ES. Preoperative single-fraction partial breast radiotherapy – a novel phase I dose-escalation protocol with radiation response biomarkers. Int J Radiat Oncol Biol Phys. 2015;92(4):846–55.
74. O'Sullivan B, Davis AM, Turcotte R, Bell R, Catton C, Chabot P, Wunder J, Kandel R, Goddard K, Sadura A, Pater J, Zee B. Preoperative versus postoperative radiotherapy in soft-tissue sarcoma of the limbs: a randomised trial. Lancet. 2002;359(9325):2235–41. doi:10.1016/s0140-6736(02)09292-9.
75. Vandenbrouck C, Sancho H, Le Fur R, Richard JM, Cachin Y. Results of a randomized clinical trial of preoperative irradiation versus postoperative in treatment of tumors of the hypopharynx. Cancer. 1977;39(4):1445–9.
76. Sassler AM, Esclamado RM, Wolf GT. Surgery after organ preservation therapy. Analysis of wound complications. Arch Otolaryngol Head Neck Surg. 1995;121(2):162–5.
77. Chaudhry H, Hanlon AL, Kesmodel SB, Bellavance EC, Tkaczuk KH, Drogula CL, Citron WK, Cohen RJ, Regine WF, Feigenberg SJ. A prospective trial of preoperative accelerated partial breast irradiation (APBI): predictors of asymptomatic and symptomatic seroma formation. Int J Radiat Oncol Biol Phys. 2013;87(2):S215–6. doi:10.1016/j.ijrobp.2013.06.558.
78. Feigenberg SJ, Christenson E, Staats P, Webb T, Chumsri S, Tkaczuk K, Nichols E, Kesmodel S, Bellavance E, Regine W. Preoperative accelerated partial breast radiation is associated with

decreased Cd8+ cells in patients with early breast cancer. Int J Radiat Oncol Biol Phys. 2012;84(3):S243. doi:10.1016/j.ijrobp.2012.07.630.
79. Zellars RC, Lange JR, Habibi M, Fetting JH, Stearns V. Preoperative PARPi and irradiation (POPI) for women with an incomplete response to neoadjuvant chemotherapy (NAC) for breast cancer: a phase I trial. J Clin Oncol. 2014;32(5s):abstr TPS1142.
80. Bondiau PY, Courdi A, Bahadoran P, Chamorey E, Queille-Roussel C, Lallement M, Birtwisle-Peyrottes I, Chapellier C, Pacquelet-Cheli S, Ferrero JM. Phase 1 clinical trial of stereotactic body radiation therapy concomitant with neoadjuvant chemotherapy for breast cancer. Int J Radiat Oncol Biol Phys. 2013;85(5):1193–9. doi:10.1016/j.ijrobp.2012.10.034.

Chapter 28
Hypofractionated Regional Nodal Irradiation for Breast Cancer

Matthew Poppe, Chirag Shah, and Atif J. Khan

Contents

28.1 Introduction to Hypofractionated Regional Nodal Radiation

Research from the 1950s and 1960s out of the UK and Australia pioneered work in hypofractionated RNI for breast cancer but resulted in unacceptable toxicity given their limited knowledge of radiobiology [1–4]. The 1970s and 1980s brought us

M. Poppe, MD (✉)
Department of Radiation Oncology, Huntsman Cancer Hospital, University of Utah, Salt Lake City, UT, USA
e-mail: Matthew.Poppe@hci.utah.edu

C. Shah, MD
Department of Radiation Oncology, Summa Health System, Akron, OH, USA

A.J. Khan, MD
Department of Radiation Oncology, Rutgers Cancer Institute of New Jersey, New Brunswick, NJ, USA

D.W. Arthur et al. (eds.), *Short Course Breast Radiotherapy: A Comprehensive Review of Hypofractionation, Partial Breast, and Intra-Operative Irradiation*,
DOI 10.1007/978-3-319-24388-7_28

well-known randomized (postmastectomy radiation therapy) PMRT data from Canada and the development of the UK Start trials, both revealing safe delivery of hypofractionated RNI for breast cancer after chemotherapy [5, 6]. The 1990s and 2000s include a follow-on UK Start trial, as well as several small prospective trials from Pakistan, Greece, and Belgium, all demonstrating safe hypofractionated RNI for breast cancer [7–10].

Treatment of locally advanced breast with hypofractionated radiation is not currently an accepted standard in the United States but is the standard in many other countries. This situation occurs in both breast conservation and mastectomy (+/– reconstruction) patients in which radiation delivered to regional lymph nodes is required. While there has been a relative reduction in the incidence of locally advanced breast cancer, the utilization of RNI will increase in response to emerging data suggesting a benefit for those with limited nodal involvement (1–3 nodes positive) [11]. Radiation treatment that incorporates RNI is typically prescribed over 5 to 5 ½ weeks, utilizing a standard fractionation schedule of 1.8–2 gray (Gy) per day, to a total dose of 46–50 Gy. Hypofractionated radiation (HRT) is given in doses of greater than 2 Gy per day, either in the standard 5–6 weeks or more commonly in an accelerated course, usually over 3–4 weeks. In the last 5–10 years, there has been a significant shift in the radiation of women with intact breast cancer to shorter, more cost-effective and convenient treatment courses when RNI is not incorporated [12]. Decreasing the time required for women to undergo radiation improves treatment compliance, decreases health care costs, and allows patients to spend more time out side of the healthcare setting, ultimately improving patient, employer and payer satisfaction. Through the work of several prospective published trials, this concept has been found to be safe and effective in women undergoing breast-conserving therapy [7, 12–14]. As for breast cosmesis, both data from Canada and the combined 10-year UK Start trials have demonstrated equivalent, if not superior breast cosmesis utilizing hypofractionated radiation in women undergoing breast conservation [5, 14]. The move to hypofractionation is built upon evidence of a radiobiological model which finds the radiosensitivity of breast cancer, much like normal tissue, to be more dependent on dose per fraction than previously thought, allowing a lower total dose for similar efficacy [15]. Some of the strongest data comes from Canada and the United Kingdom where phase III trials have demonstrated no difference in local control with hypofractionated whole breast irradiation (WBI) with long-term follow-up [5, 7, 13, 16, 17].

Given this demand for shorter courses of radiation, this chapter will explore the data behind hypofractionated regional nodal radiation. Historically, RNI was reserved for stage III breast cancer, but based on the National Cancer Institute of Canada Clinical Trials Group (NCIC-CTG) MA.20 and The European Organisation for Research and Treatment of Cancer (EORTC) 22922 preliminary results, most patients with stage II disease are now being considered for RNI [18, 19]. In the setting of postmastectomy breast cancer, nodal positivity remains the main indication for PMRT; therefore, the vast majority of PMRT includes RNI [20]. While the use of PMRT was routinely reserved for T4, N2, and N3 patients, a 2014 Early Breast Cancer Trialists' Collaborative Group (EBCTCG) updated meta-analysis now demonstrates a survival advantage for PMRT even in N1 patients, with the addition of PMRT decreasing the 10-year risk of local recurrence from 20 to 4 % (p <0.0001) and improving the 20-year breast cancer mortality from 50 to 42 % (p=0.01) [21].

The main concern regarding hypofractionated schedules treating regional lymph nodes is the potential for increased short- and long-term toxicities, including injury to the heart, lungs, axilla, and brachial plexus. As toxicity from RNI can be influenced by surgical axillary management, it's important to review the surgical changes that have occurred over the last few years. The American College of Surgical Oncology Group (ASOCOG) Z011 trial, published in 2010, demonstrated that in the setting of 1 or 2 positive sentinel lymph nodes in breast conservation, patients can forgo axillary dissection with standard breast radiation [22]. Although patients on this trial were prescribed breast only radiation, a retrospective analysis of 228 patients reveals that 50 % of treated patients received "high tangents," defined as the cranial tangent border less than or equal to 2 cm from the humeral head, and an additional 18.9 % received 3 or more treatment fields specifically directed at the regional lymph nodes [23]. Comparison of Complete Axillary Lymph Node Dissection with Axillary Radiation Therapy in Treating Women with Invasive Breast Cancer (AMAROS) was a prospective trial from the EORTC randomizing T1/T2 clinically node-negative patients from 2001 at 2010 in 34 European centers [24]. In this trial 1,425 patients with a positive sentinel node at surgery were randomized to axillary node dissection or axillary radiation (axilla levels I–III and medial supraclavicular fossa). With a median follow-up of 6 years, axillary recurrence occurred in 4 out of 744 patients in the axillary dissection group versus 7 out of 681 patients in the axillary radiotherapy group. The 5-year axillary recurrence rate was 0.43 % with axillary node dissection versus 1.19 % with axillary radiation therapy, which is not statistically significant. Of note, the lymphedema in the ipsilateral arm was significantly worse in patients undergoing axillary lymph node dissection.

Which patients are optimally treated with breast only radiation, axillary radiation, or axillary + internal mammary radiation continues to be debated. The NCIC-CTG MA.20 Trial tried to answer this question, randomizing patients to breast only versus breast with RNI RT. Patients were eligible with node-positive disease, or high-risk node-negative disease, which is defined as a tumor size greater ≥5 cm or ≥2 cm with <10 lymph nodes removed and one of the following risk factors: ER negative, grade 3 histology, or lymphovascular space invasion (LVSI). Radiation was prescribed as 50 Gy to the whole breast and 45 Gy to the regional lymph nodes, both in 25 daily fractions. At 10 year analysis, there was no difference in overall survival, but there was a 5 % improvement in disease free survival, from 77 % to 82 % with the addition of RNI (p=0.01). This came at a cost of higher rates of grade 2 or greater pneumonitis (1.2 % vs. 0.2 %) and lymphedema (8.4 % vs. 4.5 %) [19]. EORTC 22922 enrolled 4,004 women with intermediate-risk disease, defined as node positive or node negative with a central or medial tumor, randomizing them to standard breast or chest wall radiation plus or minus internal mammary (IM) and medial supraclavicular (MS) radiation. All radiation was delivered to 50 Gy in 2 Gy fractions. Results were presented in abstract at the ESTRO conference in 2014 [18]. With a median follow-up of 7 years, overall survival was 78 % versus 75 %, favoring the group receiving internal mammary and medial supraclavicular radiation, HR = 0.86 (95 % CI (0.75; 0.99), $p = 0.04$). Of note, the number of patients who developed cardiac disease was comparable between the two groups.

28.2 Lymphatic Drainage in Breast Cancer

The first route of spread in breast cancer is usually through the regional lymphatic system. The risk of lymphatic spread depends on the location, size, and grade of the tumor [25–27]. The axillary, medial, and lateral supraclavicular and internal mammary lymph nodes are considered regional draining lymphatics (Fig. 28.1). The axilla is divided into 3 levels based on their relation to the pectoralis minor muscle. Level I nodes lie lateral, level II nodes beneath, and level III nodes are medial to the pectoralis minor. The majority of level I axilla is treated in standard breast tangents. The superior aspect of the level I axilla, levels II and III of the axilla, and the lateral supraclavicular nodes are covered by a standard matching 3rd field, usually referred to as a supraclavicular field. The superior axillary apex is covered by high tangents or by extending the supraclavicular field to the lateral aspect of the humeral head (Fig. 28.2). Radiation coverage to the internal mammary lymph nodes (IMNs) requires increased complexity in treatment planning (Fig. 28.3) [28]. The at-risk IMNs occur in the first 3 intercostal spaces [29–31]. There are several different

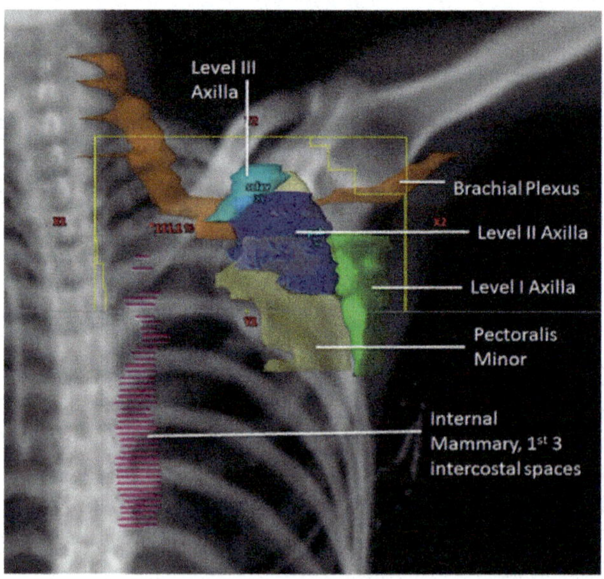

Fig. 28.1 Contours of the regional lymphatics, from an anterior-posterior digitally reconstructed radiograph. An AP supraclavicular axillary apex field is superimposed showing the structures contained within

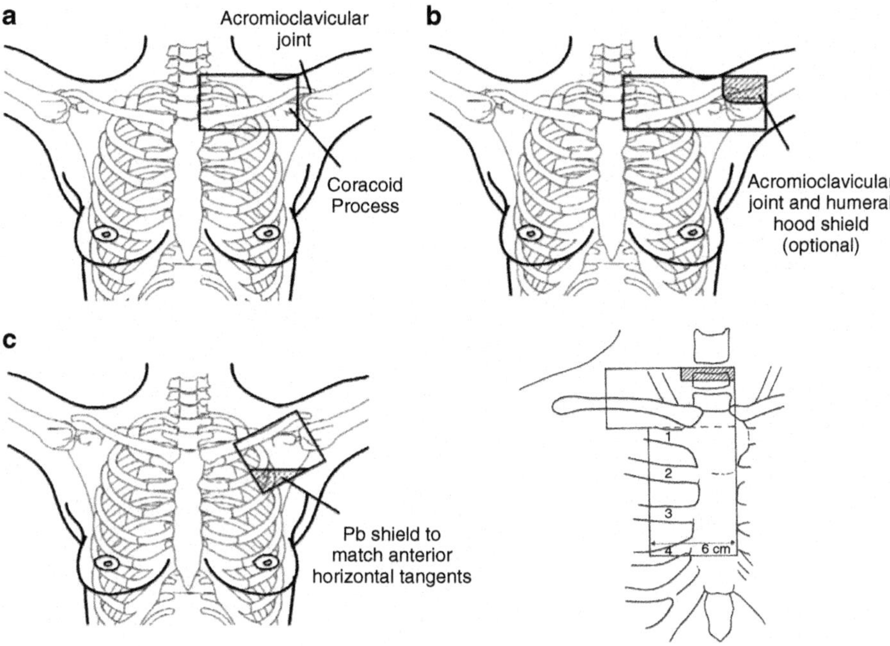

Fig. 28.2 NCIC-CTG MA.20 standard anterior supraclavicular field (**a**), anterior supraclavicular with axillary apex field (**b**), and posterior axillary boost field (**c**), optionally used when needing a greater dose at depth [69]. Anterior treatment fields, covering the medial supraclavicular and IMN on EORTC 22922

techniques to provide coverage to the IMN while minimizing the dose to the heart and lung, including partially wide tangents, matched IM-tangent fields, and intensity modulated radiation (IMRT). Each can have a dosimetric advantage based on an individual patient's anatomy. Due to ease of setup, we prefer the use of partial wide tangents.

28.3 Biological Equivalent Dose

A detailed review of the radiobiology of breast cancer has been discussed in a separate chapter. A comparison of various hypofractionation schedules requires a conversion into biological equivalent doses (BED). The rationale for conventional fractionation and the relationship between fraction size and tissue response are well described by the α/β ratio in the linear quadratic model of fractionation sensitivity [32]. In this model "late-reacting" normal tissues, such as fibroblasts and neurons, have a low α/β ratio (2–5 Gy) and are more affected by an α/β increase in fraction size. Whereas, "acutely reacting" normal tissues, such as the skin and hematopoietic cells, have a higher α/β ratio (>7 Gy), closer to that of tumor cells (estimated to have

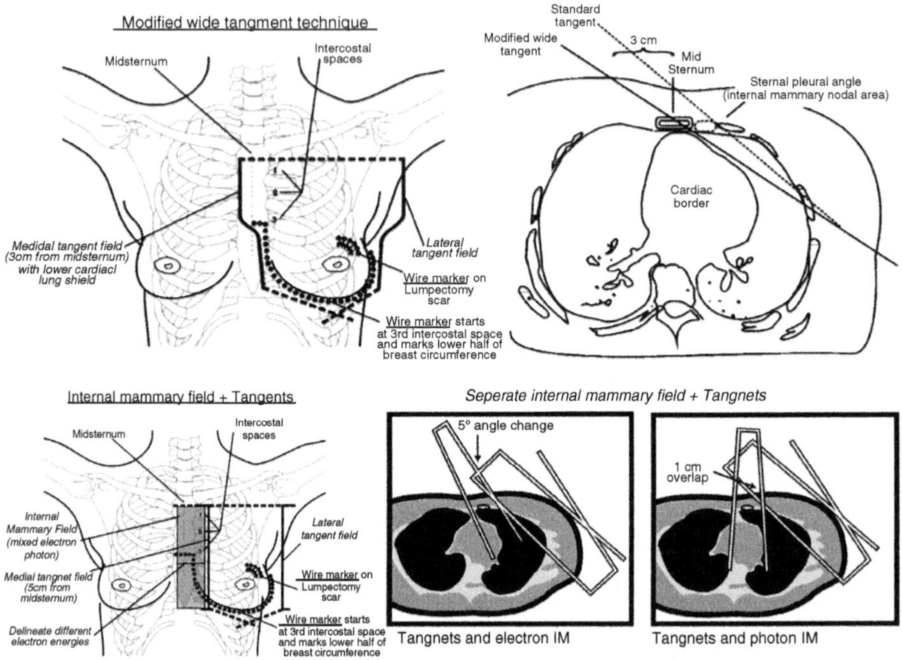

Fig. 28.3 NCIC-CTG MA.20 partially wide (modified) tangents [68]. NCIC-CTG MA.20 separate IMN field and matched tangents [69]

an α/β ratio of 10). Both types of tissue are less sensitive to changes in fraction size. In vitro experiments in human breast carcinoma cell lines have suggested an α/β ratio of about 4 Gy, which is lower than traditionally estimates used for epithelial malignancies [33, 34]. This has been confirmed in vivo using Cox proportional hazard regression modeling comparing outcomes of patients treated with different dose fractionations [13, 15, 35]. As we compare hypofractionated RNI dose schedules, an α/β ratio of 2 will be conservatively used to represent late effects, such as arm edema, brachial plexopathy, pneumonitis, shoulder stiffness, etc. [15]. Figure 28.4 gives a comparison of hypofractionation breast radiation to regional nodes with BEDs calculated in currently reported literature.

28.4 Hypofractionated Regional Nodal Radiation Experience

Some of the earliest prospective hypofractionated RNI data come from Australia and Europe. Stoll et al. from Melbourne, Australia, reported on 117 patients treated between 1958 and 1962, postmastectomy with 4 MeV LINAC therapy to 6300 rad (~63 Gy) in 12 fractions, including regional nodes. Their 1966 publication entitled "Radiation-Induced Peripheral Neuropathy," highlights their unacceptable

Study	Time Period	Patients	IMNs radiated?	RNI dose (Gy)	Fractions	BED $\alpha/\beta = 4$ (tumor control)	BED $\alpha/\beta = 2$ (late effects)	EQD2 tumor	EQD2 normal tissue
Standard (50 Gy)				50	25	75.0	100.0	50.0	50.0
Standard (45 Gy)				45	25	65.3	85.5	43.5	42.8
Melbourne, Australia [4]	1958–1962	117, PMRT	Yes	63	12	145.7	228.4	97.1	**114.2**
Sweden [37]	1963–65	71, PMRT	Maybe	57	17	104.8	152.6	69.9	**76.3**
St. Thomas, London [1]	1968–1974	411, PMRT	Yes, 28–35Gy	35	6	86.0	137.1	57.4	**68.5**
			Yes, 42–52Gy	50	12	102.1	154.2	68.1	**77.1**
Western General Hospital, Edinburgh [39]	1979–1982	484, PMRT and RNI	Yes	42.5	10	87.7	132.8	58.4	**66.4**
	1982–1984	289, PMRT and RNI	Yes	42.5	20	65.1	87.7	43.4	43.8
Vancouver,BC [6]	1979–1986	318, PMRT and RNI	Yes, 37.5Gy	35.0	16	54.1	73.3	36.1	36.6
Hamburg, Germany [44]	1980–1993	140, SCL	No	52.0	20	85.8	119.6	57.2	**59.8**
Necker,Paris [40]	1984–1989	230, RNI use uncertain	Unknown	23	4	56.1	89.1	37.4	44.6
RMH/UK Start A [14]	1986–1999	2236, mainly BCS, only 21 % RNI	No	39	13	68.3	97.5	45.5	48.8
			No	42.9	13	78.3	113.7	52.2	**56.8**
Nice, France [46]	1987–1999	150, RNI 32 % RNI	Yes	27.5	5	65.3	103.1	43.5	**51.6**
Vancouver,BC [43]	1990–1996	1028, RNI	10%	37.5	16	59.5	81.4	39.6	40.7
Pakistan [9]	1998–2004	300, PMRT and RNI	No	27	5	63.5	99.9	42.3	50.0
			No	35	10	65.6	96.3	43.8	48.1
			No	40	15	66.7	93.3	44.4	46.7
UK Start B [7]	1999–2001	2215, mainly BCS, only 7 % RNI	No	40	15	66.7	93.3	44.4	46.7
Greece [8]	2003–2010	112, PMRT and RNI	No	38.5	11	72.2	105.9	48.1	**52.9**
Thailand [47]	2004–2006	148, PMRT, 31 % RNI	No	47.7	18	79.3	110.9	52.9	**55.5**
Brussels, Belgium [10]	2007–2011	70, helical IMRT, 35 % RNI	No	42	15	71.4	100.8	47.6	50.4
Utah/NJ [71]	2011–2014	68, PMRT and RNI	Variable	36.3	11	66.2	96.2	44.2	48.1

Fig. 28.4 Table of BED comparisons from the published PMRT hypofractionated trials

neuropathy rate of 73 % [4]. A 34-year follow-up from Sweden on patients treated from 1963 to 65 also sheds light on the risk of plexopathy with high BED hypofractionation [36, 37]. Records were reviewed from 71 patients treated with Cobal-60 teletherapy using 3 matching fields to the axilla, supraclavicular fossa, and parasternum (no chest wall radiation). The dose prescribed was 44 Gy in 11 daily fractions; however, there were noted field overlaps with doses to the brachial plexus estimated to be 54–57 Gy. At 34 years, the risk of fibrosis was 86 %, and neuropathy was 63 %. These two reports highlight the hazards of overdosing critical structures rather than any condemnation of the hypofractionation concept itself. In the Melbourne experience, the equivalent dose in 2 Gy fractions (EQD2) for their fractionation would be estimated at 114 Gy and in the Swedish study 76 Gy, which likely explains the high neuropathy rate.

Bates et al. retrospectively reviewed 1,200 patients treated at the St. Thomas' Hospital in London from 1953 to 1962 and discovered that radiation treatment delivered 3 times per week resulted in similar survival, local recurrence, and morbidity to radiation administered over 5 fractions per week [1]. This was followed by a prospective trial initiated in 1968 comparing two different fractionation schemes after a simple mastectomy (some with axillary dissection) [38]. In one arm the chest wall received 37 Gy in 12 fractions (3.08 Gy/fraction) over 28 days (with 70 kVp x-rays) along with 45–51 Gy to the cervico-axillary areas (with Co-60) in 12 fractions and 42 Gy to internal mammary (IMs) nodes at a depth of 3 cm, over 12 fractions (with mixed beam (1:1) Co-60 and Cs-137 teletherapy). The other randomized arm treated the chest wall to 31.5 Gy in 6 fractions (5.25 Gy/fx) over 18 days, the cervico-axillary areas were treated to 31–35 Gy and the IMNs to 28 Gy at depth of 3 cm with an identical technique. The 10-year results of 411 randomized patients demonstrated no significant difference in local control, 12.5 % vs 12.8 %. Acute effects were equal in the two groups, including dysphagia and acute skin reactions. The 12-fraction treatment group had a greater late fibrosis (0.8 vs 1.2 average scores), higher shoulder restriction, and more lymphedema (29.5 % vs 12 %). No statistics were reported on the toxicity endpoints. Many factors could have contributed to the results, including the non-controlled use of axillary dissections. Nonetheless, a simple bioequivalent dose calculation shows that with an α/β ratio of 2 to represent late effects, the nodal regions received an EQD2 of 69 Gy and 77 Gy for the 6 and 12-fraction regimens, respectively. It's therefore not surprising that the 12-fraction regimen had a greater fibrosis and lymphedema rate.

Rodger et al. at Western General Hospital, Edinburgh, UK, published a retrospective review of late effects in postmastectomy patients before and after a policy change in their department, changing from 4.5 Gy times 10 fractions over 4 weeks to 2.25 Gy times 20 fractions over 4 weeks, after a simple mastectomy [3]. Dose was prescribed to a maximum point, and the cervico-axillary area received 42.5 Gy. They reviewed 484 patients who were treated with the 10-fraction regimen between January 1979 and March 1982 and 289 patients who were treated with the 20 fraction regimen between April 1982 and December 1984. Grade 2–3 arm edema was higher in the hypofractionated group, 29 % vs 14 %, as were rib fractures, 52 % vs 11 %. Two radiation-induced plexopathies were found in the 10-fraction cohort, and 2 others were indeterminate (radiation vs. recurrence). There were no cases of brachial plexopathy in the 20 fraction cohort. Although not a randomized comparison, the outcomes reported in this study are useful in reviewing the fractionations in terms of BED. Again, using an α/β ratio of 2 to model late effects, the Edinburgh patients received a regional nodal EQD2 of 73 Gy with the 45 Gy/10 (45 Gy in 10 fractions) schedule and 43.8 Gy when using the 42.5 Gy/20 schedule (42.5 Gy in 20 fractions). Similar to the St. Thomas hospital experience, we see that the linear quadratic equation would predict an increase in late effect toxicity. Therefore, it is not hypofractionation itself, but rather the combination of all the dosimetric specifics combined that may lead to a higher BED and it is this higher BED that likely explains the toxicity experienced. Other efforts at hypofractionated RNI include the report from the Department of Radiation Therapy of the Necker Hospital in Paris, France [39]. These investigators randomized 230 women from 1982 to 1984 to 45 Gy in 25 fractions or 23 Gy in 4 fractions (5 Gy on days 1 and 3 and 6.5 Gy on days 15 and 17). They included patients with intact breasts and postmastectomy chest walls. Seventy-nine percent had surgery (mastectomy or lumpectomy + Ir-192 implant [20 Gy]), while the rest had RT alone with chemotherapy (21 %). With a minimum follow-up of 4 years, the local failure rates were 4 out of 56 (7 %) in the conventional arm vs 2 out of 45 (4 %) in the hypofractionation arm. They reported more fibrosis (18 % vs 9 %) and telangiectasia (14 % vs 9 %) in the hypofractionation arm, but no statistics were reported. The EQD2 for their hypofractionation schedule would be 45 Gy, and therefore no increase in late effects was expected. Given the heterogeneity of the patient population, outdated radiation techniques, lack of formal statistics, and information about regional nodal radiation, the results are difficult to interpret in the modern context.

The prospective British Columbia trial by Ragaz et al. enrolled 318 node-positive premenopausal breast cancer patients from 1979 to 1986 and randomized them after modified radical mastectomy to either radiation therapy or no additional locoregional therapy [6, 41]. Both groups received adjuvant cyclophosphamide, methotrexate, and fluorouracil (CMF) chemotherapy for 12 months with the first 80 patients and then changed to 6 months. Radiation therapy was delivered to the chest wall to a dose of 37.5 Gy in 16 daily fractions through opposed tangential photon fields. The supraclavicular and axilla nodes were treated with an anterior and a posterior axillary boost field, with a target dose to the mid-axilla of 35 Gy. Bilateral IMNs were treated with an anterior field to a dose of 37.5 Gy in 16 fractions, prescribed to a maximum point dose. All treatments were delivered with cobalt-60, between cycle 4 and 5 of chemotherapy. The 20-year survival-free of locoregional disease, before systemic relapse, was reported as 61 % in the chemotherapy alone arm and 87 % in the irradiated group. There were 3 cardiac deaths (2 %) in the irradiated group versus one (0.6 %) in the control group ($p=0.62$) and 9 % of patients in the irradiated group developed arm edema compared with 3 % in the control group ($p=0.035$). Symptomatic arm edema requiring a compression sleeve was 3.7 % in the irradiated group compared with 0.6 % in the control group. All patients in the irradiation group were found to have asymptomatic apical lung fibrosis, but only 1 (0.6 %) patient developed interstitial pneumonitis requiring steroids. The EQD2 for this fractionation, in evaluating late toxicity ($\alpha/\beta=2$), would be 36.6–40 Gy in 2 Gy fractions to the regional lymphatics. This appears to be a lower dose to regional lymphatics than is currently used with conventional fractionation. At 20 years, the chemo + RT group had a 13 % risk of locoregional disease any time before systemic disease with almost 90 % of patients having T1–2 disease and 60 % having N1 disease. This local recurrence rate is similar to that seen in the Danish PMRT trials that occurred during the same era and used conventional fractionation of 50 Gy in 25 fractions [42]. It appears that the standard RNI fraction size in Vancouver, British Columbia, was increased to 40 Gy in 16 fractions, as a study demonstrates reviewing the BC population database from 1990 to 1996 [42]. With an EQD2 of 45 Gy, no cases of brachial plexopathy were reported in the 4,929 women.

Investigators from Hamburg, Germany, reviewed patients from 1980 to 1993 treated with cobalt-60 through an anterior supraclavicular fossa field [43]. The extent of the treatment field and the radiation to the breast or chest wall are not described. Radiation was prescribed at 60 Gy in 20 fractions, 4 days a week. The prescription point was $d=0.5$ cm which was estimated to correspond to a 3 cm depth of 52 Gy, which would represent the brachial plexus. With this fractionation, the EQD2 of 60–75 Gy resulted in a rate of grade 1 (LENT-SOMA) or greater brachial plexopathy of 4 % at 5 years but increasing to 64 % at 19 years (Fig. 28.5).

In 1986, the Royal Marsden Hospital and the Gloucestershire Oncology Centre collaborated in a prospective trial evaluating 3 breast fractionation schedules: 50 Gy in 25 fractions, 39 Gy in 13 fractions (3.0 Gy/fx), or 42.9 Gy in 13 fractions (3.3 Gy/fx)

Grade 1	Mild sensory deficits, no pain, no treatment required
Grade 2	Moderate sensory deficits, tolerable pain, mild arm weakness
Grade 3	Continuous paresthesia with incomplete paresis, pain medication required
Grade 4	Complete paresis, excruciating pain, muscle atrophy, regular pain medication required

Fig. 28.5 Caption (Modified LENT-SOMA scale for brachial plexopathy)

over 5 weeks [44]. In 1999, after over 1,400 patients had been enrolled, the trial design was expanded into a multi-institutional trial. Patient data from the earlier study was rolled into what became UK START A trial, with the 13-fraction regimen changed to 3.2 Gy/day for 41.6 Gy. A total of 2,236 women were randomized to one of three arms between 1986 and 1999, treating patients with 2D planning and cobalt-60. The overall treatment time of 5 weeks was kept constant in all three arms. The primary endpoint was late breast change; local control was a secondary endpoint. Locoregional relapse was not significantly different in the 3 arms at 10 years with results of 7.4 %, 6.3 %, and 8.8 %, respectively [5]. There were 290 (20.6 %) patients who received regional nodal radiation to the supraclavicular and axillary nodes which included 1 reported case of brachial plexopathy with a median of 10 years follow-up (Fig. 28.6). Fourteen percent of patients received CMF chemotherapy. Using Cox proportional hazards regression models, they estimated an α/β for shoulder stiffness of 1.8 (CI 1.0–3.6) and for arm edema of 2.2 (CI 1.0–7.9) [15].

Running in parallel to START A, the UK START B trial was an accelerated hypofractionation trial comparing 50 Gy in 2 Gy daily fractions for 5 weeks versus 40 Gy delivered in 2.67 Gy daily for 3 weeks [7]. This trial accrued 2,215 stage I and II breast cancer patients between 1999 and 2001, treating most patients with 6 MV photons. Although patients were predominantly treated after lumpectomy with breast tangents only, 8 % of the patients were radiated after mastectomy, and 7 % received radiation to the regional nodes. With either fractionation, there were no reported cases of brachial plexopathy at 10 years. Twenty-three percent of patients received chemotherapy +/− tamoxifen (Fig. 28.7).

Ortholan et al. conducted a prospective single-arm study between 1987 and 1999 of whole breast hypofractionation for elderly patients in Nice, France [45]. The authors acknowledge the uncertainty of the α/β ratio, estimating a range of 4–10 Gy; they used 6.3 Gy for their calculations. Based on this, a single weekly fraction of 6.5 Gy was presumed to equal 5 fractions of 2 Gy. There were 150 patients with a median age of 78 years who received a total dose of 32.5 Gy in 5 weekly fractions of 6.5 Gy delivered via tangent fields using cobalt or 6 MV photons. Of the patients, 31.8 % were treated to the IMNs and supraclavicular areas (due to positive axillary nodes or location of the primary tumor). The regional nodes received 5.5 Gy × 5 weekly fractions, with 3 fractions given through photon beams and 2 with electrons. No RNI-specific toxicity has been reported to date, but the EQD2 for late effects based on this fractionation would be estimated to be 51.6 Gy; therefore, it is not likely to have an excess risk of toxicity.

RMH/START A @ 10 yrs.[5]	50 Gy/25	42.9 Gy/13	39 Gy/13
Arm edema (moderate)	16.3 %	22.5 %	8.2 %
Shoulder stiffness (moderate)	17.5 %	14.8 %	11 %
Symptomatic lung fibrosis (reported)	0.8 %	1.2 %	1.1 %
Ischemic heart disease	0.9 %	0.7 %	0.8 %
BED $_{\alpha/\beta = 2}$	100	113.7	97.5

Fig. 28.6 Toxicity rates reported from UK Start A

STARTB @ 10 years [5]	50 Gy/25	40 Gy/15
Arm edema (moderate)	13.5 %	4.7 %
Shoulder stiffness (moderate)	8.2 %	3.1 %
Symptomatic lung fibrosis (reported)	1.7 %	1.7 %
Ischemic heart disease	2.1 %	1.5 %
BED α/β =2	100	93.5

Fig. 28.7 Toxicity rates reported from UK Start B

A prospective randomized trial from Pakistan, conducted between 1998 and 2004, enrolled 300 patients with T2–3 breast cancer postmastectomy to treatment plans of 27 Gy in 5 fractions (1 week), 35 Gy in 10 fractions (2 weeks) and 40 Gy in 15 fractions (3 weeks) [9]. Radiation was delivered through cobalt-60 with 2 tangential fields matched to the anterior supraclavicular and posterior axillary boost fields. Reporting 5-year event rates, the complications were not found to be statistically different with G2/G3 lymphedema at 21 %, 22 %, and 27 %, respectively. Cardiac and pulmonary toxicity was between 4 and 6 % and not statistically different in the treatment groups. A comparison of these regimens shows roughly equivalent BEDs, with an EQD2 46–50 Gy.

A prospective phase II study from Greece treated 112 patients after mastectomy with hypofractionated accelerated radiation with cytoprotective amifostine (HypoARC) [8]. Patients received 10 consecutive 3.5 Gy fractions with a 2-fraction 4 Gy scar boost and 1-fraction 3.5 Gy RNI boost for cases of extensive nodal disease. The IMNs were not part of the RNI treatment field. Eighty-six percent of the women received adjuvant pre-radiation chemotherapy. With a median follow-up of 44 months, no cases of clinical pneumonitis were noted, although 3.6 % (4 out of 112) had intense radiographic evidence. There was a 1.8 % rate of brachial plexopathy, described as minor pain recorded in 2 of 112 patients. The EQD2 for this fractionation would be estimated at 53 Gy, slightly higher than we've seen in studies finding no cases of plexopathy. Clinical outcomes were consistent with previous series. Three of the 112 patients developed a locoregional relapse over a 5-year period with a projected rate of 97 % local relapse-free survival and 84 % disease-specific survival.

A retrospective review from Thailand compared conventional and hypofractionated (2.65 Gy × 16–18 fx) PMRT. This series of 215 patients found no difference in clinical outcomes and no difference in chest wall appearance, skin fibrosis, brachial plexopathy, arm edema, pulmonary and cardiac events, or rib fractures with a 39-month follow-up [46].

A recent prospective trial from Brussels, Belgium, included postmastectomy and regional patients in a hypofractionated schema of 42 Gy in 15 fractions. Of the 69 patients treated with RNI and reported, 32 patients were treated with conventional fractionation and 37 patients with hypofractionated approach using tomotherapy. Of the total, 40 % ($n=28$) received PMRT, and 60 % ($n=41$) were treated after breast-conserving surgery, and 50 % ($n=35$) received chemotherapy [10]. Although not stratified by surgery type, there was no increase in chronic fibrosis or lymphedema and no change in cardiac function. A reduction in the diffusing capacity of the lungs for carbon monoxide (DLCO) was noted to be significant with the hypofractionated technique. Of these women with a reduction in DLCO, 78 % received concomitant chemotherapy, 33 % received RNI, and 44 % had a smoking history.

At this time, the data are promising with regard to hypofractionated PMRT and RNI. All reported outcomes appear to report similar rates of local control and equivalent toxicity profiles in which the BED can be compared using the linear quadratic formula.

28.5 Cardiac and Cerebrovascular Toxicity

Cardiac toxicity with breast radiation is considered to be a late toxicity and is important to consider with hypofractionation. The Early Breast Cancer Trialists Cooperative Group (EBCTCG), as well as population studies, has demonstrated modestly increased risk of cardiac mortality in women undergoing left-side breast cancer [47–49]. Late radiation injuries that have been attributed to radiation include pericarditis, congestive heart failure (CHF), ischemic disease, coronary artery disease (CAD), and myocardial infarction (MI), valvular disease, and arrhythmias. Small portions of the heart can be exposed to radiation with breast only coverage but may increase significantly with IMN radiation. Adding supraclavicular and axillary apex radiation fields does not increase heart dose [50, 51]. Since only a small volume of the heart (usually left apex near the LAD artery) is exposed to radiation in breast cancer, the most commonly reported toxicity is CAD or cardiac-related death. The heart is sensitive to dose fraction with an estimated α/β ratio of 2.5–3.0 [52]. Investigators at the University of Pennsylvania evaluated 961 consecutive early stage breast patients treated between 1977 and 1994 for cardiac morbidity and mortality, with 12.7 % of patients who received IMN radiation [53]. There was no significant difference in cardiac death at 20 years comparing left- versus right-sided patients, but there was a significant increase in chest pain, CAD, and MI for left-sided patients. In specifically looking at the impact of IMN fields, CAD occurred in 18 % of patients with IMN radiation compared to 7 % without (P <0.001). Myocardial infarctions were also more common with IMN radiation (9 % with versus 3 % without [$P=0.01$]). The incidence of other cardiac abnormalities has rarely been reported. The majority of investigations into cardiac injury from breast cancer radiation come from standard fractionation schedules [53]. Ten-year follow-up data from START A and B failed to demonstrate an increase in ischemic heart disease at currently reported follow-up with their hypofractionated schedules [5]. Left-side breast cancer deaths accounted for 15 out of 392 deaths in START A and 17 out of 351 deaths in START B (Fig. 28.8) [5].

The UK START trials did not deliver radiation to the IMNs, although they did allow approximately 450 patients to receive supraclavicular and axillar radiation. Stokes et al. performed a retrospective population-based retrospective analysis in British Columbia of 4,929 women that had received adjuvant radiation to the breast/chest wall + regional nodes in 22 % of patients and IMNs in 9 % of patients. The majority of these patients received daily fraction sizes of greater than 2 Gy, including those treated with RNI and IMN radiation. After a median follow-up of 11.7 years, they found that fraction sizes greater than 2 Gy and the use of RNI were not associated with increased cardiac events [42]. Although fraction size was not associated with increased risk, RNI was found to increase the risk of cardiac and cerebrovascular death by 1.5 % over breast RT alone, with the inclusion of IMNs having no effect.

Similar to conventional fraction with RNI, the study from Pakistan cited earlier of 300 patients receiving postmastectomy radiation on three sequential hypofractionated protocols found a 5 % rate of cardiac toxicity [9]. These findings have been confirmed on a larger scale in a retrospective study of over 7,000 patients

	Left Side BC Cardiac Death	Left Side Ischemic Heart Disease (Confirmed)
START A 50/25	0.53%	0.8 %
START A 42.9/41.6/13	1.3 %	0.1 %
START A 39/13	0.14 %	0.5 %
START B 50/25	1.1 %	0.5 %
START B 40/15	0.45 %	0.4 %

Fig. 28.8 Cardiac Toxicity rates reported on the combined analysis of UK Start A and B

which found no increase in cardiac toxicity for fractions greater than 2 Gy with an 8-year follow-up [55].

Based on standard RNI planning and the limited data available, it seems fair to say that the modestly increased cardiac risk observed in older data sets (if still true in the modern context) is unlikely to be modified by hypofractionation that is calibrated for bioequivalence. There is simply no compelling reason to believe hypofractionated radiation, given with an EQD2 of ≤50 Gy ($\alpha/\beta = 2$), would significantly increase the risk of cardiac injury over a standard fractionated radiation schedule. Advanced radiation delivery techniques, including intensity modulation and breath holding, may even further reduce the risk of cardiac toxicity in the future [55].

28.6 Pulmonary Toxicity

The primary concern with regard to pulmonary toxicity is the potential for sub-acute pneumonitis and subsequent fibrosis leading to impaired respiratory function and decreased quality of life. The addition of RNI does potentially increase the rate of pneumonitis, as a greater volume of the lung is exposed in both supraclavicular and IMN treatment fields. Normal lung is sensitive to dose per fraction, perhaps to a lesser degree than the heart, with a described ratio of $\alpha/\beta = 4.0$ +/− 0.9 Gy [56]. NCIC-CTG MA.20 was a standard fractionation trial randomizing node-positive or high-risk node-negative patients to whole breast only radiation versus breast plus radiation with a regional trial. At 10 years, the rate of grade 2 or greater was 1.2 % with RNI and 0.2 % with WBI alone ($p = 0.01$) [19]. Randomized data from START A and B and other prospective series have found the rates of pulmonary fibrosis to be less than 2 % for hypofractionated radiation; however, a separate analysis has not been described on the approximately 11 % of patients receiving RNI [5]. Patients in the randomized PMRT trial from Vancouver, BC, received hypofractionated radiation with RNI (37.5 Gy/16 fx, EQD2 = 41 Gy) [6]. One hundred percent of patients treated with radiation were noted to have asymptomatic pneumonitis that was seen on follow-up CXR imaging, but only 1 of the 164 irradiated patients (0.6 %) developed symptomatic pneumonitis, and it resolved after a course of steroids. The aforementioned radiation was delivered with cobalt-60 teletherapy, utilizing an average energy of 1.25 MV, much lower than the 6–10 MV that we routinely use today. This lower energy would have resulted in a greater absorbed dose in the lung, likely explaining such high pneumonitis seen on imaging. In a prospective randomized study from Pakistan, 300 patients were treated with 3 hypofractionated PMRT schedules covering RNI (no IMs) to biological equivalent fractionations and were also treated using cobalt-60. An incidental pneumonitis rate of 4–5 % of patients was reported and only 1 patient developing symptoms, which were resolved with steroids [9].

The study from Belgium is difficult to interpret, as the hypofractionated group received helical IMRT and the conventional fraction group received conventional 3D radiation planning. This trial demonstrated that hypofractionation was able to reduce the change in DLCO occurring postradiation, but the reduction is likely an effect of radiation technique, rather than dose fractionation [10]. The prospective trial from Greece is also difficult to interpret. While all patients received hypofractionated radiation, they were randomized to the radiation protector, amifostine [8]. No patient in this trial experienced symptomatic pneumonitis; however 3.6 % did experience intense radiographic pneumonitis, and another 21.4 % barely demonstrated any evidence of pneumonitis. In the group of patients receiving amifostine, no patient experienced pneumonitis. In the retrospective trial from Thailand, grade I CTCAE pneumonitis (asymptomatic, seen on diagnostic evaluation only) was described in 32.5 % of hypofractionated patients vs. 23.7 % of patients in the conventional arm [8]. No statistics were given in the paper to describe the impact of this difference.

The reported rates of asymptomatic pneumonitis are difficult to compile into a single estimate, given heterogeneous reporting time periods, methods of detection, and reporting scales. Based on the summary of the limited data for hypofractionated RNI, the more important rate of symptomatic pneumonitis may be estimated at 0.5–1 %. This number compares favorably with the 1.3 % reported in the NCIC MA.20 trial in which RNI was delivered with conventional fractionation. Based on standard RNI planning from the data, hypofractionation with an EQD2 of ≤50 Gy ($\alpha/\beta = 2$) is unlikely to significantly increase the risk of significant pneumonitis over standard fractionation.

28.7 Lymphedema

RNI can increase the potential for breast cancer-related lymphedema. Data presented from NCIC-CTG MA.20 found at 10 years RNI resulted in a lymphedema rate of 8.5 % vs. 4.5 % with WBI alone ($p = 0.001$) [19]. The most significant risk of lymphedema is attributable to the extent of axillary dissection. Patients in MA.20 could have an axillary dissection or sentinel node biopsy alone, with the median number of 12 lymph nodes removed. The AMAROS trial demonstrated the risk of lymphedema. In this study, lymphedema is defined as an arm circumference increased to ≥10 % from the baseline. For axillary radiation versus dissection, the study found that the circumference was 6 % vs. 13 % at 5 years, respectively [24]. Limited data exists on the radiobiology of the lymphatic system, but Cox regression modeling allowed Yarnold et al. to estimate, based on the START data, the α/β ratio for lymphedema to be 2.2 with a wide confidence interval of 1.0–7.9 [15]. The 10-year toxicity review from the START A and B trials failed to identify higher rates of lymphedema in patients undergoing hypofractionated WBI compared with standard WBI, with a trend toward less lymphedema in the hypofractionated group. The 11 % of their patients who received RNI and lymphedema rates were not reported separately [5]. Review of the remaining literature, based on hypofractionated RNI publications, shows no significant difference in the rate of lymphedema with hypofractionated radiation. Lymphedema is reported using either a LENT-SOMA or CTCAE scale (or slight variation), with a focus on an increase in arm

Grade 1	2-4 cm increase
Grade 2	4-6 cm increase
Grade 3	>6 cm increase
Grade 4	Useless arm or angiosarcoma

Grade 1	
Grade 2	Elastic stocking/elevate arm
Grade 3	Intensive physiotherapy, compression wrapping
Grade 4	Surgical intervention/amputation

Fig. 28.9 Caption (Modified LENT-SOMA grading scale for arm lymphedema; Modified LENT-SOMA grading scale for management of arm lymphedema)

Grade 1	Trace thickening or faint discoloration
Grade 2	Marked discoloration,leathery skin texture,limiting instrumental ADLs
Grade 3	Severe symptoms,limiting self-care ADL
Grade 4	

Fig. 28.10 CTCAE v3.0 grading scale for arm lymphedema

circumference or impaired function (Figs. 28.9 and 28.10). Estimating the true rate of lymphedema with hypofractionated RNI is difficult, as the toxicity scales vary with each publication.

The older series, utilizing RNI fractionations with EQD2 values greater than 50 Gy, show greater rates of lymphedema, but these would be expected compared to modern conventional fractionation at similar doses. Data from 1960 by Bates et al. uses 45–51 Gy in 12 fractions (EQD2 77) versus 31.5 Gy in 6 fractions (EQD2 69). They found a 10-year risk of lymphedema necessitating a sleeve or causing incapacity in 29.5 % vs. 12 %. These results favor the 6 fraction, lower BED fractionation [38]. These high lymphedema numbers are mostly from the high BED radiation, as the majority of patients had simple mastectomies. However, the full extent of nodal dissection and the median number of removed nodes is not available. In the 1970s, Roger et al. used 42.5 Gy in 10 fractions (EQD2 66) versus 42.5 Gy in 20 fractions (EQD2 44) and found no significant different in severe lymphedema with a rate of 7 % vs. 4 % [3]. These numbers are lower than expected for that BED of radiation. This is likely because patients only underwent axillary sampling, and almost a quarter of patients had no axillary staging. Ragaz et al., with a median of 12 nodes dissected and 37.5 Gy in 16 fractions delivered (EQD2 41 Gy), had a 20-year rate of lymphedema of 9.1 % vs. 3.2 % in the no-RT arm [6]. The percentage of patients requiring intervention for lymphedema was 3.7 % after RT and 0.6 % in the chemo only cohort. In a paper out of Pakistan by Shahid et al., patients were treated with or without axillary dissection, without further details available. 5-year rates of lymphedema (LENTA-SOMA ≥grade 1) were 13–14 % in all treatment arms, with an EQD2 of 46–50 Gy [9]. Patients in the Greece experience by Koukourakis et al. had mixed axillary surgery, with 30 % having ≤3 nodes removed and 60 % with >3 nodes removed, with no description of median or range [8]. At 3.5 years, 9.8 % had a LENT-SOMA grade 1 lymphedema, and 1.8 % had grade 2. Van Parijs et al. found no significant difference in their conventional versus hypofractionated (EQD2 50 Gy) cohorts with a 12.5 % LENT-SOMA ≥G1 rate in both groups [10]. In this group 50 % had sentinel node biopsy alone, with the remaining 50 % undergoing an axillary dissection with no available median number of nodes removed.

In summary of the lymphedema hypofractionation data, toxicity based on a change in arm measurement is difficult to interpret, due to the variations in scales being used and interobserver variability [57–59]. In the heterogeneous hypofractionation data that we have available, utilizing a EQD2 ≤50 Gy, RNI, and various axillary surgical managements, the risk of measurable lymphedema ≥2 cm is estimated to around 10 % at 5–10 years. The risk of lymphedema that requires interventions is estimated to be 4–5 %, with the longest data from the Vancouver, BC, dataset. These rates are similar to those reported with RNI and conventional fractionation.

28.8 Brachial Plexopathy

Brachial plexopathy is one of the chief concerns that radiation oncologists express when considering hypofractionated RNI. Brachial plexopathy is a potential toxicity associated with RNI, as the brachial plexus crosses the supraclavicular and axillary treatment field (Fig. 28.2). Injury to the brachial plexus can significantly impair arm/shoulder function and quality of life (pain, motor function, paresthesia) and is related to dose, volume, and fractionation [60–62]. Review of the literature for rates of brachial plexopathy in breast cancer radiation finds that the majority of publications do not define the extent of plexopathy. Brachial plexopathy includes a spectrum of neurological change, ranging from complete loss of arm function, weakness, pain, or asymptomatic (only clinically diagnostically detected). Several grading scales have been devised for standardized reporting, including the LENT-SOMA and CTCAE, but the majority of publications give no graded definition (Fig. 28.11). Without knowing the cut-off to define the event, it is difficult to define the true risk of brachial plexopathy that affects quality of life. Older historical series describing hypofractionated breast radiation often prescribed higher biological effective doses, which resulted in an increased risk of brachial plexopathy [36, 43]. Data from the 1950s by Stoll et al. out of Melbourne, Australia, demonstrated the risk of brachial plexopathy as high as 70 % when radiated to 63 rads in 12 fractions, EQD2 of 114 Gy [4]. Even data from the 1970s and 1980s with cobalt-60 RT using conventional fraction to 50 Gy reported higher rates of plexopathy that we routinely see now. The PMRT

Grade 1	Mild sensory deficits, no pain, no treatment required
Grade 2	Moderate sensory deficits, tolerable pain, mild arm weakness
Grade 3	Continuous paresthesia with incomplete paresis, pain medication required
Grade 4	Complete paresis, excruciating pain, muscle atrophy, regular pain medication required

Grade 1	Asymptomatic, detected on diagnostic or clinical exam
Grade 2	Moderate symptoms, not interfering with ADL
Grade 3	Severe symptoms, interfering with ADL
Grade 4	Disabling

Fig. 28.11 Caption (Modified LENT-SOMA grading scale for brachial plexopathy; CTCAE v3.0 grading scale for brachial plexopathy)

Danish series reported a 50-month follow-up with 5 % disabling and 9 % mild cases of brachial plexopathy with conventional fractionation of 50 Gy in 25 fractions to regional nodes compared with no cases of plexopathy reported from the Vancouver, BC, series using 37.5 Gy in 15 fractions [63]. Data from Hamburg, Germany, in the 1980s, using a cobalt teletherapy, revealed a persistent risk of any brachial plexopathy after radiation to 60 Gy in 20 fractions, EQD2 for this regimen would be 60–75 Gy [43]. An important finding in this publication is a continual risk in brachial plexopathy over time, with an incidence of 3.9 % at 5 years, 24.5 % at 10 years, 27.9 % at 15 years, and 64 % at 19 years. The risk of continued paresthesia requiring pain medication (grade ≥3, LENT-SOMA) was 2 % at 5 years, 4.5 % at 10 years, 11.8 % at 15 years, and 19.1 % at 19 years. The initial Edinburgh data from 1987 did not report any cases of plexopathy at around 10 years; however, in the 1996 publication at least 2 confirmed radiation-associated plexopathy were documented with another 2 possible [3, 38]. This series, and others, serves as a reminder that plexopathy can be a late event, often showing up 15–20+ years after the completion of therapy [64, 65]. Data in head and neck cancer radiotherapy, in which the brachial plexus was contoured with 3-dimensional imaging, demonstrates the risk in brachial plexopathy rises significantly after an EQD2 of 60 Gy, in addition to an important volumetric effect (Fig. 28.12) [61, 66, 67]. Data by Pierce et al., from the Joint Center for Radiation Therapy in Boston, reviewed 1,624 women with stage I or II breast cancer treated with breast-conserving therapy with standard fractionation between 1968 and 1995 [68]. They described a 1.8 % risk of brachial plexopathy with supraclavicular radiation at 6 years compared to a 0 % rate in women who received breast tangents only. Brachial plexopathy was defined as new numbness, paresthesia, pain, or weakness in the ipsilateral arm after radiation. Of the cases identified, 80 % were considered both transient and mild and resolved in 1 year. The risk of severe brachial plexopathy causing impairment was 0.25 %. Looking at the hypofractionated RNI patients from UK START trials, the initial 5- and 8-year

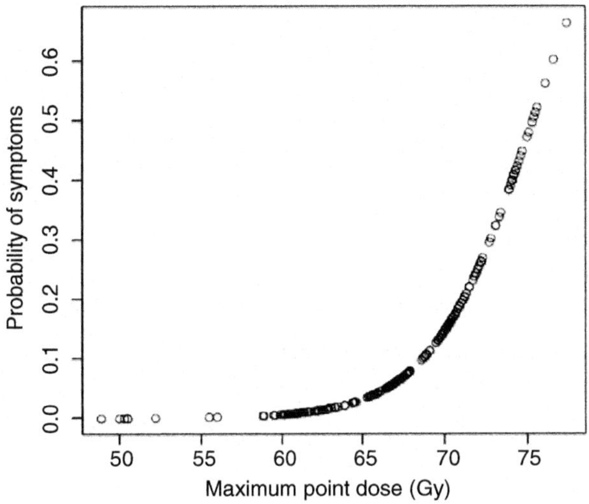

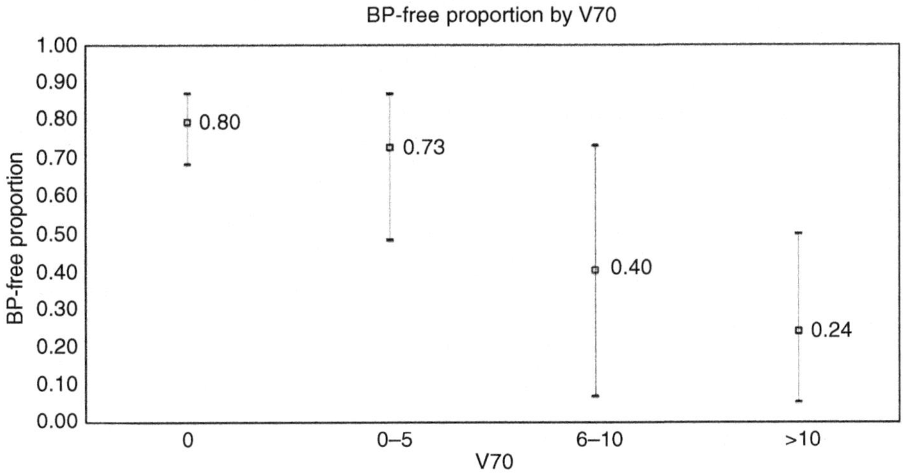

Fig. 28.12 Caption (Data from Chen et al. showing the relationship between developing brachial plexopathy and maximum dose to the plexus [66]; Data from Chen et al. showing the relationship between developing brachial plexopathy and volume of the brachial plexus getting ≥70 Gy of radiation [67])

publications showed no evidence of brachial plexopathy [7, 13, 15]. In the combined 10-year publication, 1 case was recorded in the 41.6 Gy arm with no described severity [5]. Although the START A publication does not describe the number of patients treated with RNI in the 41.6 Gy arm. If we assume an equal distribution of RNI in the 3 treatment arms, this would reveal an estimated risk of 1 % for brachial plexopathy with hypofractionated RNI at an EQD2 of 54 Gy (Fig. 28.13). There were no cases of brachial plexopathy at 10 years in patients

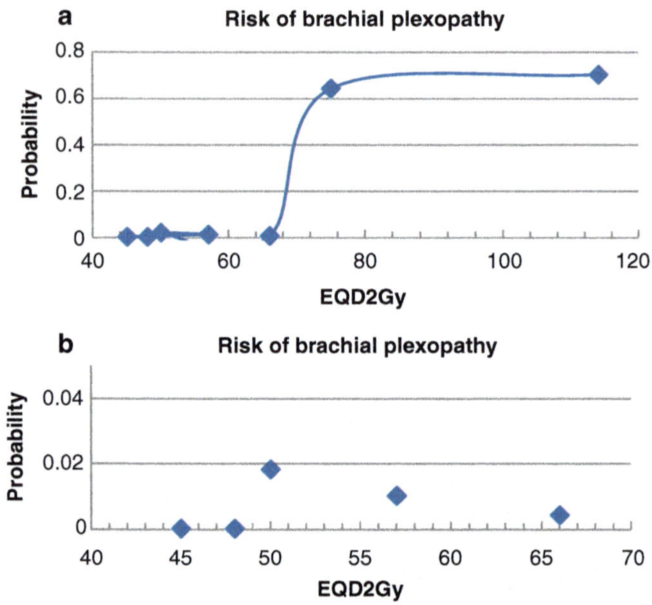

Fig. 28.13 (**a**) Hypofractionated radiation equivalent dose in 2 Gy fractionation. Incidence of brachial plexopathy based on published literature (**b**) shows the low end of the chart magnified

receiving RNI with 40 Gy in 15 fractions or 39 Gy in 13 fractions. Hypofractionated RNI would therefore appear to cause about the equivalent rate of brachial plexopathy as conventional fractionation, assuming a BED delivered of an EQD2 ≤50 Gy.

28.9 Conclusion

Hypofractionated RNI is an area that is sure to be explored in the next decade of breast cancer radiation research. Although the data presented above demonstrates that toxicity of RNI is greater than for breast only radiation, there does not appear to be an increased toxicity for hypofractionation schedules in which the BED (EQD2) is ≤50 Gy.

References

1. Bates T, Fleming JA, Wiernik G. Carcinoma of the breast. The effect of dose fractionation and radiotherapeutic technique on survival. Clin Radiol. 1969;20:278–86.
2. Bates TD, Fleming JA, Wiernik G. The treatment of carcinoma of the breast. The effect of dose fractionation on survival rate. Br J Radiol. 1968;41:480.

3. Rodger A, Jack WJL, Kerr G. A change in postmastectomy radiotherapy fractionation: an audit of tumour control, acute and late morbidity. Breast. 1996;5:244–50.
4. Stoll BA, Andrews JT. Radiation-induced peripheral neuropathy. Br Med J. 1966;1:834–7.
5. Haviland JS, Owen JR, Dewar JA, et al. The UK Standardisation of Breast Radiotherapy (START) trials of radiotherapy hypofractionation for treatment of early breast cancer: 10-year follow-up results of two randomised controlled trials. Lancet Oncol. 2013;14:1086–94.
6. Ragaz J, Olivotto I, Spinelli J, et al. Locoregional radiation therapy in patients with high-risk breast cancer receiving adjuvant chemotherapy: 20 year results of the British Columbia randomized trial. J Natl Cancer Inst. 2005;97:116–26.
7. Group ST, Bentzen SM, Agrawal RK, et al. The UK Standardisation of Breast Radiotherapy (START) Trial B of radiotherapy hypofractionation for treatment of early breast cancer: a randomised trial. Lancet. 2008;371:1098–107.
8. Koukourakis MI, Panteliadou M, Abatzoglou IM, Sismanidou K, Sivridis E, Giatromanolaki A. Postmastectomy hypofractionated and accelerated radiation therapy with (and without) subcutaneous amifostine cytoprotection. Int J Radiat Oncol Biol Phys. 2013;85:e7–13.
9. Shahid A, Athar MA, Asghar S, Zubairi T, Murad S, Yunas N. Post mastectomy adjuvant radiotherapy in breast cancer: a comparison of three hypofractionated protocols. J Pak Med Assoc. 2009;59:282–7.
10. Van Parijs H, Miedema G, Vinh-Hung V, et al. Short course radiotherapy with simultaneous integrated boost for stage I-II breast cancer, early toxicities of a randomized clinical trial. Radiat Oncol. 2012;7:80.
11. Society AC. Brease cancer facts and figures 2013–2014. Atlanta; 2014.
12. Haffty BG, Buchholz TA. Hypofractionated breast radiation: preferred standard of care? Lancet Oncol. 2013;14:1032–4.
13. Group ST, Bentzen SM, Agrawal RK, et al. The UK Standardisation of Breast Radiotherapy (START) Trial A of radiotherapy hypofractionation for treatment of early breast cancer: a randomised trial. Lancet Oncol. 2008;9:331–41.
14. Whelan TJ, Pignol JP, Levine MN, et al. Long-term results of hypofractionated radiation therapy for breast cancer. N Engl J Med. 2010;362:513–20.
15. Yarnold J, Ashton A, Bliss J, et al. Fractionation sensitivity and dose response of late adverse effects in the breast after radiotherapy for early breast cancer: long-term results of a randomised trial. Radiother Oncol. 2005;75:9–17.
16. FAST Trialists group, Agrawal RK, Alhasso A, et al. First results of the randomised UK FAST Trial of radiotherapy hypofractionation for treatment of early breast cancer (CRUKE/04/015). Radiother Oncol. 2011;100:93–100.
17. Whelan T, MacKenzie R, Julian J, et al. Randomized trial of breast irradiation schedules after lumpectomy for women with lymph node-negative breast cancer. J Natl Cancer Inst. 2002;94:1143–50.
18. Poortmans P, Struikmans H, Collette S, Bartelink H. Lymph node RT improves survival in breast cancer: 10 years results of the EORTC ROG and BCG phase III trial 22922/10925. In: ESTRO; 2014; Vienna, Austria; 2014.
19. Whelan TJ et al. N Engl J Med. 2015;373:307–16.
20. Truong PT, Olivotto IA, Whelan TJ, Levine M. Steering Committee on Clinical Practice Guidelines for the C, Treatment of Breast C. Clinical practice guidelines for the care and treatment of breast cancer: 16. Locoregional post-mastectomy radiotherapy. Can Med Assoc J = journal de l'Association medicale canadienne. 2004;170:1263–73.
21. Ebctcg MP, Taylor C, et al. Effect of radiotherapy after mastectomy and axillary surgery on 10-year recurrence and 20-year breast cancer mortality: meta-analysis of individual patient data for 8135 women in 22 randomised trials. Lancet. 2014;383:2127–35.
22. Giuliano AE, McCall L, Beitsch P, et al. Locoregional recurrence after sentinel lymph node dissection with or without axillary dissection in patients with sentinel lymph node metastases: the American College of Surgeons Oncology Group Z0011 randomized trial. Ann Surg. 2010;252:426–32; discussion 32–3.
23. Jagsi R, Chadha M, Moni J, et al. Radiation field design in the ACOSOG Z0011 (Alliance) Trial. J Clin Oncol. 2014;32:3600–6.

24. Donker M, van Tienhoven G, Straver ME, et al. Radiotherapy or surgery of the axilla after a positive sentinel node in breast cancer (EORTC 10981–22023 AMAROS): a randomised, multicentre, open-label, phase 3 non-inferiority trial. Lancet Oncol. 2014;15:1303–10.
25. Gann PH, Colilla SA, Gapstur SM, Winchester DJ, Winchester DP. Factors associated with axillary lymph node metastasis from breast carcinoma: descriptive and predictive analyses. Cancer. 1999;86:1511–9.
26. Mustafa IA, Cole B, Wanebo HJ, Bland KI, Chang HR. Prognostic analysis of survival in small breast cancers. J Am Coll Surg. 1998;186:562–9.
27. Voogd AC, Coebergh JW, Repelaer van Driel OJ, et al. The risk of nodal metastases in breast cancer patients with clinically negative lymph nodes: a population-based analysis. Breast Cancer Res Treat. 2000;62:63–9.
28. Dogan N, Cuttino L, Lloyd R, Bump EA, Arthur DW. Optimized dose coverage of regional lymph nodes in breast cancer: the role of intensity-modulated radiotherapy. Int J Radiat Oncol Biol Phys. 2007;68:1238–50.
29. Fowble B, Solin LJ, Schultz DJ, Goodman RL. Frequency, sites of relapse, and outcome of regional node failures following conservative surgery and radiation for early breast cancer. Int J Radiat Oncol Biol Phys. 1989;17:703–10.
30. Haffty BG, Fischer D, Fischer JJ. Regional nodal irradiation in the conservative treatment of breast cancer. Int J Radiat Oncol Biol Phys. 1990;19:859–65.
31. Halverson KJ, Taylor ME, Perez CA, et al. Regional nodal management and patterns of failure following conservative surgery and radiation therapy for stage I and II breast cancer. Int J Radiat Oncol Biol Phys. 1993;26:593–9.
32. Fowler JF. The linear-quadratic formula and progress in fractionated radiotherapy. Br J Radiol. 1989;62:679–94.
33. Matthews JH, Meeker BE, Chapman JD. Response of human tumor cell lines in vitro to fractionated irradiation. Int J Radiat Oncol Biol Phys. 1989;16:133–8.
34. Steel GG, Deacon JM, Duchesne GM, Horwich A, Kelland LR, Peacock JH. The dose-rate effect in human tumour cells. Radiother Oncol. 1987;9:299–310.
35. Bentzen S, Baumann M. The linear-quadratic model in clinical practice. In: Steel G, editor. Basic clinical radiobiology. London: Arnold; 2002. p. 134–46.
36. Johansson S, Svensson H, Denekamp J. Timescale of evolution of late radiation injury after postoperative radiotherapy of breast cancer patients. Int J Radiat Oncol Biol Phys. 2000;48:745–50.
37. Westling P, Svensson H, Hele P. Cervical plexus lesions following post-operative radiation therapy of mammary carcinoma. Acta Radiol Ther Phys Biol. 1972;11:209–16.
38. Bates TD. The 10-year results of a prospective trial of post-operative radiotherapy delivered in 3 fractions per week versus 2 fractions per week in breast carcinoma. Br J Radiol. 1988;61:625–30.
39. Baillet F, Housset M, Maylin C, et al. The use of a specific hypofractionated radiation therapy regimen versus classical fractionation in the treatment of breast cancer: a randomized study of 230 patients. Int J Radiat Oncol Biol Phys. 1990;19:1131–3.
40. Ragaz J, Jackson SM, Le N, et al. Adjuvant radiotherapy and chemotherapy in node-positive premenopausal women with breast cancer. N Engl J Med. 1997;337:956–62.
41. Danish Breast Cancer Cooperative G, Nielsen HM, Overgaard M, Grau C, Jensen AR, Overgaard J. Study of failure pattern among high-risk breast cancer patients with or without postmastectomy radiotherapy in addition to adjuvant systemic therapy: long-term results from the Danish Breast Cancer Cooperative Group DBCG 82 b and c randomized studies. J Clin Oncol. 2006;24:2268–75.
42. Stokes EL, Tyldesley S, Woods R, Wai E, Olivotto IA. Effect of nodal irradiation and fraction size on cardiac and cerebrovascular mortality in women with breast cancer treated with local and locoregional radiotherapy. Int J Radiat Oncol Biol Phys. 2011;80:403–9.
43. Bajrovic A, Rades D, Fehlauer F, et al. Is there a life-long risk of brachial plexopathy after radiotherapy of supraclavicular lymph nodes in breast cancer patients? Radiother Oncol. 2004;71:297–301.

44. Owen JR, Ashton A, Bliss JM, et al. Effect of radiotherapy fraction size on tumour control in patients with early-stage breast cancer after local tumour excision: long-term results of a randomised trial. Lancet Oncol. 2006;7:467–71.
45. Ortholan C, Hannoun-Levi J, Ferrero J, Largillier R, Courdi A. Long-term results of adjuvant hypofractionated radiotherapy for breast cancer in elderly patients. Int J Radiat Oncol. 2005;61:154–62.
46. Pinitpatcharalert A, Chitapanarux I, Euathrongchit J, Tharavichitkul E, Sukthomya V, Lorvidhaya V. A retrospective study comparing hypofractionated radiotherapy and conventional radiotherapy in postmastectomy breast cancer. J Med Assoc Thai = Chotmaihet thangphaet. 2011;94 Suppl 2:S94–102.
47. Favourable and unfavourable effects on long-term survival of radiotherapy for early breast cancer: an overview of the randomised trials. Early Breast Cancer Trialists' Collaborative Group. Lancet 2000;355:1757–70.
48. Paszat LF, Mackillop WJ, Groome PA, Boyd C, Schulze K, Holowaty E. Mortality from myocardial infarction after adjuvant radiotherapy for breast cancer in the surveillance, epidemiology, and end-results cancer registries. J Clin Oncol. 1998;16:2625–31.
49. Paszat LF, Mackillop WJ, Groome PA, Schulze K, Holowaty E. Mortality from myocardial infarction following postlumpectomy radiotherapy for breast cancer: a population-based study in Ontario, Canada. Int J Radiat Oncol Biol Phys. 1999;43:755–62.
50. van der Laan HP, Dolsma WV, van't Veld AA, Bijl HP, Langendijk JA. Comparison of normal tissue dose with three-dimensional conformal techniques for breast cancer irradiation including the internal mammary nodes. Int J Radiat Oncol Biol Phys. 2005;63:1522–30.
51. Zhang Q, Chen JY, Hu WG, Guo XM. Modified partially wide tangents technique in postmastectomy radiotherapy for patients with left-sided breast cancer. Chin Med J (Engl). 2010;123:2825–31.
52. Gagliardi G, Constine LS, Moiseenko V, et al. Radiation dose-volume effects in the heart. Int J Radiat Oncol Biol Phys. 2010;76:S77–85.
53. Harris EE, Correa C, Hwang WT, et al. Late cardiac mortality and morbidity in early-stage breast cancer patients after breast-conservation treatment. J Clin Oncol. 2006;24:4100–6.
54. Marhin W, Wai E, Tyldesley S. Impact of fraction size on cardiac mortality in women treated with tangential radiotherapy for localized breast cancer. Int J Radiat Oncol Biol Phys. 2007;69:483–9.
55. Bartlett FR, Colgan RM, Donovan EM, et al. Voluntary breath-hold technique for reducing heart dose in left breast radiotherapy. J Vis Exp. 2014;89.
56. Bentzen SM, Skoczylas JZ, Bernier J. Quantitative clinical radiobiology of early and late lung reactions. Int J Radiat Biol. 2000;76:453–62.
57. Erends M, van der Aa T, de Grzymala AP, van der Hulst R. Validity and reliability of three-dimensional imaging for measuring the volume of the arm. Lymphat Res Biol. 2014;12:275–81.
58. Galiano-Castillo N, Ariza-Garcia A, Cantarero-Villanueva I, Fernandez-Lao C, Sanchez-Salado C, Arroyo-Morales M. Agreement between telerehabilitation involving caregivers and face-to-face clinical assessment of lymphedema in breast cancer survivors. Support Care Cancer. 2014;22:253–8.
59. Ohberg F, Zachrisson A, Holmner-Rocklov A. Three-dimensional camera system for measuring arm volume in women with lymphedema following breast cancer treatment. Lymphat Res Biol. 2014;12:267–74.
60. Galecki J, Hicer-Grzenkowicz J, Grudzien-Kowalska M, Michalska T, Zalucki W. Radiation-induced brachial plexopathy and hypofractionated regimens in adjuvant irradiation of patients with breast cancer – a review. Acta Oncol. 2006;45:280–4.
61. Amini A, Yang J, Williamson R, et al. Dose constraints to prevent radiation-induced brachial plexopathy in patients treated for lung cancer. Int J Radiat Oncol Biol Phys. 2012;82:e391–8.
62. Delanian S, Lefaix JL, Pradat PF. Radiation-induced neuropathy in cancer survivors. Radiother Oncol. 2012;105:273–82.

63. Olsen NK, Pfeiffer P, Johannsen L, Schroder H, Rose C. Radiation-induced brachial plexopathy: neurological follow-up in 161 recurrence-free breast cancer patients. Int J Radiat Oncol Biol Phys. 1993;26:43–9.
64. Fathers E, Thrush D, Huson SM, Norman A. Radiation-induced brachial plexopathy in women treated for carcinoma of the breast. Clin Rehabil. 2002;16:160–5.
65. Johansson S, Svensson H, Denekamp J. Dose response and latency for radiation-induced fibrosis, edema, and neuropathy in breast cancer patients. Int J Radiat Oncol Biol Phys. 2002;52:1207–19.
66. Chen AM, Hall WH, Li J, et al. Brachial plexus-associated neuropathy after high-dose radiation therapy for head-and-neck cancer. Int J Radiat Oncol Biol Phys. 2012;84:165–9.
67. Chen AM, Wang PC, Daly ME, et al. Dose – volume modeling of brachial plexus-associated neuropathy after radiation therapy for head-and-neck cancer: findings from a prospective screening protocol. Int J Radiat Oncol Biol Phys. 2014;88:771–7.
68. Pierce SM, Recht A, Lingos TI, et al. Long-term radiation complications following conservative surgery (CS) and radiation therapy (RT) in patients with early stage breast cancer. Int J Radiat Oncol Biol Phys. 1992;23:915–23.
69. Whelan T. MA. 20: A Phase III study of regional radiation therapy in early breast cancer. In: (CTG) NCIoCCTGN, ed.; 2013.
70. Poppe M. Phase II trial of hypofractionated post mastectomy radiation. In: San Antonio Breast Conference 2014; San Antonio; 2014.

Part VI
Hypofractionation for Metastatic Disease

Chapter 29
Stereotactic Treatment for Oligometastatic Breast Cancer

Steven J. Chmura and Joseph K. Salama

Contents

29.1 Rationale of Oliometastatic Cancer

Patients with solid tumor malignancies are staged as M0 or M1 – with or without metastatic disease. In most situations, metastatic disease in solid malignancies is traditionally considered incurable. Oligometastasis (OM) was first defined by Weichselbaum and Hellman in 1995, as an intermediate state in the spectrum of metastatic disease. From clinical observations of patients presenting with metastatic

S.J. Chmura, MD, PhD (✉)
Department of Radiation and Cellular Oncology, University of Chicago, Chicago, MC9006, IL 60611, USA

Cancer Research Center, University of Chicago, Chicago, IL USA

Ludwig Center for Metastasis Research, Chicago, IL USA
e-mail: schmura@radonc.uchicago.edu

J.K. Salama, MD
Department of Radiation Oncology, Duke University, Durham, NC, USA

D.W. Arthur et al. (eds.), *Short Course Breast Radiotherapy: A Comprehensive Review of Hypofractionation, Partial Breast, and Intra-Operative Irradiation*,
DOI 10.1007/978-3-319-24388-7_29

disease, they proposed a framework including the idea that in newly diagnosed metastatic disease, some patients have cancer spread limited to a few organs and radiographically visible lesions (≤5) [1] and that a subset of these oligometastatic patients may be curable through metastasis-directed therapy (surgery or ablation via radiation or other techniques) [2]. They reasoned that in patients where these few metastases were responsible for subsequent dissemination of disease, aggressive metastasis-directed therapy would limit further progression and be potentially curative.

Clinical outcome data supporting the oligometastatic state comes from promising, better than expected long-term outcomes of patients with few metastases treated with metastasis-directed therapies. These outcomes are seen in several cancer types, including breast cancer, non-small cell lung cancer, and prostate cancer [3], among the most common cancers and in whom clinical study is of particular importance. Most series demonstrating long-term disease-free survival are from patients undergoing surgical metastasectomy. These data are the most well established, supporting long-term survivorship [4]. Large series of pulmonary metastasectomy [4–6] and hepatic resection for limited metastasis [7] and multiorgan metastases all demonstrate approximately 25 % of treated patients are long-term survivors and subsets remaining disease-free and potentially cured [8, 9]. While metastasectomy series demonstrate long-term survivors, not all women are eligible for surgery due to comorbid factors or the location of the metastases. An emerging technology called stereotactic body radiation therapy (SBRT) or stereotactic ablative radiotherapy (SABR) [10] differing radiation planning and delivery hardware and software combine to deliver a conformal dose of radiation directed at the metastases with relative sparing of normal tissues nearby. SBRT has an established role in the management of early stage lung cancer [11–13], and it has emerged as a noninvasive, ablative therapy with high rates of local control and a potential role in the treatment of OM patients, similar to surgical metastasectomy [14–17]. Compared with resection, SBRT offers the advantage of targeting sites difficult or impossible to resect surgically and may extend the benefit of metastasis-directed therapies to patients unfit for surgical resection. Retrospective and single-institution series demonstrate promising local control, disease-free, and overall survival with metastasis-directed SBRT [18–21]. SBRT has also been shown to be feasible and tolerated for large volume metastases [22], extending the advantages of ablative therapies to larger tumors as well. These series suggest that SBRT or surgical resection may be considered equivalent when testing a hypothesis that demands high rates of tumor cell kill and local control.

Due to the belief that SBRT will lead to high rates of treated metastasis control, it is increasingly employed as an ablative technique in patients with oligometastatic disease. Salama et al. demonstrated the widespread adoption of this technique worldwide in a 2014 international survey of radiation oncologists [23] (Fig. 29.1). Over 60 % of physicians had used SBRT to treat oligometastases. More than half of the remainder were initiating programs utilizing SBRT despite the lack of level 1 evidence. SBRT has also been included in many guidelines for the treatment of metastatic breast, NSCLC, colon cancer, thyroid cancer, and other malignancies.

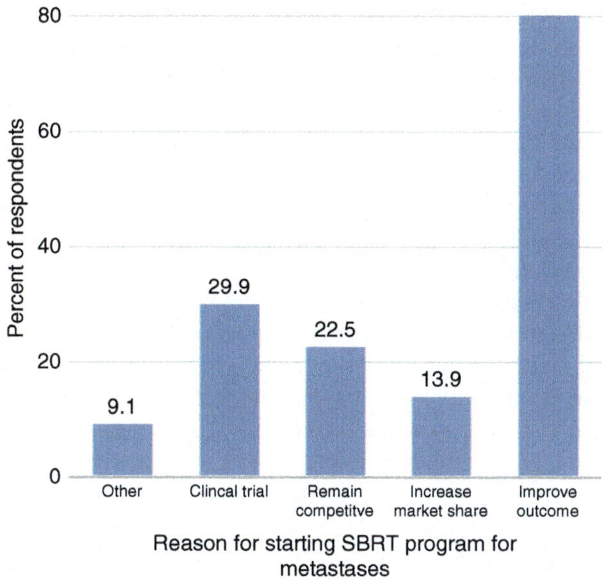

Fig. 29.1 Percentage of respondents from an international survey when asked the rationale for starting a metastasis-directed SBRT program in the next 3 years (Adapted from Salama et al. [57])

While the concept of curing metastatic disease with SBRT is exciting for both physicians and their patients, there is a lack of level 1 evidence yet to support the conclusion that metastasis-directed ablative intervention in patients with oligometastatic disease is predictive of overall survival. Rather, the biology of the disease itself in this patient population may simply be determining the better than expected outcomes. In this chapter we will review the evidence supporting the continued investigation of oligometastatic breast treatment, the patient selection, and outcome data from the largest series and summarize the rationale and design of the ongoing NCI-sponsored clinical trials. Finally, we will review the initial studies investing biology that may be driving the oligometastatic state and relatively good overall survival compared to most metastatic disease presentations.

29.2 Rationale of Oligometastatic Breast Cancer

Metastatic breast cancer has been commonly used as a model to appreciate the underlying molecular mechanisms of metastatic cancer. Halstead in the late nineteenth century, based on clinical observations in his surgical patients, hypothesized that breast cancer metastasized in an orderly fashion from the primary tumor, through regional lymphatics, to defined nodal groups, and finally to systemic dissemination [24]. This popular view of metastases drove the adoption of increasingly radical en bloc operations. By removing all microscopic local disease, proponents of these surgeries hoped survival and cure rates would improve. However, continued death due to metastatic breast cancer despite aggressive surgeries suggested a need for alternative hypotheses. The systemic hypothesis of metastasis was best articulated by Fisher [25]. Contrary to the Halstead hypothesis, Fisher held that in patients ultimately succumbing to widespread metastases, the dissemination likely occurred *before* clinical detectable disease was appreciated in the breast or regional nodes. Therefore, increasing aggressive surgeries to the primary tumor and regional lymphatics would not improve patient outcomes as a whole, since those destined to develop metastatic disease already had microscopic dissemination. In order to improve overall survival and reduce breast cancer mortality, effective systemic therapies were needed to eliminate clinically undetectable distant metastases. Despite the simplicity of these two hypotheses, clinical observations suggested a more complex picture. This complexity is reflected by the fact that not all breast cancers were widely metastatic at initial presentation and that some patients with metastases had long disease-free intervals following metastasectomy without systemic therapy.

The spectrum hypothesis held some breast cancers behave in a Halstead-like manner and remain locoregionally confined. Others, like Fisher suggested, are metastatic at presentation. However the remaining and potentially largest set of women progress from only locoregional disease to widespread metastases [26]. This hypothesis correctly suggested that prevention of locoregional recurrence would lead to fewer breast cancer deaths as seen in the first modern postmastectomy trials [27].

Soon thereafter, Hellman and Weichselbaum advocated the oligometastatic state. Oligometastases would be a necessary part of the spectrum hypothesis where metastases limited in number and destination organ are unlikely to progress rapidly [1]. This hypothesis predicted that if some metastases are the source of future metastases in other organs, then successful ablation of the limited disease may be curative. Support for this idea was based on successful surgical removal of metastases, reported by Weinlechner as early as 1882 [28], and long-term survival (1939) and cure (1947) following metastasectomy [29] in the absence of systemic chemotherapy. With improvements in the efficacy of adjuvant systemic chemotherapy in eradicating microscopic metastatic disease, increasing number of patients may have a reduction in tumor burden where ablative metastasis-directed therapy represents a potential means to impact the natural history of metastatic breast cancer. Demonstrating that intervention with metastasis-directed ablative therapy produced long-term progression-free survival and freedom from breast cancer mortality could modify treatment standards in an analogous way to curative intent treatment of women with breast cancer supraclavicular metastases.

Advances in breast cancer awareness and screening may account for many of the differing hypotheses of the underlying mechanisms responsible for metastatic breast cancer. Most breast cancers in the modern era are radiographically detected when relatively small. Often there is no palpable adenopathy. Positive lymph nodes are found commonly with only microscopic cells with the aid of immunohistochemistry. As breast cancer presentation has changed significantly since the original Halstead hypothesis, so might the behavior of the resulting metastatic disease in the era of increasingly effective systemic regimens.

Similar to the impact that imaging has had on detection of primary breast tumors, improvements in imaging the whole body with CT/bone scan or PET/CT may significantly improve our threshold for detecting metastases. Proponents of the aggressive treatment of oligometastases advocate that just as locoregional treatments have evolved, so must those currently used for the treatment of metastatic disease.

29.3 Incidence of Oligometastasis in Breast Cancer in the Modern Era

The hypothesis of an oligometastatic state is compelling to physicians as can be demonstrated the increase in publications on PubMed.org for articles published from 1995 to 2014 (Fig. 29.2). Despite this academic interest, the actual number of women presenting each year with this clinical scenario is unknown. Up until recently, large clinical trials were designed to report metastatic disease as a binary event. Data on the number of metastases or even the number of organs initially affected was not collected, as it would not influence the initial treatment. One must therefore mainly rely on secondary analyses of clinical trial and outcomes data to give an indication of the frequency of oligometastatic breast cancer.

When looking at data from modern first-line metastatic breast cancer trials, it appears that many of patients present with limited metastatic disease. Data from first-line metastatic breast cancer (MBC) trials published between 2003 and 2012 imply that a large proportion of patients present with oligometastases. In addition, patients presenting with fewer metastases demonstrate improved progression-free survival. As shown in Table 29.1, approximately 50 % of patients enrolling in recent first-line MBC trials with differing ER and HER2 status had <2 metastatic sites. In one trial, greater than 75 % presented with had <4 metastatic sites. The difficulty in interpreting these data is twofold. First, these data are from patients consenting to mainly randomized prospective trials. Due to eligibility criteria and other factors driving which patients enroll, these trials may not be representative of the metastatic breast cancer population. The second difficulty using these data is the meaning of

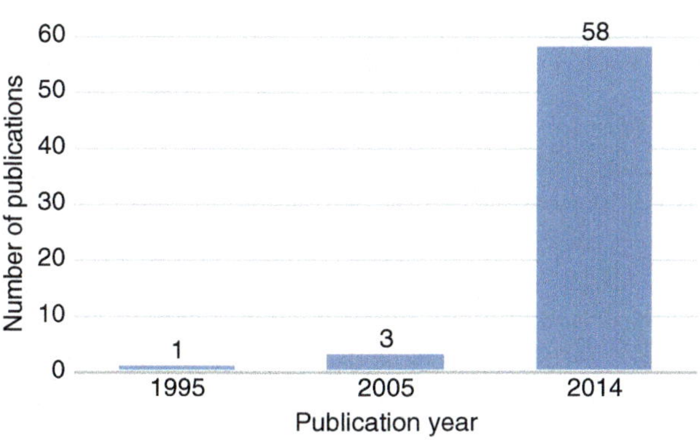

Fig. 29.2 Number of publications on pubmed.org whose keywords include "oligometastases" or "oligometastatic" or "oligometastasis"

Table 29.1 Frequency of patients enrolled on first-line metastatic breast cancer trials with limited number metastatic sites who appear potentially eligible for ablative therapy

Author	Year	Phase	*n*	ER/ PR +	HER2+	<2 met sites	<4 met sites	Arms	PFS
Sledge	2003	III	739	45	–	**49**	–	1. Doxorubicin 2. Paclitaxel 3. Doxorubicin +paclitaxel	6 6.3 8.2
Albain	2008	II	599	32	–	**57**	91	1. Gem+paclitaxel 2. Paclitaxel	9.89 8.4
Bergh	2012	III	593	72	Pos.	**52**	–	1 Sunitinib +docetaxel 2. Docetaxel	8.6 8.3
Tawfik	2013	II	30	77	Neg.	**50**	–	1. Vinorelbine, capecitabine	8.6
Hurvitz	2013	IIR	137	54	Pos	**49.3**	–	1. Trastuz +docetaxel 2. T-DM1	9.2 14.2
Gianni	2013	III	424	51	Pos	**50**	–	1. Docetaxel +trastuz 2. Docet +tras+BEV	13.7 16.5

"metastatic sites." A metastatic site in these trials may refer to individual metastases, individual organs, or even the entire skeletal system. This is supported by analyses of large carefully followed breast cancer cohorts, where 17 % of stage I/II breast cancer patients who progressed to metastatic disease presented with 1–5 metastases [30]. Even if this is the true extent of the oligometastatic breast cancer population, this still represents a significant number of patients. Despite these limitations, these data suggest that metastases are likely limited at presentation in patients who meeting eligibility for prospective clinical trials.

29.4 Prognosis for Patients with Oligometastatic Breast Cancer

In order for any metastasis-directed therapy, to be of clinical benefit, the rate of disease progression must be slower than in patients with more widespread disease. If the limited metastases seen on imaging are simply markers of rapid progression in the near future (oligovisible), ablative therapies would be of little benefit. Limited data suggest that patients presenting with fewer metastases often live longer than those initially presenting with widespread disease.

One large series of women treated with first-line anthracycline-based therapy compared those with ≤5 metastases to those >5. Those with few metastases on multivariate analysis had significantly improved survival [31]. The median survival for women with ≤5, 6–12, and 13–20 metastases was 146, 96, and 80 weeks, respectively ($p<0.01$). In another long-term analysis of stage I–III breast cancer patients, those eventually presenting with ≤5 metastases had significantly longer overall survival (mOS 107.7 months) than patients with >5 metastases (mOS 22 months, $p=.001$). The 5-year actuarial survival for ≤5 metastases was 59.6 % compared to 11.6 % for >5 metastases [30]. Interestingly in these patients, the time from locoregional treatment to first metastatic presentation did not differ between those with <5 or >5 initial metastases. These data suggest that the clinical scenario first described by Hellman and Weichselbaum of oligometastases can be seen in large populations of breast cancer patients treated with modern local and systemic therapy. In addition, analysis such as these suggests that breast oligometastatic breast cancer patients have a slower natural history of disease progression and longer survival. Thus, aggressive local therapy in this population of patients may be of some benefit and warrants investigation in a rigorous manner.

29.5 Management of Patients with Limited Metastatic Disease

The standard of care (SOC) first-line treatment for metastatic breast cancer is systemic therapy with hormonal, cytotoxic, and/or biologics. Local therapy to the primary tumor with surgery, radiation, or radiofrequency ablation is often relegated to managing symptoms, as is treatment to symptomatic metastases as well as to those metastases that have the potential to cause catastrophic conditions.

However, systemic therapy alone *is* curative in a small number of metastatic breast cancer patients. Greenberg et al. analyzed over 1,500 women with metastatic breast cancer treated with systemic regimens containing doxorubicin and alkylating agent-based chemotherapy. With over 15 years of follow-up, 1.6 % remained in complete remission and free of relapse [32]. Patient factors that predicted for long-term progression-free survival included young age, KPS >70, premenopausal, and presenting initially with only a few metastatic sites. Interestingly, 1/3 of the long-term survivors also had some type of local ablative therapy including hepatic artery infusion, radiation, or surgery. Other similar studies in breast cancer patients demonstrate rare but consistent population with long-term progression-free survival of MBC when treated with systemic therapies alone [33, 34].

When compared to chemotherapy only series, the use of ablative therapy to radiographically eliminate metastatic disease results in a seemingly higher percentage of patients achieving long-term disease control. Resection or radiation of hepatic [35, 36], pulmonary [35, 37], CNS [38, 39], adrenal [40, 41], and multiple organ metastases [16, 42, 43] has been associated with 20–25 % long-term disease control in selected patients. These series suggest that ablation of radiographically visible disease may lead to significantly improved long-term disease-free intervals.

29.6 Combined Modality Management of Metastatic Breast Cancer Patients

When looking at series of combined modality treatment of first-line metastatic breast cancer patients, the outcomes appear to be superior to those including other metastatic diseases. Series in breast cancer patients undergoing surgical resection of liver metastases report median progression-free (14-34 months) and overall survival (24–63 months). In series with resection of pulmonary metastases, median survivals have ranged between 32 and 97 months, and 5-year survivals have ranged from 27 to 80 % [44, 45]. A pooled analysis of 460 women undergoing pulmonary resection for metastases demonstrates a median survival of 35 months. However, the cumulative 5-, 10-, and 15-year survival rate was 35 %, 20 %, and 18 %, respectively. Similar to other series, longer disease-free intervals, complete resections, and fewer metastases had improved overall survival. When looking at women with only a single metastasis that was completely resected, and a length of time from primary breast cancer treatment until development of metastases greater than 36 months, 5-year overall survival was 50 % compared to 13 % in those with multiple metastases and/or shorter disease-free intervals [44]. Similar results are seen in large analyses of metastatic breast cancer patients undergoing hepatic metastasectomy, where a longer disease-free interval, >24 months, was associated with longer overall survival (100.7 months vs 47.5 months; $p<0.001$). These data further demonstrate that a small number of breast cancer patients achieve long freedom from progression and that presentation with limited disease is again prognostic.

29.7 Stereotactic Body Radiotherapy for Breast Cancer Metastases

While surgical resection of metastatic disease is an option in select patients, most patients with MBC are not candidates for surgery. Newer radiation techniques are ideally suited for the treatment of limited metastases. Commonly termed stereotactic body radiotherapy (SBRT) or stereotactic ablative radiotherapy (SABR), the radiation techniques typically deliver 1–5 radiation treatments under various image guidance with doses 2–10 times that of conventional radiation treatments [46]. Similar to techniques used in CNS radiosurgery, the hallmark of SBRT treatments is their confomality to the target with a steep dose gradient allowing relative sparring of nearby organs at risk (OAR). At these high doses, other mechanisms of cell death besides double-stranded DNA breaks appear to be in play including endothelial mediated [47, 48] and immune mediated [49, 50].

Generally, doses of at least 54 Gy in 3 fractions have been shown necessary when using three radiation doses to target tumors in the lung and liver [51]. McCammon et al. demonstrated in one of the largest series of 246 liver or lung oligometastases; doses >54 Gy in 3 fractions had a 3-year actuarial local control rate of over of

89.3 % compared with 59.0 and 8.1 % for those treated to 36–53.9 Gy and less than 36 Gy. On multivariate analysis, only increased nominal dose and EUD (equivalent uniform dose) retained statistical significance. Treatment was well tolerated; 5.7 % of patients experienced grade 3 or higher toxicity [51]. These data, and that from other series, suggest a dose-control relationship within the range of SBRT doses applied. These results support the use of aggressive SBRT regimens when durable tumor control is the primary objective.

Perhaps the best data with the longest follow-up in oligometastatic breast cancer patients comes from the University of Rochester [52]. A pooled analysis of 40 women with limited breast cancer metastases, 90 % of who received systemic therapy for their metastatic disease prior to SBRT, demonstrated the 2- and 4-year progression-free survival was 44 % and 38 %, respectively. At 4 years, the treated metastasis control per patient was 80 % despite an actuarial overall survival was 59 %. Similar to other studies in the surgical series, patients with a solitary metastasis had improved PFS and OS ($p=0.028$). Additionally, bone-only metastases had a remarkable rate of 85 % freedom from new metastases at a median follow-up of 50 months. Treated lesions that appeared at least stable if not responding to therapy on CT imaging demonstrated 2-year PFS 53 % vs 13 % and $P=0.026$ and 2 year OS 81 % vs 63 % ($p=0.061$).

Currently, oligometastatic patients are selected via clinical criteria in including number of lesions (<4–5), size of each lesion <5 cm, performance status, and disease-free interval from completion of primary breast cancer treatment until development of metastases. Many small series demonstrate that patients with intracranial metastases, synchronous oligometastases, male gender, and non-adenocarcinoma histology have been associated with worse outcomes l [17]. In breast cancer patients receiving ablative radiotherapy, specifically, those with bone metastases, bone-only metastases, single metastases, and stable or responding metastases have improved outcomes [52]. However, these clinical criteria are imperfect surrogates for identifying those with the true underlying biology of oligometastases.

Despite the promise of reported studies, there is a need for further prospective study of locally directed metastatic therapies in oligometastatic breast cancer. Retrospective and single-institution studies are subject to bias and limited by lack of appropriate control groups, not allowing for generalizable conclusions [53, 54]. Patients included in reported oligometastatic series are likely highly selected, with better performance status and perhaps slower growing tumors. Prospective data are needed to define which groups, if any, are likely to benefit from local therapy [55] and to establish treatment guidelines for safe, appropriate delivery of SBRT and surgery to metastases. Patterns of care data demonstrate an increase in metastasectomy rates performed over the last decade [56]. Recent evidence also finds the majority of radiation oncologists are offering SBRT for limited metastasis off protocol [57]. This illustrates the heightened interest in the treatment of oligometastases and metastasis-directed ablative therapies and reinforces that it is imperative to establish a high level of evidence through clinical trials to ensure best practices.

While these advanced radiation techniques have been shown to be effective in targeting few metastases in limited organs [35, 42, 58], the studies evaluating patients with multiple metastases have been small and limited to a few institutions [15, 16, 43]. Therefore, data are scare describing treatment and toxicity outcomes of patients with ≥3 or 2 close metastases. In particular when targeted metastases are in close proximity, the target organ and surrounding normal tissues are exposed to higher integral radiation doses. When three to four metastases are targeted, the volume of low-dose radiation in the body can be substantial in both target and normal organs. In this situation, the potential toxic effects of radiation are not well characterized. The reported toxicities of ablative radiotherapy are increasingly reported in the literature, but they are limited [42, 59–62].

As the body of evidence for an oligometastatic state grows, there is heightened interest in determining the biologic underpinnings of limited disease. Enhanced understanding of etiology could enable better selection of patients for locally aggressive treatments and potentially spare others from non-beneficial, costly treatments. Despite high local control rates are high, 60–80 % of patients in reported series will still go on to develop additional metastases [35, 63]. While certain clinical parameters, such as number of metastasis and disease-free interval [4, 17, 64], are helpful selection criteria, there are no clearly defined guidelines for patient selection. Clinical surrogates vary between series and have limited accuracy and ability to predict outcomes. Biological study could lead to identification of OM with greater accuracy and opportunity to advance clinical care through enhanced selection and prioritization of treatment.

29.8 Current Clinical Trials of Breast Cancer Oligometastases

Taken together, the single-institution series of both surgery and SBRT that suggest long-term survival following metastasis-directed therapy in patients with limited breast cancer metastases is possible. The benefits these patients derive may come from delaying progression in known metastases, as well as preventing known metastases from seeding new metastases. Furthermore, ablative radiation has been shown to have an abscopal effect, which may improve outcomes by inhibiting progression of untreated micrometastatic foci [65, 66]. However, no study to date has demonstrated that the actual intervention – whether it be surgical resection or SBRT – is responsible for the progression-free and seemingly excellent overall survival [67].

In order to demonstrate ablation of asymptomatic metastases with surgery or SBRT impacts survival in oligometastatic breast cancer patients, randomized trials are essential. However, these trials face enrollment issues as SBRT is becoming widely adopted despite limited evidence to its efficacy [68]. NRG Oncology is conducting a streamlined randomized phase II trial (NRG BR002: NCT02364557 https://www.nrgoncology.org/Clinical-Trials/NRG-BR002) to determine if the ablation of all known metastases in addition to standard of care improves progression-free survival in women with 1–2 breast cancer metastases (Fig. 29.3). One hundred

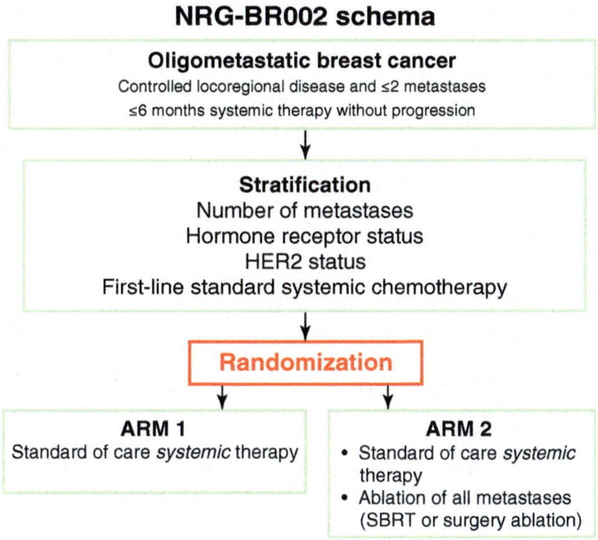

Fig. 29.3 Scheme for NRG BR002: A Phase IIR/III Trial of Standard of Care Therapy with or without Stereotactic Body Radiotherapy (*SBRT*) and/or Surgical Ablation for Newly Oligometastatic Breast Cancer

forty-six patients will be needed to demonstrate a progression-free survival improvement from 10.5 to 19 months. If the progression-free survival is met, the trial will roll directly into a phase III study requiring an additional 256 patients to demonstrate that the ablative arm improves OS from 28 to 42.5 % at 5 years. Secondary translational endpoints will be examining whether circulating tumor cells (CTC) and circulating tumor DNA (ctDNA) are prognostic or predictive in the oligometastatic breast cancer patient. Successful completion of this trial is critical to either shift the standard of care of oligometastatic breast cancer toward multimodality care or inform physicians that off protocol SBRT should stop in this population.

NRG Oncology is also conducting a phase I dose de-escalation study (NRG BR001: NCT02206334 https://www.nrgoncology.org/Clinical-Trials/NRG-BR001) in which breast, lung, and prostate cancer patients with 2 metastases in close proximity (<5 cm) or those with 3–4 metastases will receive radiation to all known sites of disease. This trial directly addresses the challenge of treating patients with multiple metastatic lesions or those with lesions in close proximity. With multiple lesions or closely related lesions, the challenges of balancing ablative doses with critical structures and normal tissue toxicity are exaggerated. Most series reporting SBRT for OM have fewer than two lesions, and the compounding toxicity of overlapping low-dose regions is not well established. Each metastasis will be assigned to one of seven regions (neck and mediastinum, lung central, lung peripheral, spinal, osseous, abdominopelvic, and hepatic) based on the potential for normal tissue toxicity. Doses for each region were selected based on all available prospective phase II data and expert consensus (Table 29.2). Doses will be de-escalated to each region should toxicity be seen. Careful analysis of adverse events combined will help to truly understand the tolerances of normal tissues to this type of ablative radiation.

Table 29.2 NRG BR001: initial starting dose and fraction schedule for the seven potential tumor treatment sites

Metastatic locations	Initial starting dose
Lung – peripheral	45 Gy (3 fractions)
Lung – central	50 Gy (5 fractions)
Mediastinal/cervical lymph node	50 Gy (5 fractions)
Liver	45 Gy (3 fractions)
Spinal/paraspinal	30 Gy (3 fractions)
Osseous	30 Gy (3 fractions)
Abdominal-pelvic metastases (lymph node/adrenal gland)	45 Gy (3 fractions)

29.9 Conclusion

The clinical presentation of oligometastatic breast cancer is usually defined as ≤5 radiographically visible metastases. This presentation, especially in patients likely to enroll in first-line metastatic breast cancer trials, is frequent. Large single-institution and pooled analysis demonstrate that breast cancer patients presenting with few or one metastases detected after a long disease-free interval from their initial local treatment have the best chance at long-term progression-free survival. In addition to systemic therapy, ablation of all metastases with either surgery or SBRT has been associated with long disease-free intervals for many tumor types, including breast cancer and appears to be superior to the chemotherapy only series. Two NCI-sponsored studies to identify the safety and efficacy of ablative therapy in oligometastatic breast cancer are currently activated and accruing patients. Completion of these clinical trials may lead to the establishment of a new paradigm in the treatment of limited metastatic disease. Metastasis-directed therapy in conjunction with systemic therapy may become the best chance for cure for a subset of metastatic breast cancers.

References

1. Hellman S, Weichselbaum RR. Oligometastases. J Clin Oncol. 1995;13(1):8–10.
2. Corbin KS, Hellman S, Weichselbaum RR. Extracranial oligometastases: a subset of metastases curable with stereotactic radiotherapy. J Clin Oncol. 2013;31(11):1384–90.
3. Ashworth A, et al. Is there an oligometastatic state in non-small cell lung cancer? A systematic review of the literature. Lung Cancer. 2013;82(2):197–203.
4. Pastorino U, et al. Long-term results of lung metastasectomy: prognostic analyses based on 5206 cases. J Thorac Cardiovasc Surg. 1997;113(1):37–49.
5. Casiraghi M, et al. A 10-year single-center experience on 708 lung metastasectomies: the evidence of the "international registry of lung metastases". J Thorac Oncol. 2011;6(8):1373–8.
6. Pfannschmidt J, Dienemann H, Hoffmann H. Surgical resection of pulmonary metastases from colorectal cancer: a systematic review of published series. Ann Thorac Surg. 2007;84(1):324–38.
7. Rees M, et al. Evaluation of long-term survival after hepatic resection for metastatic colorectal cancer: a multifactorial model of 929 patients. Ann Surg. 2008;247(1):125–35.

8. Romero Arenas MA, et al. Adrenal metastectomy is safe in selected patients. World J Surg. 2014;38(6):1336–42.
9. Wasif N, et al. Does metastasectomy improve survival in patients with Stage IV melanoma? A cancer registry analysis of outcomes. J Surg Oncol. 2011;104(2):111–5.
10. Loo Jr BW, et al. Stereotactic ablative radiotherapy: what's in a name? Pract Radiat Oncol. 2011;1(1):38–9.
11. Timmerman R, et al. Stereotactic body radiation therapy for inoperable early stage lung cancer. JAMA. 2010;303(11):1070–6.
12. Onishi H, et al. Hypofractionated stereotactic radiotherapy (HypoFXSRT) for stage I non-small cell lung cancer: updated results of 257 patients in a Japanese multi-institutional study. J Thorac Oncol. 2007;2(7 Suppl 3):S94–100.
13. Haasbeek CJ, et al. Outcomes of stereotactic radiotherapy for a new clinical stage I lung cancer arising postpneumonectomy. Cancer. 2009;115(3):587–94.
14. Milano MT, et al. A prospective pilot study of curative-intent stereotactic body radiation therapy in patients with 5 or fewer oligometastatic lesions. Cancer. 2008;112(3):650–8.
15. Salama JK, et al. Stereotactic body radiotherapy for multisite extracranial oligometastases: final report of a dose escalation trial in patients with 1 to 5 sites of metastatic disease. Cancer. 2012;118(11):2962–70.
16. Milano MT, et al. Oligometastases treated with stereotactic body radiotherapy: long-term follow-up of prospective study. Int J Radiat Oncol Biol Phys. 2012;83(3):878–86.
17. de Vin T, et al. Stereotactic radiotherapy for oligometastatic cancer: a prognostic model for survival. Ann Oncol. 2014;25(2):467–71.
18. Zhang Y, et al. Stereotactic body radiation therapy favors long-term overall survival in patients with lung metastases: five-year experience of a single-institution. Chin Med J (Engl). 2011;124(24):4132–7.
19. Chang DT, et al. Stereotactic body radiotherapy for colorectal liver metastases: a pooled analysis. Cancer. 2011;117(17):4060–9.
20. Katz AW, et al. Hypofractionated stereotactic body radiation therapy (SBRT) for limited hepatic metastases. Int J Radiat Oncol Biol Phys. 2007;67(3):793–8.
21. Rudra S, et al. Stereotactic body radiation therapy for curative treatment of adrenal metastases. Technol Cancer Res Treat. 2013;12(3):217–24.
22. Corbin KS, et al. Feasibility and toxicity of hypofractionated image guided radiation therapy for large volume limited metastatic disease. Pract Radiat Oncol. 2013;3(4):316–22.
23. Lewis S, et al. Definitive stereotactic body radiotherapy (SBRT) for extracranial oligometastases: an international survey of >1000 radiation oncologists. Int J Radiat Oncol Biol Phys. 2013.
24. Halstead W. The results of radical operations for the cure of carcinoma of the breast. Ann Surg. 1907;46(1):1–19.
25. Fisher B. Laboratory and clinical research in breast cancer – a personal adventure: the David A. Karnofsky memorial lecture. Cancer Res. 1980;40(11):3863–74.
26. Hellman S. Karnofsky Memorial Lecture. Natural history of small breast cancers. J Clin Oncol. 1994;12(10):2229–34.
27. EBCTCG, et al. Effect of radiotherapy after mastectomy and axillary surgery on 10-year recurrence and 20-year breast cancer mortality: meta-analysis of individual patient data for 8135 women in 22 randomised trials. Lancet. 2014;383(9935):2127–35.
28. van Dongen JA, van Slooten EA. The surgical treatment of pulmonary metastases. Cancer Treat Rev. 1978;5(1):29–48.
29. Alexander J, Haight C. Pulmonary resection for solitary metastatic sarcomas and carcinomas. Surg Gynecol Obstet. 1947;85:129–46.
30. Dorn PL, et al. Patterns of distant failure and progression in breast cancer: implications for the treatment of oligometastatic disease. Int J Radiat Oncol Biol Phys. 2011;81(2S):S643–3.
31. Hortobagyi GN, et al. Multivariate analysis of prognostic factors in metastatic breast cancer. J Clin Oncol. 1983;1(12):776–86.
32. Greenberg PA, et al. Long-term follow-up of patients with complete remission following combination chemotherapy for metastatic breast cancer. J Clin Oncol. 1996;14(8):2197–205.

33. Yamamoto N, et al. Clinical characteristics of patients with metastatic breast cancer with complete remission following systemic treatment. Jpn J Clin Oncol. 1998;28(6):368–73.
34. Tomiak E, et al. Characterisation of complete responders to combination chemotherapy for advanced breast cancer: a retrospective EORTC Breast Group study. Eur J Cancer. 1996;32A(11):1876–87.
35. Rusthoven KE, et al. Multi-institutional phase I/II trial of stereotactic body radiation therapy for liver metastases. J Clin Oncol. 2009;27(10):1572–8.
36. Fong Y, et al. Liver resection for colorectal metastases. J Clin Oncol. 1997;15(3):938–46.
37. Pastorino U, Buyse M, Friedel G, Ginsberg RJ, Girard P, Goldstraw P, Johnston M, McCormack P, Pass H, Putnam Jr JB, International Registry of Lung Metastases. Long-term results of lung metastasectomy: prognostic analyses based on 5206 cases. The International Registry of Lung Metastases. J Thorac Cardiovasc Surg. 1997;113(1):37–49.
38. Wronski M, et al. Survival after surgical treatment of brain metastases from lung cancer: a follow-up study of 231 patients treated between 1976 and 1991. J Neurosurg. 1995;83(4):605–16.
39. Kocher M, et al. Adjuvant whole-brain radiotherapy versus observation after radiosurgery or surgical resection of one to three cerebral metastases: results of the EORTC 22952-26001 study. J Clin Oncol. 2011;29(2):134–41.
40. Tanvetyanon T, et al. Outcomes of adrenalectomy for isolated synchronous versus metachronous adrenal metastases in non-small-cell lung cancer: a systematic review and pooled analysis. J Clin Oncol. 2008;26(7):1142–7.
41. Torok J, et al. Stereotactic body radiation therapy for adrenal metastases: a retrospective review of a noninvasive therapeutic strategy. Future Oncol. 2011;7(1):145–51.
42. Salama JK, Kirkpatrick JP, Yin FF. Stereotactic body radiotherapy treatment of extracranial metastases. Nat Rev Clin Oncol. 2012;9(11):654–65.
43. Tong CC, et al. Phase II trial of concurrent sunitinib and image-guided radiotherapy for oligometastases. PLoS One. 2012;7(6), e36979.
44. Friedel G, et al. Results of lung metastasectomy from breast cancer: prognostic criteria on the basis of 467 cases of the International Registry of Lung Metastases. Eur J Cardiothorac Surg. 2002;22(3):335–44.
45. Pockaj BA, et al. Metastasectomy and surgical resection of the primary tumor in patients with stage IV breast cancer: time for a second look? Ann Surg Oncol. 2010;17(9):2419–26.
46. Kirkpatrick JP, et al. Stereotactic body radiotherapy: a critical review for non-radiation oncologists. Cancer. 2014;120:942–54.
47. Fuks Z, Kolesnick R. Engaging the vascular component of the tumor response. Cancer Cell. 2005;8(2):89–91.
48. Garcia-Barros M, et al. Tumor response to radiotherapy regulated by endothelial cell apoptosis. Science. 2003;300(5622):1155–9.
49. Lee Y, et al. Therapeutic effects of ablative radiation on local tumor require CD8+ T cells: changing strategies for cancer treatment. Blood. 2009;114(3):589–95.
50. Liang H, et al. Radiation-induced equilibrium is a balance between tumor cell proliferation and T cell-mediated killing. J Immunol. 2013;190(11):5874–81.
51. McCammon R, et al. Observation of a dose-control relationship for lung and liver tumors after stereotactic body radiation therapy. Int J Radiat Oncol Biol Phys. 2009;73(1):112–8.
52. Milano MT, et al. Oligometastatic breast cancer treated with curative-intent stereotactic body radiation therapy. Breast Cancer Res Treat. 2009;115(3):601–8.
53. Treasure T. Pulmonary metastasectomy for colorectal cancer: recent reports prompt a review of the available evidence. Curr Colorectal Cancer Rep. 2014;10(3):296–302.
54. Treasure T, et al. Pulmonary metastasectomy: what is the practice and where is the evidence for effectiveness? Thorax. 2014;69(10):946–9.
55. Treasure T, et al. The need to determine whether lung metastasectomy improves survival in advanced colorectal cancer. BMJ. 2014;348:g4085.
56. Bartlett EK, et al. The rise in metastasectomy across cancer types over the past decade. Cancer. 2015;121:747–57.

57. Lewis SL, et al. Definitive stereotactic body radiotherapy (SBRT) for extracranial oligometastases: an international survey of >1000 radiation oncologists. Am J Clin Oncol. 2015 Feb 2. [Epub ahead of print].
58. Sahgal A, Larson DA, Chang EL. Stereotactic body radiosurgery for spinal metastases: a critical review. Int J Radiat Oncol Biol Phys. 2008;71(3):652–65.
59. Forquer JA, et al. Brachial plexopathy from stereotactic body radiotherapy in early-stage NSCLC: dose-limiting toxicity in apical tumor sites. Radiother Oncol. 2009;93(3):408–13.
60. Hoppe BS, et al. Acute skin toxicity following stereotactic body radiation therapy for stage I non-small-cell lung cancer: who's at risk? Int J Radiat Oncol Biol Phys. 2008;72(5):1283–6.
61. Sahgal A, et al. Probabilities of radiation myelopathy specific to stereotactic body radiation therapy to guide safe practice. Int J Radiat Oncol Biol Phys. 2013;85(2):341–7.
62. Sahgal A, et al. Vertebral compression fracture after spine stereotactic body radiotherapy: a multi-institutional analysis with a focus on radiation dose and the spinal instability neoplastic score. J Clin Oncol. 2013;31(27):3426–31.
63. Rusthoven KE, et al. Multi-institutional phase I/II trial of stereotactic body radiation therapy for lung metastases. J Clin Oncol. 2009;27(10):1579–84.
64. Fong Y, et al. Clinical score for predicting recurrence after hepatic resection for metastatic colorectal cancer: analysis of 1001 consecutive cases. Ann Surg. 1999;230(3):309–18; discussion 318–21.
65. Formenti S, et al. Abscopal response in irradiated patients: results of a proof of principle trial. Int J Radiat Oncol Biol Phys. 2008;72(S1):S6–7.
66. Postow MA, et al. Immunologic correlates of the abscopal effect in a patient with melanoma. N Engl J Med. 2012;366(10):925–31.
67. Treasure T. Oligometastatic cancer: an entity, a useful concept, or a therapeutic opportunity? J R Soc Med. 2012;105(6):242–6.
68. Tree AC, et al. Stereotactic body radiotherapy for oligometastases. Lancet Oncol. 2013;14(1):e28–37.

Chapter 30
Hypofractionated Palliative Radiation Therapy for Breast Cancer

Stephen T. Lutz

Contents

30.1 The Development of Palliative Radiotherapy

One of the earliest uses of radiation following its discovery in the late 1800s was exposure of anatomically superficial tumors to a small number of doses in an effort to alleviate symptoms [1]. Though fractionation experiments led to curative treatment regimens of 1.8–2.0 Gy daily doses given 30–40 times over 6–8 weeks, hypofractionated palliative regimens of 8–30 Gy in 1–10 fractions optimize patient and caregiver convenience and minimize acute toxicity. More than 50 years ago, Parker defined the goals of palliative radiotherapy (PRT) [2]:

S.T. Lutz
Department of Radiation Oncology, Blanchard Valley Health System, Findlay, OH, USA
e-mail: slutz@bvha.org

D.W. Arthur et al. (eds.), *Short Course Breast Radiotherapy: A Comprehensive Review of Hypofractionation, Partial Breast, and Intra-Operative Irradiation*,
DOI 10.1007/978-3-319-24388-7_30

> When the initial objective of radiation therapy is palliation, new ground rules must be applied. Possible serious complications or even slowly self-limiting adverse effects of treatment are no longer acceptable. Overall treatment time must be short. Cost must be minimized. Convenience of treatment must be considered.

The selection of a palliative radiotherapy fractionation scheme therefore depends upon patient factors such as performance status and comorbidities, tumor factors such as histology and stage, and treatment factors such as other available modalities and prior therapies. Properly prescribed, hypofractionated radiotherapy provides palliation for locally symptomatic and metastatic disease that is effective, efficient, and associated with minimal side effect risks.

30.2 Palliation of Symptomatic Primary Breast Cancer

While screening and treatment improvements have steadily decreased breast cancer mortality rates in the United States since the 1990s, breast cancer remains the most common malignancy and the second leading cause of death in women living in developed countries [3, 4]. Local recurrence rates following mastectomy alone may approach 45 % for patients with T3/T4 or lymph node positive disease [4, 5]. Locally advanced or recurrent disease can cause pain, ulceration, arm edema, bleeding, or brachial plexopathy. Bedwinek observed that 62 % of women with uncontrolled local disease suffered distressing symptoms for the duration of their life [6]. Though the need for PRT has diminished with improvements in systemic therapy and more options for tumor debulking or mastectomy for locally advanced disease, PRT can provide favorable anti-secretory, anti-inflammatory, and analgesic effects [7].

Limited high-quality data exists to guide the choice for the most effective fractionation schemes for women who require PRT. Treatment volumes and dose fractionation schemes must take into account the site and extent of the local disease, recent or concurrent use of systemic therapy, history of previous radiotherapy, ease of transportation, and patient wishes. Given the efficacy of currently available systemic therapies, only 2 % of women with newly diagnosed breast cancer will require palliative radiotherapy at some point during their treatment course [8]. A review of women who died from breast cancer in Alberta, Canada, between 2000 and 2004 showed that 22 % received local-regional PRT during the course of their disease [9]. For reasons that are unclear, women greater than 75 years old in this and other studies were less likely to receive PRT when compared to younger women, with all other factors taken into account [9–11].

30.2.1 Locally Advanced Disease

Locally advanced breast cancer (LABC) ranges in scope from neglected tumors to those with aggressive biological growth like inflammatory breast cancer [12]. The most common approach to women with LABC is neoadjuvant systemic therapy

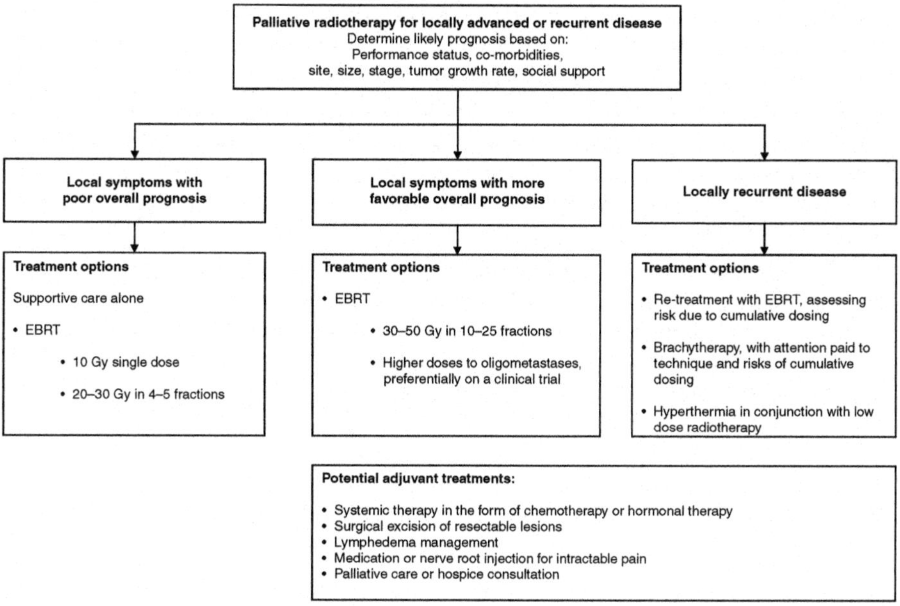

Fig. 30.1 Algorithm for use of palliative radiotherapy for patients with locally advanced or recurrent breast cancer

with the goal of cytoreduction and subsequent surgery, though women who are not fit enough for systemic treatment may respond to PRT [13, 14]. The evidence for this approach derives from older, non-randomized studies which suggest response rates of 60–80 %, though with responses maintained until death in only 27–35 % of women [15, 16]. There exists a trend toward higher local control rates with greater total doses, so the decision to offer hypofractionated treatment rests upon tumor, patient, and transportation factors [17, 18]. Those treated with purely palliative intent may receive 30–50 Gy in 10–20 fractions, while those with short life expectancy or limited travel capabilities may be more efficiently treated with 20–30 Gy in 4–5 fractions. A woman who has been admitted to hospice or who wishes to limit travel to a single trip may be treated with a 10 Gy fraction (Fig. 30.1).

30.2.2 Recurrence Within a Previously Irradiated Area

Local tumor recurrence following adjuvant radiotherapy may manifest within the breast, on the chest wall, or in the regional draining lymphatics. Re-irradiation alone or combined with chemotherapy or hyperthermia may be considered for local recurrences that are unresectable or which do not respond to salvage systemic treatment. While small series of patients have been re-treated to combined total doses of more than 100 Gy with good local control and acceptable toxicity, care should be taken to limit the irradiated volume and to assess normal tissue tolerance of structures such as skin, subcutaneous tissues and ribs, and brachial plexus [19, 20]. The heterogeneity of presentation and lack of data for external beam radiotherapy, absent concurrent systemic or hormonal therapy, create uncertainty regarding control rates and durability. Re-irradiation may be delivered by standard external beam methods, intraoperative radiotherapy, or brachytherapy. The use of electron external beam therapy rather than photon delivery can limit re-treated volumes when the disease-causing symptoms are more superficial [21]. Brachytherapy or intraoperative re-treatment can be effective but require practitioners experienced in these approaches [22, 23]. Data regarding the value of adding hyperthermia to external beam radiotherapy was pooled from 5 randomized trials and suggested a complete response of 41 % in those given radiotherapy alone versus 59 % in those whose radiotherapy was combined with hyperthermia [24]. Still, hyperthermia treatments require a high degree of expertise and the positive effects of its delivery may be short lived (Fig. 30.1).

30.3 Palliation of Symptomatic Metastatic Disease

The two most common indications for palliative radiotherapy from breast cancer are painful bone metastases and symptomatic brain metastases, each of which can be aided by hypofractionated courses.

30.3.1 Painful Bone Metastases

Local symptoms of bone metastases include pain, pathologic fracture, or spinal cord compression. Compared to bone metastases from prostate cancer that are usually osteoblastic and those from multiple myeloma that are mostly osteolytic, bone metastases due to breast cancer are most commonly mixed. Proper management of painful bone metastases requires interdisciplinary care including the appropriate use of pain medicines, surgical stabilization, systemically delivered bone-strengthening agents, radiopharmaceuticals, and vertebroplasty or kyphoplasty. Still, hypofractionated external beam radiotherapy (EBRT) is the mainstay of treatment for painful bone metastases, with extensive data showing partial pain relief of 60–80 % and complete relief of 30–50 % 3–4 weeks after initiation of EBRT [25, 26].

Numerous prospective, randomized trials have detailed pain relief equivalency following dose fractionation schemes including 30 Gy in 10 fractions, 24 Gy in 6 fractions, 20 Gy in 5 fractions, and a single 8 Gy fraction [25, 26]. The advantages of the single fraction course include convenience and decreased acute side effects, though the re-treatment rates to the same anatomic site are higher following single fraction versus multi-fraction regimens, averaging 20 % and 8 %, respectively. Long-term side effects following a single 8 Gy fraction do not appear to be higher than those associated with multi-fraction regimens, even when assessing spinal cord damage in patients treated to spine bones [27]. Patients commonly note the initial onset of pain relief 5–10 days after delivery of the first radiotherapy fraction, irrespective of the fractionation scheme. In evaluating a group of 1-year survivors, the longevity of pain relief following a single 8 Gy fraction was non-inferior to the relief provided from a longer course [28]. Also, a recently reported trial of patients with recurrent skeletal pain revealed a reasonable rate of palliation and acceptable toxicity with repeat hypofractionated treatment to the same anatomic site [26]. Given that the full beneficial effects of palliative radiotherapy may require a month to manifest, re-treatment should not be considered until at least that time frame has passed.

Malignant epidural spinal cord compression (MESCC) is an oncologic emergency with higher rates of ambulation and lower requirements for corticosteroids following decompressive surgery plus surgery versus radiotherapy alone [29]. However, patients with poor performance status, severe comorbid disease, or a limited prognosis are commonly treated with EBRT, alone. Maranzano has evaluated hypofractionated courses for MESCC patients, including phase III study that showed no difference in rates or durability of response, survival, or toxicity between 16 Gy in 2 fractions and a split course of 15 Gy in 3 fractions plus 15 Gy in 5 fractions [30]. Furthermore, a phase III trial of poor performance patients showed equivalent results following 16 Gy in 2 fractions versus a single 8 Gy fraction [31].

30.3.2 Brain Metastases

Brain metastases due to breast cancer can cause significant functional impairment and eventual death. The choice of treatment for brain metastases patients depends upon patient factors such as performance status and comorbid disease, tumor factors such as number and size of brain lesions and control of systemic disease, and treatment-related factors such as previous surgical resection or radiotherapy for metastatic brain disease. Prognostic indices using these variables can estimate patient survival and should be used to help guide treatment choice [32, 33]. Patients with excellent performance status and a limited number of brain lesions may be better treated with surgical resection or stereotactic radiosurgery. Hypofractionated, whole brain EBRT regimens are appropriate for those with a poorer prognosis. Two early fractionation studies showed no difference in outcomes between regimens of 40 Gy in 20 fractions, 30 Gy in 15 fractions, 30 Gy in 10 fractions, and 20 Gy in 5 fractions [34, 35]. For patients with a limited life expectancy, the lack of observed difference in outcomes between 30 Gy in 10 fractions and 20 Gy in 5 fractions means that the latter regimen might be preferred in situations where transportation is limited and patient convenience must be maximized [36]. Any increased durability of response or decreased toxicity risks associated with lengthier courses prove less relevant in these poor performance status patients whose life expectancy may be as little as 2–3 months. Given that the beneficial effects of whole brain treatment may not appear for 2–3 weeks, those with a poor prognosis of less than 1 month may fare as well or better with supportive care including dexamethasone and pain medicines [37].

30.4 Barriers to the Use of Hypofractionated Palliative Radiotherapy

Hypofractionated palliative radiotherapy courses are most likely underutilized because of overly optimistic survival predictions, overestimations of long-term side effect risks, and inadequate palliative care instruction during radiation oncology residency training.

30.4.1 Survival Estimation Inaccuracies

Survival estimates for patients with advanced cancer are complex and are commonly overestimated by physicians by a factor of 3 or more [38]. This disparity might lead radiation oncologists to both underestimate the inconvenience of longer palliative courses and to overestimate the risk of a patient living long enough to face long-term side effect risks that might be associated with some hypofractionated regimens. The more routine use of existing, validated prognostic tools might facilitate an easier pathway to choosing shorter-course therapy for patients whose survival estimates so demand [39, 40].

30.4.2 Inadequate Palliative Care Training

Though a large proportion of radiation oncology patients require treatment while taking into account their full list of palliative care needs, very few radiation oncology training programs include palliative care instruction. The absence of this education limits the understanding of which clinical circumstances would be better approached with hypofractionated courses, as is evidenced by the belief of hospice professionals that radiation oncologists are too reluctant to deliver short-course therapy [41]. Some programs have begun to pilot programs in which palliative radiotherapy services exist in the same way as do services that focus on specific disease sites. Only an increased dedication to this type of approach, coupled with more research funding for palliative care studies, will provide the type of training that will increase the use of hypofractionated palliative radiotherapy courses.

30.5 Guidelines and Quality Measures

The realization that bone metastases have commonly been treated with more than 100 different fractionation schemes led the American Society for Radiation Oncology (ASTRO) to author bone metastases treatment guidelines [25, 42].

In spite of evidence that a single 8 Gy fraction can be equally as efficacious as longer courses, only 3.3 % of Medicare patients receive this dose fractionation [43]. This single fraction approach decreases time spent traveling to or receiving treatment, which has led some centers to pioneer programs in which they respond quickly to bone metastases consultations and complete consultation, dosimetric calculations, and treatment delivery in the same day [44]. The National Quality Forum has developed a quality measure that evaluates the appropriateness of care in cancer centers by the provision of bone metastases treatment in a scheme of 8–30 Gy in 1–10 fractions [45]. In its first Choosing Wisely publication, ASTRO has declared [46]:

> Do not routinely use extended fractionation schemes (>10 fractions) for palliation of bone metastases.

Increasing attention to optimizing palliative care will surely lead to guidelines and quality measures that accentuate hypofractionated treatment courses in a host of clinical circumstances.

30.6 Conclusion

Breast cancer remains the most common malignancy in women in developed countries as well as the second leading cause of death among females in those locales. Palliative radiotherapy can help to alleviate symptoms due to locally advanced or recurrent disease, with hypofractionated courses effective and preferred in those with poor performance status, limited life expectancy, or difficulties traveling to the radiation oncology facility. The use of hypofractionated treatment for bone or brain metastases is standard and is recommended in an increasing number of guidelines and quality measures.

References

1. Coutard H. Principles of X-ray therapy of malignant diseases. Lancet. 1934;2:1–8.
2. Parker RG. Palliative radiation therapy. JAMA. 1964;190:1000–2.
3. Cancer Research UK. Breast Cancer – UK Mortality Statistics. Available at: http://info.cancerresearchuk.org/cancerstats/types/breast/mortality/. Most recently Accessed 17 June 2012.
4. Glück S. The prevention and management of distant metastases in women with breast cancer. Cancer Invest. 2007;25:6–13.
5. Lee MC, Jagsi R. Postmastectomy radiation therapy: indications and controversies. Surg Clin North Am. 2007;87:511–26.
6. Bedwinek JM, Lee J, Fineberg B, et al. Prognostic indicators in patients with isolated local-regional recurrence of breast cancer. Cancer. 1981;47:2232–5.
7. van Oorschot B, Beckmann G, Schulze W, et al. Radiotherapeutic options for symptom control in breast cancer. Breast Care. 2011;6:14–9.
8. Jacob S, Wong K, Delaney GP, et al. Estimation of an optimal utilisation rate for palliative radiotherapy in newly diagnosed cancer patients. Clin Oncol. 2010;22:56–64.

9. Danielson B, Winget M, Gao Z, et al. Palliative radiotherapy for women with breast cancer. Clin Oncol. 2008;20:506–12.
10. Huang J, Zhou S, Groome P, et al. Factors affecting the use of palliative radiotherapy in Ontario. J Clin Oncol. 2001;19:137–44.
11. Johnston GM, Boyd CJ, Joseph P, et al. Variation in delivery of palliative radiotherapy in persons dying of cancer in Nova Scotia, 1994–1998. J Clin Oncol. 2001;19:3323–32.
12. Rodger A, Leonard RC, Dixon JM. ABC of breast disease. Locally advanced breast cancer. BMJ. 1994;309:1431–3.
13. Specht J, Gralow JR. Neoadjuvant chemotherapy for locally advanced breast cancer. Semin Radiat Oncol. 2009;19:222–8.
14. Rodger A, Jack WJ, Hardman PD, et al. Locally advanced breast cancer: report of phase II study and subsequent phase III trial. Br J Cancer. 1992;65:761–5.
15. Griscom NT, Wang CC. Radiation therapy of inoperable breast carcinoma. Radiology. 1962;79:18–32.
16. Langlands AO, Kerr GR, Shaw S. The management of locally advanced breast cancer by X-ray therapy. Clin Oncol. 1976;2:365–71.
17. Sheldon T, Hayes DF, Cady B, et al. Primary radiation therapy for locally advanced breast cancer. Cancer. 1987;60:1219–25.
18. Price A, Kerr GR, Rodger A. Primary radiotherapy for T4 breast cancer. Clin Oncol. 1992;4:217–21.
19. Würschmidt F, Dahle J, Petersen C, et al. Reirradiation of recurrent breast cancer with and without concurrent chemotherapy. Radiat Oncol. 2008;3:1–9.
20. Harkenrider MM, Wilson MR, Dragun AE. Reirradiation as a component of the multidisciplinary management of locally recurrent breast cancer. Clin Breast Cancer. 2011;11:171–6.
21. Laramore GE, Griffin TW, Parker RG, et al. The use of electron beams in treating local recurrence of breast cancer in previously irradiated fields. Cancer. 1978;41:991–5.
22. Harms W, Krempien R, Hensley FW, et al. Results of chest wall reirradiation using pulsed-dose-rate (PDR) brachytherapy molds for breast cancer local recurrences. Int J Radiat Oncol Biol Phys. 2001;49:205–10.
23. Delanian S, Housset M, Brunel P, et al. Iridium 192 plesiocurietherapy using silicone elastomer plates for extensive locally recurrent breast cancer following chest wall irradiation. Int J Radiat Oncol Biol Phys. 1992;22:1099–104.
24. Vernon CC, Hand JW, Field SB, et al. Radiotherapy with or without hyperthermia in the treatment of superficial localized breast cancer: results from five randomized controlled trials. International Collaborative Hyperthermia Group. Int J Radiat Oncol Biol Phys. 1996;35:731–44.
25. Lutz S, Berk L, Chang E, et al. Palliative radiotherapy for bone metastases: an ASTRO evidence-based guideline. Int J Radiat Oncol Biol Phys. 2011;79:965–76. Chow E, Harris K, Fan G, et al. Palliative radiotherapy trials for bone metastases: a systematic review. J Clin Oncol. 2007;25:1423–36.
26. Chow E, van der Linden YM, Roos D, et al. Single versus multiple fractions of repeat radiation for painful bone metastases: a randomised, controlled, noninferiority trial. Lancet Oncol. 2014;15:164–71.
27. Howell DD, James JL, Hartsell WF, et al. Single fraction radiotherapy versus multifraction radiotherapy for palliation of painful vertebral bone metastases: Equivalent efficacy, less toxicity, more convenient—a subset analysis of Radiation Therapy Oncology Group trial 97–14. Cancer. 2013;119:888–96.
28. van der Linden YM, Steenland E, van Houwelingen HC, et al. Patients with a favourable prognosis are equally palliated with single and multiple fraction radiotherapy: Results on survival in the Dutch Bone Metastasis Study. Radiother Oncol. 2006;78:245–53.
29. Patchell R, Tibbs P, Regine W, et al. Direct decompressive surgical resection in the treatment of spinal cord compression caused by metastatic cancer: a randomized trial. Lancet. 2005;366:643–8.

30. Maranzano E, Bellavita R, De Angelis V, et al. Short-course versus split-course radiotherapy in metastatic spinal cord compression: results of a phase III, randomized, multicenter trial. J Clin Oncol. 2005;23:3358–65.
31. Maranzano E, Trippa F, Constantini S, et al. 8Gy single-dose radiotherapy is effective in metastatic spinal cord compression: results of a phase III randomized multicentre Italian trial. Radiother Oncol. 2009;93:174–9.
32. Gaspar LE, Scott C, Murray K, et al. Validation of the RTOG recursive partitioning analysis (RPA) classification for brain metastases. Int J Radiat Oncol Biol Phys. 2000;47:1001–6.
33. Sperduto PW, Kased N, Roberge D, et al. Summary report on the graded prognostic assessment: an accurate and facile diagnosis-specific tool to estimate survival for patients with brain metastases. J Clin Oncol. 2012;30:419–25.
34. Borgelt B, Gelber R, Kramer S, et al. The palliation of brain metastases: final results of the first two studies by the Radiation Therapy Oncology Group. Int J Radiat Oncol Biol Phys. 1980;6:1–9.
35. Borgelt B, Gelber R, Larson M, et al. Ultra-rapid high dose irradiation schedules for the palliation of brain metastases: final results of the first two studies by the Radiation Therapy Oncology Group. Int J Radiat Oncol Biol Phys. 1981;7:1633–8.
36. Tsao MN, Rades D, Wirth A, et al. Radiotherapeutic and surgical management for newly diagnosed brain metastasis(es): an American Society for Radiation Oncology evidence-based guideline. Pract Radiat Oncol. 2012;2:210–25.
37. Langley RE, Stephens RJ, Nankivell M, et al. Interim data from the Medical Research Council QUARTZ Trial: does whole brain radiotherapy affect the survival and quality of life of patients with brain metastases from non-small cell lung cancer? Clin Oncol (R Coll Radiol). 2013;25:e23–30.
38. Christakis NA, Lamont EB. Extent and determinants of error in physicians' prognoses in terminally ill patients. West J Med. 2000;172:310–3.
39. Chow E, Abdolell M, Panzarella T, et al. Predictive model for survival in patients with advanced cancer. J Clin Oncol. 2008;26:5863–9.
40. Krishnan MS, Epstein-Peterson Z, Chen YH, et al. Predicting life expectancy in patients with metastatic cancer receiving palliative radiotherapy: the TEACHH model. Cancer. 2014;120:134–41.
41. Lutz S, Spence C, Chow E, et al. Survey on use of palliative radiotherapy in hospice care. J Clin Oncol. 2004;22:3581–6.
42. Fairchild A, Barnes E, Ghosh S, et al. International patterns of practice in palliative radiotherapy for painful bone metastases: evidence-based practice? Int J Radiat Oncol Biol Phys. 2009;75:1501–10.
43. Bekelman JE, Epstein AJ, Emanuel EJ. Single- vs multiple-fraction radiotherapy for bone metastases from prostate cancer. JAMA. 2013;310:1501–2.
44. Thavarajah N, Wong K, Zhang L, et al. Continued success in providing timely palliative radiation therapy at the Rapid Response Radiotherapy Program: a review of 2008–2012. Curr Oncol. 2013;20:e206–11.
45. National Quality Forum: NQF endorses cancer measures. https://www.qualityforum.org/News_And_Resources/Press_Releases/2012/NQF_Endorses_Cancer_Measures.aspx. Accessed 20 Apr 2015.
46. Choosing Wisely: an initiative of the ABIM Foundation. ASTRO releases list of five radiation oncology treatments to question as part of national Choosing Wisely® campaign. http://www.choosingwisely.org/astro-releases-list-of-five-radiation-oncology-treatments-to-question-as-part-of-national-choosing-wisely-campaign/. Accessed 20 Apr 2015.

Index

D.W. Arthur et al. (eds.), *Short Course Breast Radiotherapy: A Comprehensive Review of Hypofractionation, Partial Breast, and Intra-Operative Irradiation*, DOI 10.1007/978-3-319-24388-7

Printed by Printforce, the Netherlands